Medical Radiology

Diagnostic Imaging

For further volumes:
http://www.springer.com/series/4354

Medical Radiology

Diagnostic Imaging

Apostolos H. Karantanas (Ed.)

Sports Injuries in Children and Adolescents

Foreword by

Albert L. Baert

Springer

Editor
Prof. Apostolos H. Karantanas
Department of Radiology
University Hospital of Heraklion
711 10 Crete
Heraklion
Greece
akarantanas@gmail.com

ISSN: 0942-5373

ISBN: 978-3-540-88589-4 e-ISBN: 978-3-540-88590-0

DOI: 10.1007/978-3-540-88590-0

Springer Heidelberg Dordrecht London New York

Library of Congress Control Number: 2011921725

Cover design: eStudio Calamar, Figueres/Berlin

Printed on acid-free paper

Springer is part of Springer Science+Business Media (www.springer.com)

To
Katerina, Alexis and Gabriella
for their great and constant support

Foreword

Modern lifestyle includes more and more active sport participation among children and adolescents leading to a substantial number of acute and overuse injuries requiring medical care. This volume highlights the role of modern imaging for problem solving and for better patient management of the wide spectrum of sport injuries including not only lesions which mirror those in adults but also others which are unique to the young age group owing to the inherent weakness of the growing skeleton at specific sites.

The specific strengths and limitations of each imaging modality are discussed in depth with a particular focus on ultrasound. The specific advantages of this modality in the examination of children are quite evident because of the absence of ionising radiation and the close interaction between examiner and patient.

The editor A.H. Karantanas is an internationally well-known academic musculoskeletal radiologist with a great dedication and interest in paediatric musculoskeletal pathology. He has published and lectured largely on his special area of expertise. The authors of individual chapters, from both sides of the Atlantic, have been invited to contribute because of their long standing experience and major contributions to the radiological literature on the topic.

I would like to thank and to congratulate most sincerely the editor and the authors for their efforts which have resulted in this comprehensive but well-balanced and very readable text, completed with a superb atlas-type final part, presenting the most common injuries in a number of popular sports.

This book will be of great value for general and paediatric radiologists, both certified and those in training, but also for paediatricians and orthopedic surgeons. It will provide them with the state-of-the-art information on our knowledge in the specific field of sports injuries.

I am confident that it will meet the same success with the readers as the previous volumes published in this series.

Leuven, Belgium — Albert L. Baert

Preface

In Western societies and industrialized countries, where athletic activity is a positive determinant of good health, sport-related injuries in the pediatric and adolescent population are becoming a common clinical entity. I am therefore honored and particularly grateful to Professor Albert L. Baert for providing me with the opportunity to edit a book on this topic. I have chosen to focus on injuries involving the musculoskeletal system because they are the most common and challenging ones.

Both acute and chronic injuries have unique characteristics because they occur in the growing skeleton. The result from an injury may occur locally but also remotely from the site of trauma. Furthermore, the spectrum of clinical appearance of various sport-related injuries may vary enormously due to the wide spectrum of the biomechanics related to each particular athletic activity. Factors which may increase the risk of injury include pressure from family and trainers, improper or absent training, and increased demands for professional performance among adolescent athletes. As the injuries in young athletes are common, imaging should be tailored to modalities not inducing ionizing radiation. Last, children commonly will not lie still or will feel uncomfortable in the magnet's bore. Thus the role of ultrasound has increased significantly.

The book consists of three parts. In the first one, general knowledge on classification, epidemiology, clinical examination, normal variants, incidental findings, and the use of ultrasonography is presented. In the second part, specific imaging findings on each joint and on spine are discussed with emphasis on the most appropriate use of each imaging modality. In the third part, common injuries in sports popular among children and adolescents, are pictorially presented.

The book aims to increase awareness among radiologists and physicians who are involved in the health care of young athletes. It further aims to provide a useful resource on the best imaging approach and appropriate management pathways. Radiologists are more and more commonly becoming members of the medical team – including sports physicians, physiotherapists, and orthopedic surgeons – which treats young athletes. In this respect, not only will prompt diagnosis be their task, but also prognosis, estimated recovery period, and occasionally treatment.

I feel fortunate to have worked with experts whose wide experience on the topic has been established with major and important publications. They have also witnessed the changes in imaging algorithms over the last two decades during which MRI and US have provided efficient ways of approaching accurate diagnosis. I am grateful to the international panel of authors for their contribution to this effort.

Heraklion, Greece | Apostolos H. Karantanas

Contents

Sports Injuries in Children and Adolescents: Classification, Epidemiology, and Clinical Examination

Ravi Mallina and Peter V. Giannoudis

Contents

Key Points

- Important issues regarding accurate diagnosis and/or differential diagnosis of sports injuries in young athletes include: a thorough history focusing on age of the athlete, type of sport, point of maximum intensity of pain, onset and timing of pain in relation to the sport, associated neurovascular symptoms, previous injuries, and presence of swelling, deformity and bruising.
- Whereas avulsion fractures occur in the growing skeleton, it is uncommon to see musculotendinous and ligamentous injuries in pediatric athletes.
- Familiarity with the classification of the musculoskeletal injuries and the limitations of the various clinical tests in each anatomic area, allow accurate referral for imaging.
- The incidence of musculoskeletal injuries largely depends on the type of sport, level of performance (competition/match vs. noncompetition/practice), intensity and technique.

1 Introduction

Over centuries and since the advent of Olympic Games by the ancient Greeks in 776 BC, sport has become an integral part of the human race. According to the data published by the United Sates National Collegiate Athletic Association (NCAA), over 7,018,709 high school students were enrolled in sports during the year

R. Mallina
Academic Department of Trauma and Orthopaedics, School of Medicine, University of Leeds, Leeds, United Kingdom

P.V. Giannoudis (✉)
Department of Trauma and Orthopaedics, Academic Unit, Clarendon Wing, Leeds Teaching Hospitals NHS Trust, Great George Street, Leeds LS1 3EX, United Kingdom
e-mail: pgiannoudi@aol.com

A.H. Karantanas (ed.), *Sports Injuries in Children and Adolescents*,
Med Radiol Diagn Imaging, DOI: 10.1007/174_2010_39,

2005. In addition to being a recreational activity, several health benefits of sports have been established. However, the rewards are not without risks, and sport related morbidity is a well recognized problem. In addition to causing severe strain on the health economics, some of these injuries have long term consequences especially those involving growth plates in children and spinal cord trauma leaving them with long-term disability. Annually, 775,000 children aged less than 15 receive emergency medical care for sport-related injuries. The Centre for Disease Control and Prevention (CDC) reported 1.4 million sports-related injuries for the year 2005–2006. Results from the same source reported that around 40% of sport-related injuries occur in children between 5 and 14 years old. In order to effectively cater this huge population, sports medicine as a speciality has expanded its horizons encompassing various disciplines. Epidemiology, General Practice, Orthopedics, Radiology, Physiotherapy and several other specialties are closely involved in providing treatment to the injured amateur or professional athlete. In this current chapter, we describe sports related injuries by region with emphasis on epidemiology, classification and clinical examination of the most common and significant injuries of the musculoskeletal system.

2 Spine

2.1 Classification

Major sport related injuries of spine although rare, when present can cause a debilitating effect on the athletes' future both socially and as sports personnel. In the extreme cases of paraplegia the athlete is rendered wheel chair bound. Cervical spine is the commonest segment to be involved in sport related trauma. For practical purposes sport related trauma can be classified into cervical and thoracolumbar injuries.

2.1.1 Cervical Spine Injuries

To date there is no universally accepted classification for sport related cervical spinal injuries. Classification by Maroon (1996) perhaps is close to an ideal system describing the whole spectrum of cervical cord injury and is shown on Table 1 (Maroon and Bailes 1996):

Table 1 Cervical cord injuries classification

Type I Injury: Permanent spinal cord injury
Complete paralysis
Anterior cord syndrome
Brown-Sequard syndrome
Central cord syndrome
Mixed incomplete syndrome
Type II Injury: Transient spinal cord injury
Spinal cord concussion
Neuropraxia
Burning hands syndrome
Type III injury: Radiological abnormality without neurological deficit
Congenital spinal stenosis
Acquired spinal stenosis
Herniated cervical disc
Unstable fracture or fracture and dislocation
Stable spinal fracture (lamina, spinous process, minor portion of vertebral body)
Ligamentous injury (unstable)
Spear tackler's spine

Type I Injury: The injuries in this group can cause immediate and complete paralysis below the level of the injured vertebra. Understanding the topographic anatomy of the sensory and motor tracts helps one to easily appreciate the clinical manifestations of syndromes in this injury group and for this purpose readers are recommended to refer to standard neuroanatomy text books. In anterior cord syndrome, the sensory tracts carrying the proprioception and light touch are intact and patients often present with complete paralysis due to the involvement of corticospinal tract. The selective central location of upper extremity motor fibers, immediately around the spinal canal, causes preferential weakness of the upper extremities in central cord syndrome. Brown-sequard syndrome referred as hemi-section of the spinal cord presents with ipsilateral paralysis and contralateral pain and temperature sensation, and is seen in unilateral facet fracture/dislocation.

Type II Injury: In this group of injuries the results of imaging and many a times neurological examination are normal. This group constitutes the majority of the sport related injuries. The sensory and /or motor deficits, if present, are transient and usually resolve within minute to hours (Zwimpfer and Bernstein 1990; Bailes and Maroon 1991). Spinal cord concussion refers to spinal cord injuries that result in complete neurological recovery within 24–48 h (Maroon and Bailes 1996). It is hypothesized that in concussion there is transient prolongation of absolute refractory period of long tract axons of the spinal cord causing a delay or failure in transmission of subsequent impulses (Zwimpfer and Bernstein 1990). In neuropraxia the peripheral nerve is macroscopically healthy, but microscopically, may have segmental demyelination resulting in physiologic block in conduction of impulses. Burning hand syndrome originally described by Maroon (1977) different from "burner or stringer," is a mild variant of central cord syndrome and is not widely reported in literature. A burner or stinger injury is a common injury pattern seen in sport-related trauma which refers to burning, dysesthetic pain radiating unilaterally into the arm or hand. Traction injury to the brachial plexus is thought to be the etiology of this condition (Poindexter and Johnson 1984).

Type III injury: Cervical spine injuries are associated with radiological abnormality suggestive of either primary or secondary cord injury, ligamentous, or bony disruption. Examples in this category include posterior ligament injury causing secondary narrowing of the cervical canal, congenital spinal stenosis, herniated intervertebral discs manifesting as radiculopathy, neck pain, and myelopathic signs. "Spear tackler's spine" refers to axial loading impact to the congenitally narrowed cervical canal and straightened cervical spine (in the absence of normal cervical lordosis) seen in athletes engaging in frequent head impact (Torg 1990; Torg et al. 1993). Any spinal injury classification is incomplete without mentioning about a unique group of spinal injuries occurring in pediatric population whereby a spinal injury can occur without a radiological abnormality on X-ray, abbreviated as SCIWORA. It is also worth mentioning the biomechanical classification of the cervical spine injuries based on the maximum injury vector which describes the resultant force, direction, and point of application that causes the final injury (Mcafee et al. 1983; White and Panjabi 1987). According to this classification cervical spine injuries are classified as follows:

Pure Distraction injury: Usually causes upper cervical spine injury, and the injury is often confined to the intervertebral disc. Ex: Atlanto-occipital dislocation, very rare in sports.

Distraction/extension injury: A variant of pure distraction and extension injury that usually results in posterior displacement of the cephalad vertebra on the caudal vertebra. Ex: classic odontoid fracture.

Extension injury: These groups of injuries are mostly ligamentous and can cause bony injuries when the force on ligaments reaches a critical point. Ex: Hangman's fracture.

Compression (axial loading) injury: The injury is usually confined to the vertebral body, and in a typical scenario the vertebra is crushed (burst fracture). This pattern is common in injuries where the athlete strikes an opponent with a straight cervical spine. Classic Jefferson's fracture with C1 burst at the ring belongs to this group of injuries.

Flexion/compression injury: Produces a fracture of the anterior vertebral body with rupture of posterior ligaments. Often the anterior vertebral body fracture will take the form of a "tear drop" off the upper corner of the vertebral body.

Flexion and distraction/flexion injury: These injuries cause dislocation of cervical facets which can be unilateral or bilateral.

2.1.2 Thoracolumbar Spine Injuries

The unique anatomy of thoracic and lumbar spine renders it susceptible to certain injury patterns. Thoracic spine due to vertically oriented facet joints, costovertebral and sternocostal joints is well suited for rotation; however, flexion and extension forces are not well adapted along the thoracic spine. On the contrary, facet joints of the lumbar spine lie slightly in a coronal plane and are less suited to withstand rotational forces. Majority of the sport-related thoracolumbar injuries are lumbar strain and sprain, and are categorized as benign. Injuries causing bony or ligamentous instability are rare, but when present may have a great impact on the career of the athlete. Injuries to this region can be divided into (1) Soft tissue, and (2) Bony injuries. Only significant injuries in these groups will be discussed:

Soft Tissue Injuries

Disc herniation: Repetitive trauma causes weakening of annular fibers which in turn predisposes to herniation of nucleus pulposus. At cellular level constituents of disc herniation differ in younger athletes and adults; in the former group proteoglycan constitutes much of herniated material as opposed to collagen in adults (Mcculloch 1997). Majority of the disc herniations are posterior or posterolateral, and are extremely lateral only in minority of the cases.

Bony Injuries

The chief bony lesions in sport-related thoracolumbar trauma pertain to injury of pars interarticularis and include pars stress fracture, spondylolysis, and spondylolisthesis. Traditionally, these three diagnostic entities were considered as a continuum, with acute form of injury, the pars stress fracture at one end, and spondylolisthesis the final outcome towards the other extreme (Wiltse 1975).

Spondylolysis: A type of overuse spinal injury, is defined as an acquired defect (stress fracture) involving either single or both pars interarticularis. Pars stress fractures and spondylolysis are rare in thoracic spine region because of very restricted flexion and extension capability, partly due to the pars arrangement in this region. An important concept in sport-related thoracolumbar injuries is to appreciate the subtle difference between (acute) pars stress fracture and spondylolysis: there is biological activity at the fracture site in pars stress fracture hence measures can be advocated at aiming the fracture to heal whereas in spondylolysis the absence of cellular milieu dismisses the chance of fracture to heal. Although this distinction is of little clinical relevance, there are practical implications for the athlete to participate in future sporting events with these two different injury patterns (Kraft 2002).

Spondylolisthesis: Is defined as anterior displacement of the cephalad vertebra in relation to the immediate caudal vertebra. L5 displacement over S1 is the commonest variant. Unlike pars stress fracture and spondylolysis, spondylolisthesis is a chronic condition. Spondylolisthesis is graded based on Meyerding system and grades spondylolisthesis as the percent of anterior displacement of the proximal vertebra relative to the lower: Grade 1: 1–25%, Grade 2: 26–50%, Grade 3: 51–75%, Grade 4: 76–100% and Grade 5: >100% slippage.

Spondylolisthesis greater than grade 1 seldom is seen in athletic population, perhaps due to early medical attention by athletes. The Taillard system of classifying spondylolisthesis is based on sacral inclination, the relationship of the plane of the sacrum to the vertical plane, and slip angle, the angle determined by a line passing across the posterior border of S1 and the inferior endplate of L5.

Vertebral body fractures: Fortunately, fractures to thoracolumbar region in sport-related trauma are very rare, but when present would require immediate attention. Combination of axial loading, flexion and extension forces are required to cause significant fractures of the vertebral body as seen in equestrian sport-related falls. Since the description of thoracolumbar fractures by Boehler in 1947, numerous classification systems have been developed and readers are referred to Sethi et al. (2009) for a comprehensive review on classification systems for thoracolumbar fractures. For the purpose of this chapter we would classify the vertebral body fractures into three major types: (1) burst (2) wedge and (3) chance fractures. *Burst* fracture involves the anterior and posterior aspects of the vertebral body, and is characterized by a vertically passing fracture line. There is higher risk of retropulsion of the fractured bony fragments into the spinal canal causing serious neurologic injury with this injury. A *wedge* fracture typically spares the posterior elements and is characterized by loss of vertebral body height anteriorly. *Seat belt (Chance)* fracture is caused by hyperflexion of the thoracolumbar junction, disrupting the middle and posterior elements of the thoracolumbar vertebral column, and is characterized by a horizontally oriented fracture line.

2.2 Epidemiology

The spinal column in an athlete is prone to several injuries of which strains and sprains are the commonest and are relatively benign. The term catastrophic spinal injury refers to unstable fractures, dislocations, or combination of both, cervical cord injury with transient quadriplegia, and disc herniation (Banerjee et al. 2004), and most of the epidemiological data in the literature refers to these injuries. Different sports are associated with sport-specific injuries and to some degree involve preferentially a particular segment of the spinal column.

NCAA data on football injuries suggests a higher rate of cervical spine trauma in 1977. The rate of fractures, subluxations, and dislocations of the cervical spine was 7.72/100,000 and 30.66/100,000 for high-school and college athletes, respectively. With the introduction of ban on spear tackling in football these figures decreased dramatically, and repeat study in 1984 recorded 2.31/100,000 and 10.66/100,000 injuries in similar athletic age groups. A year following the implementation of the ban on spearing the rate of cervical quadriplegia decreased between 1977 and 1984 from 0.40/100,000 and 0/100,000 in 1984 to 0.40/100,000 and 0/100,000 again in similar athletic age groups (Torg 1990). In ice hockey, 9% of all injuries manifested as fracture or/and dislocation between C5 and C7 (Molsa et al. 1999). Data from Canadian Sports Registry reveals an average of 17 catastrophic spinal injuries per year (Biasca et al. 2002). A review of spinal injuries sustained in Canada between 1943 and 1999 revealed a rate of 9.43 spinal injuries per 100,000 participants annually. Of this, half the injuries occurred in athletes aged 16–20 years and 83.3% injuries belonged to cervical vertebra with 47.3% injuries causing permanent spinal cord injury. In the same cohort an estimated one-third of the injuries rendered the patients wheelchair bound for the rest of the life (Tator et al. 2004).

Reports on wrestling quote a rate of 2.11 catastrophic spinal injuries annually or 1 per 100,000 participants. Two-third of these injuries were fractures or major ligamentous injuries confined to the cervical spine (Boden et al. 2002). Similar rates were reported by Kordi et al. (2008). Cheerleading, a sport with high content of gymnastic stunts is associated with high rate of cervical injuries. The United States Consumer Product Safety Commission reported that Cheerleading was the cause of 76 cervical spine fractures among 1,814 neck injuries that presented to the emergency department. Rugby, a popular collision sport has a varied injury pattern. The most common mechanism of spinal injury is hyperflexion of the cervical spine resulting in fracture dislocation of C4–5 or C5–6. Injuries are dependent on the level of the athlete, age of the athlete, and position of the player in the game (Quarrie et al. 2002). Studies from Australia quote an incidence of cervical injury causing tetraplegia or quadriparesis to be 6.5/100,100 annually during the period 1984–1996 (Rotem et al. 1998). A report from Fiji Island quotes a higher figure, where death or tetraplegia associated with rugby was 10/100,100 players. There has been steady increase in cervical spinal injuries in South Africa where rugby is a popular game. Between 1987 and 1996, the rate of admissions to Spinal Unit in that country has risen from 5.4 per year during 1981–1987, to 8.7 annually (Scher 1998).

Diving related injuries again often involve the cervical column of the spinal cord, and are attributed to the axial compression injury when divers hit head-first into the pool. A review from the German registry revealed that 7.7% traumatic injuries of the spine were caused by inappropriate diving techniques (Schmitt and Gerner 2001). Skiing and snowboarding are associated with higher rate of thoracolumbar injuries. Earlier studies reported snowboarding to be the major cause of spinal injuries with up to 80% of spinal injuries related to snowboarding (Scher 1998; Tarazi et al. 1999). Data obtained from Switzerland where skiing and snowboarding are popular, the reported prevalence of spinal injuries related to these sports is 10%. Catastrophic spinal injuries were associated with skiing (63/73 injuries), most of the injuries involving the lumbar vertebra and 53.4% injuries affecting two or more levels of the spinal column (Franz et al. 2008).

2.3 Clinical Evaluation

Evaluation of any suspected spinal injury should begin with immobilizing the spine as outlined in the ATLS guidelines; a full history including the mechanism of injury, the sports involved as certain injuries are sports-specific, and presence of extremity symptoms. History of previous injuries to spinal column or any chronic bony abnormalities should be taken into account. It is vital not to miss any associated life threatening abdominal injuries requiring urgent operative intervention. In one series of the 330 patients admitted with spinal injuries, 36 patients had significant abdominal injury requiring emergency laparotomy, highlighting the importance of concomitant life threatening injuries. Detailed description of neurological examination is out of scope of the current chapter and the readers are referred to standard neurology textbooks. For the purpose of this chapter an algorithm proposed by Banerjee et al. (2004) should aid in initial management of suspected cervical spinal injury and is illustrated in Fig. 1:

The role of repeated neurological examination in assessing a spinal injury cannot be under estimated. Neurological signs should be interpreted with great caution in the presence of spinal shock. The final

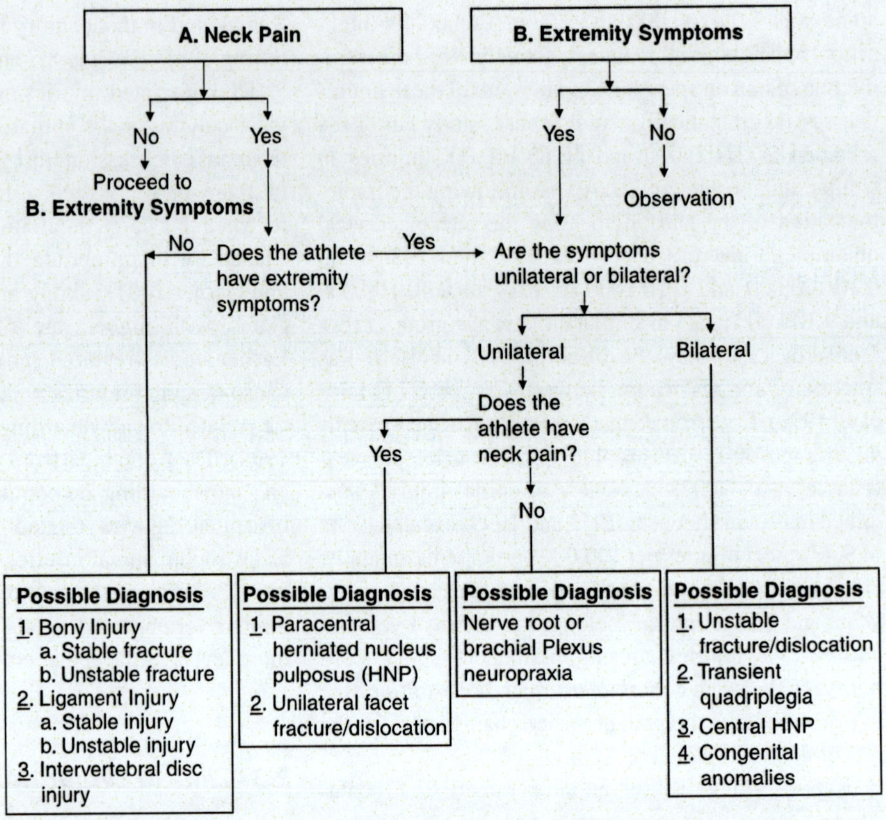

Fig. 1 Onfield-evaluation of cervical spine injury

clinical diagnosis of cord injury should be only made after the resolution of spinal shock, and one should have a very low threshold to use neuroimaging to diagnose underlying cord injury in such circumstances. In examining back injuries related to sports one has to bear in mind a possibility of any coexisting pathologies unrelated to the primary sport injury such as lumbar spinal stenosis, degenerative spondylolysis and cauda equina syndrome. Finally, one should also remember the association between head and neck injuries, and therefore a quick spinal injury assessment should also include evaluation for head injury.

3 Upper Extremity

3.1 *Shoulder Injuries*

The upper extremity is connected to the axial skeleton by a series of joints, the sternoclavicular, acromioclavicular, glenohumeral and scapulothoracic joints, collectively termed as shoulder girdle. Among these, the glenohumeral and acromioclavicular joints are commonly injured in sports and are discussed below. As there is limited epidemiological data on individual sports causing isolated injuries to a particular joint of the shoulder girdle, we herein describe overall epidemiology of shoulder injuries. Also, clinical examination of an injured shoulder is described in general, rather than a detailed review on assessment of individual joints of the shoulder girdle.

3.1.1 Acromioclavicular Injuries

The acromioclavicular (AC) joint complex is composed of bony and ligamentous structures. It includes a synovial joint between the distal third of the clavicle and acromion of the scapula, and is stabilized by static and dynamic components. The static components include the AC joint capsule surrounded by coracoclavicular and acromioclavicular ligaments, and trapezius and deltoid muscles constitute the dynamic elements (Rios and Mazzocca 2008).

Classification

Sport related acromioclavicular injuries are broadly divided into three pathological processes: (1) trauma (fracture, AC joint separation, or dislocation), (2) AC joint arthrosis (posttraumatic or idiopathic), and (3) distal clavicle osteolysis. Amongst these, AC separations represent the bulk of shoulder injuries. Rockwood's classification is commonly used to describe AC separations and includes six types. Posttraumatic osteoarthritis occurs commonly after AC disruptions and distal third clavicle fractures.

Distal clavicle osteolysis, an overuse injury, is a rare form of acromioclavicular injury. It has characteristic radiographic appearance, the presence of subchondral cysts along the distal third of the clavicle that distinguish it from AC arthritis. It is usually seen in weight lifters and athletes using bench press and push-ups. Often, the injury is bilateral and repetitive microtrauma is thought to be the underlying cause (Slawski and Cahill 1994).

3.1.2 Glenohumeral Injuries

The glenohumeral joint is frequently injured in overhead sports such as baseball, swimming, tennis, and volleyball; all these sports, apart from swimming, grouped as throwing sports. A characteristic pattern of forces along the glenohumeral joint is unique to the aforementioned sports causing specific injury pattern, termed as "shoulder instability" and "impingement." Patho-mechanical classification of sports injury to the shoulder originally described by Kvitne and Jobe, taking into account the direction of forces across the GH joint, and the arthroscopic findings will be presented below (Kvitne et al. 1995). This classification divides injuries into four major groups.

1. Pure impingement; no instability
2. Primary instability due to chronic labral injury; Secondary impingement
3. Primary instability due to generalized ligamentous hyperelasticity; Secondary impingement
4. Pure instability; no impingement

In group I, athletes have shoulder pain due to "primary impingement," in the absence of shoulder instability. Arthroscopic findings include fraying or tearing of the undersurface of rotator cuff; the glenoid labrum and glenohumeral ligaments are usually normal. Fibrosis and scarring of the subacromial bursa causes narrowing of the subacromial space. The coracoacromial ligament and an osteophyte from the acromion can be observed causing impingement on the superior surface of the rotator cuff. This injury pattern is seen only in small number of athletes, and most of them are over 35 years of age, and seldom seen in pediatric and adolescent athlete.

In group II, "primary" instability (subluxation) and "secondary subacromial impingement" is the result of repetitive microtrauma to the capsule and glenoid labrum. Arthroscopic findings include anterior glenoid labral damage, attenuation of the inferior GH ligament and anterior translation of the humeral head, in addition to rotator cuff findings similar to those seen in group I injuries.

In group III injuries there is attenuation of the inferior GH ligament and anterior joint capsule in the presence of normal glenoid labrum. In these injuries the humeral head is easily subluxated anteriorly. Usually these athletes show bilateral symmetrical increase in shoulder laxity.

In group IV injuries, there is a history of trivial or significant blow to the shoulder either by a fall on to the shoulder or collision against a fellow athlete, subluxating or dislocating the glenohumeral joint anteriorly. Typically, the arthroscopic findings include a normal rotator cuff, anterior glenoid labral damage (Bankart lesion), posterior humeral head defect (Hill-Sachs lesion), and the humeral head can be easily dislocated. Classification of sport-related shoulder injuries is incomplete without mentioning a unique group of injury type called SLAP (superior labrum, anterior to posterior) lesions. In a pure SLAP lesion, the biceps tendon is avulsed from its origin, the superior glenoid tubercle and the anterior and posterior labrum. However, there appears to be paucity in the data on the true incidence of pure SLAP lesion in throwing sports, and often only labral tears are noticed on arthroscopy (Tomlinson and Glousman 1995).

3.1.3 Miscellaneous: Clavicle and Humerus Fractures

Clavicular fractures typically result from direct blow in contact sports, fall on to the shoulder or outstretched hand. Eighty percent of the fractures usually occur in the middle third of the clavicle. In children there is high propensity of green stick type fracture due to increased plasticity of the periosteum.

Humerus fractures traditionally have been classified into proximal, shaft and distal, also called as supracondylar fractures. The latter group will be discussed in the elbow injury section. It is estimated that approximately 20% of proximal humerus fractures in the pediatric age group occur during sports. Two-thirds of these fractures are confined to the proximal humeral physis, with vast majority of the fractures belonging to Salter-Harris type I or II (Kohler and Trillaud 1983). Neers classification of proximal humerus fractures and AO classification for humerus fractures are the widely used classification systems, and readers are referred to standard orthopedic text books for an overview of these classification systems.

3.1.4 Epidemiology of Shoulder Injuries

A comprehensive review of published studies in competitive young (12–18-year-old) players revealed that shoulder injuries represented 25–47% of all arm injuries and 7–16% of all reported injuries, ranking it second among anatomic areas (Kibler 1995). However, most of the available studies do not clearly differentiate the injuries into specific diagnostic entities, so the true incidence of specific shoulder injuries is not known. Under reporting appears to be a major issue in sport-related shoulder injury. For example, it is difficult to evaluate the true incidence of acute rotator-cuff tears that may occur during sport, because some athletes sustain full-thickness tears but remain very functional (Burkhart et al. 1994; Ticker and Warner 1997). As a result the injury may go undiagnosed. After the initial pain and acute symptoms subside, these patients may return to full activity without ever seeking medical advice. In spite of these pitfalls, one can still say that shoulder injuries are common in contact and collision sports such as ice hockey (15%), rugby league (10%) and Australian Rules football (8%) and throwing sports (Orchard et al. 2002; Gabbett 2003). In a series by Headey et al. (2007), reporting shoulder injuries in professional rugby union, the incidence of shoulder injuries sustained during matches was 8.9/1,000 player-hours, with acromioclavicular joint injury (32%) being the leading shoulder injury followed by rotator cuff injury/shoulder impingement (23%), and shoulder dislocation/instability (14%). The results in the same study for injuries sustained during training sessions was 0.10/1,000 player-hours, a difference attributed to the degree of tackles per player per match in training session and the actual match. In football, the yearly incidence of shoulder injuries range between 10 and 20% (Delee and Farney 1992; Karpakka 1993). Epidemiological study on shoulder injuries in American football quotes 1.3 shoulder injuries per injured player, again, AC joint separation being the commonest (41.2%) injury followed by shoulder instability (20.9%), and rotator cuff injury (10.2%).Direct contact with fellow player or ground is responsible for 80% of AC injuries, and noncontact shoulder injuries are often responsible for rotator cuff injuries. In volleyball, an overhead sport, the injury pattern is slightly different. In one study, the incidence of chronic shoulder injury and reinjury was 2.98/1,000 player hours and 9.29/1,000 player hours respectively. The overall incidence, which included diagnosis of new shoulder injury in the study was 13.27/1,000 player hours, with rotator cuff injury being the leading cause of the injury (Wang and Cochrane 2001).

Skiing and snowboarding appear to be associated with mixed injury pattern. In a review of 7,430 snowboarding injuries, 32% of the injuries pertained to acromioclavicular joint and 29% of the shoulder injuries were fractures, mostly to the clavicle. Glenohumeral dislocations accounted for 20% of the injuries (Idzikowski et al. 2000). There seems to be lesser involvement of AC joint in skiing. A study on upper extremity injuries in skiing by Kocher et al. (1998) revealed glenohumeral dislocation to be the leading cause of shoulder injury (22%) followed by clavicle fracture (11%). A similar study on skiing injuries by quotes a much higher figure with 52% of shoulder trauma pertaining to glenohumeral dislocations. Improved skiing facilities are thought to be partly responsible for this decreased incidence of glenohumeral dislocations between the 80s and 90s (Weaver 1987). A study analyzing humerus fractures in skiers and snowboarders revealed an incidence of 0.041 and 0.062 humerus fractures per 1,000 skier-days with a prevalence of 1.5 and 2.2% respectively. In both these groups the proximal humerus constituted majority of the humerus fractures (Bissell et al. 2008).

3.1.5 Clinical Evaluation of Shoulder Injuries

Shoulder examination perhaps is one of the few joint examinations in the body that is associated with a long list of clinical tests helping to identify the etiology of shoulder pain. However, it should be said at the outset of this section that in clinical practice there is clearly a lack of absolute evidence as to whether these common orthopedic special bed side tests help clinician to differentiate the pathologies arising from shoulder (Hegedus et al. 2008).

Examination of the shoulder begins with a good history focusing on onset of symptoms, history of overuse with sports like base ball and tennis, presence of clicks or popping. Special emphasis should be placed on neurovascular symptoms, subjective evidence of instability during play, previous injuries to the shoulder girdle, and a recent change of sport or sporting technique. A thorough history should follow the actual examination of the shoulder which broadly is divided into (1) Inspection, (2) Palpation, and (3) Movement of the joint including special tests. This pattern is pertinent to any joint examination and will not be mentioned here after in the chapter. A recent review on Examination of the Shoulder in the Overhead and Throwing Athlete is an excellent resource for clinicians involved in treating sports injuries (Mcfarland et al. 2006; Mcfarland et al. 2008). It should be appreciated that the reliability of the clinical tests are highly dependent on the experience of the examiner. For the purpose of this chapter we list only a few of the several special tests which would aid the clinician to reach to a possible clinical diagnosis of the shoulder injury.

1. *The active compression test* (O'Brien et al. 1998): to detect labral tear (Sensitivity: 100%, Specificity: 98.5%, Positive Predictive Value (PPV): 94.6%, Negative Predictive Value (NPV): 100%).

This is performed with patient standing; the shoulder flexed at 90°, the arm adducted by 10° crossing the body and thumb facing down. In a positive test, the patient experiences pain deep in the shoulder when the examiner applies downward pressure with the patient resisting it. Next, with the arm position unchanged the palm is turned up, and again the examiner pushes down on the arm, and now the pain should be abolished or diminished.

2. *The anterior slide test* (Kibler 1995): to detect SLAP lesion (sensitivity: 78.4%, Specificity: 91.5%, PPV: 66.7%, NPV: 80.8%).

This is performed with the patient standing; the affected arm of the patient is placed on the ipsilateral hip. Examiner stands to the side and applies axial load up the arm toward the shoulder, and the test is considered positive if patient experiences deep pain or a click within the shoulder when resisting this maneuver of the examiner.

Special tests for Rotator Cuff Pathology: Again, the usefulness of the tests listed below is highly variable, but are still commonly used in evaluating a shoulder injury. Several authors have reported a wide range of sensitivity, specificity, NPV and PPV values in individual series for the tests described below.

1. *The Neer impingement test* (Neer 1983): The patient is either standing or sitting, and the examiner stabilizes the scapula and lifts the arm into flexion. The test is positive if patient experiences pain in the anterior shoulder or deltoid region as the arm is raised in full flexion.
2. *The Kennedy–Hawkins test* (Hawkins and Kennedy 1980): The patient is either seated or standing. The examiner elevates the arm to approximately 90° in flexion and then internally rotates the arm. The test is positive if it produces pain in the anterior shoulder with this maneuver.
3. *The painful arc test*: The patient is asked to elevate the arm overhead to full elevation. The test is positive if patient has pain between 70° and 120°, or at terminal flexion.
4. *The Whipple test* (Savoie et al. 2001): Is intended to detect rotator cuff tears. This test is performed with the patient standing. The arm is forward-flexed at 90°, and the hand placed opposite the other shoulder. The examiner pushes down on the arm and the patient resists this movement of the examiner. The test is positive if there is weakness or pain in the deltoid region or anterior shoulder.

Finally, the laxity of the shoulder joint is evaluated by the anterior ad posterior drawer tests and the load and the shift tests. The stability of the shoulder joint is assessed by apprehension test, the relocation test, and the "surprise" maneuvers (Mcfarland et al. 2006; 2008).

3.2 Elbow Injuries

3.2.1 Classification

Elbow is a complex synovial joint between the humerus, radius and ulna via three articulations: the ulnotrochlear joint, the radiocapitellar joint, and the proximal radioulnar joints. The soft tissue structures chiefly the radial collateral ligament and the ulnar collateral ligament provide approximately half of the stability to the elbow joint. Throwing and racquet sports are commonly implicated in elbow injuries with vast majority of the injuries being overuse injuries. There is no universally accepted classification of sport-related elbow injuries. The injuries can be either grouped into soft tissue and bony injuries or enthesopathies (lateral and medial epicondylitis and other rare similar conditions), valgus stress injuries, and nerve compression syndromes. Herein, we present classification of injuries to the common structures of the elbow joint inflicted in a sport-related injury. It should be noted that most of these classification systems are based on radiological findings.

Supracondylar Fractures

Supracondylar fractures of the humerus in general are the second most common fractures in children. Often the fracture is secondary to hyperextension forces around the elbow, say for example as a result of fall on an outstretched arm. In its typical form the distal fragment is displaced posteriorly in 90% of cases. Gartland's classification, modified by Wilkins is the most accepted classification system for these fractures and is divided into three main types:

Type I: The fracture is undisplaced or minimally displaced, and the anterior humeral line passes through the capitellum.

Type II: The distal fragment is displaced with the direction of displacement being posterior, or angulated medially or laterally depending on the direction of forces at the time of the initial impact on the elbow. In general, the posterior angulation is hinged on an intact posterior cortex.

Type III: The distal segment is completely displaced posteriorly with absolutely no cortical contact. Wilkins subdivided type III fractures into "A" and "B" depending on whether the posteriorly displaced fragment is rotated medially or laterally, respectively.

Radial Head and Neck Fractures

Radial head and neck fractures are common in athletes and often are the result of a fall on an outstretched hand with the forearm held in pronation, an action which results in approximately 90% of the body weight being transmitted across the radial head (Morrey et al. 1988). Radial head fractures are classified according to Mason's classification, modified by Morrey and Johnston into four major types based on the degree of displacement of the radial head (Mason 1954). In the original description Mason described only three types, did not include radial neck fractures, and did not quantify displacement, a feature added by Morrey. According to him displacement is defined as a fragment involving 30% or more of the articular surface and is displaced by more than 2 mm.

Type I: Non displaced radial head.

Type II: Minimally displaced radial head with depression, angulation and impaction.

Type III: Comminuted and displaced radial head.

Type IV: Radial head fractures involving the neck and associated with dislocation of the elbow.

Overall, athlete's radial fractures are usually type I and II.

Olecranon Fractures

An olecranon fracture can occur following a direct impact on the ulna or rarely as a result of the forceful pull of triceps. Morrey classified olecranon fractures based on the degree of communition, stability, and displacement into three types:

Type I: Nondisplaced fracture. The fractured fragments are displaced less than 2 mm.

Type II: Displaced, stable. This pattern accounts for about 85% of olecranon fractures and olecranon fractures in athletes are usually of this type. Type II is further divided into "A" (noncommunited) and "B" (communited).

Type III: Displaced, unstable. This pattern accounts for 5% of all olecranon fractures and is again divided into "A" (noncommunited) and "B" (communited). This type is very rare in athletes. Associated radial head fractures are often seen with this type of olecranon fractures.

Coronoid Fractures

Fortunately coronoid fractures are rare in athletes; nevertheless deserve a mention, as, if missed could affect the stability of the elbow joint. Based on the stability of the joint and the articular surface involved Regan and Morrey classified coronoid fractures into three types

(Regan and Morrey 1989): type I: avulsion fracture of the tip of the coronoid process; type II: fractured fragment is ≤50% of the coronoid process; and type III: fractured fragment is ≥50% of the coronoid process. Recently, a more comprehensive classification system based on anatomical location of the fracture was introduced and is described below (O'Driscoll et al. 2003):

Type I: Transverse fracture of the tip of the coronoid process
- Subtype 1: ≤2 mm of coronoid bony height (usually referred as flake fracture)
- Subtype 2: >2 mm of coronoid bony height

Type II: Fracture of anteromedial facet of the coronoid process
- Subtype 1: Anteromedial rim
- Subtype 2: Anteromedial rim + tip
- Subtype 3: Anteromedial rim + sublime tubercle (±tip)

Type III: Fracture of the coronoid process is at the base
- Subtype 1: Coronoid body and base
- Subtype 2: Transolecranon basal coronoid fractures

Elbow Dislocation

The elbow is the second most common joint prone to dislocation in the adults and is the most commonly dislocated joint in the pediatric population. It often is the result of fall on an outstretch hand which creates hyperextension at the elbow joint. Elbow dislocations are linked to higher percentage of associated injuries around the elbow joint, namely fractures of radial head and neck, coronoid process, and medial epicondyle fractures.

Original elbow dislocation pattern described by O'Driscoll is based on mechanical forces acting across the elbow joint in stages, ultimately resulting in dislocation (O'Driscoll et al. 1992). According to this classification, an elbow joint is considered as a "stable ring" of soft tissue elements which is disrupted in stages. Stage I causes disruption of ulnar component of lateral collateral ligament causing posterolateral rotatory subluxation of the elbow that reduces spontaneously. With increase in the magnitude of forces, the ring is disrupted anteriorly and posteriorly resulting in an incomplete posterolateral dislocation, also termed as "perched dislocation" (Stage II); some authors use the term subluxation. In Stage III A, all soft tissue structures are disrupted except the anterior band of the medial collateral causing posterior dislocation. The final event (Stage III B) would include damage to the entire medial collateral ligament complex making the dislocated elbow highly unstable.

In clinical practice, classifying dislocations simply into posterior, anterior, and divergent is more relevant. Over 95% of the dislocations are posterior, and only about 2% are anterior dislocations. A divergent dislocation fortunately is rare in athletic injuries to the elbow. It is the result of high velocity trauma resulting in separation of the radius from ulna, completely disrupting the interosseous membrane, annular ligament, and distal radioulnar joint capsule (Cohen and Hastings 1998).

Overuse Injuries

Overuse injuries of the elbow are very common in athletes participating in throwing sports. The structures around the elbow joint namely ligaments (mainly ulnar collateral ligament), musculotendinous structures (flexor-pronator muscle complex: pronator teres, flexor carpi radialis, palmaris longus, flexor digitorum superficialis and flexor carpi ulnaris), and nerves (e.g., ulnar nerve) are all involved in throwing sports (Rettig 2004). Safran (1995) in his elaborative review on elbow injuries in athletes arbitrarily divided elbow pain into four regions associated with possible underlying etiologies (Safran 1995):

1. Anterior elbow pain
   Biceps tendinitis and rupture
   Ectopic bone
   Pronator teres syndrome
2. Posterior elbow pain
   Traction apophysitis
   Triceps tendinitis and rupture
   Olecranon stress fractures and spurs
3. Medial elbow pain
   Medial epicondylar physeal fracture
   Medial epicondylitis
   Flexor-pronator tendinosis (golfer's elbow) or rupture
   Ulnar neuritis
   Medial elbow instability
4. Lateral elbow pain
   Osteochondritis dissecans
   Lateral epicondylitis
   Loose bodies secondary to radiocapitellar overload syndrome
   Radial nerve entrapment

A more clinical approach would be classifying the elbow overuse injuries into postero-medial and lateral elbow conditions and few of the common conditions are described below.

Postero-Medial Elbow Conditions

Ulnar collateral ligament (UCL) rupture is by far the commonest ligamentous injury of the elbow seen in throwing sports. Often microtears of the UCL occur when the valgus forces generated during the throwing action exceeding the tensile strength of the UCL. Repetitive abnormal stresses eventually result in the rupture of the UCL causing valgus instability of the elbow joint.

Flexor-pronator tendinosis although commonly referred as golfer's elbow is more common than tennis elbow in tennis players. Improper serving techniques as seen in tennis and abnormal throwing action, and excessive fatigue cause inflammation of flexor-pronator complex. Often flexor carpi radialis and pronator teres are implicated in the inflammatory process (Vangsness and Jobe 1991).

Ulnar nerve compression, causing ulnar neuritis can occur at several sites along its path across the elbow: (1) at the entrance into the cubital tunnel, (2) in the cubital tunnel, (3) exiting the cubital tunnel where it passes between the two heads of the origin of the flexor carpi ulnaris. Ulnar neuritis in the throwing athlete develops as a result of excessive traction due to valgus stress, compression from adhesions and osteophytes, flexor muscle hypertrophy, or subluxation of the nerve around the medial epicondyle (Bozentka 1998).

Posterior impingement of the elbow is the end result of valgus-extension overload syndrome caused by repetitive hyperextension, extension, valgus, and supination movements. A repetitive valgus force leads to weakening of UCL, which in turn causes posteromedial olecranon impingement within the shallow olecranon fossa. Subsequently the tip of the olecranon is inflamed, eventually resulting in chondromalacia and osteophytes. The osteophytes with continued elbow motion detach and become loose bodies, the terminal outcome of the valgus-extension syndrome (Safran 1995).

Lateral Elbow Conditions

Lateral epicondylitis and osteochondritis dissecans are the two most common affecting the lateral elbow of athletes. Lateral epicondylitis, also called as tennis elbow, occurs 10 times more frequently than medial epicondylitis. It is defined as chronic tendinitis of the extensor muscles, chiefly the extensor carpi radialis brevis, usually at its origin. Although encountered more often in tennis players, this injury can occur in an athlete participating in any throwing sport. Necrosis of capitellar ossific nucleus, also called as osteochondritis dissecans of the capitellum is often confined to the pediatric athletic population. The current hypothesis suggests that chronic radiocapitellar compression due to repetitive trauma results in arterial injury causing necrosis of the capitellum. Other less frequent condition of the lateral elbow is the radial tunnel syndrome. It is a type of entrapment neuropathy of the posterior interosseous nerve within the radial tunnel, and often can be confused with lateral epicondylitis (Roles and Maudsley 1972).

3.2.2 Clinical Evaluation of Elbow Injuries

A thorough history focusing on age of the athlete, type of sport, point of maximum intensity of pain around the elbow, onset and timing of pain in relation to the sport, associated neurovascular symptoms, previous injuries to the elbow, evidence of delayed skeletal maturity, presence of swelling, deformity and bruising.

Age of the athlete gives a clue about the underlying diagnosis. In a skeletally immature adult recurrent microtrauma suggests the presence of apophyseal injury in the medial or lateral epicondyle. However, similar injury mechanism in an adolescent can cause avulsion fractures. Similarly, it is uncommon to see musculotendinous and ligamentous injuries in pediatric athletes.

Throwing sports that produce excessive valgus stress are usually associated with ligamentous injuries, whereas contact sports resulting in fall on an outstretched hand are more commonly implicated in fractures/dislocations of the elbow. As mentioned earlier in the classification section, point of maximum pain/tenderness would narrow the differential diagnosis of the elbow pain. Sudden onset of pain is usually typical of avulsion injuries, as opposed to recurrent bouts of acute pain which suggests a chronic overuse injury. Ecchymosis, gross deformity and swelling around the elbow are indicative of bony injury. Symptoms of peripheral nerve injury along the distribution of ulnar nerve and rarely the radial nerve point out to an underlying entrapment syndrome of these nerves.

Adequate history should follow inspection, palpation and assessment of the elbow joint for range of movement. Presence of crepitus and pain while assessing the range of motion indicates the presence of an osteochondral lesion or loose bodies. In a normal subject the end-feel in extension is usually firm, as opposed to a soft feel at the extremes of flexion. However, in a throwing athlete with an osteophyte or loose body the end-feel in terminal flexion is bony. Palpations should involve bony structures, ligaments, tendon insertions, muscle mass, and nerves. Tenderness along medial epicondyle suggests an injury to the growth plate or avulsion fracture. Pain on palpation of the lateral olecranon border is suggestive of olecranon stress fracture, and similarly pain about the radial head on its palpation as the forearm is rotated passively implies a possible radial head and/or neck fracture, osteochondritis dissecans of the capitellum or rarely injury to the annular ligament of the radial collateral ligament. A gap in the tendinous insertions of triceps and biceps suggests their rupture. Ulnar nerve should be palpated for any evidence of subluxation of the nerve and gently percussed around the medial epicondyle and along the cubital cannel to observe for paresthesia along the distribution of ulnar nerve (tinnel's sign) suggestive of ulnar neuritis.

Muscle strength of chief muscles around the elbow: biceps and triceps by flexion and extension of the elbow, and long flexors and extensors of the forearm through wrist flexion and extension should be assessed and compared with the contralateral side. Assessment of valgus instability of the elbow is assessed to check for the integrity of the UCL complex. This is best performed with the athlete sitting and the examiner securing the athletes wrist between his (examiner's) forearm and trunk and then with elbow flexed between 20° and 30°, valgus stress is applied. An opening of the medial joint space by more than 1 mm and loss of firm end point with this maneuver in the presence of tenderness along the distribution of UCL would suggest a ruptured UCL (Heim 1999). It should be noted that approximately 50% of the patients with an UCL injury have associated symptoms of ulnar neuritis, and therefore care should be taken to establish a firm diagnosis of UCL injury in such cases. An essential differential diagnosis of UCL injury is flexor-pronator tendinosis. In the later there is increased pain posterior to the flexor origin on wrist flexion. Unlike its medial counterpart, instability due to insufficiency of radial collateral ligament is rare and is usually seen in elbow dislocations.

3.2.3 Epidemiology of Elbow Injuries

As with any sports the incidence of elbow injuries largely depends on the type of sport, level of performance of the sports (competition/match vs. noncompetition/practice), intensity and technique of the sport. Annually, more than two million people participate in Little League baseball in the US and the elbow is the most frequently injured joint in the adolescent baseball pitcher (Klingele and Kocher 2002). It was noticed that the frequency of the injury is higher in players with poor sporting technique (52%) vs. in players with proper technique (6%) (Albright et al. 1978). Overall, 25–52% of all baseball players report elbow pain (Lyman et al. 2002; Hang et al. 2004). Avulsion of the medial epicondyle is the most common fracture in adolescent and preadolescent overhead throwing athletes. A single season study in Little League baseball players reported that approximately half of the boys aged 9–12 years had avulsion of medial epicondyle causing elbow pain (Hang et al. 2004). In a comprehensive review on epidemiology of pediatric and adolescent elbow injuries, Magra et al. (2007) quote an incidence of elbow injuries in American football and rugby as 2–6% and 2.6% respectively. Sports like gymnastics which require higher athletic maneuvers are associated with much higher rates of elbow trauma: 3.7–8.5% (Caine et al. 1989). Conditions under which a sport is played also influence the injury rates. For example, there is higher rate of elbow injuries in women's gymnastics in competition than practice. On the contrary, the incidence of elbow injuries in two major wrestling competitions was 3.6% as opposed to a rate of 7% in wrestling played at noncompetitive level (Lorish et al. 1992; Pasque and Hewett 2000).

Studies from different countries depict varying rates of elbow injuries in snow sports. Approximately 2% of all snowboarding accidents in Austrian children were confined to the elbow, as opposed to 5% in Canadian snowboarders (Machold et al. 2000). Cumulative figures for the incidence of skiing and snowboarding injuries around the elbow in Canadian population in athletes <18 years was just under 1.5% (Hagel et al. 1999). In ice hockey 2–6% of the total injuries sustained pertain to the elbow (Stuart and Smith 1995;

Pinto et al. 1999). The rates of elbow pain in tennis players varied according to the study. Tennis elbow constituted 5.6% of all injuries in adolescents playing competitive tennis. There is a difference in prevalence of tennis related sport injuries depending on the age of the athlete. In the US less than 10% of boys and girls playing tennis at national level reported lateral elbow symptoms as opposed to 22–25% of adolescents reporting of similar elbow injury pattern with the same sport (Hutchinson and Ireland 2003).

In children, fractures around the elbow form a significant proportion of sport-related injuries. Approximately 40% of elbow dislocations occur during sports such as gymnastics, wrestling, baseball and football. Some authors quote a still higher figure: Houshian et al. (2001) report that about 50% of elbow fractures in pediatric population are the results of sports.

3.3 Wrist and Hand Injuries

Hand and wrist injuries although are very common in athletes there is no universal classification that describes whole spectrum of injuries. There is a wealth of literature describing individual injuries of the hand and wrist by eponyms, e.g., gamekeepers thumb (injury to UCL of thumb), deQuervain's tendonitis, Bennett's fractures (fracture first metacarpal) are a few to name. Injuries in this region can be divided into (1) traumatic: fractures, dislocations, and ligamentous injuries, and (2) overuse injuries. Overuse injuries are predominantly confined to wrist, and traumatic injuries are equally common at both hand and wrist.

3.3.1 Overuse Injuries of the Wrist

(a) *De Quervain's syndrome*: Is defined as tenosynovitis of the tendons of the first extensor compartment of the wrist: the abductor pollicis longus and extensor pollicis brevis. The underlying etiology is thought to be microtrauma to these structures due to repetitive gliding of the above tendons over the styloid as seen in racquet sports such as squash, tennis, and badminton.

(b) *Extensor carpi ulnaris (ECU) tendonitis*: Is defined is inflammation of ECU tendon in the wrist and is the second most common overuse injury following De Quervain's tendonitis. It is seen in rowing and racquet sports. Interestingly, this overuse injury is seen in tennis players in the nondominant wrist.

(c) *Extensor carpi ulnaris subluxation*: This condition, in addition to overuse of the wrist, can also occur following a single traumatic episode as in a fall on an outstretch hand. The pathology involves rupture to medial wall of the ECU tendon sheath secondary to sudden or repetitive flexion and ulnar deviation, causing subluxation of ECU.

(d) *Intersection syndrome*: Is defined as an inflammation at the crossing points of the tendons of the first dorsal compartment and the extensor radialis longus and brevis. This point is typically 2–3 in. proximal to the radio-carpal joint. This entity is seen in sports involving repetitive wrist extension.

Ligamentous Injuries of the Wrist

(a) *Scapholunate injuries*: Are considered to be the most common ligamentous injury of the wrist. In its typical pattern, the injury is the result of abnormally large forces causing wrist extension, ulnar deviation and supination at the carpal bones. In extreme situations seen with complete scapholunate rupture, the normal alignment between scaphoid, lunate and triquetrum is lost: a characteristic appearance of scapholunate dissociation is seen on plain radiographs. This injury pattern is seen in collision with the fellow sports personnel and fall on an outstretched hand, with the hand held in the above position at the time of the impact in both instances.

(b) *Lunotriquetral injuries*: Are less common compared to scapholunate injuries and usually do not progress to arthrosis and collapse of the architecture of proximal row of carpal bones. These injuries occur as the result of forces that cause wrist extension, radial deviation and pronation at the carpal bones. Unlike scapholunate ruptures, insufficiency of lunotriquetral ligament does not disrupt the normal alignment of the lunate and triquetrum due to presence of extrinsic dorsal and volar ulnar ligaments stabilizing these carpal bones.

(c) *Triangular fibrocartilage complex (TFCC) injuries*: The TFFC transmitting about one fifth of the axial load from the wrist to the forearm plays a pivotal role as a stabilizer of the distal radioulnar joint. TFFC is a ligamento-cartilagenous complex separating the proximal row of the carpus and ulna. It is made up of a centrally located relatively avascular biconcave, fibrocartilage, and peripheral ligamentous anchor: the dorsal and palmar distal radioulnar ligaments, and the ulnolunate and ulnotriquetral ligaments. The TFCC is completed on the ulnar side by the ulnar collateral ligament, and the extensor carpi ulnaris sheath. Principally, TFCC injuries are divided into traumatic (class I) and degenerative tears (class II), the former being more common in athletes. Each class is further subdivided into A, B, C, and D, with IB being the commonest type of injuries in the athletes. In IB injuries there is a tear in the peripheral ligamentous complex at its ulnar insertion. Injuries to the TFCC complex may develop either secondary to repetitive stress on the ulnar border of the wrist as seen in racquet sports, or acutely, following a fall on an outstretched hand in contact sports, transmitting abnormally high degree of rotational forces.

Bony Injuries of the Wrist

Distal Radius Fractures

The distal radius fractures in the athletes typically differ from the osteoporotic Colle's fracture. The fracture pattern in the later is usually extra-articular and is the result of relatively low energy trauma, whereas in athletes the fracture usually involves the articular surface and is often caused by severe axial load. The compressive forces created by the axial load are transmitted across the lunate on to the radial articular fossa causing various fracture patterns of the distal radius involving the radial shaft, radial styloid, dorsal medial fragment and palmar medial fragment (Melone 1993). Much of the literature on distal radius fractures in athletes is based on Melone's classification:

TypeI: Undisplaced, stable and noncommunited fracture.

Type II: Displaced, unstable, communited fracture with radial shortening and/or angulation.

Type III: Displaced, unstable, communited, additional spike fragment either from the anterior or posterior cortex of the radial metaphysis.

Type IV: Displaced, unstable, communited, wide separation or rotation of the dorsal and/or palmar medial fragment.

Carpal Fractures

(a) *Scaphoid* fracture: Scaphoid is the most frequent carpal bone sustaining a fracture. The precarious blood supply to the scaphoid renders it more prone to vascular necrosis more than any other carpal bone. The proximal two third of the scaphoid, demarcated anatomically from the distal third at the waist of the scaphoid, receives its blood supply in a retrograde fashion: distal to proximal. The more proximal from the waist the fracture is, the higher the chance of avascular necrosis. Typically, forces resulting in severe hyperextension and ulnar deviation of the wrist may cause scaphoid fracture.

(b) *Triquetral* fracture: This is the second most common carpal bone fracture in sport-related injuries. Fractures are secondary to a fall on an outstretched with the wrist held in dorsiflexion and ulnar deviation. The two most common mechanisms underlying the fractures of triquetrum in the athletes are impaction of ulnar styloid or the hamate on the triquetrum, and avulsion of the soft tissue attachments, chiefly the radiotriquetral and scaphotriquetral ligaments from the dorsal cortex of the triquetrum. The later injury mechanism is seen in hyperflexion wrist injuries (Hocker and Menschik 1994).

(c) *Hamate* fracture: The hook of the hamate being the most superficial structure at the hypothenar eminence is prone to fractures in sports more often than the body of the hamate. Direct pressure against the hook of the hamate by the racquet and severe pull of the hypothenar muscles arising from the hook of the hamate and nearby flexor tendons contribute to its fractures (Stark et al. 1989). In contrast, fractures of the body of the hamate are usually the result of axial load along the little finger metacarpal. Underlying ulnar neurovascular bundle in the Guyon's canal can be injured in severely displaced fractures of the hamate.

(d) *Lunate* fractures: Fortunately, fractures of the lunate in the athletes are rare, partly due to its safe position in the large congruent radial fossa. Severe compressive axial forces directed along the distally located capitate on to the lunate results in the fracture across the body of the lunate. In hyperextension injuries of the wrist the dorsal lip of the lunate close to the distal radius can be fractured. In the opposite mechanism of injury the volar lip is frequently fractured in which case it may be associated with volar subluxation. In severe scapholunate injuries there can be associated scapholunate dissociation. In the presence of a peri-lunate dislocation one has to consider any damage to median nerve that is in close proximity to the lunate.

One of the major concerns in the athletic population more than a fracture, is the avascular necrosis of lunate, also referred as Kienbock's disease. It is thought that repetitive microtrauma predisposes to avascular necrosis in some athletes with inherently compromised blood supply to the lunate. The other theory is that presence of a shortened ulna, also known as ulnar minus variance, causes shearing forces across the lunate, again predisposing to avascular necrosis (Beckenbaugh et al. 1980). Staging of Kienbock's disease is based on sequential radiographic appearances ranging from sclerotic and cystic changes to lunate collapse.

(e) *Pisiform* fractures: Pisiform is a sesamoid bone in the tendon of the flexor carpi ulnaris. Its superficial relationship at the hypothenar eminence makes it susceptible to fracture on a direct blow as seen in racquet sports. Similar to the hook of the hamate, the pisiform is an origin for strong ligaments, thereby rendering it susceptible to avulsion injuries. A strong association of concomitant injuries to the distal radius and other carpal bones in the presence of fractured pisiform is well documented (Ruby 1992).

(f) *Trapezium* fractures: Trapezium fractures are divided into fractures of the body and the ridge, the former being the commonest type. Axial forces along the thumb metacarpal cause vertical shear fracture across the radial aspect of the body of the trapezium, a fracture pattern usually associated with dislocation of the thumb carpometacarpal joint. Trapezial ridge fractures are divided into two types based on the alignment of the fracture line. In type I fracture the fracture line runs across the base of the ridge, and type II fracture is the avulsion fracture of the tip of the ridge. Chronic injuries in the form of repetitive microtrauma around the trapezium can sometimes present as carpal tunnel syndrome and tendonitis of flexor carpi radialis which runs in the grove formed by the trapezial ridge and the transverse carpal ligament (Palmer 1981).

(g) *Trapezoid* fractures: Trapezoid is the least common fractured carpal bone, and constitutes about less than 1% of all carpal fractures. The common mechanism of the fracture is axial compressive forces directed along the index finger metacarpal on to the trapezoid (Ruby 1992). A combination of avulsion fracture of the trapezoid and dorsal subluxation of the index finger metacarpal can be seen.

(h) *Capitate* fractures: The most common site of the fractures of the capitate are at the junction of body and neck. In addition to this isolated fracture pattern, fractures of the capitate can also occur as a part of scaphoid perilunar fracture dislocation as result of a high-energy fall on an outstretched hyperextended and radially deviated wrist. The forces generated from such a mechanism of injury typically cause fractures of the scaphoid at the waist, and of the capitate at the neck (Vance et al. 1980).

Common Injuries of the Hand

Injuries to the hand can be broadly classified into extraarticular fractures of the metacarpals and phalanges, joint injuries, and closed tendon injuries (Rettig 2004).

Extra Articular Fractures of the Metacarpal and Phalanges

Majority of the metacarpal and phalangeal fractures in athletes, unlike those from high energy trauma, are stable injuries. Distal phalanges fractures are usually the result of crush injuries and may be accompanied by an underlying nail-bed injury. Middle phalangeal fractures are often caused by direct blows, as in by a forceful strike with a cricket ball, and are usually transverse in nature. Rotational forces on the flexed digits are implicated in the spiral fractures of the proximal phalanx or the metacarpal which are often unstable. Each of these fractures can have an associated tendon injury. Metacarpal neck and shaft fractures are common injuries in contact sports and the volar pull of the interosseous muscles causes dorsal angulation of the neck (Brunet and Haddad 1986). Individual metacarpal can tolerate a varying degree of angulation beyond which the fracture is classified as unstable requiring surgical fixation.

Joint Injuries

(a) Proximal interphalangeal joint injuries

The proximal interphalangeal joint (PIPJ) a functionally hinged joint and is held in place by soft tissue structures namely: the radial and ulnar collateral ligaments, the volar plate, and the capsule. Disruption of these soft tissue constraints at PIPJ level is common in sport-related injuries. The collateral ligaments, often on the radial side, are disrupted partially or completely by axial loading and dorsiflexion forces across the PIPJ. In severe injuries, in addition to the disruption of collateral ligaments, the volar plate is often severed causing dislocation of the PIPJ. The PIPJ dislocations can be dorsal, volar, or lateral depending on the direction of forces. As these injuries are often seen in ball-handling sports the direction of the impact of the ball over the PIPJ determines the type of PIPJ dislocation (Rettig 2004). In the extreme situations the volar plate may avulse the base of the articular surface of the middle phalanx. The involvement of the articular surface by more than one-third of the surface area may render the fracture unstable. Isolated condylar fractures of the proximal phalanx: unicondylar, bicondylar or communited are common injuries.

(b) Thumb carpometacarpal (CMC) and metacarpophalangeal (MCP) joint injuries

Dislocations of the thumb CMC joint are rare. Bennet's fracture, the commonest thumb metacarpal fracture is seen in several sport-related injuries, the injury occurs as a result of a severe adductor pull on a semiflexed thumb. Typically, the fracture is two part intra-articular: volar-ulnar and the dorsal-radial displaced/dislocated metacarpal fragments. Common thumb MCP joint injuries are MCP joint dislocations and ulnar collateral ligament ruptures. Among the MCP joint dislocations, dorsal dislocation is the commonest type, and typically is the result of hyperextension injury involving volar plate tear.

Ulnar collateral ligament injury of the thumb MCPJ, also referred as *skier's* or *gamekeepers thumb* is a very common injury in sport-related injuries of the thumb seen in collision sports and skiing. Typically, the injury is secondary to radially directed force on an abducted thumb causing partial or complete tear of the UCL. In majority of the cases UCL rupture occurs at its insertion into the proximal phalanx (Isani and Melone 1986). *Sterner lesion*, a unique type of UCL injury is described as interposition of the thumb adductor muscle aponeurosis between the two ends of the ruptured UCL. The interposed adductor aponeurosis impedes the healing of the UCL requiring surgical fixation of the UCL.

Closed Tendon Injuries of the Hand

(a) Mallet finger: Is defined as avulsion of extensor tendon from its insertion at the base of the distal phalanx, a common injury seen in ball-handling sports. The axial compressive forces along the extended distal phalanx cause forceful flexion of distal interphalangeal joint (DIPJ) avulsing the extensor tendon from its insertion. The other mechanisms are forceful hyperextension at the DIPJ or a direct blow over the dorsum of the finger at the level of the DIPJ (McCue and Wooten 1986). The disruption of the extensor mechanism can occur through the extensor tendon itself, or may develop secondary to avulsion of the bone fragment. The bony avulsion on plain radiographs can be of varying degrees: (1) avulsion of the fleck of bone, (2) avulsion of up to one-third of the articular surface, and (3) avulsion of the bony fragment resulting in palmar subluxation of the larger portion of the distal phalanx (Wehbe and Schneider 1984).

(b) Boutonniere deformity: Is defined as an avulsion of the central slip from its insertion into the base of the middle phalanx causing flexion deformity of the PIPJ. This deformity is secondary to a blow over the dorsum of the middle phalanx causing forced flexion at the PIPJ. The other common mechanism of boutonniere deformity is palmar dislocation of the PIPJ that is spontaneously reduced or is reduced by the athlete himself on field (Leddy 1998). Immediately following the injury the associated extension at the DIPJ is not usually seen, and only with time when the lateral bands migrate palmar to the axis of rotation at the PIPJ, the typical appearance of extension of the DIPJ in addition to the primary flexion of PIPJ ensures (Aronowitz and Leddy 1998).

(c) Subluxation/dislocation of the MCPJ extensor tendon mechanism: Subluxation or dislocation of the extensor tendon, a rare injury in athletes usually is secondary to radial sagittal band tears of the extensor hood. The sagittal bands secure the extensor tendon over the metacarpal heads, the tears causing dislocation or subluxation of the extensor tendon between the two heads of metacarpals. A similar injury, the boxer's knuckle secondary to repetitive microtrauma is a tear of sagittal bands of the extensor tendon in the absence of subluxation or dislocation of the extensor tendon.

(d) Avulsion of the flexor digitorium profundus (FDP) tendon: This is a relatively common injury in athletes with the avulsion usually occurring at the base of the insertion of distal phalanx. Interestingly, two-thirds of these injuries are confined to the ring finger. The injury occurs when an athlete forcibly extends the finger. Avulsion of FDP is classified into three types based on the level of the retraction of the FDP tendon and the presence of bony fragment (Leddy 1985). In type I injuries the avulsion of FDP tendon retracts it into the palm. Type II injuries result in retraction of the tendon up to the level if the PIPJ, occasionally with a small fleck of the avulsed bone lying at the level of the PIPJ. Type III injuries are associated with avulsions of a large bony fragment that lies just proximal to the PIPJ.

3.3.2 Clinical Evaluation of Wrist and Hand Injuries

Evaluation of hand injuries comprises of a through history and physical examination. The later encompassing the principles of standard orthopedic examination of any joint: look, feel, and move. A thorough understanding of the several surface bony landmarks is imperative in conducting a successful wrist examination. Herein, we describe only the salient features of examination of the wrist and hand. History should focus on onset of the pain, location of pain, sport involved, evidence of snapping or clicking, mechanism of injury and preexisting wrist or hand pathologies. Certain sports are associated with a specific injury pattern. For example, UCL injuries are often seen in skiers compared to other athletic groups, mallet finger is associated with ball-handling sports, overuse injuries often accompany racquet sports, and contact sports resulting in fall on an outstretched hand would involve bony injuries.

Inspection should always involve comparison with the contralateral side in the anatomical position, with particular emphasis on the presence of any muscle wasting and deformities. Loss of muscle mass over the hypothenar and thenar area would suggest chronic entrapment of ulnar and median nerve from a racquet sport. A mallet finger is indicative of an injury from ball-handling sport. Classic appearance of FDP avulsion is manifested as loss of the cascade seen on tackling injuries seen in rugby. Shortening or over-riding of the fingers on making a fist point to an underlying metacarpal or ring fracture secondary to fall on an outstretched hand in contact sports.

Several structures of the wrist joint located superficially means an easy access to these structures on palpation. Floor of the anatomic snuff box which is more pronounced on ulnar deviation of the wrist is an important bony landmark, and is tender on deep palpation in fracture and avascular necrosis of the scaphoid. Tenderness proximal to the head of the third metacarpal or distal to the Lister's tubercle of the radius is suggestive of a scapholunate injury (Watson and Weinzweig 1997). Tenderness between ulnar styloid and FCU suggests an injury to TFCC (Buterbaugh et al. 1998). Similarly tenderness along the bony landmarks of the hook of the hamate suggests an underlying fracture of the hamate as seen in racquet sports. Tenderness, swelling and crepitance proximal to the radial styloid along the tendons of the first extensor compartment are indicative of deQuervain's tenosynovitis (Eathorne 2005).

Range of movements at wrist and hand should be evaluated both actively and passively, and again comparing it with the contralateral side and observing for pain or discomfort at a particular point on movement of the joint. For example, pain in the distal forearm on pronation and supination in the appropriate clinical setting raises suspicion of the distal radioulnar joint injury. Feeling for end points on moving the joint gives a clue to the underlying injury as in UCL injuries. In UCL injury on abducting the thumb there is appreciable loss of end-point to this movement, which becomes more obvious on comparing the same maneuver with the contralateral side. There is a list of specific maneuvers to establish the diagnosis of the underlying wrist or hand injury, the sensitivity and specificity of which are highly examiner and athlete dependent and only a few are listed below. Often, these maneuvers should be compared with the uninjured contralateral side.

(a) *Finkelstein's test*: Pain on flexion of the patient's thumb into the palm, and passive ulnar deviation of the wrist is referred as positive Finkelstein's test and is suggestive of deQuervain's tenosynovitis.

(b) *Tinel's and Phalen's test*: These are the tests for compressive neuropathy of the median nerve. A positive test would involve paresthesia and/or pain over the distribution of the median nerve on percussing the median nerve in the carpal tunnel, with the wrist slightly dorsiflexed. The presence of similar neurological symptoms on full flexion of the wrist for at least 30 s, with the back of the wrists facing each other is referred as positive Phalen's test.
(c) *Watson's test*: Is used to assess the scapholunate instability. The examiner holds the radial side of the wrist one hand and gently applies counter pressure with the thumb of the other hand over the scaphoid tubercle. The wrist is then passively moved slowly from ulnar to radial deviation. Pain, or laxity, appreciated as a clunk as the scaphoid is moved dorsally over the dorsal rim of the radius suggests underlying scapholunate instability.
(d) *Reagen's test*: Is used to assess the lunotriquetral integrity. This test is performed with the examiner applying pressure on the lunate dorsally using the thumb, and simultaneously exerting counter force from the volar surface on the triquetrum using the index finger (Reagan et al. 1984).
(e) *Supination lift test*: Is used to diagnose peripheral tears of the TFCC. The athlete places arms supinated with palms facing the undersurface of the table, ulnar wrist pain wit this maneuver is indicative of a peripheral tear of the TFCC (Buterbaugh et al. 1998).

3.3.3 Epidemiology of Wrist and Hand Injuries

There is limited epidemiological data in the literature on sport-related injuries of the hand and wrist in young athletes, and when available the data is difficult to interpret due to heterogeneity of the study population and nature of injury. Overall, the incidence of sport-related hand and wrist injuries is between 3 and 9% (Rettig 1998). Gymnastics is associated with higher rate of wrist injuries. Approximately 46–87% of gymnasts develop significant wrist pain at least once in their career, with majority of the injuries pertaining to the radial physis (Caine et al. 1992; Difiori et al. 1997). Sports related hand fractures occur in 22.4% with football, rugby and snow-sports accounting for over two-thirds of these injuries (Court-Brown et al. 2008).

4 Lower Extremity

4.1 Hip and Groin Injuries

4.1.1 Classification of Hip and Groin Injuries

Traditionally, injuries to the groin and hip were considered to be relatively rare, compared to the other regions of the lower limb. The peculiarities of pediatric athlete's growing skeleton with a wide range of pathologies pertaining to the hip joint compounds to the difficulties in reaching to an accurate diagnosis of the relevant sport injury. However, increased awareness among athletes and innovation of newer imaging techniques, including invasive procedures like arthroscopy has immensely contributed towards establishing an accurate etiology of the hip and groin injuries. Injuries in this region can be divided into soft tissue and bony injuries, although injury to one component may lead to damage of the other. For example, muscular strain, a soft tissue injury, in extreme situations can cause avulsion of the bony fragments of the pelvis or the femur.

Soft Tissue Injuries

(a) *Muscular strains*: These groups of injuries by far include the bulk of sports-related groin and hip injuries. Often the injuries occur when the external load generated by the activity of the athlete exceeds the intrinsic muscle force. These injuries are seen frequently in football and hockey players, with the adductor muscles and hamstrings frequently sustaining the strain at the myotendinous junction or within the belly (Gilmore 1998). It is not uncommon for muscular strains to coexist with other soft tissue injuries as seen in "sports hip triad": a combination of labral tear, adductor strain and rectus femoris strain noticed in football players (Feeley et al. 2008).
(b) *Contusions*: Are often the results of a direct blow or a fall on to the thigh or the iliac crest from which several large muscles arise. Contusions can cause hemorrhage within the muscle tissue, and when large enough can cause compression of neurovascular structures. One such common condition is meralgia paraesthetica, compression of the lateral cutaneous femoral nerve in the region of

the inguinal ligament. Occasionally, repetitive microtrauma at the region of the contusion can lead to the development of myositis ossificans. Athletes with significant contusions sometimes are prone to gluteal and thigh compartment syndromes requiring emergency intervention.

(c) *Groin hernias*: This injury for years has been surrounded with several controversies in terms of the precise underlying etiology. Currently, the most prevalent definition of groin hernia is weakening of the posterior wall of the inguinal canal in the absence of a palpable inguinal hernia causing chronic groin pain. More recently, it has been suggested that the term groin hernia should perhaps be renamed as "athletic pubalgia" due to the absence of hernia (Meyers et al. 2008). Tears in the transversalis fascia or conjoined tendon or avulsion of the internal oblique muscle from the pubic tubercle due to repetitive microtrauma is thought to be the underlying cause of the chronic pain in groin hernias (Taylor et al. 1991). Often, athletes in several reported series returned to play following open or laparoscopic herniorrhaphy, implicating that surgery is beneficial in the treatment of this condition.

(d) *Labral tears*: The acetabular labrum is a triangular fibrocartilaginous structure that encases the acetabulum increasing the congruency of the hip joint. Labral tears once thought to be the consequence of high energy trauma are now seen frequently in athletic trauma. Labral tears can develop denovo due to repetitive microtrauma, or may arise secondarily in a hip with the background history of acetabular dysplasia or femoroacetabular impingement, commonly abbreviated as FAI in sports literature (Philippon et al. 2007). The commonest variant of labral tear is of the antero-superior type. Labral tears are classified into four categories based on arthroscopic findings (Lage et al. 1996): (1) radial free margin flap tears, (2) radial fiberlated labrum, (3) peripheral longitudinally oriented tears, (5) highly "mobile" tears, with the first two types constituting over two-thirds of the labral tears.

Several associated intra-articular lesions are observed in athletes with labral tears, making the precise etiology of the groin pain difficult. Chondromalacia, chondral flap tears, loose bodies, and partial tears to ligmanetum teres are a few to name. Based on the associated pathological changes in the acetabulum and femoral head they are divided into four major stages, a classification bearing prognostic significance.

Stage 1: marginal tear of the labrum in the presence of an intact articular cartilage of the femoral head and acetabulum.

Stage 2: labral tear with articular damage to the femoral head only.

Stage 3: labral tear with acetabular articular damage, with or without femoral head articular cartilage damage.

Stage 4: extensive labral tear with osteoarthritic changes of the hip.

(e) *Other soft tissue injuries*: The hip joint is surrounded by various soft tissue structures that are prone to repetitive trauma. Due to relatively sparse data in sports literature, conditions such as piriformis syndrome, hip pointers, bursitis, snapping hip syndrome have gained relatively less attention. However, as majority of these conditions often can be successfully managed by appropriate rehabilitation techniques, accurate diagnosis is vital.

(i) Piriformis syndrome: It is caused by the entrapment of the sciatic nerve within the bulk of the hypertrophied piriformis. Occasionally, myositis ossificans within piriformis can cause piriformis syndrome. Prolonged seating as in bike and cycle sports and gymnastic maneuvers frequently involving repetitive hip flexion, internal rotation, and adduction can aggravate the symptoms of piriformis syndrome.

(ii) Bursitis: Is defined as inflammation of bursa, the iliopsoas and greater trochanteric bursa being commonly affected in the athlete. Iliopsoas bursitis is seen in sports involving rigorous hip flexion: soccer, sprinting, ballet, and rowing. It is believed that women with a prominent greater trochanter are more prone to greater trochanter bursitis. Dancers who frequently adduct the hip medial to the midline and runners with a cross-over-style gait are more prone to this condition (Toohey et al. 1990).

(iii) Snapping hip syndrome: This syndrome refers to the sensation of snapping felt around the hip joint associated with repetitive use. Only a minority of athletes experience pain requiring intervention. Based on the origin of snapping, this syndrome can be classified as intra-articular and extra-articular. The common cause of extraarticular snapping syndrome is repetitive movement of the iliotibial band, tensor fascia lata, or gluteus medius over the greater trochanter that results in thickening of connective tissue within these structures. Subsequently, these tissue bands give a sensation of catching when moving across the bony surface that is felt similar to a snap. The underlying bursa in extreme cases may result in inflammation. The intra-articular snapping syndrome is secondary to labral tear, damage to articular cartilage, or loose bodies.

4.1.2 Bony Injuries

(a) *Avulsion or apophyseal injuries*: Are common injuries in the pediatric and the adolescent athletes and often result from violent eccentric contraction of the muscle. Typically, any muscle attachment can be avulsed from the apophysis of the growing skeleton. However, the commonly encountered avulsions are from the origin of the hamstrings: ischial tuberosity, rectus femoris: anterior inferior iliac spine, adductors: pubic symphysis, and sartorius: anterior superior iliac spine. In the milder form, the physis can undergo repetitive microtrauma causing apophysitis which can be difficult to differentiate on clinical examination alone. The type of the avulsion injury is sport-dependent. For example, kicking in soccer players results in avulsion injury of the rectus femoris, whereas in gymnasts avulsions are at ischial tuberosity.

(b) *Stress fractures*: Are common injuries in runners and are caused by repetitive overuse, the femoral neck and pubic ramus being the common structures involved. Less frequently the proximal third of the femoral diaphysis is also subjected to stress fractures. These injuries are seen in female athletes more commonly than men. Femoral neck stress fractures are thought to be the result of muscle fatigue, principally in the abductors. In normal circumstances stresses and strains along the femoral neck are counteracted by abductor muscles, chiefly the gluteus medius. In the presence of fatigued abductors, this neutralizing force is lost and the femoral neck experiences tensile strains resulting in stress fractures. Fullerton and Snowdy classified femoral neck stress fracture into three types: tension, compression, and displaced (Fullerton and Snowdy 1988). Tension stress fractures are believed to occur on the supero-lateral aspect of the femoral neck and compression fractures in the infero-medial side. The former groups of fractures are notorious for fracture displacement, mandating surgical fixation. Often the heterogeneity in the etiology of the groin and hip pain leads to a delay in diagnosis of the femoral neck stress fractures, increasing the risks of avascular necrosis and nonunion of the hip.

(c) *Hip subluxation and dislocations*: These injuries although rare in sports deserve a mention because of the seriousness of the injury. The commonest mechanisms of dislocations in sport are (1) fall on the knee with the hip flexed, and (2) athlete in the hand-and-knees position is stuck from behind by the fellow player, in both the situations the posterior dislocation being the commonest type. Levin's classification described for dislocations caused by high energy trauma can also be applied to athletic trauma. Based on the presence of associated injuries to the hip joint five major types of dislocations were described:

Type I: No associated fracture, no instability
Type II: Irreducible dislocation, no fracture
Type III: Unstable after reduction, incarcerated fracture fragments
Type IV: Associated acetabular fracture requiring repair
Type V: Associated neck of femur or head injury

Often athletic dislocations are without any major acetabular fractures that require surgical fixation. Hip subluxation in sports perhaps is more common than dislocation, but because of less prominent clinical features compared to dislocation this injury appears to be under reported. The mechanisms of injury are similar to those causing dislocation, however in subluxation, the femoral head spontaneously returns into the acetabulum. Recurrent subluxation or dislocation although rare at the hip compared to the shoulder joint, its presence may suggest an underlying chronic instability. This entity, when diagnosed requires further investigation of the underlying etiology of the instability.

(d) Other bony injuries

Slipped capital femoral epiphyses (SCFE) and *Legg-Calve-Perthes* (LCP) disease of the hip joint are two conditions pertaining to the pediatric population which should be considered in the differential diagnosis of pediatric athletic trauma. SCFE involves the posterior slippage of the proximal femoral epiphysis caused by mechanical shear stress, causing mechanical instability of the hip joint. LCP is a self-limiting idiopathic condition affecting the femoral head and is defined as avascular necrosis of the femur. Although a direct sport related etiology is not associated with these injuries, these pathologies when coexist, can sometimes be masked by the sport injury causing long term growth abnormalities if not diagnosed and managed promptly.

4.1.3 Clinical Evaluation of Hip and Groin Injuries

The primary aim of hip examination is to exclude a lumbar spine pathology that might be causing the hip pain. The principles of a general orthopedic hip examination are applicable to the athlete presenting with a groin and hip pain, bearing in mind the above mentioned differential diagnosis of hip and groin pathology. This often can be accomplished by a few targeted questions at the outset such as the onset, radiation, aggravating and relieving factors, and precise location of pain. Onset of the pain provides clues to the origin of the pain. Acute onset of pain is usually the result of muscular strain, contusions, avulsion injuries, hip subluxation, and acetabular tears. On the other hand sports hernias, overuse syndromes and snapping hip syndrome are associated with insidious onset of pain. It should be noted that athlete's symptoms can be caused solely by the hip, groin or a concomitant spinal pathology. As majority of the athletic injuries appear to be arising from the hip joint, this section focuses primarily on the examination of the hip.

Examination of the hip begins with brief examination of the athlete standing and then observing for changes in gait. Loss of the normal alignment of the iliac crests suggests the presence of lordosis, scoliosis or an underlying true and functional leg length discrepancy. Principle gait abnormalities include trendelenburg and antelgic gait implying weakness of the hip abductors or an underlying primary hip pathology respectively. It is essential to observe for snapping or clicking, particularly of the iliotibial tract and iliopsoas tendon.

The hip examination is carried out with the athlete in supine, lateral and prone positions. Ideally, internal and external rotation of the hip is examined with the athlete seated, and flexion, extension, abduction and adduction in the supine position. There is wealth of literature on examination findings of the hip and their significance. For the purpose of this chapter, however, only some special tests relevant to sports injuries of the hip will be presented:

1. *Patrick FABER* (Flexion Abduction External Rotation) test characterizes the pain in the abducted position of the hip. The ankle of the affected limb is placed across the contralateral thigh, resembling a figure of "4"position and pressure applied on the knee of the affected limb. Pain in the groin with this maneuver is indicative of iliopsoas pathology, over lateral hip joint implies FAI.
2. *McCarthy* test is used to diagnose acetabular tears. The hip joints are bought into full flexion and the affected hip is extended both in external and internal rotation one after the other observing for reproducible pain associated with these two movements.
3. *Ober* test is used to assess the tightness associated of the abductor mechanism of the hip. This test is performed with the athlete lying laterally on the nonaffected limb and involves abducting the hip and then allowing it to move to the neutral position with the knee and hip being either flexed or extended during this maneuver. Pain on moving the hip from abducted to neutral position with the knee and hip held in flexion is suggestive of contracture or tightness of the iliotibial tract. Similarly, pain with the same maneuver, but now with the knee and hip held in flexion and neutral respectively, is suggestive of gluteus medius contracture, tightness or tear.
4. *Ely* test is used to assess the rectus femoris tightness, or contractures. This test is performed with the patient lying prone. The injured leg is flexed at the knee joint until the lower leg is as near as possible to the thigh. Upward tilt of the pelvis and buttock with this maneuver is indicative of rectus femoris pathology.

Any hip examination is incomplete without clinical evaluation of the lumbar spine and complete neurovascular examination of the affected side. Neurological examination should be specifically aimed at eliciting motor or sensory signs of radiculopathy. Also, the athletic hip examination is slightly different from the standard orthopedic examination of the hip. It includes a brief examination of the groin and external genitalia either to exclude nonathletic related causes of groin pain or to diagnose sports-related injuries such as avulsion injuries and stress fractures of the pubis, or groin hernias.

4.1.4 Epidemiology of Hip and Groin Injuries

Epidemiological data on hip injuries in pediatric and adolescent athletes is sparse in the literature. The incidence and prevalence of injuries at this joint is different among athletes who sustain injuries first time compared to those sustaining recurrent injuries. The United States National Football League which analyzed 23806 injuries of which the prevalence of hip injuries was 3.1% (Feeley et al. 2008). Muscle strains were the most common overall hip injury, contributing to 59% of all injuries about the hip and 1.7% of all injuries in the NFL. Hip flexor strains accounted for nearly 63% of all strains. Intraarticular injuries accounted for only about 5% of all injuries about the hip. In the same study contusions (53%) and strains (36%) dominated amongst the injuries sustained due to contact while strains (93%) dominated the noncontact injury group. Among swimmers the technique adopted influenced the rate of hip injury. Breaststroke swimmers were more likely to have groin pain (6.9%) compared to medley swimmers who do not compete in pure breast stroke (0%) (Grote et al. 2004).

A study on basketball injuries recruiting 780,651 athlete exposures reported the injury rate of hip and pelvis injuries as 8.4% with majority of the injuries occurring in competition than in practice (Borowski et al. 2008). Apophyseal avulsion fractures of the hip and pelvis are common in adolescent athletes playing soccer and gymnastics. Analysis of 203 avulsion fractures in this group of individuals revealed that avulsion of the ischial tuberosity (109 cases) was the commonest followed by anterior inferior iliac spine (45 cases) (Rossi and Dragoni 2001).

4.2 *Knee Injuries*

4.2.1 Classification of Knee Injuries

The knee joint is a complex synovial joint of hinge type and is surrounded by several soft tissue structures which are responsible for the stability of the knee joint. The soft tissue structures can be divided into intra, and extra-articular components: menisci, capsule, and ligaments. The close proximity of several major neurovascular components to the bony structures of the knee joint renders them susceptible to secondary damage in sport-related injuries. Athletic knee injuries can be divided into soft tissue and bony injuries.

Soft Tissue Injuries

(a) *Meniscal injuries*: Menisci are fibro-cartilaginous C- shaped or semicircular structures providing congruity and stability to the knee joint. In children, meniscal injuries are encountered less frequently compared to adolescents, perhaps due to the abundant blood supply and the unique biochemical composition of the menisci in the former. The classical mechanism of injury described by the athlete is one of a twisting injury to the knee: flexion of the knee associated with tibio-femoral compression and rotation, subjecting the menisci to shear stress. This causes injury to the menisci in isolation or with concomitant injury to the ligamentous structures. The most commonly prevalent classification of meniscal tears is based on the pattern and location of tear seen on arthroscopy or MRI, and the arthroscopic classification is presented in this chapter.

Meniscal tears can occur in a normal or a degenerative meniscus, although the later is rare in adolescent athletes. Cooper's classification divides meniscal tears based on location and type of the tear (Cooper et al. 1991). According to this system the meniscus in regards to the location of the tear is divided into three radial (measuring one-third each: anterior, posterior and lateral) and four circumferential zones. The radial zones are designated as A, B, C and D, E, F for the medial and lateral meniscus, respectively. The four circumferential zones are: 0- menisco-capsular junction, 1-outer third, 2-middle third, 3-inner third of the meniscus. Based on the type of tear, meniscal tears are divided into vertical longitudinal, oblique, complex (degenerative), transverse (radial) and horizontal, with 80% of the tears being either vertical longitudinal or oblique type. Vertical longitudinal tears are more often seen in younger athletes and can be complete, referred as bucket handle tears, or incomplete. The medial meniscus is often involved vertical longitudinal tears because of its strong attachments to the tibial plateau subjecting it to shear stress. Oblique tears referred as parrot beak or flap tears, are often found at the junction of middle and posterior thirds of the meniscus. These tears have a propensity to migrate if untreated.

The uniqueness of a meniscal injury in children and adolescent is that it is often associated with ligamentous injury, usually the anterior cruciate ligament (ACL). In children and adolescents presenting with a history of meniscal injury one has to consider benign pathologies such as the discoid meniscus and meniscal cyst as the cause of the pain as these entities are approached by the treating clinician differently. Meniscal cyst is defined as focal collection of synovial fluid within the meniscus (intrameniscal) or adjacent (parameniscal) to the meniscus, lateral meniscus being the commonest site of such cysts. It is hypothesized that intrameniscal cysts are formed by accumulation of fluid within a torn or degenerated meniscus, and parameniscal cysts arise due to extravasation of the fluid into parameniscal soft tissues through a meniscal tear (Beaman and Peterson 2007). Discoid meniscus is thought to arise secondary to failure of resorption of the central portion of the meniscus during its embryological development. The other proposed theory is that discoid meniscus is secondary to failure of the attachment of the menisco-tibial ligament leading to subsequent instability of the meniscus. This eventually results in the development of hypertrophic and discoid changes in the meniscus.

(b) *Ligament injuries*: The four major ligaments protecting the knee from rotational and axial forces are anterior and posterior cruciate ligaments (PCL), and the medial and lateral collateral (MCL and LCL) ligaments. Among these, LCL injuries are very rare and when present in the pediatric or adolescent population they form part of the injuries of the posterolateral complex. Similar to adults, injuries to the ligaments in children and adolescents often occur in combination with meniscal injuries.

In children, relatively stronger strength of ACL causes avulsion of ACL from the tibial spine more often than through the midsubstance of the ligament and mid-substance tears are thought to occur in older adolescents. Avulsion of the ACL at its insertion on the femoral condyle is relatively rare. ACL injury often is the result of sudden deceleration with an externally rotated tibia on a relatively fixed foot. A simultaneous valgus force applied to an extended knee in such circumstances causes rupture of MCL too. Isolated injuries to ACL occur with internal rotation of the tibial relative to the femur or hyperextension of the knee (Fehnel and Johnson 2000). Classification of ACL rupture is based on whether the tear is intra-articular or at their origin from the tibial spine; the later classification is described in the section on tibial spine fractures.

Anatomically, ACL consists of two main bundles based on their orientation of their tibial insertion: anteromedial (AM) and posterolateral (PL) bundles. The midsubstance tear or the intraarticular rupture of the ACL is based on tears associated within these individual bundles and are represented by numbers 1–5 (for AM bundle) and alphabets A-E (for PM bundle) as follows:

Grade 1: Femoral rupture
Grade 2: Mid-substance rupture
Grade 3: Tibial rupture
Grade 4: An elongated functional insufficient AM bundle
Grade 5: Intact AM bundle
Grade A: Femoral rupture
Grade B: Mid-substance rupture
Grade C: Tibial rupture
Grade D: An elongated functional insufficient PM bundle
Grade E: Intact PM bundle

According to this classification, for example, code 1A denotes femoral rupture of the AM and PM bundles.

Injuries to the PCL compared to the ACL are rare. Typically, isolated tears in PCL develop secondary to hyperflexion injuries, avulsing the PCL from the femoral insertion (Fowler and Messieh 1987). This is typically seen in adolescents sustaining football injuries when an athlete lands forcefully on a flexed knee with the foot held in plantar flexion. Rotational or varus forces applied to such a flexed knee can also cause LCL rupture or if forces are strong enough, will result in a unique group of injury called the posterolateral corner injury (Cooper et al. 2006). Classification of PCL injuries is based on the relationship between the tibial plateau and femoral condyles with the knee in 90° and damage to the associated ligaments and is described below (Janousek et al. 1999).

Type	Definition	Laxity (mm)	Tibial plateau
I	PCL stretched	<5	5–10 mm anterior to femoral condyle
II	PCL torn, intact MF ligaments	5–9	0–5 mm anterior to femoral condyle
III	PCL torn, MF ligaments torn	>10	Flush with femoral condyle
IVa	PCL and LCL torn	>12	>2 mm posterior to femoral condyle
IVb	PCL and MCL torn	>12	>2 mm posterior to femoral condyle
IVc	PCL and ACL torn	>15	>5 mm posterior to femoral condyle

Grades I–III are isolated PCL injuries, grade 4 are combined injuries
Grade IVa and IVb comprise posterolateral and posteromedial injuries respectively
MF meniscofemoral ligament

MCL injuries are common in contact and noncontact sports that subject the knee to valgus load, sudden changing of direction, twisting and pivoting as seen skiing. Additional rotation forces can cause concomitant disruption of the ACL or tear of the posteromedial corner, a much serious injury than MCL tear alone (Indelicato 1995). There is considerable controversy surrounding the classification of the MCL injuries and no single classification system described below is universally accepted. In general, the classification of MCL injuries is based on the degree of joint space opening with valgus stress and degree of laxity. Fetto (1978) grades the MCL injury into three grades and assesses the degree of stability in both knee extension and 30° of flexion(Fetto and Marshall 1978):

Grade I: Injury is clinically stable both in extension and 30° flexion, but painful with valgus stress

Grade II: Increased medial joint space opening in 30° flexion but not in full extension

Grade III: Unstable both in 30° flexion and full extension

The original classification of MCL tears was later modified to include both the degree of laxity and severity of the MCL tear:

Grade I: tear in few fibers of MCL without instability of the knee

Grade II: Incomplete tear of the MCL without instability of the knee

Grade III: Complete tear of the MCL with resultant instability of the knee

Grade III injuries are further divided into grade 1+, 2+, 3+ laxities, based on the degree of medial opening that is assessed with knee held in 30° of flexion: grade 1+: 3–5 mm of opening, grade 2+: 6–10 mm of opening, grade 3+: >10 mm opening. Grade III with 3+ laxity is associated with higher incidence of ACL injuries.

Bony Injuries

(a) *Distal femoral epiphyseal and proximal tibial epiphyseal fractures*: Fractures of these regions are classified based on the system proposed by Salter and Harris (Salter 1992). This classification is based on the orientation of the fracture line in relation to the physis of the growing skeleton, and five major types of fracture patterns are described below:

Type I: The fracture line passes through the physis without involving the adjacent metaphysis or epiphyses.

Type II: Is the commonest fracture pattern involving the physes of the growing skeleton. The fracture line passes through the physis and crosses obliquely at one end of the metaphysis.

Type III: The fracture line passes through the physes and then crosses the epiphyses vertically extending into the joint.

Type IV: Is again an intra-articular fracture, with a vertical fracture line extending across the metaphysis, physis, and epiphysis.

Type V: This fracture pattern is described as crush injury to the physis and is often difficult to diagnose.

Type III and IV fractures are notorious for growth abnormalities if improperly reduced, and often require internal fixation to maintain the reduction and joint congruity.

(b) *Tibial tubercle fractures*: Are common in the skeletally immature adolescents and typically is seen in sports involving violent contraction of quadriceps muscle as seen in competitive jumping, basketball or in football during a tackle when the knee is passively flexed against a contracted quadriceps muscle. Tibial tubercle fractures are classified according to Watson-Jones classification that was later modified by Ogden (Ogden et al. 1980). According to this classification there are three major fracture patterns subdivided into "A" and "B" based on the degree of displacement and communition.

(i) Type IA and IB: In type IA, the fracture line crosses distal to the junction of the ossification centers of the proximal end of the tibia and its tuberosity. In type IB, the fragment is displaced or hinged.
(ii) Type IIA and IIB: In type IIA, the fracture line crosses the junction of the ossification centers of the proximal end of the tibia and its tuberosity. In type IIB, the fragment is communited.
(iii) Type IIIA and IIIB: In type III, the fracture pattern is similar to that seen in type II, but in addition extends into the knee joint; IIIA being noncommunited and IIIB being communited.

(c) *Tibial spine fractures*: The anterior tibial spine is the distal attachment of the ACL. Sport injuries that result in ACL ruptures usually involve the avulsion of the anterior tibial spine particularly in the skeletally immature athlete. Based on the degree of displacement of the tibial spine, Meyers and McKeever classified these injuries into three main types.

(i) Type I: The fractured tibial spine is minimally displaced, with only slight elevation of its anterior margin.
(ii) Type II: The fractured anterior portion of the avulsed tibial spine is elevated and hinges on the posterior portion.
(iii) Type III: The fractured tibial spine is completely displaced and sometimes may be rotated.

(d) *Patellar fractures*: Fortunately, patellar fractures are rare in children as the patella is predominantly a cartilaginous structure. They tend to occur in adolescents when the ossification of the patella is nearing completion. The most common fracture pattern is avulsion injury secondary to violent forces caused by the quadriceps across the patella. Four types of injuries across the patella have benn described: superior, inferior, medial, and lateral. The medial injuries to the patella are often accompanied by lateral dislocation of the patella. The lateral injury to the patella is thought to be an overuse injury secondary to the repetitive pull of vastus lateralis muscle (Grogan et al. 1990).

(e) *Instability of proximal tibiofibular joint*: This injury once thought to be the result of high energy trauma, now appears to be one of the several common etiologies of lateral knee pain in the adolescent athletes. It is seen in athletes involving in violent twisting motions such as gymnastics, skiing, football, and roller skating. Ogden (1974) originally described four types of instability of the proximal tibiofibular joint: atraumatic subluxation that is commonly seen in individuals with generalized ligamentous laxity, anterolateral dislocation, posteromedial dislocation, and superior dislocation. An anterolateral dislocation is by far the commonest instability pattern, and usually involves concomitant injury to the LCL of the knee and typically results from a fall on a hyperflexed knee with the foot inverted and plantar flexed (Falkenberg and Nygaard 1983; Giachino 1986). Superior dislocation is usually the result of high energy trauma to the ankle and is seldom seen in sports injuries.

4.2.2 Clinical Evaluation of Knee Injuries

Examination of the knee involves obtaining a thorough history, focusing on the mechanism of the injury and development of swelling immediately, or after several hours following the injury, history of delayed skeletal maturity, and previous knee injuries. It should, however be noted that children often are not able to give a precise history relating to the position of the knee or the foot at the time of the injury, a vital point in predicting injury patterns sustained to the knee. In such circumstances symptoms such as intensity, location of the pain, and swelling of the knee will guide the clinician to assess the severity of the injury. Swelling immediately following the injury indicates haemarthrosis and usually suggests the presence of a significant injury to the ligamentous structures. Haemarthrosis due to injury to relatively avascular structures such as menisci manifests later, usually 24–48 h after the injury.

Although presence of pain and swelling is an important symptom, their absence does not necessarily rule out a significant knee injury. For example, PCL injuries are sometimes associated with minimal pain and swelling that is sometimes difficult to appreciate; emphasizing the fact that it is not always necessary to have a full constellation of signs and symptoms pointing out towards an underlying meniscal or ligamentous injury. History of acute locking of the knee suggests underlying meniscal pathology. The type of sport provides a clue to underlying knee injury as discussed above in the section on specific knee injuries. Gait abnormalities provide a clue to the underlying etiology of the knee injury. Athletes walking with a limp or vaulting-type gait involving the active recruitment of quadriceps helping to stabilize the knee joint may suggest a complete or partial tear of MCL tear. On the other hand, athletes with a ACL or meniscal injury walk with a slightly flexed knee.

Examination of the knee should begin with general inspection of the joint, looking for alignment, swelling, deformities, and shortening and follows the general principles of orthopedic joint examination. Point of maximum tenderness should be elicited by gently palpating across the joint line and bony landmarks around the knee joint. Attention should be focused on any obvious palpable gaps in the joint line, as seen with patellar fractures. It is vital that the varus and valgus stress maneuvers be performed with the knee in both full extension and 30° flexion to isolate the relevant structures being examined. For example, when assessing the knee for MCL injuries in full extension, participation of the ACL will mask any laxity due to MCL injury. Examining the knee joint in slight flexion at 30° in such circumstances would negate the effect of ACL, increasing the sensitivity and specificity of the valgus stress test. Clinical examination of the knee joint can be hampered by severe pain which would not allow the athlete to adequately relax the knee joint. In such cases, it is prudent to re-examine the knee 48–72 h following the acute injury. As with any joint injuries, there is an exhaustive list of special tests pertaining to knee injuries helping the clinician to make a relevant clinical diagnosis, or at least narrow the differential diagnosis of the knee pathology. Only a few clinical tests, that we believe from our experience as useful are discussed below:

1. *Lachman test*: Is more sensitive in diagnosing an ACL injury compared to the conventional anterior draw test. We recommend performing the Lachman's test with the patient in supine position and the knee held in 20–30° of flexion. Examiner places one hand on the thigh of the athlete and presses it against his own thigh, and simultaneously grasps the upper third of the leg and pulls it forward. This maneuver helps the examiner appreciate the end point and the amount of anterior tibial displacement that is directly related to the degree of ACL rupture.
2. *Reverse Lachman test*: This test is to diagnose PCL injury and is performed similar to the Lachman's test. However, the proximal third of the leg is displaced posteriorly evaluating the end point and the amount of posterior displacement. In both the Lachman and reverse Lachman test the anterior or posterior displacement of the tibia should be compared with the normal knee.
3. *Thessaly test*: In recent reports Thessaly test for meniscal injury appears to be more sensitive and specific than the traditional McMurray's and Apley grinding test (Karachalios et al. 2005; Konan et al. 2009). The examiner supports the standing athlete by holding his or her outstretched hands. The athlete then rotates his or her knee and body internally and externally, three times, with the knee held in a flexion of 5°. The same maneuver is repeated with the knee flexed at 20° and athletes with suspected medial or lateral meniscal tears experience medial or lateral joint-line discomfort or pain and may have a sense of locking or catching.
4. *External rotation recurvatum test*: This test is used to diagnose posterolateral corner injuries of the knee and is performed with the athlete lying supine. The examiner holds the athlete's great toes and lifts his or her heels off the examination couch simultaneously. The presence of a significant posterolateral corner injury is indicated by hyperextension, external rotation and tibia vara of the affected limb; the examiner should observe the tibial tuberosities to watch for the external rotation.
5. *Dial test*: This is a test to diagnose posterolateral corner injuries and can be performed with the examiner in prone or supine. In supine position the legs are allowed to hang off by the end of the examining couch, and thighs are stabilized by an assistant. Gently, the examiner externally rotates both legs simultaneously and the amount of

external rotation is compared with the other side. An increase of approximately 15° of external rotation suggests a significant posterolateral corner injury.

4.2.3 Epidemiology of Knee Injuries

Knee injuries are the second most common joint involved in athletic injuries. In a large systematic review in adolescent sports the global prevalence of knee injury was quoted as 10–25% with higher prevalence of these injuries noticed in the recent studies (Louw et al. 2008). Both higher injury rates and better definition of knee injuries appeared to be partly responsible for the increase in prevalence. In the same study higher prevalence of the knee injuries was observed in female adolescent athletes. A large epidemiological study on knee injuries in high-school athletes in the United States reported a rate of 3.89 knee injuries per 10,000 athlete exposures (Ingram et al. 2008). On the contrary to the above study, in the study by Ingram et al, boys had higher rate of knee injury. However, girls were twice as likely to sustain knee injuries that required surgery than boys. Athletes sustained Knee injuries three times more often during competition than in practice. The higher rates of knee injuries were reported for football at 6.91 per 10,000 athlete exposures followed by girls' soccer (5.08), wrestling (3.81), and girls' basketball (3.80). Baseball and softball were associated with lowest knee injury rates of 1.05 and 1.41 per 10,000 athlete exposures.

Commonest knee injuries in pediatric and adolescent athletes are ligament tears. In US a study evaluating 1,383 knee injuries reporting 3,551,131 athlete exposures incomplete ligament tears was the commonest knee injuries (32%) followed by contusions(15.2%), complete ligament tears (13.2%), torn cartilages (8%) and fracture/dislocations (5.8%). Muscle tears, inflammation and tendinitis are the other relatively rare injuries in this series (Ingram et al. 2008). Forty-two percent of all football knee injuries constituted incomplete ligament tears. Baseball and wrestling were associated with highest rates of contusions: 35.6% and 17.8% respectively. Injuries to the cartilage were most frequently seen in wrestling (16.1%). Gender differences are found in many of the knee injuries sustained. Complete ligament tears are seen 2.5 times more likely in girls compared to boys. Injury rates are higher in boys than in girls: 4.29 vs. 3.11 per 10,000 athlete exposures.

Knee injuries constituted 29% of the overall sport injuries in a series of 1,378 athletic injuries (Darrow et al. 2009). It is well known that sporting conditions influence the injury rates. A large number of knee injuries were the result of competition (34.6%) compared to 21.3% sustained during practice, with ligamentous injuries constituting 81.8% of knee injuries. In this series soccer was associated with the highest rate of knee injuries followed by football: 38.9% vs. 25.8%. Again distinct gender difference was noticed in this study. Girls sustained greater proportion of knee injuries compared to boys: 49.7% vs. 23.3%, the most common diagnosis being fractures (30.3%) and incomplete ligament sprains (20.3%).

4.3 Foot and Ankle Injuries

4.3.1 Classification of the Foot and Ankle Injuries

Foot and ankle being the major weight bearing joint of the body is prone to various sports related injuries. Similar to other injuries described in this chapter, injuries sustained to the foot and ankle depends on the mechanism of injury, type of sport and age of the athlete. The unique structure of the growing bone predisposes to fractures around the growth plates in the children more often than adults, in whom a similar mechanism would result in ligamentous injuries. A thorough understanding of developmental variations existing in the skeletally immature athlete is required before a particular injury is labeled as pathological. There is no universally accepted classification of the sport-related injuries pertaining to the foot and ankle. For practical purposes the injuries at this region are divided into: (1) injuries related to growth, (2) overuse injuries and, (3) acute injuries (Chambers 2003; Pontell et al. 2006; Malanga and Ramirez-Del Toro 2008). Injuries that cause pain from coalitions and accessory ossicles belong to the first group. Osteochondroses, apophysitis and stress fractures are grouped under overuse injuries. Acute injuries to ligaments, tendons, muscles and bones of the foot and ankle constitute the third group.

Injuries Related to Growth

Coalitions: Coalition is defined as a bony, cartilaginous or fibrous connection or fusion of two or more bones (Omey and Micheli 1999). Although coalitions are present in approximately 1% of the population they are seldom the cause of foot pain in nonathletes. The coalition site can act as secondary ossification centre and when these connections undergo ossification excessive stress around this bony architecture causes pain in adolescent athletes. In the foot and ankle region the commonest coalitions are: (1) Talocalcaneal and (2) Calcaneonavicular. These two constitute nearly 90% of all the coalitions seen in the foot and ankle region. Athletes often have more than one coalition in the same foot and the coalition is bilateral. In talocalcaneal coalition, the middle facette is most commonly involved followed by the posterior and anterior facettes. The presence of coalition results in limited motion between the bones of the triple joint complex (the subtalar, talonavicular and calceneaocuboidal joints) causing excessive stresses in the hind foot joints. This predisposes to chronic inflammatory process and premature joint degeneration (Bohne 2001). Pain in 'coalesced joints' usually coincides with strenuous physical activity and ossification of the fibro-cartilagenous bridge. Athletes with tarsal coalition may often have an associated peroneal spastic foot which is the result of the action of peroneal tendons attempting to overcome the limited subtalar motion. In addition, athletes with tarsal coalition suffer from recurrent ankle sprains secondary to increased stress on the ankle joint which compensates for the absent subtalar motion(Bohne 2001).

Accessory ossicles: Accessory ossicles or sesamoid bones are defined as extrachondral ossification centers. The accessory ossicles appear at the age of 8–10 years and usually fuse by 1 year after their formation. Although by and large these structures are asymptomatic, repetitive stress around accessory ossicles prior to fusing can result in their avulsion. The three common sites for accessory ossification centers are os trigonium (over the posterior aspect of the talus), medial malleolus, and the navicular bone (Malanga and Ramirez-del Toro 2008).

Overuse Injuries

Overuse injuries in adolescents around foot and ankle can present as apophysitis, osteochondral injury and stress fractures depending on the structures involved in the repetitive movements. Apophysis, the junction between the tendon and the epiphyses can be under constant stress in various sports causing inflammation at the physis of the bone: *apophysitis*. The most common site of apophysitis is at os calcis at the insertion of Achilles tendon (Sever's disease) and at the base of the fifth metatarsal (Iselin's disease) corresponding to the level of insertion of peroneus brevis tendon. Sever's disease is often referred as the "ankle equivalent" of Osgood-Schlatter's disease at the knee.

Osteochondral injury/Osteochondroses: These are group of injuries related to osteonecrosis of ossification centers as a result of overuse. Eventually, the areas of osteonecrosis undergo recalcification. The commonest osteochondral injuries are *Kohler's disease* (osteochondrosis of the tarsal navicular) and *Freiberg's infarction* (osteochondrosis/osteonecrosis of the second or third metatarsal head). Although some authors group osteochondral lesions of the dome of the talus (also known as osteochondritis dissecans of the talus) under osteochondrosis, in strict sense they are more aptly referred as complication of ankle sprains and talar fractures (Farmer et al. 2001).

Stress fractures: The terms "insufficiency fractures," "march fractures," "stress fractures "or" fatigue fractures" are synonymous and the result of overuse. In adolescents, metatarsals and navicular bones are the frequent sites of stress fractures. In pediatric population, however stress fractures in foot and ankle are less common. Several risk factors are implicated in the development of stress fractures: type of sporting activity, repetitive forceful muscle contractions, footwear, terrain, age, gender and race, nutrition, bone mineral density and skeletal alignment and mass (Pommering et al. 2005). Often the stress fracture is the result of combination of one or more of these risk factors.

Acute Injuries

Epiphyseal fractures: The Salter-Harris classification system described in the hand and wrist section can also be applied to the physeal plate injuries of the distal tibia and fibula. This classification system not only describes the orientation of the fracture line, but also predicts the association of certain fracture patterns with growth disturbances and also the need for operative intervention. Salter-Harris type I fracture of the distal fibula is the commonest fractures type in the adolescent foot and ankle. The two "subtypes" of Salter-Harris type fractures: the Tillaux and the triplane fracture deserve a special mention. These two fractures are almost always confined to the adolescent athletic population.

Tillaux fracture is essentially an avulsion injury of anterolateral tibial physis as a result of the forceful pull of the strong anterior tibiofibular ligament in an external rotation injury of the foot relative to the leg. In severe cases, the ankle mortice is disrupted requiring operation. Some authors consider tillaux fracture as a subtype of Salter-Harris type III injury and is one of the commonest fractures seen in adolescent athletes. *Triplane fracture* is similar to the tillaux fractures in two aspects: It is the fracture of anterolateral distal tibia and is the resultant of the similar deforming forces causing the tillaux fracture. However, in triplane fracture the fracture pattern is "multiplanar": the fracture line extends along the growth plate, epiphysis, and distal tibial metaphysis with these patterns corresponding to the transverse, sagittal and coronal planes respectively. *Lisfranc injury*: Lisfranc joint of the midfoot is the articulation between the bases of the first and second metatarsals and the medial and middle cuneiforms. Several dorsal, plantar and interosseous ligaments arranged in various directions support this joint. Lisfranc ligament the strongest interosseous ligament consists of dorsal and plantar bands. The dorsal band is narrow and extends from medial cuneiform to base of second metatarsal whereas the plantar band is wider and extends from the base of the medial cuneiform to the most plantar and lateral aspect of the second metatarsal and in between the second and third metatarsal bases. It is believed that axial loading through the Lisfranc joint with forceful plantar flexion and rotation (either external or internal) of the foot results in disruption of this ligament. Based on the degree of deforming forces Lisfranc injury can be graded as follows: Grade I injuries are analogs to simple sprains without interruption of ligamentous and capsular structures of the Lisfranc joint. Grade II injuries are characterized by partial tear in the ligament(s). It is generally agreed that these two groups of injuries usually have no clinical or radiological evidence of instability of the Lisfranc joint. Grade III injuries are associated with complete disruption of the capsule and several ligaments of the Lisfranc joint rendering the joint grossly instable. Grade III injuries include nondisplaced fractures at one end and frank fracture-dislocation of the osseous structures of the Lisfranc joint in extreme cases (Nunley and Vertullo 2002).

Fifth metatarsal fractures: The commonest site of fractures of the fifth metatarsal is at the base and three major types are identified: (1) stress fractures at the base of the fifth metatarsal, which is usually the result of overuse, (2) acute avulsion fractures, and (3) Jones fractures. Avulsion fractures from the base of the fifth metatarsal are the result of forceful contraction of peroneus brevis tendon following inversion type of injury. Jones fracture is described as fracture of the metaphyseal-diaphyseal junction.

Miscellaneous

Tendon injuries: The two common tendons of the foot and ankle region involved in sports-related injuries are the Peroneal and Achilles tendon. The major etiopathogenesis of peroneal tendon injuries are: (1) tendonitis and tenosynovitis and (2) tendon subluxation and dislocation (Heckman et al. 2009). Sobel et al coined the term painful os peroneum syndrome (POPS) to describe a range of posttraumatic conditions of the peroneal tendons. The following categories are included in this syndrome :(1) acute fracture of os perineum, (2) "chronic" fracture of the os perineum associated with stenosing tenosynovitis of the peroneus longus, (3) partial or complete rupture of the peroneus longus tendon near the os peroneum, or (4) entrapment of the peroneus longus tendon and the os peroneum by a hypertrophied peroneal tubercle (Sobel et al. 1994). *Peroneal tendon subluxation* is the result of displacement of one or both tendons from the retromalleolar groove. The most common mechanism of subluxation and dislocation is forceful, sudden contraction of the peroneal muscles either during an active inversion injury to the dorsiflexed ankle or as a result of forced dorisflexion of the everted foot (Maffulli et al. 2006). Often the superior peroneal retinaculum is injured or attenuated in peroneal tendon subluxation and dislocations. Peroneal tendon ruptures result from acute ankle inversion injuries or occasionally is seen in chronic conditions such as lateral ankle instability and anatomic variations that lead to stenosis within the retromalleolar groove (Sobel et al. 1993; Bonnin et al. 1997). Peroneal brevis tendon tears arise within the vicinity of retromalleolar sulcus whereas peroneal longus tears are found at the level of cuboid tunnel, at the os peroneum, at the peroneal tubercle, or at the tip of the lateral malloeolus; all these regions correspond to the regions of high shear stress (Hyer et al. 2005). In addition, peroneal longus tears can also occur as part of the POPS.

Achilles tendon injuries: Achilles tendon disorders resulting from various sports include a spectrum of degenerative and inflammatory disorders affecting the Achilles tendon along its course. The most acceptable classification of Achilles tendon injuries divides the injuries into two zones (Puddu et al. 1976). Zone I: Noninsertional area injuries. Injuries of this zone include Achilles paratenonitis, adhesive tendinopathy, Achilles tendinosis, and Achilles tendon rupture. Zone II: Insertional area injuries. Injuries of the region include retrocalcaneal bursitis, Achilles insertional calcific tendinosis, Retro-Achilles bursitis, and avulsion fracture of the calcaneus.

Ankle sprains: Ankle sprains constitute nearly 25% of all athletic injuries. They can be arbitrarily divided into syndesmotic, lateral, and medial ankle sprains. Medial ankle sprains are less common and when present are associated with a higher incidence of syndesmosis sprains. Children often sustain distal fibular physis injury (Salter-Harris type I) and usually are not prone to lateral ankle sprains. However, because of the presence of stronger bone in the more skeletally matured adolescents, lateral ankle sprains are more frequently encountered. The commonest mechanism of lateral ankle sprain is forceful inversion and internal rotation with the foot in plantar flexion in relation to the leg (Bennett 1994). The anterior talofibular ligament (ATFL) and calcaneofibular ligament (CFL) preventing lateral translation of the ankle are involved in lateral ankle sprain, with ATFL being the first ligament to be injured. The CFL is more frequently damaged if the ankle is dorsiflexion at the time of the injury. Ankle sprains are graded into three grades based on the severity of the ligamentous injury. Grade 3 injuries involve the interosseous membrane in addition to the lateral ligaments predisposing to chronic instability and osteochondral injuries to the talar dome (Farmer et al. 2001). Syndesmosis sprains results from external rotation of the ankle with the foot held in dorsiflexion and pronated position (Xenos et al. 1995). Grading scheme described for lateral ankle sprains is also applicable to syndesmosis sprains, with grade 3 injuries resulting in profound distal fibulotibular diastases.

4.3.2 Clinical Evaluation of Foot and Ankle Injuries

Clinical evaluation of sport injuries pertaining to foot and ankle injuries begins with focusing on the mechanism of injury, the age of the athlete, and the sport involved. Particular emphasis should be placed on the position of the foot relative to the leg at the time of the injury. A complete foot and ankle evaluation should include examination of the contralateral uninjured foot and assessment of the foot in both weight-bearing and nonweight bearing positions. Evaluation of foot and ankle injuries should include paying attention to the footwear or any orthotic device used by the athlete to correct the biomechanical abnormalities of the foot that may be contributing to the injury. It is imperative to focus on previous minor injuries in diagnosing the etiology of the presenting complaint. For example, sprain of the hallux metatarsophlangeal joint ("jammed great toe"- a stable joint contusion without ligamentous injury) can shift the weight to the lateral metatarsals that may result in stress fractures of the second metatarsal. Prior injury or weakness of the peroneal tendon can shift the biomechanics of the foot and ankle resulting in fifth metatarsal or cuboid or medial malleolus stress fractures (Schon 2009).

Injuries or deformities unique to a specific sport are also seen in foot and ankle injuries and examination should focus on the appearance of the toes. In dancers the hallux valgus may result from excessive rearfoot varus with increased pronation and increased abduction at the first metatarsophalangeal joint (Khan et al. 1995). Similarly, ballet dancers with repetitive plantar flexion are prone to flexor hallucis longus tendonitis. Turf toe, sprain of the plantar capsule ligament of the first metatarsalphalangeal joint is seen in young athletes playing on synthetic surfaces and using flexible footwear. Both hyperextension and hyperflexion of the first metatarsal phalangeal joint believed to result in turf toe and this injury is seen in soccer and basketball players (Omey and Micheli 1999). Basket ball, tennis, soccer, and ice hockey are associated with increased incidence of posterior tibialis tendonitis due to increased stress on this tendon associated with rapid changes in direction (Conti 1994).

Examination of the plantar aspect of the foot is often missed in assessment of foot and ankle injuries which can provide some vital diagnostic clues. For example in an appropriate context severe bruising over the plantar surface may suggest the diagnosis of a Lisfranc injury. Similarly, one has to observe for skin changes. In case of chronic injuries one should look for dorsal callus over the first metatarsophalangeal joint as seen in hallux limitus or presence of plantar callus may indicate prior fracture resulting in transfer of the load to the adjacent metatarsals. Impingement between adjacent toes can result in soft or hard callus in elite dancers which eventually may result in skin break down (Schon 2009).

Observing the appearance of the feet, gait, mobility, and stance is the corner stone of the clinical examination of foot and ankle injuries. Special emphasis should be placed on the position of the iliac crests, alignment of the knee and foot arches, abnormal alignment of the structures is indicative of certain overuse injuries or their presence may predispose the athlete to specific foot and ankle injuries (Wilder and Sethi 2004). A low medial arch, also referred as pes planus, may be congenital or the result of posterior tibial tendon dysfunction or contraction of the Achilles tendon. The low medial arch once diagnosed should be confirmed upon weight bearing. Significant loss of the height of medial arch upon weight bearing and restoration of normal arch when non weight bearing is suggestive of flexible flat foot. In a normal feet examiner should be able to visualize the lateral two toes from behind. However, seeing more than two lateral toes bilaterally is suggestive of pes planus. Presence of such a finding unilaterally is diagnostic of posterior tibial tendon rupture. On the other hand, high medial arch (pes cavus) can result in peroneal tendinopathy, fifth metatarsal stress fractures, lateral ankle instability, and medial malleolar stress fractures (Schon 2009). Haglund's deformity an abnormal prominence of the posterosuperior surface of the calcaneus is seen in ice skaters, soccer players and runners and on physical examination is palpated as a "bump" on lateral side of the heel (Stephens 1994).

A positive *Single-leg heel raise test* as opposed to asking the athlete walking on the toes: normal individuals can raise their heels several centimeters off the floor, indicates the presence of subtle weakness in plantar flexors, indicative of Achilles tendon injury or dysfunction of either sciatic or tibial nerve (Young et al. 2005). Tibialis posterior tendon dysfunction is assessed by a heel rise test. Absence of heel inversion on raising the heel suggests tibialis posterior dysfunction.

Ankle sprains, the commonest injury in athletes can be sometimes difficult to diagnose due to the immediate diffuse swelling and/or tenderness of the ankle joint following injury. Specific tests should be performed to diagnose ATFL and CFL. The *anterior drawer test* is useful to test the integrity of ATFL. This is performed by asking the patient to relax the ankle while the examiner stabilizes the leg with one hand and pulls the heel forward with the other hand. The difference of 3–5 mm laxity of the ankle joint compared to the contralateral side is suggestive of ATFL injury. The *talar tilt test* is useful to test the integrity of ATFL and CFL. The examiner stabilizes the leg and subjects the dorsiflexed ankle to the varus stress at the heel. A difference of more than 10° compared to the contralateral side is suggestive of tears of both the CFL and ATFL. *Squeeze test* is performed by squeezing the tibia and fibula together along the midshaft. Pain at the distal ankle is suggestive of syndesmotic sprain. Similarly, pain on application of external rotation force on a dorsiflexed ankle also is suspicious of syndesmosis sprain (*external rotation test*). Subtalar joint motion is assessed by grasping the heel and maximally inverting and everting it. On an average, there is a normal eversion of 20° and inversion of 40° at the subtalar joint, restriction of this movement is seen in tarsal coalition. In addition, in athletes with tarsal coalition there is a history of recurrent ankle sprain.

A positive *Thompson test* suggests an injury to the Achilles tendon. This test is performed with the athlete lying in prone position. The knee is flexed to 90° and the calf is gently squeezed. In normal circumstances this maneuver induces passive plantar flexion of the foot. In the presence of a complete tear of the Achilles tendon the foot will not move passively. A negative test however does not exclude a partial tear of the tendon. In addition, on physical examination there is a palpable gap at the calcaneal insertion of the tendon. Positive *Tinel's test* on percussion of the potential entrapment sites involving lateral plantar, posterior tibial and sural nerve is suggestive entrapment neuropathy. Displacement of the peroneal tendons around the posterior border of the lateral malleolus on eversion of the dorsiflexed foot against resistance is indicative recurrent subluxation of the peroneal tendons. Athletes with Morton's "neuroma" (mechanical entrapment of interdigital nerve under the intermetatarsal ligament) present with symptoms of forefoot burning, tingling, and numbness in the toes of the involved interdigital space affected. The commonest affected nerve is the third interdigital nerve, between the third and fourth metatarsal heads (Wu 1996).

4.3.3 Epidemiology of Foot and Ankle Injuries

The incidence and prevalence of foot and ankle injuries is dependent on the type of sport involved and specific data on the epidemiology of ankle injury is difficult to obtain due to variable methodology and recording systems in each individual studies. Foot and ankle injuries account for nearly 30% of visits attributed to sport-related injuries. In a large systemic review on epidemiology of sports injuries revealed that ankle sprain was the commonest sport related foot and injury with a prevalence rate of 76% (Fong et al. 2007). In the same study it was concluded that ankle sprain was the only injury (100%) in Australian foot ball, field hockey, orienteering and squash. The highest incidence of ankle injuries was noticed in hurling and camogie at 32.88 per 1,000 person-hour. In competitive sports soccer was associated the highest incidence (38.43/1,000 person-hour). Rugby had the highest incidence of ankle sprains followed by soccer; 4.20 and 2.52 per 1,000 person-hour. During competitive sports soccer was associated with the highest incidence of ankle sprains (11.68) followed by Australian football (4.86) and soccer (4.59) per 1,000 person-year. In another study from the United States which evaluated ankle sport injuries in high-school athletes revealed a total ankle injury rate of 5.23 injuries per 10,000 athlete-exposures and constituted 22.6% of all sport-related injuries (Nelson et al. 2007). Soccer was the leading cause of ankle injury which accounted for 33.6% of all ankle injuries, contact with other person being the commonest mechanism of the injury. Ankle injuries were higher during competition than practice session: 9.35 vs. 3.63 per 10,000 athlete-exposures. A highest rate of ankle injury was seen in boys' basket ball: 7.74 per 10,000 athlete exposures. Overall in this study, ligament sprains with incomplete tears was the common injury (83.4%) seen in high school athletes. A national study in United Kingdom revealed that soccer accounted for 28.9% of sport-related injuries with most injuries being sprains and strains of the lower limbs and 11.5% of injuries were confined to the ankle (Nicholl et al. 1995). There is variable data on foot and ankle soft tissue and bony injuries depending on the country of origin of the epidemiological data and the study population under evaluation. Osteochondral lesions of the talus believed to be a complication of the lateral ankle sprain are seen in up to 6.5% of ankle sprains (Farmer et al. 2001). Sever's disease one of the most common oversue injuries in adolescent athletes accounts for nearly 8% of all overuse injuries (Pommering et al. 2005). The fifth metatarsal fracture accounts for nearly 45% of all metatarsal fractures in the pediatric athlete (Omey and Micheli 1999). Fractures of the distal tibial and fibular physes constitute 4% of all ankle injuries in the pediatric population. Ninety percent of acute dislocation and subluxation of peroneal tendons is the result of winter sports, basketball, or football. Certain foot and ankle disorders have sex preponderance. For example, Freiberg's infarction is typically seen in an adolescent female aged 11–17 years, the female to male ratio of this condition being 5:1 (Katcherian 1994). Studies on military recruits have identified adolescent women to be more vulnerable to stress fractures (Brudvig et al. 1983). Methods used in diagnosing the foot and ankle injuries can influence the epidemiology data. For example, use of bone scan and/or MRI can increase the accuracy of the diagnosis of stress fractures. In a study of 320 athletes where bone scan was used to diagnose stress fractures, 69% of these injuries were seen in runners (Matheson et al. 1987). A study on 51 consecutive military recruits undergoing MRI to diagnose stress injuries to the talus revealed an incidence of 4.4/10,000 person-years (Sormaala et al. 2006). In another study evaluation of seventy-four individuals with history and physical examination consistent of stress injuries, diagnosis was confirmed in 61 cases using MRI and only in six athletes the diagnosis was made on the basis of the plain radiograph findings (Arendt et al. 2003). A similar recent study quoted the incidence of stress fractures in the foot and ankle region as 126 per 100,000 person-years based on MRI findings of which 57.7% injuries were confined to the tarsal bones and 35.7% to the metatarsal bones. In 63% of the cases multiple stress injuries were seen in a single foot (Niva et al. 2007).

Conflict of Interest The authors declare that there is no conflict of interest

Acknowledgments Academic Unit, Trauma and Orthopaedic Surgery, Clarendon Wing, Leeds General Infirmary, Great George Street, Leeds, LS1 3EX, UK.

References

Albright JA, Jokl P, Shaw R, Albright JP (1978) Clinical study of baseball pitchers: correlation of injury to the throwing arm with method of delivery. Am J Sports Med 6:15–21

Arendt E, Agel J, Heikes C, Griffiths H (2003) Stress injuries to bone in college athletes: a retrospective review of experience at a single institution. Am J Sports Med 31:959–968

Aronowitz ER, Leddy JP (1998) Closed tendon injuries of the hand and wrist in athletes. Clin Sports Med 17:449–467

Bailes JE, Maroon JC (1991) Spinal cord injuries in athletes. N Y State J Med 91:44–45

Banerjee R, Palumbo MA, Fadale PD (2004) Catastrophic cervical spine injuries in the collision sport athlete, part 1: epidemiology, functional anatomy, and diagnosis. Am J Sports Med 32:1077–1087

Beaman FD, Peterson JJ (2007) MR imaging of cysts, ganglia, and bursae about the knee. Radiol Clin North Am 45:969–982, vi

Beckenbaugh RD, Shives TC, Dobyns JH, Linscheid RL (1980) Kienbock's disease: the natural history of Kienbock's disease and consideration of lunate fractures. Clin Orthop Relat Res (149):98–106

Bennett WF (1994) Lateral ankle sprains. Part I: Anatomy, biomechanics, diagnosis, and natural history. Orthop Rev. 1994;23(5):381–7

Biasca N, Wirth S, Tegner Y (2002) The avoidability of head and neck injuries in ice hockey: an historical review. Br J Sports Med 36:410–427

Bissell BT, Johnson RJ, Shafritz AB, Chase DC, Ettlinger CF (2008) Epidemiology and risk factors of humerus fractures among skiers and snowboarders. Am J Sports Med 36: 1880–1888

Boden BP, Lin W, Young M, Mueller FO (2002) Catastrophic injuries in wrestlers. Am J Sports Med 30:791–795

Bohne WH (2001) Tarsal coalition. Curr Opin Pediatr 13:29–35

Bonnin M, Tavernier T, Bouysset M (1997) Split lesions of the peroneus brevis tendon in chronic ankle laxity. Am J Sports Med 25:699–703

Borowski LA, Yard EE, Fields SK, Comstock RD (2008) The epidemiology of US high school basketball injuries, 2005–2007. Am J Sports Med 36:2328–2335

Bozentka DJ (1998) Cubital tunnel syndrome pathophysiology. Clin Orthop Relat Res (351):90–94

Brudvig TJ, Gudger TD, Obermeyer L (1983) Stress fractures in 295 trainees: a one-year study of incidence as related to age, sex, and race. Mil Med 148:666–667

Brunet ME, Haddad RJ Jr (1986) Fractures and dislocations of the metacarpals and phalanges. Clin Sports Med 5: 773–781

Burkhart SS, Nottage WM, Ogilvie-Harris DJ, Kohn HS, Pachelli A (1994) Partial repair of irreparable rotator cuff tears. Arthroscopy 10:363–370

Buterbaugh GA, Brown TR, Horn PC (1998) Ulnar-sided wrist pain in athletes. Clin Sports Med 17:567–583

Caine D, Cochrane B, Caine C, Zemper E (1989) An epidemiologic investigation of injuries affecting young competitive female gymnasts. Am J Sports Med 17:811–820

Caine D, Roy S, Singer KM, Broekhoff J (1992) Stress changes of the distal radial growth plate. A radiographic survey and review of the literature. Am J Sports Med 20:290–298

Chambers HG (2003) Ankle and foot disorders in skeletally immature athletes. Orthop Clin North Am 34:445–459

Cohen MS, Hastings H 2nd (1998) Acute elbow dislocation: evaluation and management. J Am Acad Orthop Surg 6:15–23

Conti SF (1994) Posterior tibial tendon problems in athletes. Orthop Clin North Am 25:109–121

Cooper DE, Arnoczky SP, Warren RF (1991) Meniscal repair. Clin Sports Med 10:529–548

Cooper JM, McAndrews PT, LaPrade RF (2006) Posterolateral corner injuries of the knee: anatomy, diagnosis, and treatment. Sports Med Arthrosc 14:213–220

Court-Brown CM, Wood AM, Aitken S (2008) The epidemiology of acute sports-related fractures in adults. Injury 39: 1365–1372

Darrow CJ, Collins CL, Yard EE, Comstock RD (2009) Epidemiology of severe injuries among United States high school athletes: 2005-2007. Am J Sports Med 37:1798–1805

DeLee JC, Farney WC (1992) Incidence of injury in Texas high school football. Am J Sports Med 20:575–580

DiFiori JP, Puffer JC, Mandelbaum BR, Dorey F (1997) Distal radial growth plate injury and positive ulnar variance in non-elite gymnasts. Am J Sports Med 25:763–768

Eathorne SW (2005) The wrist: clinical anatomy and physical examination-an update. Prim Care 32:17–33

Falkenberg P, Nygaard H (1983) Isolated anterior dislocation of the proximal tibiofibular joint. J Bone Joint Surg Br 65:310–311

Farmer JM, Martin DF, Boles CA, Curl WW (2001) Chondral and osteochondral injuries. Diagnosis and management. Clin Sports Med 20:299–320

Feeley BT, Powell JW, Muller MS, Barnes RP, Warren RF, Kelly BT (2008) Hip injuries and labral tears in the national football league. Am J Sports Med 36:2187–2195

Fehnel DJ, Johnson R (2000) Anterior cruciate injuries in the skeletally immature athlete: a review of treatment outcomes. Sports Med 29:51–63

Fetto JF, Marshall JL (1978) Medial collateral ligament injuries of the knee: a rationale for treatment. Clin Orthop Relat Res (132):206–218

Fong DT, Hong Y, Chan LK, Yung PS, Chan KM (2007) A systematic review on ankle injury and ankle sprain in sports. Sports Med 37:73–94

Fowler PJ, Messieh SS (1987) Isolated posterior cruciate ligament injuries in athletes. Am J Sports Med 15:553–557

Franz T, Hasler RM, Benneker L, Zimmermann H, Siebenrock KA, Exadaktylos AK (2008) Severe spinal injuries in alpine skiing and snowboarding: a 6-year review of a tertiary trauma centre for the Bernese Alps ski resorts, Switzerland. Br J Sports Med 42:55–58

Fullerton LR Jr, Snowdy HA (1988) Femoral neck stress fractures. Am J Sports Med 16:365–377

Gabbett TJ (2003) Incidence of injury in semi-professional rugby league players. Br J Sports Med 37:36–43, discussion 43–34

Giachino AA (1986) Recurrent dislocations of the proximal tibiofibular joint. Report of two cases. J Bone Joint Surg Am 68:1104–1106

Gilmore J (1998) Groin pain in the soccer athlete: fact, fiction, and treatment. Clin Sports Med 17:787–793, vii

Grogan DP, Carey TP, Leffers D, Ogden JA (1990) Avulsion fractures of the patella. J Pediatr Orthop 10:721–730

Grote K, Lincoln TL, Gamble JG (2004) Hip adductor injury in competitive swimmers. Am J Sports Med 32:104–108
Hagel BE, Meeuwisse WH, Mohtadi NG, Fick GH (1999) Skiing and snowboarding injuries in the children and adolescents of Southern Alberta. Clin J Sport Med 9:9–17
Hang DW, Chao CM, Hang YS (2004) A clinical and roentgenographic study of Little League elbow. Am J Sports Med 32: 79–84
Hawkins RJ, Kennedy JC (1980) Impingement syndrome in athletes. Am J Sports Med 8:151–158
Headey J, Brooks JH, Kemp SP (2007) The epidemiology of shoulder injuries in English professional rugby union. Am J Sports Med 35:1537–1543
Heckman DS, Gluck GS, Parekh SG (2009) Tendon disorders of the foot and ankle, part 1: peroneal tendon disorders. Am J Sports Med 37:614–625
Hegedus EJ, Goode A, Campbell S, Morin A, Tamaddoni M, Moorman CT 3rd, Cook C (2008) Physical examination tests of the shoulder: a systematic review with meta-analysis of individual tests. Br J Sports Med 42:80–92, discussion 92
Heim D (1999) The skier's thumb. Acta Orthop Belg 65: 440–446
Hocker K, Menschik A (1994) Chip fractures of the triquetrum. Mechanism, classification and results. J Hand Surg Br 19: 584–588
Houshian S, Mehdi B, Larsen MS (2001) The epidemiology of elbow fracture in children: analysis of 355 fractures, with special reference to supracondylar humerus fractures. J Orthop Sci 6:312–315
Hutchinson MR, Ireland ML (2003) Overuse and throwing injuries in the skeletally immature athlete. Instr Course Lect 52:25–36
Hyer CF, Dawson JM, Philbin TM, Berlet GC, Lee TH (2005) The peroneal tubercle: description, classification, and relevance to peroneus longus tendon pathology. Foot Ankle Int 26:947–950
Idzikowski JR, Janes PC, Abbott PJ (2000) Upper extremity snowboarding injuries. Ten-year results from the Colorado snowboard injury survey. Am J Sports Med 28:825–832
Indelicato PA (1995) Isolated medial collateral ligament injuries in the knee. J Am Acad Orthop Surg 3:9–14
Ingram JG, Fields SK, Yard EE, Comstock RD (2008) Epidemiology of knee injuries among boys and girls in US high school athletics. Am J Sports Med 36:1116–1122
Isani A, Melone CP Jr (1986) Ligamentous injuries of the hand in athletes. Clin Sports Med 5:757–772
Janousek AT, Jones DG, Clatworthy M, Higgins LD, Fu FH (1999) Posterior cruciate ligament injuries of the knee joint. Sports Med 28:429–441
Karachalios T, Hantes M, Zibis AH, Zachos V, Karantanas AH, Malizos KN (2005) Diagnostic accuracy of a new clinical test (the Thessaly test) for early detection of meniscal tears. J Bone Joint Surg Am 87:955–962
Karpakka J (1993) American football injuries in Finland. Br J Sports Med 27:135–137
Katcherian DA (1994) Treatment of Freiberg's disease. Orthop Clin North Am 25:69–81
Khan K, Brown J, Way S, Vass N, Crichton K, Alexander R, Baxter A, Butler M, Wark J (1995) Overuse injuries in classical ballet. Sports Med 19:341–357
Kibler WB (1995) Specificity and sensitivity of the anterior slide test in throwing athletes with superior glenoid labral tears. Arthroscopy 11:296–300
Klingele KE, Kocher MS (2002) Little league elbow: valgus overload injury in the paediatric athlete. Sports Med 32: 1005–1015
Kocher MS, Dupre MM, Feagin JA Jr (1998) Shoulder injuries from alpine skiing and snowboarding. Aetiology, treatment and prevention. Sports Med 25:201–211
Kohler R, Trillaud JM (1983) Fracture and fracture separation of the proximal humerus in children: report of 136 cases. J Pediatr Orthop 3:326–332
Konan S, Rayan F, Haddad FS (2009) Do physical diagnostic tests accurately detect meniscal tears? Knee Surg Sports Traumatol Arthrosc 17:806–811
Kordi R, Akbarnejad A, Wallace AW (2008) Catastrophic Injuries in the Olympic styles of wrestling in Iran. Br J Sports Med 44:168–174
Kraft DE (2002) Low back pain in the adolescent athlete. Pediatr Clin North Am 49:643–653
Kvitne RS, Jobe FW, Jobe CM (1995) Shoulder instability in the overhand or throwing athlete. Clin Sports Med 14:917–935
Lage LA, Patel JV, Villar RN (1996) The acetabular labral tear: an arthroscopic classification. Arthroscopy 12:269–272
Leddy JP (1985) Avulsions of the flexor digitorum profundus. Hand Clin 1:77–83
Leddy JP (1998) Soft-tissue injuries of the hand in the athlete. Instr Course Lect 47:181–186
Lorish TR, Rizzo TD Jr, Ilstrup DM, Scott SG (1992) Injuries in adolescent and preadolescent boys at two large wrestling tournaments. Am J Sports Med 20:199–202
Louw QA, Manilall J, Grimmer KA (2008) Epidemiology of knee injuries among adolescents: a systematic review. Br J Sports Med 42:2–10
Lyman S, Fleisig GS, Andrews JR, Osinski ED (2002) Effect of pitch type, pitch count, and pitching mechanics on risk of elbow and shoulder pain in youth baseball pitchers. Am J Sports Med 30:463–468
Machold W, Kwasny O, Gassler P, Kolonja A, Reddy B, Bauer E, Lehr S (2000) Risk of injury through snowboarding. J Trauma 48:1109–1114
Maffulli N, Ferran NA, Oliva F, Testa V (2006) Recurrent subluxation of the peroneal tendons. Am J Sports Med 34: 986–992
Magra M, Caine D, Maffulli N (2007) A review of epidemiology of paediatric elbow injuries in sports. Sports Med 37:717–735
Malanga GA, Ramirez-Del Toro JA (2008) Common injuries of the foot and ankle in the child and adolescent athlete. Phys Med Rehabil Clin N Am 19:347–371, ix
Maroon JC (1977) 'Burning hands' in football spinal cord injuries. JAMA 238:2049–2051
Maroon JC, Bailes JE (1996) Athletes with cervical spine injury. Spine (Phila Pa 1976) 21:2294–2299
Mason ML (1954) Some observations on fractures of the head of the radius with a review of one hundred cases. Br J Surg 42:123–132
Matheson GO, Clement DB, McKenzie DC, Taunton JE, Lloyd-Smith DR, MacIntyre JG (1987) Stress fractures in athletes. A study of 320 cases. Am J Sports Med 15:46–58
McAfee PC, Yuan HA, Fredrickson BE, Lubicky JP (1983) The value of computed tomography in thoracolumbar fractures.

An analysis of one hundred consecutive cases and a new classification. J Bone Joint Surg Am 65:461–473
McCue FC 3rd, Wooten SL (1986) Closed tendon injuries of the hand in athletics. Clin Sports Med 5:741–755
McCulloch JA (1997) The lumbar spine-small is beautiful: the 3d Annual Ian Macnab Memorial Lecture. J Spinal Disord 10:260–271
McFarland EG, Selhi HS, Keyurapan E (2006) Clinical evaluation of impingement: what to do and what works. Instr Course Lect 55:3–16
McFarland EG, Tanaka MJ, Papp DF (2008) Examination of the shoulder in the overhead and throwing athlete. Clin Sports Med 27:553–578
Melone CP Jr (1993) Distal radius fractures: patterns of articular fragmentation. Orthop Clin North Am 24:239–253
Meyers WC, McKechnie A, Philippon MJ, Horner MA, Zoga AC, Devon ON (2008) Experience with "sports hernia" spanning two decades. Ann Surg 248:656–665
Molsa JJ, Tegner Y, Alaranta H, Myllynen P, Kujala UM (1999) Spinal cord injuries in ice hockey in Finland and Sweden from 1980 to 1996. Int J Sports Med 20:64–67
Morrey BF, An KN, Stormont TJ (1988) Force transmission through the radial head. J Bone Joint Surg Am 70:250–256
Neer CS II (1983) Impingement lesions. Clin Orthop Relat Res (173):70–77
Nelson AJ, Collins CL, Yard EE, Fields SK, Comstock RD (2007) Ankle injuries among United States high school sports athletes, 2005-2006. J Athl Train 42:381–387
Nicholl JP, Coleman P, Williams BT (1995) The epidemiology of sports and exercise related injury in the United Kingdom. Br J Sports Med 29:232–238
Niva MH, Sormaala MJ, Kiuru MJ, Haataja R, Ahovuo JA, Pihlajamaki HK (2007) Bone stress injuries of the ankle and foot: an 86-month magnetic resonance imaging-based study of physically active young adults. Am J Sports Med 35:643–649
Nunley JA, Vertullo CJ (2002) Classification, investigation, and management of midfoot sprains: lisfranc injuries in the athlete. Am J Sports Med 30:871–878
O'Brien SJ, Pagnani MJ, Fealy S, McGlynn SR, Wilson JB (1998) The active compression test: a new and effective test for diagnosing labral tears and acromioclavicular joint abnormality. Am J Sports Med 26:610–613
O'Driscoll SW, Morrey BF, Korinek S, An KN (1992) Elbow subluxation and dislocation. A spectrum of instability. Clin Orthop Relat Res 35(1):186–197
O'Driscoll SW, Jupiter JB, Cohen MS, Ring D, McKee MD (2003) Difficult elbow fractures: pearls and pitfalls. Instr Course Lect 52:113–134
Ogden JA (1974) Subluxation and dislocation of the proximal tibiofibular joint. J Bone Joint Surg Am 56:145–154
Ogden JA, Tross RB, Murphy MJ (1980) Fractures of the tibial tuberosity in adolescents. J Bone Joint Surg Am 62:205–215
Omey ML, Micheli LJ (1999) Foot and ankle problems in the young athlete. Med Sci Sports Exerc 31:S470–S486
Orchard J, James T, Alcott E, Carter S, Farhart P (2002) Injuries in Australian cricket at first class level 1995/1996 to 2000/2001. Br J Sports Med 36:270–274, discussion 275
Palmer AK (1981) Trapezial ridge fractures. J Hand Surg Am 6:561–564
Pasque CB, Hewett TE (2000) A prospective study of high school wrestling injuries. Am J Sports Med 28:509–515
Philippon MJ, Maxwell RB, Johnston TL, Schenker M, Briggs KK (2007) Clinical presentation of femoroacetabular impingement. Knee Surg Sports Traumatol Arthrosc 15:1041–1047
Pinto M, Kuhn JE, Greenfield ML, Hawkins RJ (1999) Prospective analysis of ice hockey injuries at the Junior A level over the course of one season. Clin J Sport Med 9:70–74
Poindexter DP, Johnson EW (1984) Football shoulder and neck injury: a study of the "stinger". Arch Phys Med Rehabil 65:601–602
Pommering TL, Kluchurosky L, Hall SL (2005) Ankle and foot injuries in pediatric and adult athletes. Prim Care 32: 133–161
Pontell D, Hallivis R, Dollard MD (2006) Sports injuries in the pediatric and adolescent foot and ankle: common overuse and acute presentations. Clin Podiatr Med Surg 23:209–231, x
Puddu G, Ippolito E, Postacchini F (1976) A classification of Achilles tendon disease. Am J Sports Med 4:145–150
Quarrie KL, Cantu RC, Chalmers DJ (2002) Rugby union injuries to the cervical spine and spinal cord. Sports Med 32:633–653
Reagan DS, Linscheid RL, Dobyns JH (1984) Lunotriquetral sprains. J Hand Surg Am 9:502–514
Regan W, Morrey B (1989) Fractures of the coronoid process of the ulna. J Bone Joint Surg Am 71:1348–1354
Rettig AC (1998) Epidemiology of hand and wrist injuries in sports. Clin Sports Med 17:401–406
Rettig AC (2004) Athletic injuries of the wrist and hand: part II: overuse injuries of the wrist and traumatic injuries to the hand. Am J Sports Med 32:262–273
Rios CG, Mazzocca AD (2008) Acromioclavicular joint problems in athletes and new methods of management. Clin Sports Med 27:763–788
Roles NC, Maudsley RH (1972) Radial tunnel syndrome: resistant tennis elbow as a nerve entrapment. J Bone Joint Surg Br 54:499–508
Rossi F, Dragoni S (2001) Acute avulsion fractures of the pelvis in adolescent competitive athletes: prevalence, location and sports distribution of 203 cases collected. Skeletal Radiol 30:127–131
Rotem TR, Lawson JS, Wilson SF, Engel S, Rutkowski SB, Aisbett CW (1998) Severe cervical spinal cord injuries related to rugby union and league football in New South Wales, 1984–1996. Med J Aust 168:379–381
Ruby LK (1992) Wrist biomechanics. Instr Course Lect 41:25–32
Safran MR (1995) Elbow injuries in athletes. A review. Clin Orthop Relat Res 257–277
Salter RB (1992) Injuries of the epiphyseal plate. Instr Course Lect 41:351–359
Savoie FH III, Papendik L, Field LD, Jobe C (2001) Straight anterior instability: Lesions of the middle glenohumeral ligament. Arthroscopy 17:229–235
Scher AT (1998) Rugby injuries to the cervical spine and spinal cord: a 10-year review. Clin Sports Med 17:195–206
Schmitt H, Gerner HJ (2001) Paralysis from sport and diving accidents. Clin J Sport Med 11:17–22
Schon LC (2009) Assessment of the foot and ankle in elite athletes. Sports Med Arthrosc 17:82–86
Sethi MK, Schoenfeld AJ, Bono CM, Harris MB (2009) The evolution of thoracolumbar injury classification systems. Spine J 9:780–788

Slawski DP, Cahill BR (1994) Atraumatic osteolysis of the distal clavicle. Results of open surgical excision. Am J Sports Med 22:267–271

Sobel M, Geppert MJ, Warren RF (1993) Chronic ankle instability as a cause of peroneal tendon injury. Clin Orthop Relat Res 187–191

Sobel M, Pavlov H, Geppert MJ, Thompson FM, DiCarlo EF, Davis WH (1994) Painful os peroneum syndrome: a spectrum of conditions responsible for plantar lateral foot pain. Foot Ankle Int 15:112–124

Sormaala MJ, Niva MH, Kiuru MJ, Mattila VM, Pihlajamaki HK (2006) Bone stress injuries of the talus in military recruits. Bone 39:199–204

Stark HH, Chao EK, Zemel NP, Rickard TA, Ashworth CR (1989) Fracture of the hook of the hamate. J Bone Joint Surg Am 71:1202–1207

Stephens MM (1994) Haglund's deformity and retrocalcaneal bursitis. Orthop Clin North Am 25:41–46

Stuart MJ, Smith A (1995) Injuries in Junior A ice hockey. A three-year prospective study. Am J Sports Med 23:458–461

Tarazi F, Dvorak MF, Wing PC (1999) Spinal injuries in skiers and snowboarders. Am J Sports Med 27:177–180

Tator CH, Provvidenza CF, Lapczak L, Carson J, Raymond D (2004) Spinal injuries in Canadian ice hockey: documentation of injuries sustained from 1943-1999. Can J Neurol Sci 31:460–466

Taylor DC, Meyers WC, Moylan JA, Lohnes J, Bassett FH, Garrett WE Jr (1991) Abdominal musculature abnormalities as a cause of groin pain in athletes. Inguinal hernias and pubalgia. Am J Sports Med 19:239–242

Ticker JB, Warner JJ (1997) Single-tendon tears of the rotator cuff. Evaluation and treatment of subscapularis tears and principles of treatment for supraspinatus tears. Orthop Clin North Am 28:99–116

Tomlinson RJ Jr, Glousman RE (1995) Arthroscopic debridement of glenoid labral tears in athletes. Arthroscopy 11:42–51

Toohey AK, LaSalle TL, Martinez S, Polisson RP (1990) Iliopsoas bursitis: clinical features, radiographic findings, and disease associations. Semin Arthritis Rheum 20:41–47

Torg JS (1990) Cervical spinal stenosis with cord neurapraxia and transient quadriplegia. Clin Sports Med 9:279–296

Torg JS, Sennett B, Pavlov H, Leventhal MR, Glasgow SG (1993) Spear tackler's spine. An entity precluding participation in tackle football and collision activities that expose the cervical spine to axial energy inputs. Am J Sports Med 21:640–649

Vance RM, Gelberman RH, Evans EF (1980) Scaphocapitate fractures. Patterns of dislocation, mechanisms of injury, and preliminary results of treatment. J Bone Joint Surg Am 62:271–276

Vangsness CT Jr, Jobe FW (1991) Surgical treatment of medial epicondylitis. Results in 35 elbows. J Bone Joint Surg Br 73:409–411

Wang HK, Cochrane T (2001) A descriptive epidemiological study of shoulder injury in top level English male volleyball players. Int J Sports Med 22:159–163

Watson HK, Weinzweig J (1997) Physical examination of the wrist. Hand Clin 13:17–34

Weaver JK (1987) Skiing-related injuries to the shoulder. Clin Orthop Relat Res (216):24–28

Wehbe MA, Schneider LH (1984) Mallet fractures. J Bone Joint Surg Am 66:658–669

White AA III, Panjabi MM (1987) Update on the evaluation of instability of the lower cervical spine. Instr Course Lect 36:513–520

Wilder RP, Sethi S (2004) Overuse injuries: tendinopathies, stress fractures, compartment syndrome, and shin splints. Clin Sports Med 23:55–81, vi

Wiltse LL (1975) Spondylolisthesis. West J Med 122:152–153

Wu KK (1996) Morton's interdigital neuroma: a clinical review of its etiology, treatment, and results. J Foot Ankle Surg 35:112–119, discussion 187–118

Xenos JS, Hopkinson WJ, Mulligan ME, Olson EJ, Popovic NA (1995) The tibiofibular syndesmosis. Evaluation of the ligamentous structures, methods of fixation, and radiographic assessment. J Bone Joint Surg Am 77:847–856

Young CC, Niedfeldt MW, Morris GA, Eerkes KJ (2005) Clinical examination of the foot and ankle. Prim Care 32:105–132

Zwimpfer TJ, Bernstein M (1990) Spinal cord concussion. J Neurosurg 72:894–900

Normal Anatomy and Variants that Simulate Injury

Filip M. Vanhoenacker, Kristof De Cuyper, and Helen Williams

Contents

F.M. Vanhoenacker (✉)
Department of Radiology, University Hospital Antwerp, Wilrijkstraat 10, 2650 Edegem, Belgium and
Department of Radiology, General Hospital Sint-Maarten Duffel-Mechelen, Rooienberg 25, 2570 Duffel, Belgium
e-mail: filip.vanhoenacker@telenet.be

K. De Cuyper
Department of Radiology, General Hospital Sint-Maarten Duffel-Mechelen, Rooienberg 25, 2570 Duffel, Belgium

H. Williams
Department of Radiology, Birmingham Children's Hospital, Steelhouse Lane, Birmingham, B4 6NH, UK

Key Points

- The immature skeleton differs fundamentally from the adult skeleton.
- The interpretation of imaging studies in young athletes requires a thorough expertise in the normal developmental musculoskeletal anatomy and its spectrum of variations.
- Knowledge of the normal anatomy variants and other pitfalls avoids overinterpretation and unnecessary and harmful treatment.
- There are many mimickers of acute and chronic musculoskeletal trauma in sportive children and adolescents on imaging studies. Most of these mimickers are related to normal developmental variations whereas others are due to artifacts.
- Most variants are asymptomatic but some variants may become symptomatic or predispose to pathology.
- Plain radiography is the mainstay in the correct diagnosis but MRI and ultrasound may be helpful in the differential diagnosis of normal variants vs. traumatic disorders in selected cases.
- Rare congenital bone diseases may mimic acute or chronic trauma of the musculoskeletal system.

1 Introduction

As the immature skeleton differs fundamentally from the adult skeleton, the interpretation of imaging studies in young athletes requires a thorough expertise in the normal developmental musculoskeletal anatomy

A.H. Karantanas (ed.), *Sports Injuries in Children and Adolescents*,
Med Radiol Diagn Imaging, DOI: 10.1007/174_2010_10, © Springer-Verlag Berlin Heidelberg 2011

and its spectrum of variations for proper diagnosis, classification, and management of sports injuries. This chapter intends to cover the general principles of normal imaging anatomy of the immature skeleton, potential misinterpretation due to artifacts, anatomical variations, and preexisting disease. For a complete and exhaustive review of normal variants that may simulate disease, the reader is referred to encyclopedic textbooks (Slovis 2008) and the atlases of Theodore Keats, Keats and Kahn, and Kohler and Zimmer (Kahn et al. 2008; Keats and Anderson 2006; Freyschmidt et al. 2002).

This chapter will focus primarily on the appendicular skeleton. For a more-in-depth discussion of the normal variants of the spine, we refer to dedicated textbooks (Swischuk 2002) and book chapters on the subject (Williams 2008).

We will emphasize those variants that may mimic acute and chronic musculoskeletal trauma encountered in pediatric sports-related injuries.

Finally, some symptomatic variants and some differential diagnostic considerations will be discussed.

2 Normal Developmental Anatomy on Imaging

The skeletal immature patient differs from the adult in that secondary cartilaginous growth centers are present around joints (epiphyses) and at the attachments of tendons and ligaments to bone (apophyses) (Barron et al. 2008).

Whereas the epiphysis contributes to the longitudinal growth of the bone, the apophysis does not and acts primarily as the insertion site for a tendon or ligament. Both the apophysis and epiphysis are separated from the adjacent bone by a physeal plate (Figs. 1 and 2), which may be mistaken for a fracture, particularly if visualized obliquely (Fig. 3) (Williams 2008).

Other normal developmental changes that may cause interpretation errors are synchondroses, accessory ossicles, and sesamoid bones (Williams 2008).

A synchondrosis is a type of cartilaginous joint in which the cartilage is usually converted into bone before or during early adult life and that serves to allow growth e.g., spheno-occipital synchondrosis at the skull base. A synchondrosis that may cause

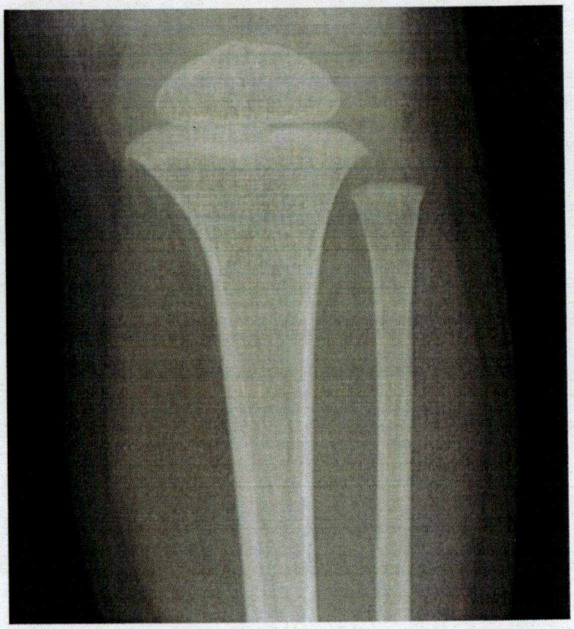

Fig. 1 Example of a normal epiphysis of the tibia in a 2-year-old child

confusion in the sportive child is the ischiopubic synchondrosis.

Differences in size and shape of ischiopubic synchondrosis in childhood may present problems in diagnosis and differential diagnosis (Kozlowski et al. 1995). The ossification of the cartilage between the ischium and pubis is highly variable in both temporal and radiologic appearance. Whereas an asymptomatic swollen ischiopubic synchondrosis represents a normal ossification process (Fig. 4), painful swelling is a symptom of underlying pathology (stress reaction or osteomyelitis, see Sect. 5).

Accessory ossicles are considered to be normal anatomical variants, which should not be mistaken for avulsion fractures. They occur most commonly in the foot and ankle, and carpus and vary in size. Accessory ossicles may persist in adult life, and occasionally, they may fuse with the adjacent bone (Bernaerts et al. 2004) (Fig. 5). Some ossicles may be the result of previous trauma. Usually, these ossicles are of no clinical significance, but they can cause symptoms in some instances (Williams 2008) (see Sect. 5).

A sesamoid bone is a bone embedded within a tendon. Sesamoid bones are typically found in locations where a tendon passes over a joint, such as the hand and the foot. Functionally, they act to protect the tendon and to increase its mechanical effect. Small

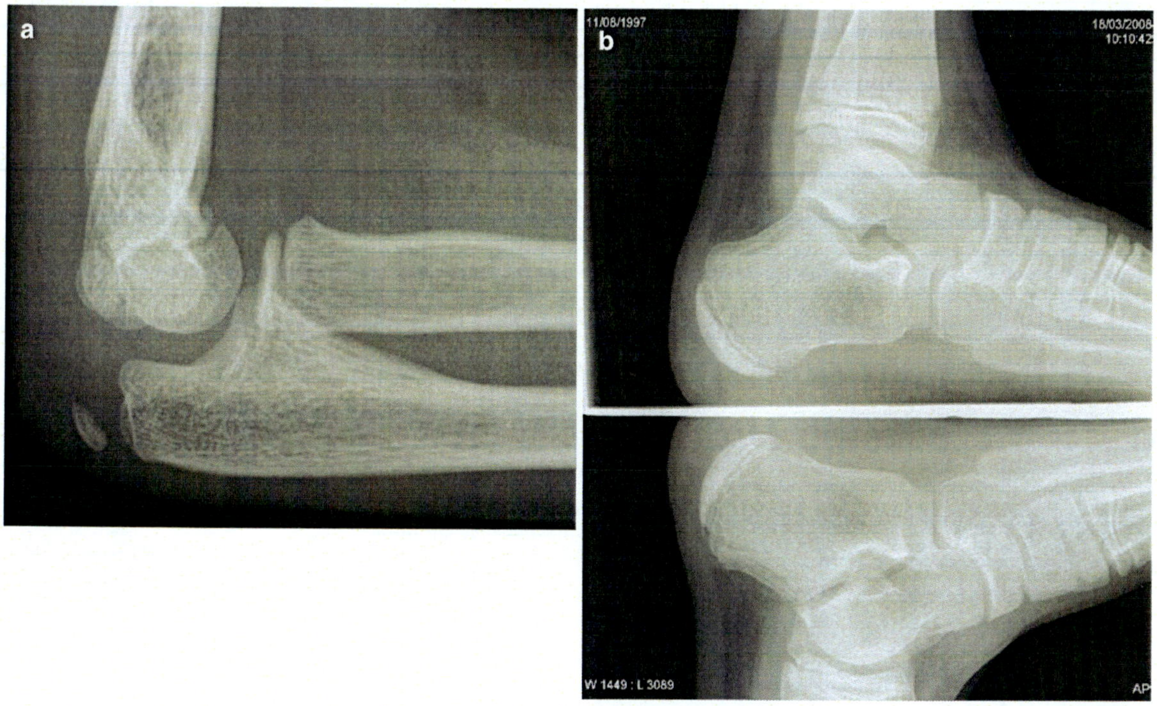

Fig. 2 Example of a normal apophysis. (**a**) Apophyseal ossification center of the olecranon at the attachment of the triceps tendon in a 9-year-old girl. (**b**) Apophyseal ossification center of calcaneus at the attachment of the Achilles tendon in a 10-year-old girl

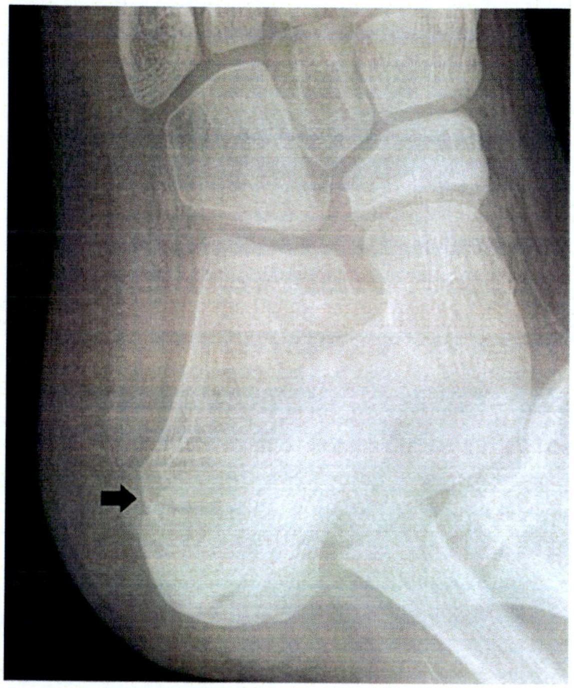

Fig. 3 Unfused calcaneal apophysis simulating a fracture in oblique projection (*arrow*)

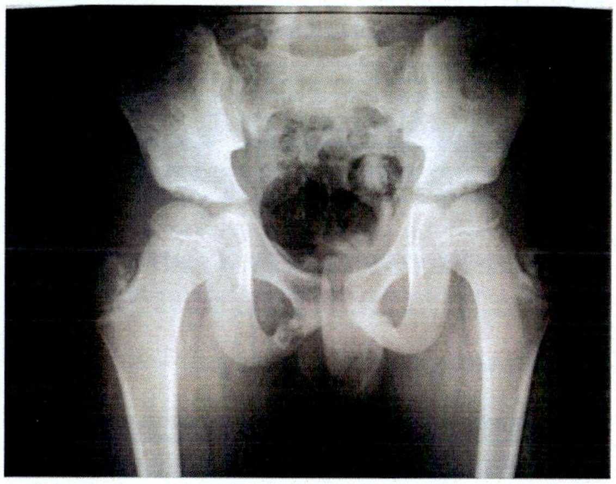

Fig. 4 Asymmetric ossification of the ischiopubic synchondrosis in an 11-year-old girl. In asymptomatic patients, variation in size and shape should be regarded as a normal variant. In this patient, the right ischiopubic synchondrosis is larger than the left one

sesamoid bones resemble sesame seeds. Sesamoid bones are well corticated and may be bipartite (Fig. 6). A bipartite sesamoid is larger overall than a fractured nonpartite sesamoid (Williams 2008; Miller 2002).

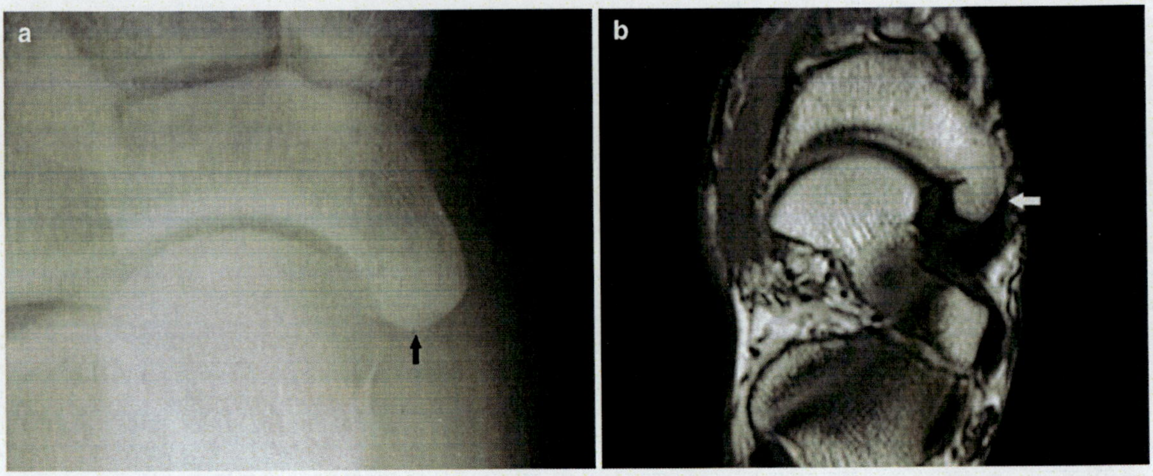

Fig. 5 Cornuate navicular in an adult patient, due to incorporation of the accessory navicular bone into the main portion of the navicular bone (*arrows*). (**a**) Plain radiograph. (**b**) Axial T1-w MR image of the left foot

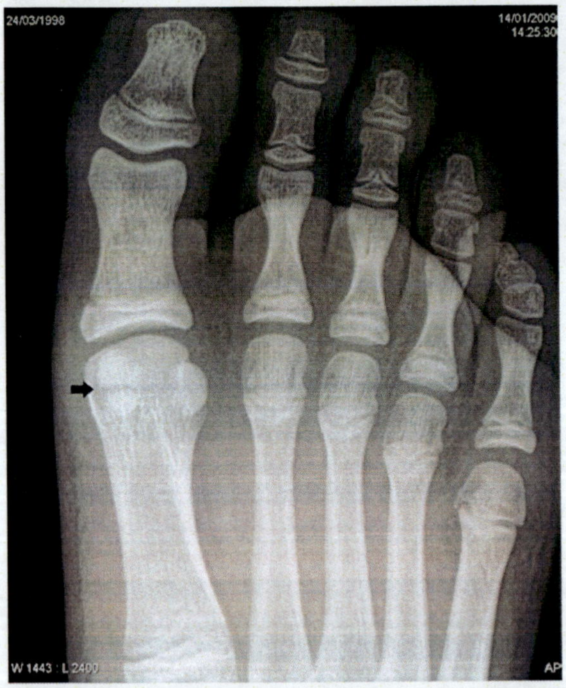

Fig. 6 Bipartite medial sesamoid bone of the first toe in a 10-year-old girl (*arrow*)

This paragraph will review very briefly normal developmental anatomy of the immature skeleton on different imaging modalities, relevant to sport-related skeletal trauma. Only the most frequent locations where sport injuries occur are discussed here.

2.1 Plain Radiography and CT Scan

Cartilage is radiolucent on plain films and CT scan. Whereas the diaphyses of the long bones are visible in the newborn, the epiphyses become only visible after ossification. The growth plates between the epiphyses/apophyses and the metaphyses are seen as radiolucent lines. As the growth plate fuses (Fig. 7), it becomes progressively narrower (Foster 2008).

2.1.1 Pelvis

In children and adolescents, ligaments and tendons can withstand more force than bones, but the growth plates at the apophyses are more prone to trauma, especially to avulsion (Vandervliet et al. 2007). In particular, the apophyses of the pelvis and hip are common sites of acute avulsions, as they tend to appear and fuse later than many other apophyseal centers (El-Khoury et al. 1996). Knowledge of the age of the patient and familiarity with the normal developmental anatomy of the pelvic apophyses is mandatory in order to distinguish normal findings from acute or chronic avulsive injuries of the pelvis (Fig. 8).

Figure 9 summarizes the radiographic appearance of the secondary ossification centers in the immature pelvis.

A bifid appearance or irregularity of the capital femoral epiphysis and irregularity of the ossification

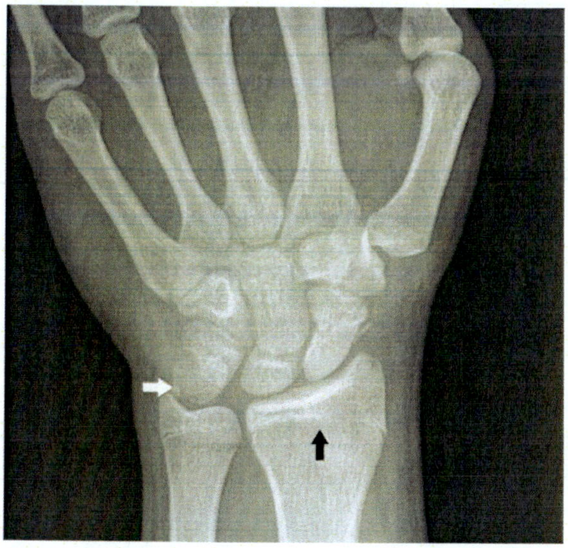

Fig. 7 Partial fusion of the growth plate. Seventeen-year-old boy presenting with a scaphoid fracture. Note partial closure of the growth plate at the central part of the distal radius (*black arrow*), whereas the ulnar and radial portions are still visible as a radiolucent line (pseudofracture). Note also the presence of an accessory ossicle at the ulnar styloid (os styloideum) (*white arrow*)

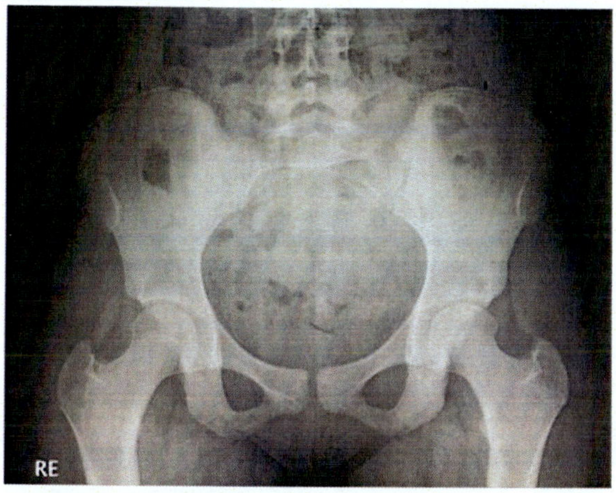

Fig. 8 Normal ossification centers of the iliac crest in a 15-year-old patient (*arrows*)

centers of the greater and lesser trochanters may exist as normal variants (Williams 2008).

Os acetabuli consists of an accessory ossicle at the acetabular rim (Fig. 10).

Previously, an os acetabuli was believed to represent a normal ossification variant. It is, however, a matter of debate whether an os acetabuli may be secondary

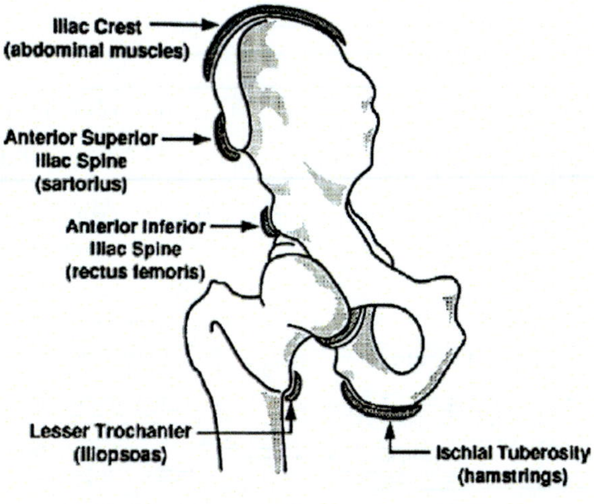

Fig. 9 Schematic drawing of the secondary ossification centers of the pelvis (used with permission from El-Khoury et al. (1996))

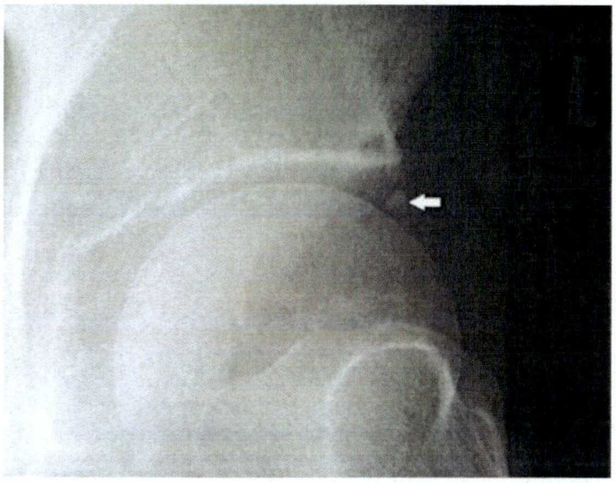

Fig. 10 Os acetabuli. Note a small ossicle at the left acetabular rim (*arrow*)

to femoro-acetabular impingement. According to the latter hypothesis, an os acetabuli may represent a stress fracture, resulting from a constant jamming of the femoral head against the acetabulum (Peeters et al. 2009).

2.1.2 Ankle and Foot

Accessory ossicles at the ankle and foot joints are very common and are estimated to occur in 5.2% of the population at each of the malleoli (Carty 1992). They should not be confused with fractures. Signs suggestive

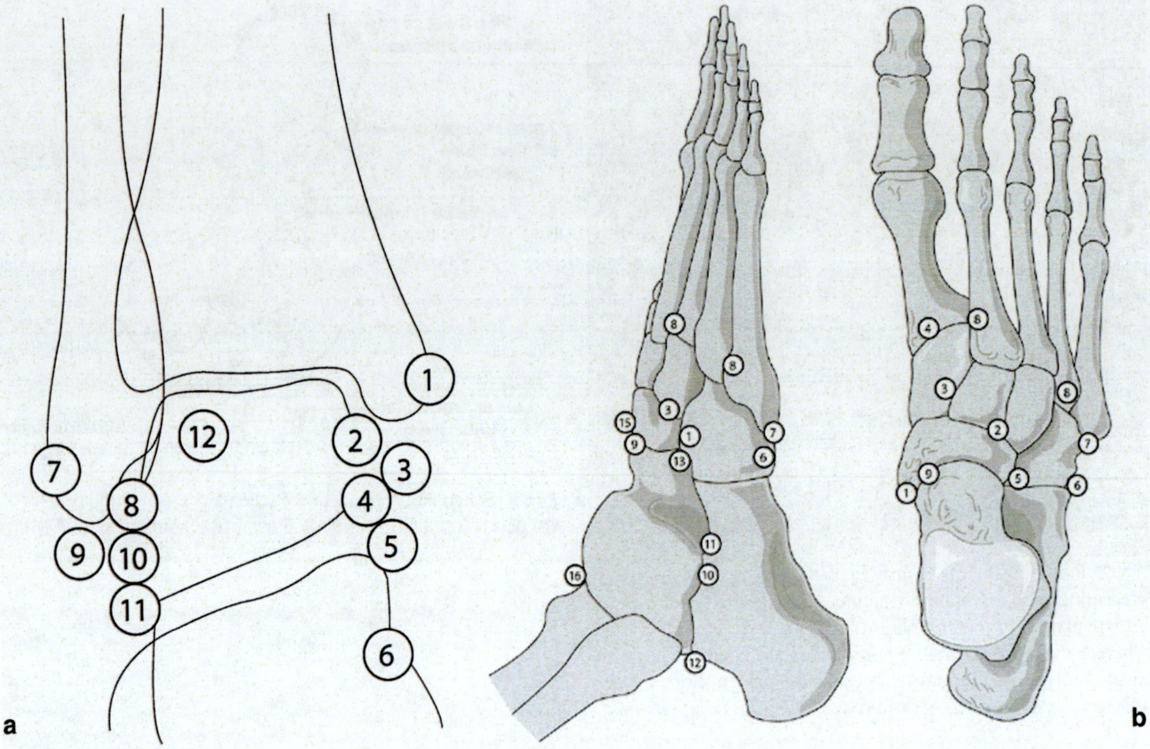

Fig. 11 Schematic drawing of accessory ossicles of the ankle and foot (used with permission from Williams (2008))

of an ossicle rather than a fracture are the absence of soft tissue swelling over the malleolus and no periosteal reaction on delayed radiographs (Vanhoenacker et al. 2002a). In relation to the lateral malleolus, one should look for a fibular groove in which an accessory ossicle would fit (Ramsden 1999).

Figure 11 shows a line drawing of accessory ossifications centers of the ankle and foot.

2.1.3 Shoulder Girdle

The proximal humeral epiphysis arises from two or three separate ossification centers (Fig. 12). In young children, the appearance of these ossification centers on different radiographic positioning should not be mistaken for a fracture. In slightly older children who may present with sports injuries (generally over 7 years), the normal radiolucent proximal physis of the humerus is "tented" and in various oblique positions can be mistaken for a fracture (Fig. 13). One side of the proximal humeral epiphyseal plate frequently projects below the other. The normal bicipital groove in the proximal humerus may simulate new bone formation (Fig. 14).

Three ossification centers of the scapula may be mistaken for a fracture (Williams 2008).

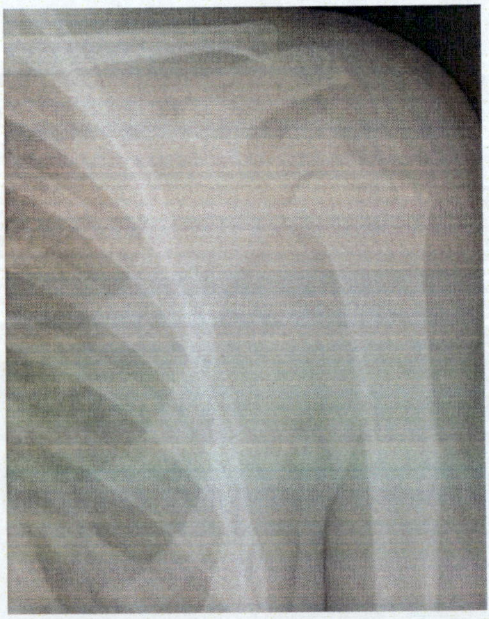

Fig. 12 Normal proximal humeral epiphysis in a 3-year-old boy, consisting of two separate ossification centers

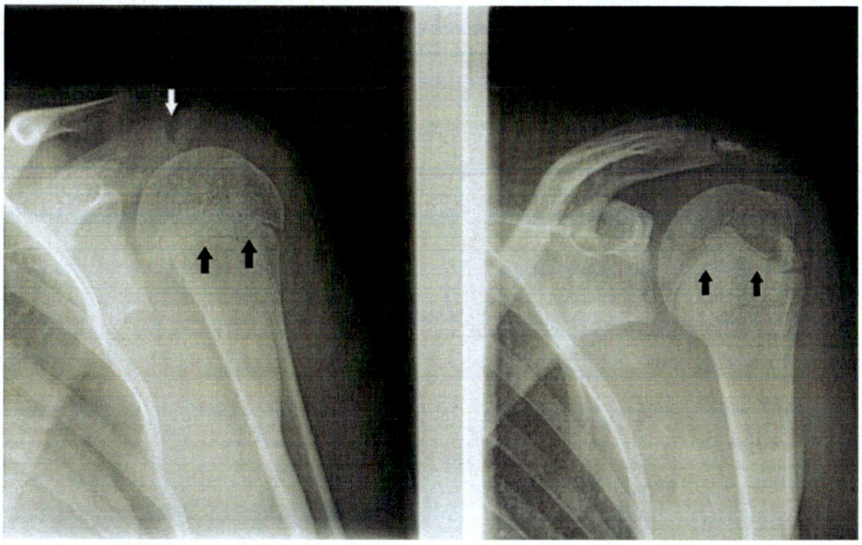

Fig. 13 Normal tented appearance of the proximal physis of the humerus (13-year-old patient) not to be mistaken for a fracture (*black arrows*). Note also the presence of a secondary ossification center of the acromion (*small white arrow*)

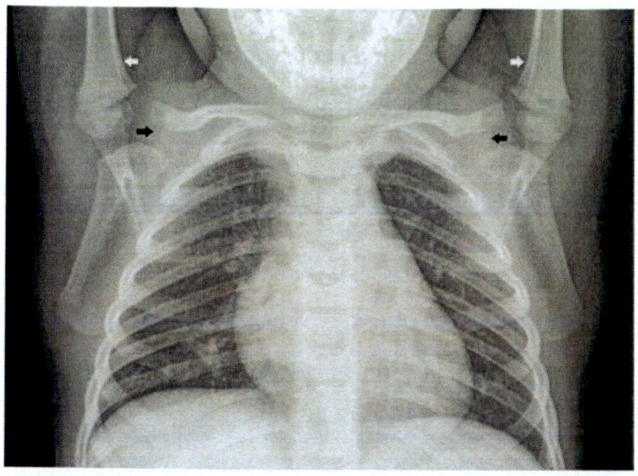

Fig. 14 Secondary ossification centers of the coracoid process (*black arrows*) in a 4-year-old boy. Note also the presence of a normal bicipital groove simulating periosteal bone formation on a chest radiograph with the upper limbs extended above the head (*white arrows*)

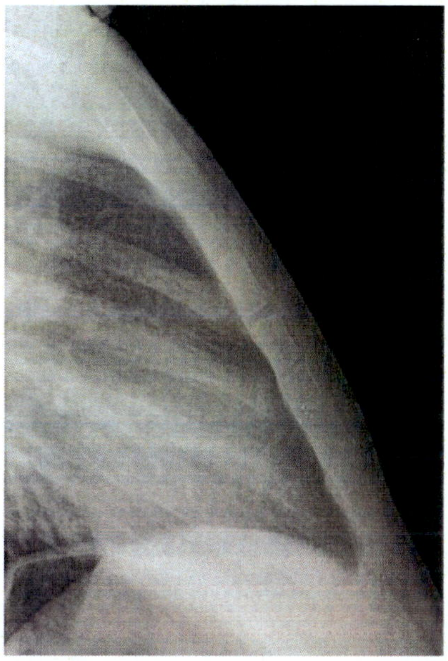

Fig. 15 Separate ossification segments or sternebrae in a 4-year-old boy. Radiographic image taken from a lateral chest radiograph

The acromion process may develop in two parts. The secondary acromial ossification center appears usually at the age of 10–12 years of age. Delineation is variable and often irregular (Fig. 13). The acromion fuses often at 15–20 years. Persistence of this center in adult life is known as an os acromiale.

Other separate ossification centers may be found at the coracoid process (Fig. 14) and at the tip of the scapula. They fuse by 20 years of age (Keats and Anderson 2006).

Ossification of the sternum is highly variable, and ossification variants should not be confused with fractures. The normal sternum forms from between four and five separate cartilaginous segments or sternebrae (Fig. 15).

2.1.4 Elbow

The appearance and fusion of the secondary ossification centers follow a set pattern, which is illustrated in Fig. 16 (Ramsden 1999). Knowledge of the expected sequence of ossification should allow acute and chronic

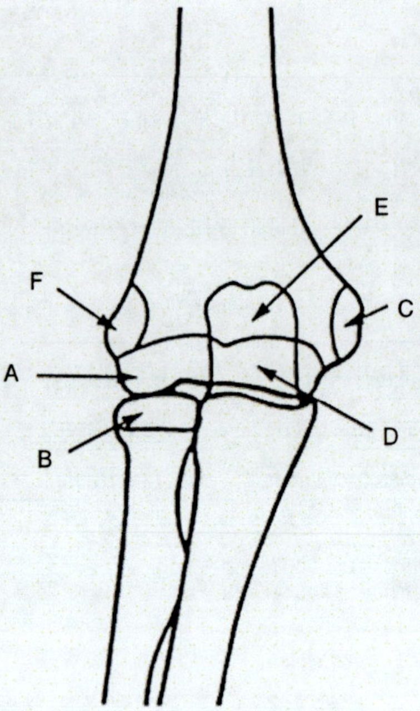

	Appears	Fuses
A. Capitellum	1–3 yrs	17–18 yrs
B. Radial Head	5–6 yrs	16–19 yrs
C. Medial Epicondyle	5–8 yrs	17–18 yrs
D. Trochlea	11 yrs	18 yrs
E. Olecranon	10–13 yrs	16–20 yrs
F. Lateral Epicondyle	10–12 yrs	17–18 yrs

Fig. 16 Normal ossification sequence of the secondary ossification centers of the elbow Ramsden (1999)

avulsion and fractures of the elbow to be accurately diagnosed. The order of ossification should follow the mnemonic "CRITOE" (capitellum, radial head, internal (medial) epicondyle, trochlea, olecranon, external (lateral) epicondyle) (Johnson and Marcus 2008). Furthermore, ununited ossification centers may persist unfused into adult life (Fig. 17) and can simulate avulsion fractures (see also Sect. 5).

2.1.5 Other Joints

Variations in ossification of the bones in the wrist and the hand (accessory ossicles and irregularity during normal development, pseudoepiphyses, developmental notches etc) are commonly seen and may cause confusion with traumatic disorders. Clinical correlation is very helpful, including absence of pain and swelling on the area in question (Williams 2008).

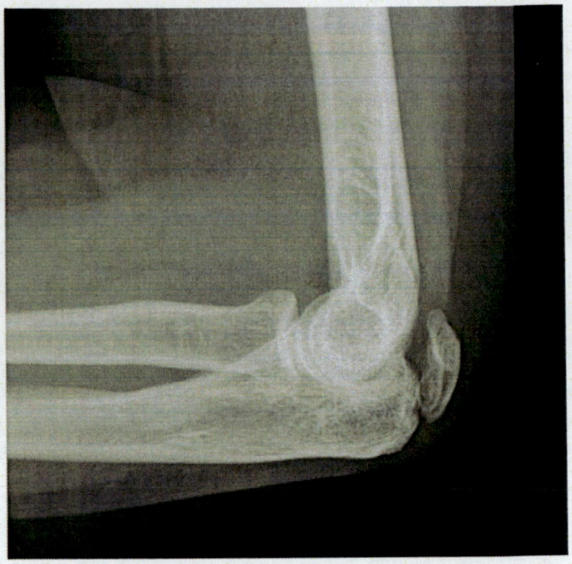

Fig. 17 Persistent unfused apophyses of the olecranon in a middle-aged woman (*arrow*)

Figures 18–21 illustrate some examples of ossification variants of the wrist and hand.

Variations around the knee joint include irregular ossification of the femoral condyle, ossification variants of the patella (Fig. 22) and tibial tubercle, notches or

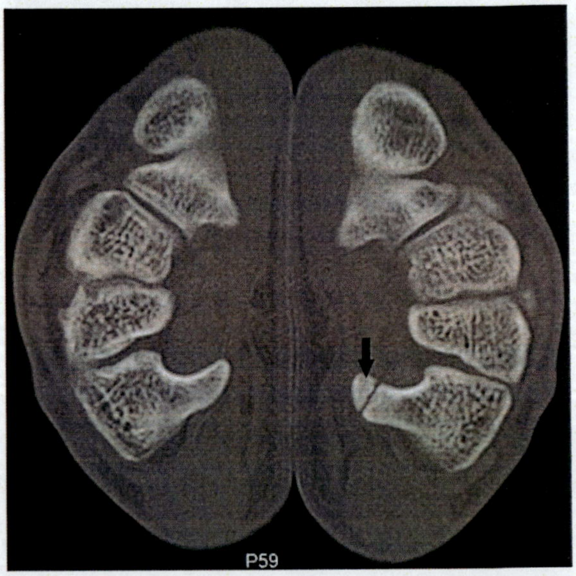

Fig. 18 Accessory ossicle at the tip of the hamate bone (*black arrow*) of the right wrist (os hamuli proprium) in an 18-year-old adolescent. Accessory ossicles are usually well corticated allowing them to be distinguished from recent fracture fragments. Moreover, the patient suffered from posttraumatic pain at the left side, whereas the right carpus was asymptomatic

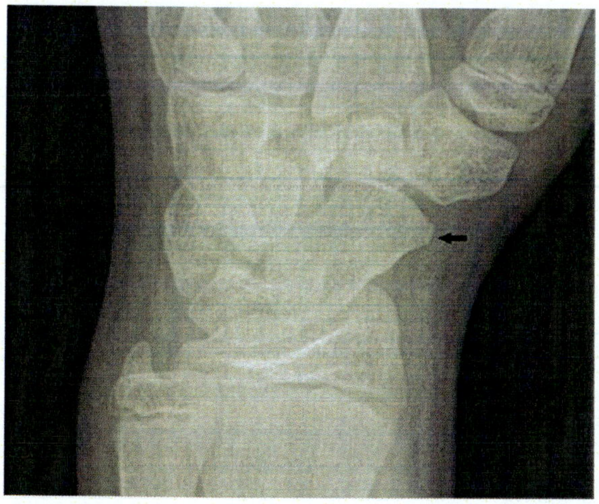

Fig. 19 Small accessory ossification center for the tuberosity of the scaphoid (*arrow*) in an 11-year-old girl, not to be mistaken for an avulsion fracture

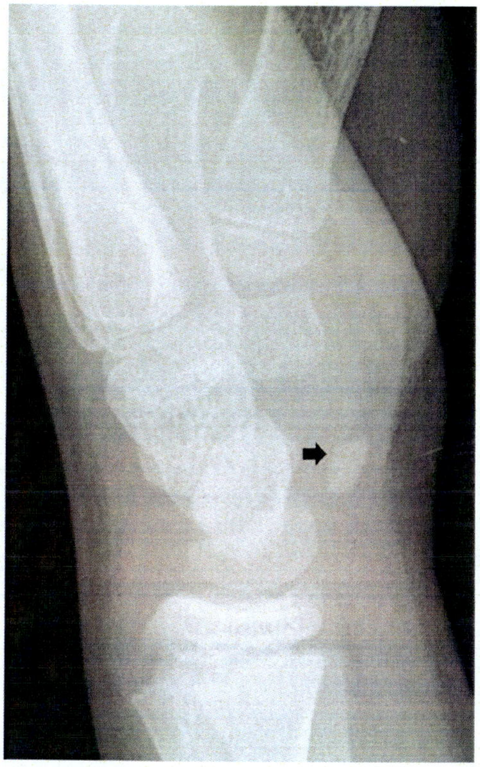

Fig. 20 Example of normal irregular ossification of the pisiform (*arrow*)

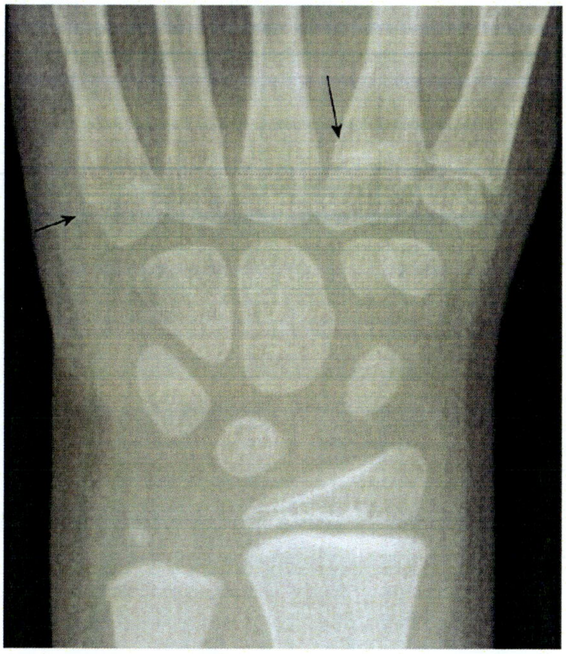

Fig. 21 Accessory ossification centers at the bases of the index and little finger metacarpals (*arrows*) that can simulate fractures Williams (2008)

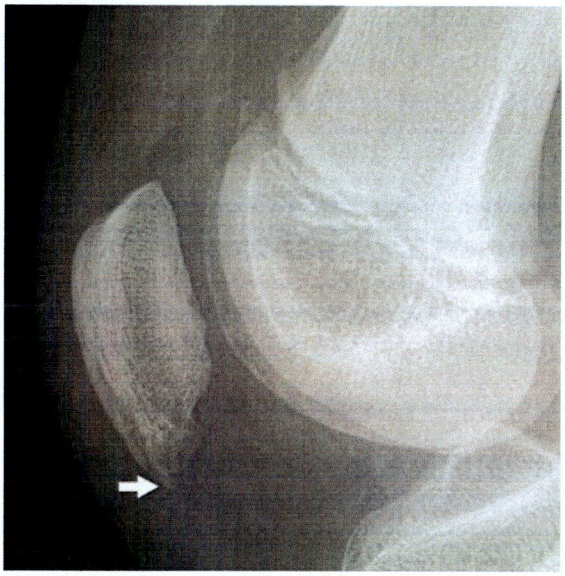

Fig. 22 Accessory ossification center at the lower pole of the patella in an 11-year-old boy (*arrow*)

grooves of the popliteus muscle, fibrous defects, and sesamoid bones (fabella and cyamella). They rarely cause difficulties in differential diagnosis with acute fractures, but some variants may simulate chronic trauma (see Sect. 4) or may be symptomatic (see Sect. 5).

2.1.6 Spine and Skull

For a more in-depth discussion of the normal variants of the spine and skull, we refer to dedicated textbooks and atlases (Swischuk 2002; Keats and Anderson

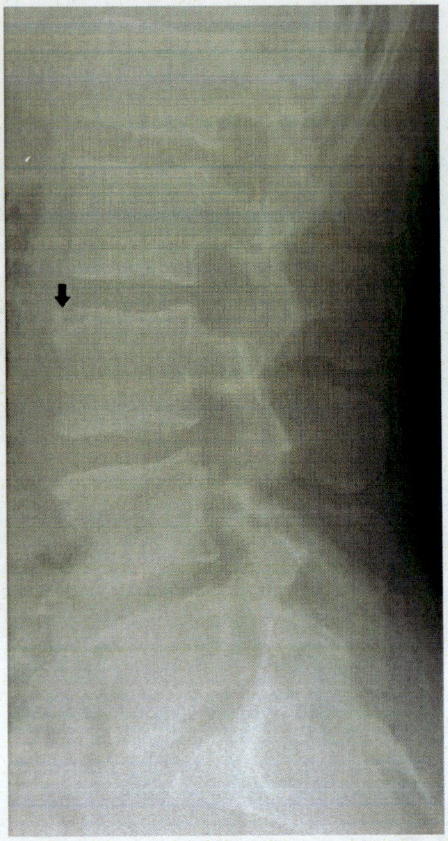

Fig. 23 Ununited secondary ossification center (limbus vertebra), simulating a fracture of L5. A limbus vertebra results from an intravertebral disc herniation

2006; Freyschmidt et al. 2002) and book chapters on the topic (Williams 2008). Moreover, most variants of the skull that may simulate fractures consist of accessory sutures and synchondroses. These are most commonly seen in the infant skull and are far less common at the age of a sportive child.

Figures 23 and 24 illustrate some examples of variants of the spine, which should not be confused with fractures.

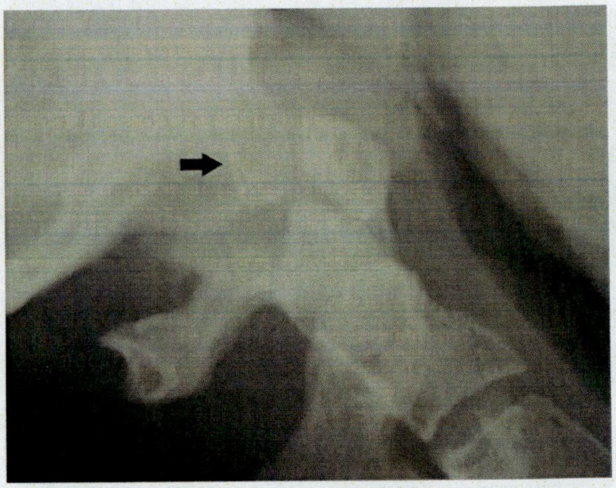

Fig. 24 Os odontoideum (*arrow*). Failure of union of the odontoid should be differentiated from an acute dens fracture. Clues to the correct diagnosis are the corticated margins of the accessory ossicle and the hypertrophy of the anterior arch of C-1

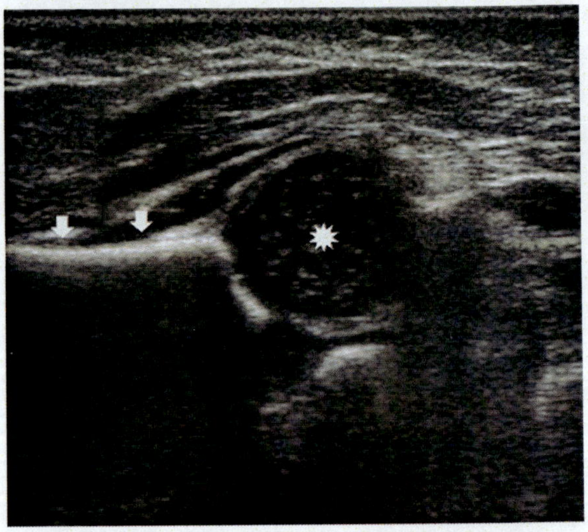

Fig. 25 Ultrasound of a normal epiphysis of the proximal femur in 5-week-old girl. The epiphysis is hypoechoic with internal echogenic stipples (*asterisk*). Note the thick hyperechoic line of the cortical bone of the ilium (*white arrows*), with distal acoustic shadowing

2.2 Ultrasound

The articular cartilage appears as a smooth anechoic area, whereas the nonossified epiphysis is relative hypoechoic to muscle and usually contains echogenic speckles (Fig. 25). The central ossification center is echogenic, whereas the cortical bone is highly hyperechoic, with associated distal acoustic shadowing (Foster 2008).

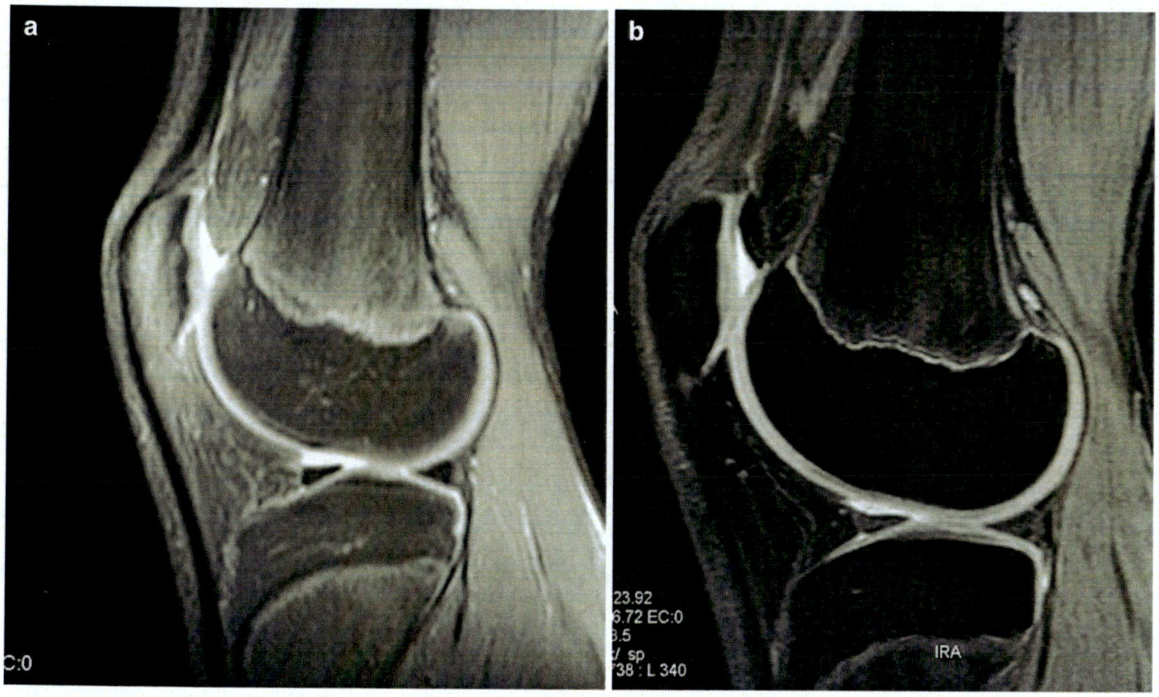

Fig. 26 MRI appearance of the immature bone in a 14-year-old boy. (**a**) Sagittal fat-suppressed PD-w image of the knee. (**b**) Sagittal fat-suppressed 3D gradient-recalled image of the knee. The epiphysis appears hypointense relative to the physis

2.3 Magnetic Resonance Imaging

The epiphyseal articular cartilage and the physis both are composed of hyaline cartilage. However, due to the different biochemical composition of cartilage, the epiphyseal cartilage appears hypointense relative to the physeal cartilage on T2-w images (Jaramillo et al. 1998). Gradient-recalled echo proton density sequences depict cartilage well, with excellent differentiation from bone. The differentiation from bone can be maximized by using fat saturation, suppressing signal of bone marrow fat (Fig. 26). Jaramillo et al. (2004) reported that differentiation between the zones of the cartilage can be more clearly seen on gadolinium enhanced sequences. This is because the physis and the juxtaphyseal cartilage enhance more than the epiphyseal cartilage which is relatively hypovascular. The number of vascular channels in the germinal layer of the physis decreases with age, as well as the degree of enhancement of the epiphysis.

Morphologically, the physis is smooth and flat at birth, but becomes progressively undulating at puberty. Physeal closure occurs first at the areas of greatest undulation.

3 Normal Variants Simulating Acute Trauma

3.1 Companion and Overlap Artifacts

3.1.1 Mach Effect

The "mach effect" is a physiological form of edge enhancement created when there is an abrupt change from light to dark (radiopaque to radiolucent) or vice versa at a concave or convex interface of a subject. Its presence at the interface of structures can simulate a fracture line (Williams 2008).

3.1.2 Overlap of Superimposing Structures

Overlap of the skin, soft tissue folds or adjacent bones may simulate acute fracture lines (Fig. 27). Unfused apophyseal ossification centers may mimic a fracture in oblique projections (Fig. 3).

3.2 *Variations in Developmental Anatomy*

3.2.1 Foramen Nutricium

Nutrient vessels passing through the cortex of the diaphysis of the long bones should not be confused with a fracture line (Fig. 28a). They are usually well defined and not associated with localized pain and soft tissue swelling. Particularly at the tibia, they should not be mistaken for a toddler's fracture (Fig. 28b). The classic toddler's fracture is a non displaced oblique fracture of the distal tibia, which is often only demonstrated on one view.

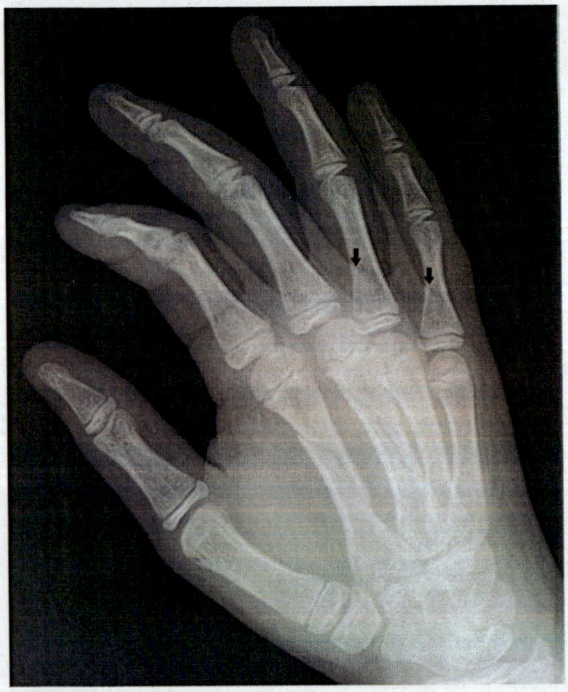

Fig. 27 Thirteen-year-old boy presenting with spiral fractures of the diaphyses of metacarpal 2 and 3. Overlapping soft tissues of the fingers may simulate additional fracture lines at the phalanges of the fourth and fifth finger (*arrows*)

3.2.2 Bipartite Patella

Several secondary ossification centers of the patella may be mistaken for a fracture. Bipartite patella is a normal variant where there is a small accessory ossification center that may remain unfused into adulthood. This is most often located at the superolateral aspect of the patella (Fig. 29). It is usually asymptomatic, but symptomatic cases have been reported (see Sect. 5). Other similar ossification variants include tripartite patella and accessory ossicles at the upper, lower, and medial borders of the patella (Williams 2008).

3.2.3 Dorsal Patellar Defect

The typical dorsal patellar defect is a round, radiolucent lesion surrounded by a zone of sclerosis located on the superolateral aspect of the dorsal surface of the patella. The typical location and radiographic appearance distinguish this variant from other lesions of the patella. In the context of knee trauma, the lesion should not be mistaken for a posttraumatic osteochondral defect.

MRI shows a cortical defect at the superolateral aspect of the patella, which is compensated by overgrowing articular cartilage (Fig. 30).

This variant is usually asymptomatic, but occasionally it may be associated with chondromalacia of the patella (see Sect. 5) (Snoeckx et al. 2008).

3.2.4 Accessory Ossicles

As previously discussed, many small supernumerary ossicles may mimic both acute and chronic trauma. Some examples of accessory ossicles mimicking acute trauma have been discussed in Sect. 2 of this chapter.

4 Normal Variants Simulating Chronic Trauma

4.1 *Irregular Epiphyses and Apophyses*

Normal irregularity of the margins of the epiphyses may be mistaken for pathological conditions such as

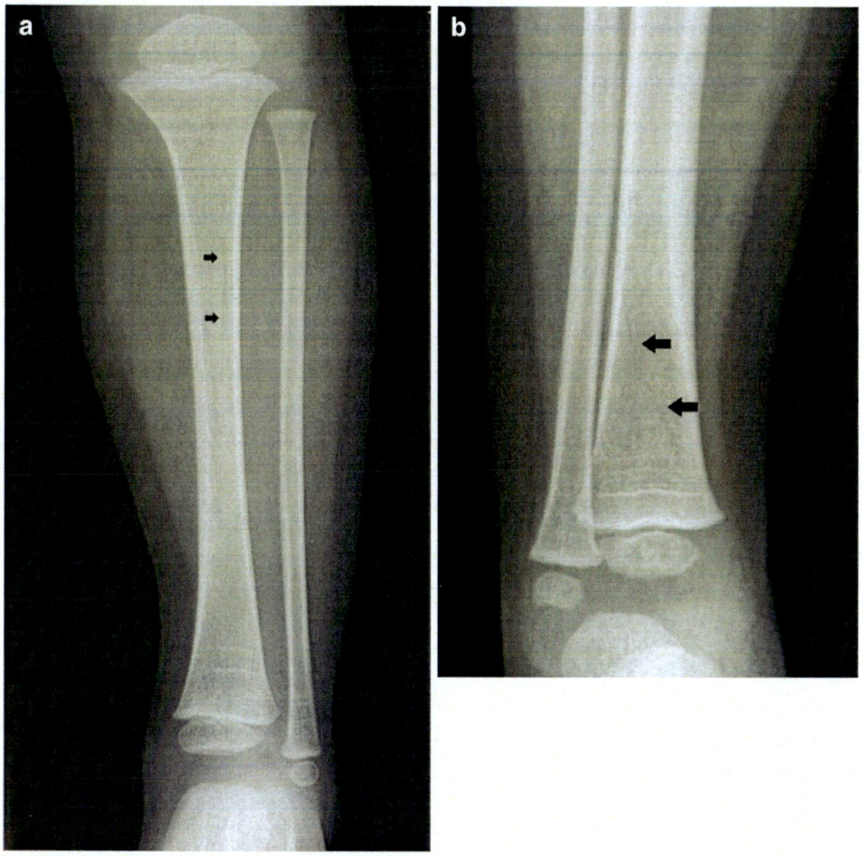

Fig. 28 Nutrient canal vs. toddler's fracture. (**a**) Nutrient canal in the tibial diaphysis (*arrows*). (**b**) Toddler's fracture. Note the oblique fracture line in the diaphysis of the right tibia in a 2-year-old boy

Perthes' disease of the hip or osteochondritis dissecans of the knee and elbow (Figs. 31–33). MRI or ultrasound may be very useful to demonstrate normal overlying cartilage, excluding pathologic conditions.

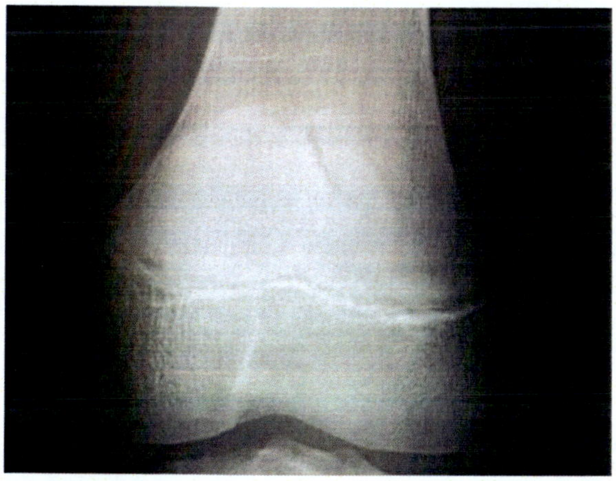

Fig. 29 Bipartite patella in a 13-year-old boy. Note the presence of a secondary ossification center at the superolateral aspect of the left patella

Irregular delineation of the apophyses may be seen as a normal variant or as result of a traction injury of the apophysis. Typical examples of traction injuries are Osgood–Schlatter disease or Sinding–Larsen–Johansson disease at the insertion of the distal and proximal patellar tendon, respectively. Both ultrasound and MRI may be useful to distinguish these chronic traction injuries from normal variants. In pathologic conditions, ultrasound may show a thickened hypoechoic tendon with hypervascularity on power Doppler. On MRI, a high signal is seen within the tendon and adjacent bone marrow in case of chronic traction injuries (Fig. 34).

4.2 Pseudoperiostitis

The normal bicipital groove of the proximal humerus may simulate periosteal new bone formation, particularly on a chest radiograph when the arms are extended (Fig. 14).

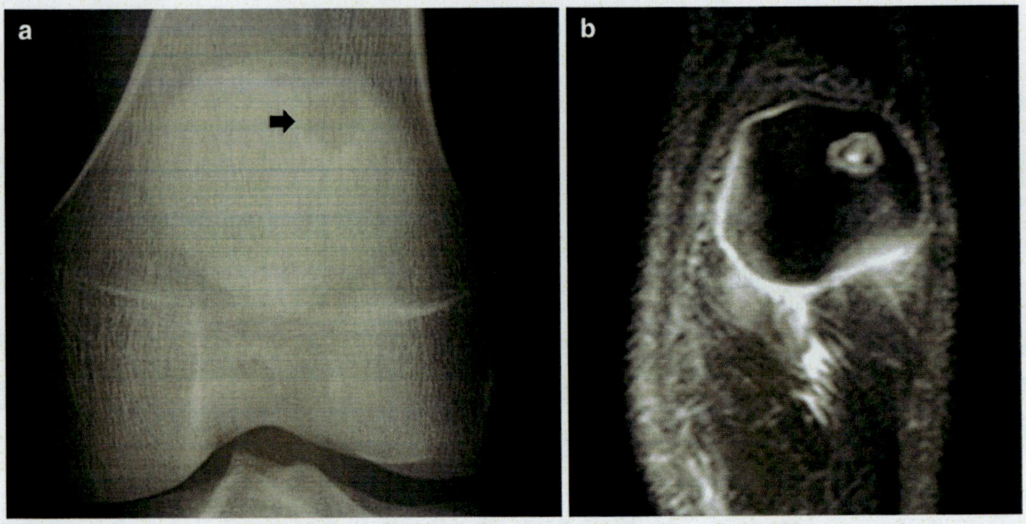

Fig. 30 Dorsal patellar defect. (**a**) Plain radiograph (AP view of the left knee). There is a cortical lucency at the superolateral aspect of the patella. (**b**) Coronal T2-w MR image shows a high signal intensity of the cartilage within the defect

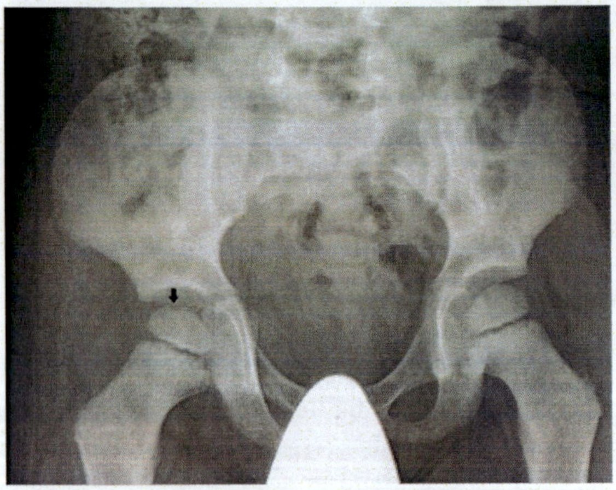

Fig. 31 Irregular ossification of the proximal epiphysis of the right hip in a 4-year-old boy, mimicking Perthes disease on a plain radiograph (*arrow*)

Physiologic "periostitis" may be seen at the femora, medial aspect of the tibiae and the humeri in the newborn, but this phenomenon is not seen in older children presenting with sporting injuries.

4.3 Accessory Bones

Some accessory bone may show an irregular delineation, simulating posttraumatic pseudarthrosis (Fig. 35).

4.4 Abnormal Density of Secondary Ossification Centers

The normal secondary ossification centers of the calcaneus may be relatively dense compared to the adjacent calcaneus (Fig. 2b). In the absence of clinical findings (pain and local swelling), this variant should not be mistaken for Sever's disease.

In case of clinical symptoms, an MRI can demonstrate bone marrow edema (BME) within the pathologic apophysis (Fig. 36).

4.5 Growth Arrest Lines of Park and Harris

Growth arrest lines of Park and Harris (Fig. 37) are dense trabecular transversely orientated lines within the long bones, commonly seen on radiographs in children of all ages. They may follow a period of immobilization or generalized illness and are related to a temporary slowdown of normal longitudinal growth. They become radiographically visible following a subsequent period of normal growth. These lines are usually symmetrical and are most prominent in rapidly growing long bones e.g., distal femur and proximal tibia. With further growth they become incorporated into the diaphysis and disappear with endosteal remodeling. Although

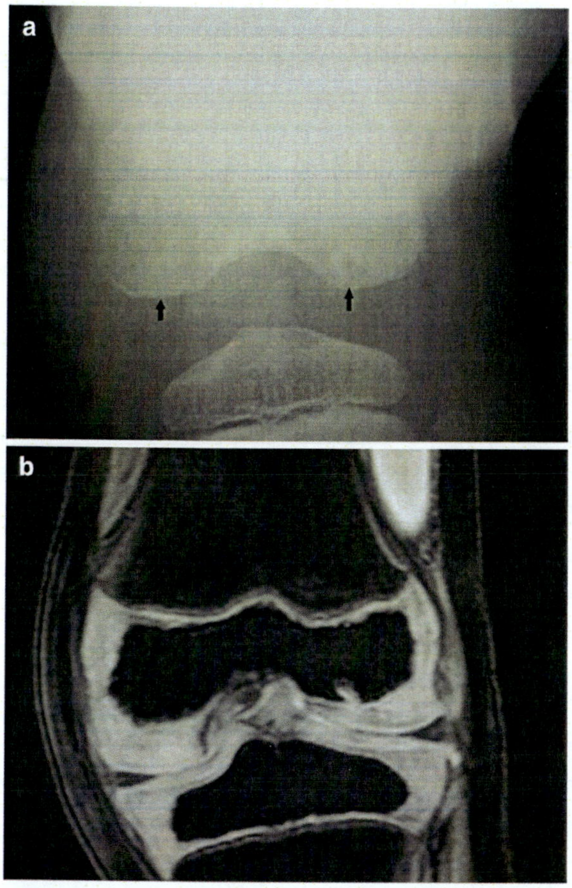

Fig. 32 Simulated osteochondrosis dissecans. (**a**) Plain radiograph of the left knee. Lateral and medial femoral condylar irregularity simulating osteochondrosis dissecans (*arrows*). (**b**) Coronal fat-suppressed T2-w image demonstrating normal articular cartilage, excluding true osteochondritis dissecans

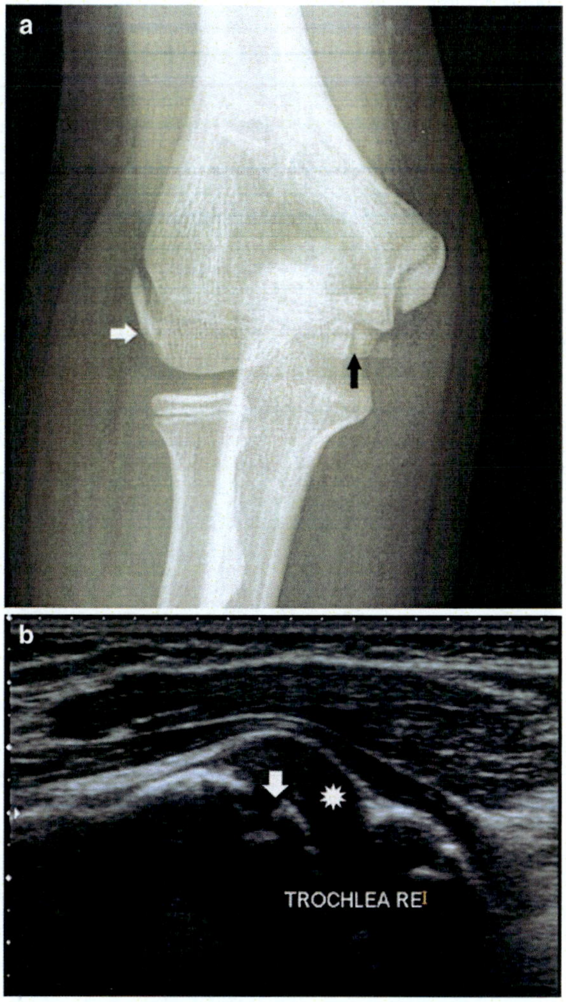

Fig. 33 Normal developmental irregularity of the trochlea of the distal humerus in a 12-year-old water polo player. (**a**) Plain radiograph shows multiple ossification centers in the developing trochlea of the humerus (*black arrow*). Note also partial fusion of the ossification center for the lateral epicondyle with the capitellum prior to closure (*white arrow*). The medial epicondyle fuses directly with the humeral diaphysis. (**b**) Ultrasound confirms irregularity of the ossification center for the trochlea (*white arrow*), but shows normal articular cartilage of the trochlea (*white asterisk*), excluding true osteochondritis dissecans

frequently associated with disease states, these lines are often seen in patients without a contributory history (Keats and Anderson 2006). These lines should not be mistaken for a stress fracture.

4.6 Dense Zones of Provisional Calcification

Dense zones of provisional calcification should not be mistaken for heavy metal poisoning or chronic trauma (Fig. 38). These zones may vary considerably in thickness in healthy children and in the same child at different ages. They tend to be proportionately thicker during the second to fifth year (Slovis 2008).

4.7 Coalition and Bone Marrow Edema on MRI

Coalition between two adjacent bones (e.g., carpal bones, tarsal bones) is rarely mistaken for acute trauma. However, many patients with tarsal coalition may present with pain of insidious onset at the ankle

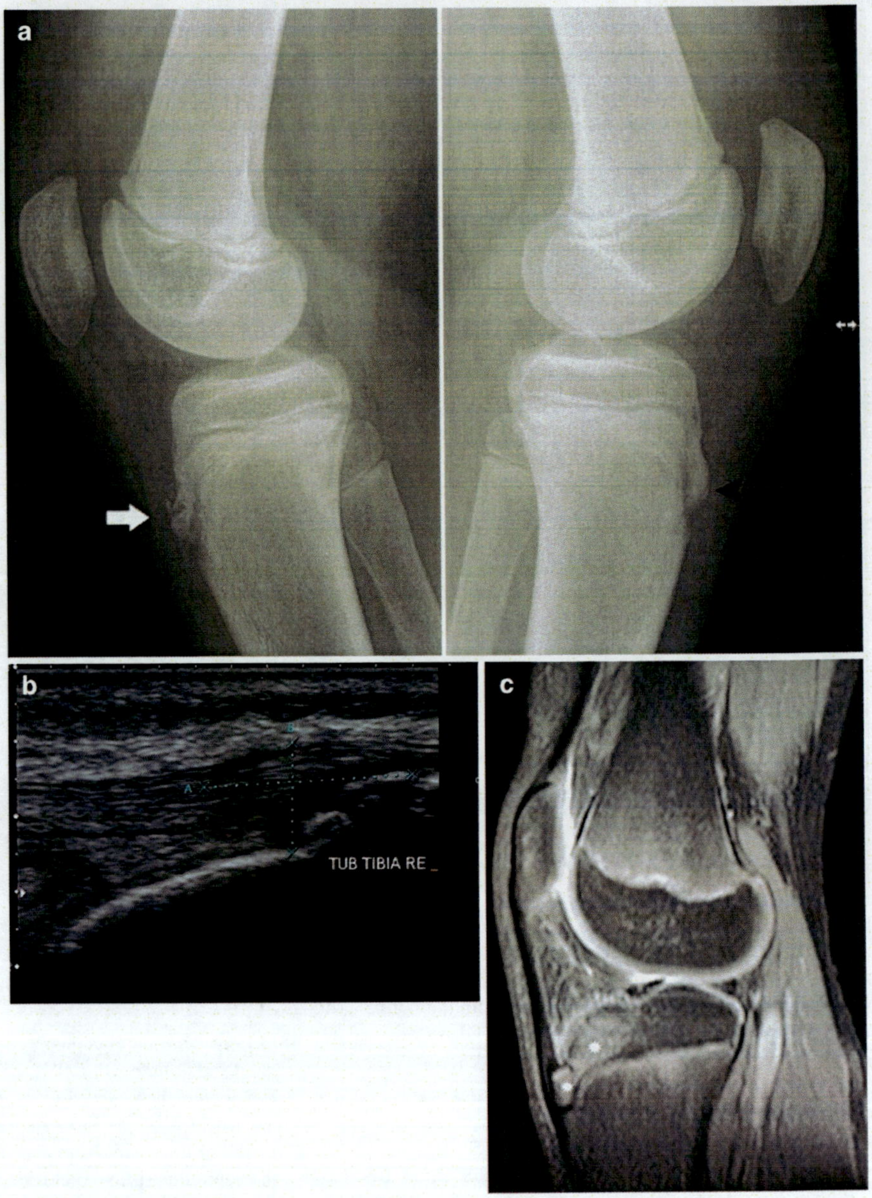

Fig. 34 Normal tibial tuberosity vs. Osgood–Schlatter disease. (**a**) Plain radiograph of an 11-year-old female basketball player showing a normal tibial tubercle on the left side (*black arrow*), whilst there is fragmentation of the ossification center of the tibial tubercle on the right side (*white arrow*). (**b**) Ultrasound shows fragmentation of the right tibial tubercle and a widened and hypoechoic distal patellar tendon. These findings are indicative of Osgood–Schlatter disease on the right side. (**c**) Sagittal fat-suppressed T2-w MR image in another patient with Osgood–Schlatter disease. Note bone marrow edema (BME) in the proximal tibia (*asterisks*)

and foot. MRI may show BME of the bones adjacent to the coalition as the most prominent abnormality (Fig. 39). This finding may simulate chronic stress reaction. Therefore, in young patients with unexplained BME at the tarsus, underlying tarsal coalition should be suspected and the bony margins should be analyzed meticulously. Repeated radiographic or CT evaluation is often required for definitive diagnosis of symptomatic coalition, as these modalities are superior at depicting ossification, including the bony edges.

4.8 Surface Lesions of Bone

Some normal variants (e.g., upper humeral notches; Fig. 40) and tug lesions at the insertion of tendons or ligaments (Fig. 41) may simulate traumatic or tumoral periosteal reaction.

The distinction between a normal variant and a developmental abnormality, be it trauma related or not, may in some instances be blurred. The cortical irregularity syndrome (Fig. 42) of the posteromedial distal femur (previously designated by the misnomer "periosteal

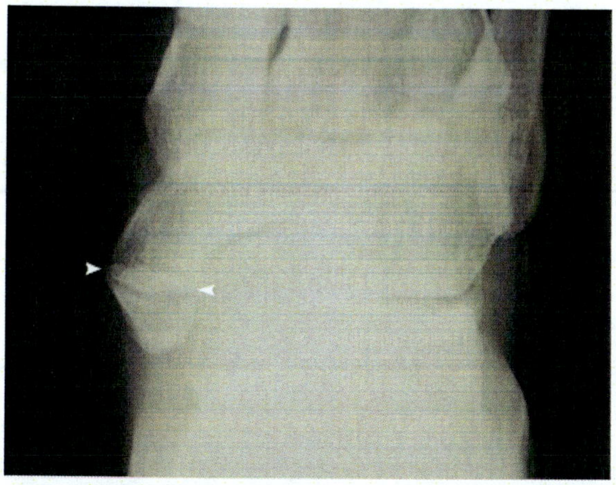

Fig. 35 Irregular delineation of the synchondrosis (*white arrowheads*) between the navicular bone and the os naviculare (type II), simulating pseudarthrosis of an avulsion fracture

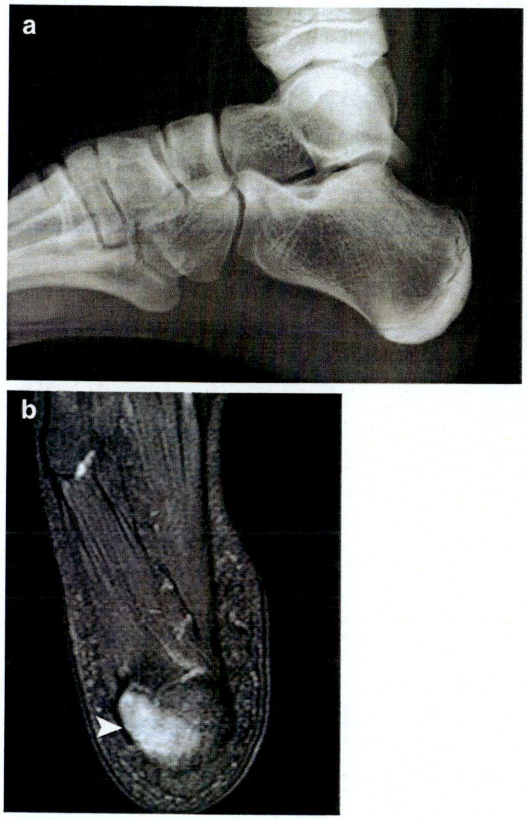

Fig. 36 Sever's disease of secondary ossification center of the os calcaneus in a young female presenting with pain at the posterior aspect of the right heel. (**a**) Plain radiograph. Note increased density of the secondary ossification center of the calcaneus. In absence of clinical symptoms, this finding is difficult to distinguish from normal variants (compare with Fig. 2b). (**b**) Axial fat-suppressed T2-w image. Note hyperintense BME in the secondary ossification center (*arrowhead*). This finding is in favor of Sever's disease

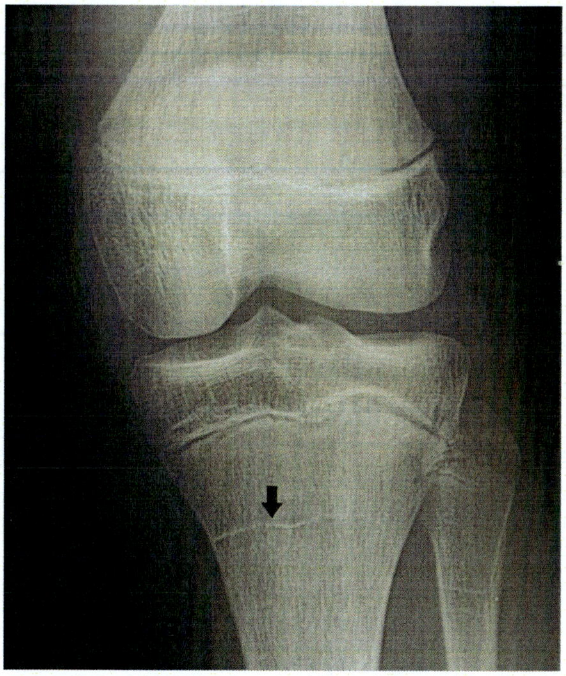

Fig. 37 Growth arrest line of Park and Harris in the proximal tibia (*arrow*). Note the dense trabecular line orientated transversely at the proximal tibia

desmoid"), is frequently attributed to mechanical stresses applied to the insertion of the adductor magnus or the origin of the medial head of the gastrocnemius muscle (Bufkin 1971; Seeger et al. 1998). The presence of focal BME on MRI at the posteromedial aspect of the distal femur as well as minor associated soft tissue edema favors a chronic microtraumatic etiology (Vanhoenacker and Snoeckx 2007). Whatever the precise etiology, the important thing to note is that the process is self-limiting and of no immediate clinical consequence (Davies and Anderson 2007).

4.9 Spotty BME on MRI

Bone marrow heterogeneity in the feet can be a normal finding in the growing skeleton and may be present in asymptomatic feet.

In younger individuals up to the age of 25 years, foci or more confluent areas of high signal are commonly seen on STIR or fat-suppressed T2-w images. They may represent isolated islands of hemopoietic marrow. These changes occur bilaterally. The multiple, small, focal

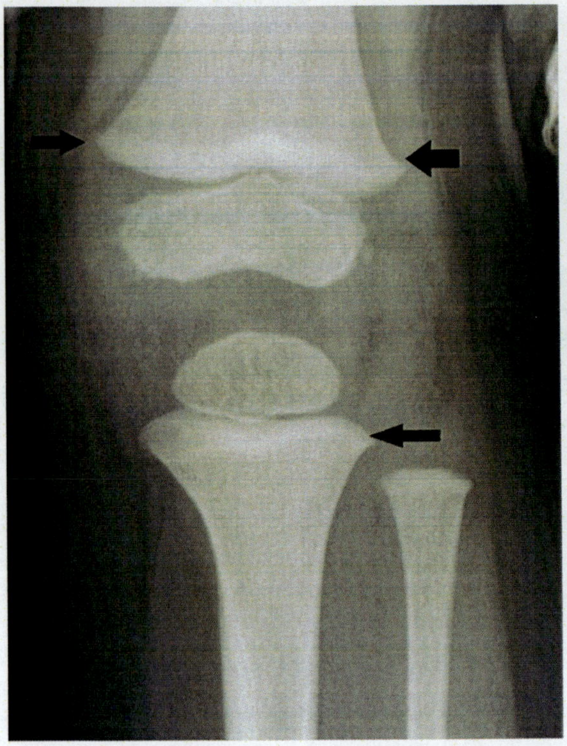

Fig. 38 Dense zones of provisional calcification at the left distal femur and proximal tibia (*arrows*) in a 2-year-old girl. Note also irregular delineation of the distal epiphysis of the femur. Both findings should be regarded as normal variants

nature of these changes makes (stress)-trauma or osteomyelitis unlikely. Transient osteoporosis and regional migratory osteoporosis can manifest as high signal on fat-suppressed T2-w or STIR images, but these conditions are usually present in adults and the foot is an unusual site (Pal et al. 1999; Zanetti 2008).

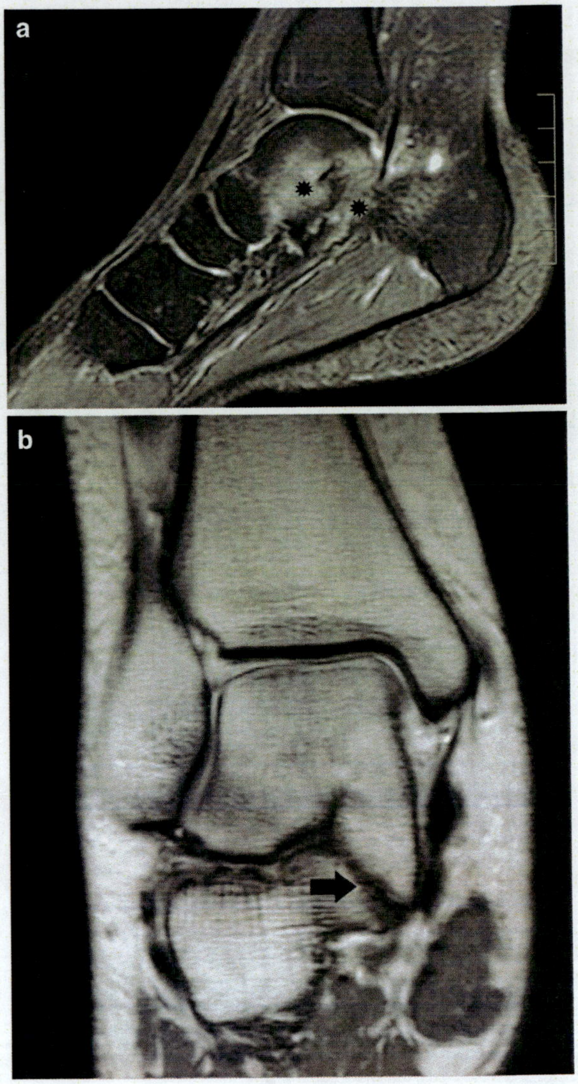

Fig. 39 Talocalcaneal coalition. (**a**) Sagittal fat-suppressed T2-w MR image showing BME at the talus and calcaneus (*asterisks*). (**b**) Coronal proton density image shows better the presence of a fibro-osseous coalition between the calcaneus and talar bone (*arrow*)

5 Symptomatic Variants

Although normal variants are often encountered as incidental findings on imaging studies, some variants may become symptomatic or predispose to pathology.

Standard radiographs are not useful in distinguishing asymptomatic from symptomatic variants (Snoeckx et al. 2008).

MRI is the imaging modality of choice as it may demonstrate bone marrow and/or soft tissue edema, which is often associated with symptomatic variants.

There are numerous reports of accessory bones that may persist into adulthood leading to friction with adjacent bone and soft tissue structures and thus cause symptoms. Examples (Figs. 43 and 44) are painful accessory navicular bone (Bernaerts et al. 2004), os trigonum syndrome (Lee et al. 2008), os peroneum friction syndrome (Bashir et al. 2009; Vancauwenberghe et al. 2009), painful os subfibulare syndrome, and painful bipartite patella (Vanhoenacker et al. 2009; Snoeckx et al. 2008).

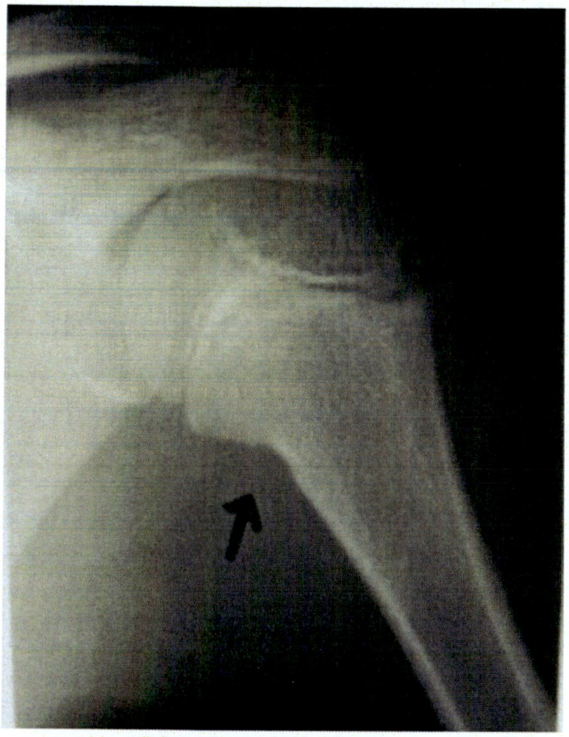

Fig. 40 Upper humeral notch (*arrow*), a normal developmental variant which may be seen in children between the age of 10 and 16 years

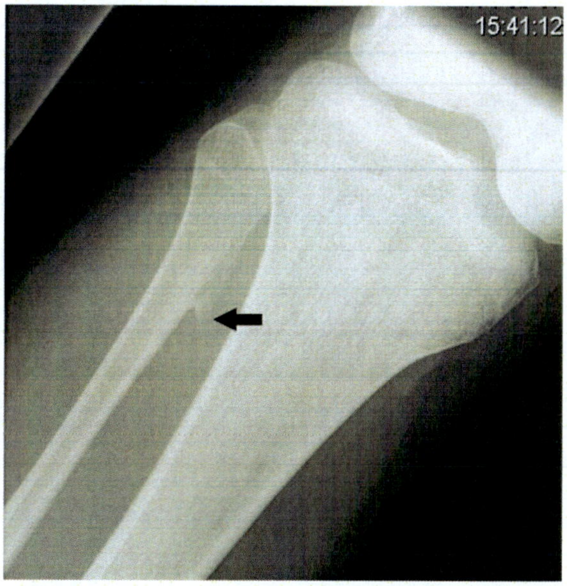

Fig. 41 Example of a tug lesion at the insertion of the soleus muscle at the proximal fibula (*arrow*). This bony overgrowth should not be mistaken for an old avulsion fracture or osteochondroma

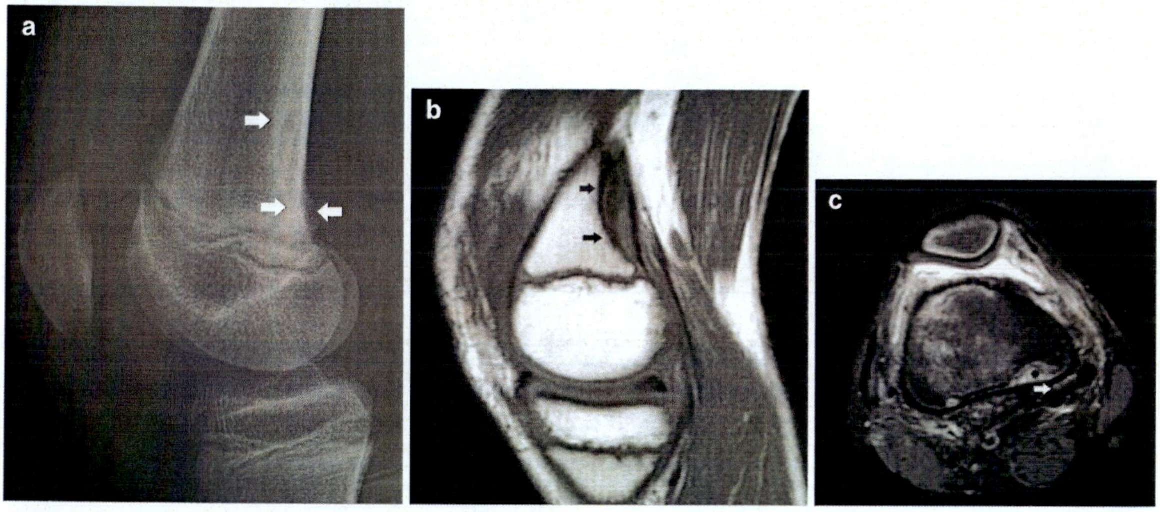

Fig. 42 Cortical avulsive irregularity syndrome at the posteromedial aspect of the right knee in a 14-year-old boy. (**a**) Plain radiograph of the right knee (lateral view). The lesion (*arrows*) is developmental in origin and should not be mistaken for a malignant or traumatic periosteal new bone formation. (**b**) Sagittal T1-w MR image. The lesion is isointense to hypointense compared to muscle (*arrows*). (**c**) Axial fat-suppressed T2-w image. The intramedullary portion of the lesion is relatively hyperintense (*asterisk*). Note also a faint hyperintense signal (soft tissue edema) at the proximal insertion of the medial gastrocnemius tendon (*white arrow*), which may suggest that the lesion is due to chronic traction of the tendon at its insertion at the posteromedial cortex of the distal femur

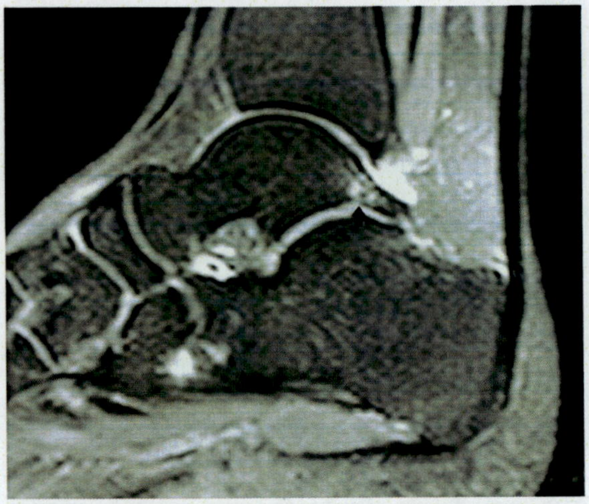

Fig. 43 Os trigonum syndrome. Sagittal fat-suppressed T2-w image showing BME either side of the synchondrosis between the os trigonum and the posterior aspect of the talus

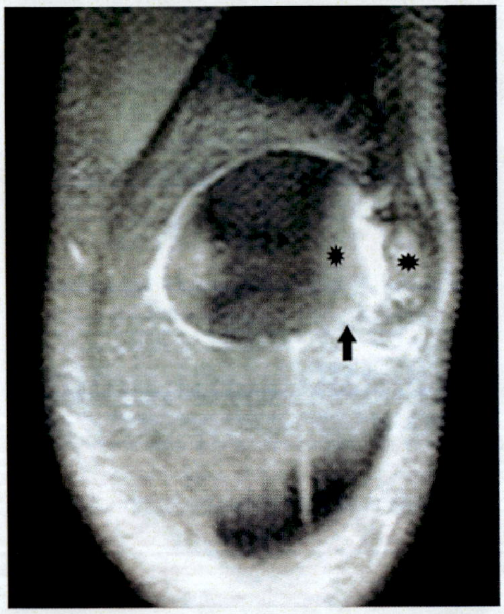

Fig. 44 Symptomatic bipartite patella. Coronal fat-suppressed T2-w image showing a bipartite patella (*arrow*) with edema either side of the division between the accessory ossification center and the main body of the patella (*asterisks*)

The os trigonum syndrome is a commonly reported source of pain in young gymnasts and dancers. This is thought to be due to repetitive impaction of the os trigonum between the calcaneus and the posterior malleolus during plantar flexion (Barron et al. 2008).

The association of patellofemoral symptoms and a dorsal defect of the patella suggests an abnormality of the cartilage overlying the defect (Monu and De Smet 1993).

A painful ischiopubic synchondrosis may be encountered in sportive children (Ceroni et al. 2004; Herneth et al. 2004; Van Hul et al. 2008). The ischiopubic synchondrosis is susceptible to mechanical stress, which may cause delayed ossification of this temporary joint. During certain athletic activities, such as jumping or kicking, mechanical forces exerted on the ischiopubic synchondrosis of the weight-bearing standing leg are increased compared with those of the swinging leg. The standing leg is in general the nondominant leg, which is the left leg in most humans. Thus, unevenly applied mechanical forces during common athletic activities may cause the prolonged persistence of the enlarged ischiopubic synchondrosis in the nondominant limb. Osteomyelitis of the ischiopubic synchondrosis is rare (Kozlowski et al. 1995). MRI will demonstrate bone and soft tissue edema in symptomatic cases about the synchondrosis (Fig. 45).

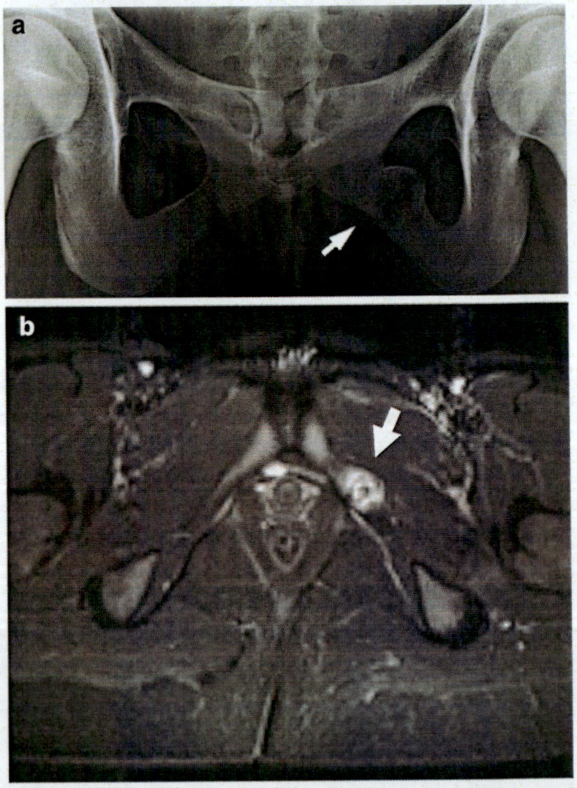

Fig. 45 Symptomatic left ischiopubic synchondrosis in a right-footed 14-year-old athlete. (**a**) Plain radiograph shows radiolucent enlargement of the left ischiopubic synchondrosis (*white arrow*) indicating delayed closure of this temporary joint, which is presumably due to asymmetrically applied mechanical strain. (**b**) Axial fat-suppressed T2-w image shows bone marrow and soft tissue edema surrounding the left ischiopubic synchondrosis (*arrow*) (Used with permission from: van Hul et al. (2008)

6 Differential Diagnosis

Many congenital disorders may be confused with acute or chronic trauma. Some examples are shown in Figs. 46–49 (Vanhoenacker and Fabry 2007).

Further discussion of these rare disorders is beyond the scope of this chapter. For a more complete and exhaustive discussion of these disorders, we refer to the textbook of Taybi and Lachman (Lachman 2006).

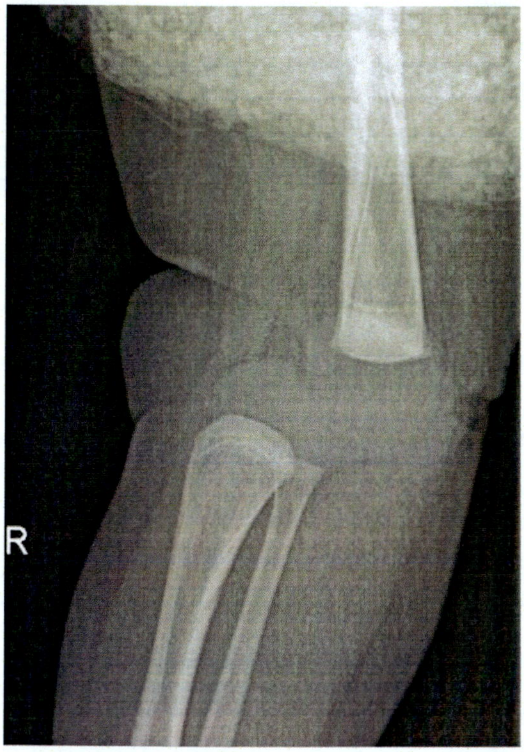

Fig. 46 Joint dislocation in an infant with Larsen syndrome. Plain radiograph of the right knee (lateral view) shows dislocation of the knee joint

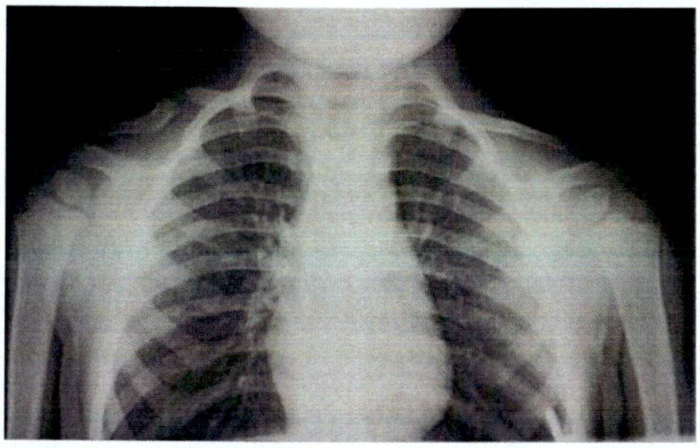

Fig. 47 Congenital pseudarthrosis of the right clavicle, simulating old trauma

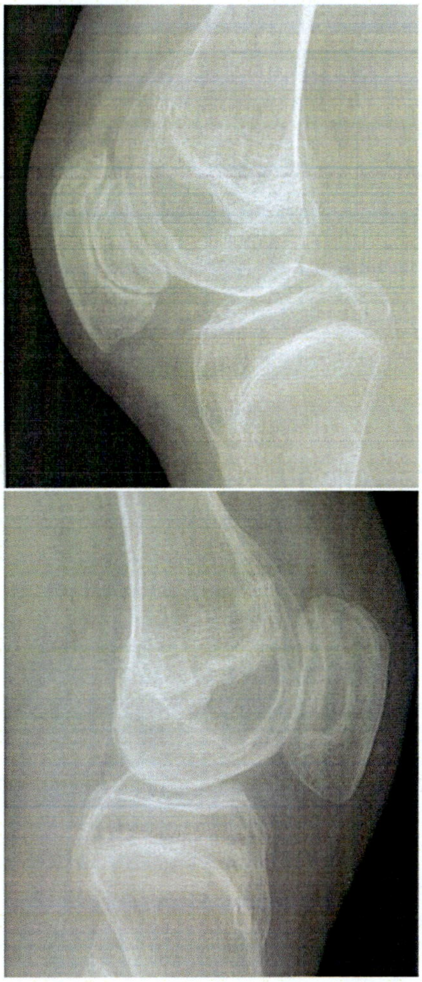

Fig. 48 Example of a bilateral double layered patella, which is highly suggestive of multiple epiphyseal dysplasia. (Used with permission from: Vanhoenacker and Fabry (2007a))

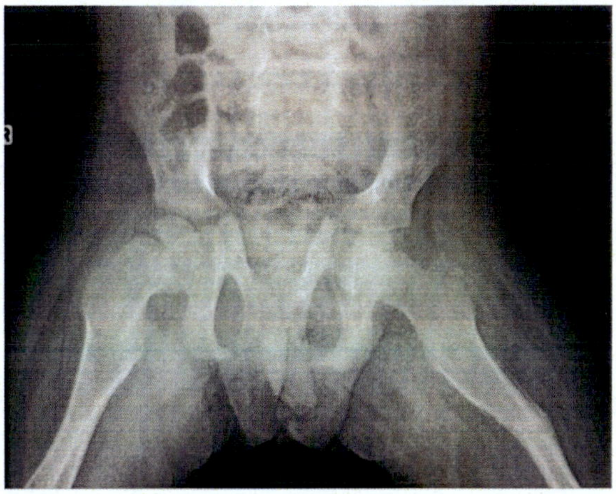

Fig. 49 Osteogenesis imperfecta in a 4-year-old child. Plain radiograph of the pelvis and proximal femora. Note the presence of multiple old fractures of both femora

7 Conclusion

A thorough knowledge of the normal anatomy, variations, and pitfalls is a prerequisite for the correct interpretation of imaging studies in sportive children and adolescents.

This will avoid overdiagnosis and unnecessary and harmful treatment.

References

Barron D, Farrant J, O'Connor P (2008) Lower extremity injuries in children (including sports injuries). In: Pope T, Bloem JL, Beltran J, Morrison W, Wilson DB (eds) Imaging of the musculoskeletal system. Saunders-Elsevier, Philadelphia, pp 916–955

Bashir WA, Lewis S, Cullen N, Connell DA (2009) Os peroneum friction syndrome complicated by sesamoid fatigue fracture: a new radiological diagnosis? Case report and literature review. Skeletal Radiol 38(2):181–186

Bernaerts A, Vanhoenacker FM, Van de Perre S, De Schepper AM, Parizel PM (2004) Accessory navicular bone: not such a normal variant. JBR-BTR 87:250–252

Bufkin WJ (1971) The avulsive cortical irregularity. AJR Am J Roentgenol 112(3):487–492

Carty H (1992) Accessory ossicles at the lateral malleolus: a review of the incidence. Eur J Radiol 14(3):181–184

Ceroni D, Mousny M, Anooshiravani-Dumont M, Buerge-Edwards A, Kaelin A (2004) MRI abnormalities of the ischiopubic synchondrosis in children: a case report. Acta Orthop Belg 70(3):283–286

Davies AM, Anderson SE (2007) Special considerations in the immature skeleton. I In: Vanhoenacker FM, Gielen JL, Maas M (eds). Imaging of Orthopedic Sports Injuries. Springer, Berlin, pp 433–447

El-Khoury GY, Brandser EA, Kathol MH et al (1996) Imaging of muscle injuries. Skeletal Radiol 25:3–11

Foster K (2008) Growth plate (physeal) injuries. In: Johnson KJ, Bache E (eds) Imaging of pediatric skeletal trauma. Springer, Berlin, pp 147–157

Freyschmidt J, Brossmann J, Wiens J et al (2002) Köhler/Zimmer Borderlands of Normal and Early Pathologic Findings in Skeletal Radiography, 5th edn. Thieme, Stuttgart

Herneth AM, Philipp MO, Pretterklieber ML, Balassy C, Winkelbauer FW, Beaulieu CF F (2004) Asymmetric closure of ischiopubic synchondrosis in pediatric patients: correlation with foot dominance. AJR Am J Roentgenol 182(2):361–365

Jaramillo D, Connolly SA, Mulkern RV, Shapiro F (1998) Developing epiphysis: MR imaging characteristics and histologic correlation in the newborn lamb. Radiology 207(3): 637–645

Jaramillo D, Villegas-Medina OL, Doty DK et al (2004) Age-related vascular changes in the epiphysis, physis, and metaphysis: normal findings on gadolinium-enhanced MRI of piglets. AJR Am J Roentgenol 182(2):353–360

Johnson AM, Marcus MA (2008) Upper extremity injuries in children (including sports injuries). In: Pope T, Bloem JL, Beltran J, Morrison W, Wilson DB (eds) Imaging of the musculoskeletal system. Saunders-Elsevier, Philadelphia, pp 879–915

Kahn LS, Gaskin CM, Sharp VL (2008) Keats and Kahn's Roentgen atlas of skeletal maturation, DVD. Lippincott Williams & Wilkins, Philadelphia

Keats TE, Anderson MW (2006) Atlas of normal roentgen variants that may simulate disease, 8th edn. Mosby, St. Louis

Kozlowski K, Hochberger O, Povysil B (1995) Swollen ischiopubic synchondrosis: a dilemma for the radiologist. Australas Radiol 39:224–227

Lachman R (2006) Taybi and Lachman's radiology of syndromes, metabolic disorders and skeletal dysplasias, 5th edn. Mosby, St. Louis

Lee JC, Calder JD, Healy JC (2008) Posterior impingement syndromes of the ankle. Sem Musculoskelet Radiol 12(2): 154–169

Miller TT (2002) Painful accessory bones of the foot. Semin Musculoskelet Radiol 6:153–161

Monu JU, De Smet AA (1993) Case report 789: dorsal defect of the left patella. Skeletal Radiol 22(7):528–531

Pal CR, Tasker AD, Ostlere SJ, Watson MS (1999) Heterogeneous signal in bone marrow on MRI of children's feet: a normal finding? Skeletal Radiol 28(5):274–278

Peeters J, Vanhoenacker FM, Marchal P et al (2009) Imaging of femoroacetabular impingement: pictorial review. JBR-BTR 92(1):35–42

Ramsden W (1999) Fractures and musculoskeletal trauma. In: Carty H (ed) Emergency pediatric radiology. Springer, Berlin, pp 313–345

Seeger LL, Yao L, Eckardt JJ (1998) Surface lesions of bone. Radiology 206(1):17–33

Slovis TL (2008) Caffey's pediatric diagnostic imaging with website, 11th edn. Mosby, St. Louis

Snoeckx A, Vanhoenacker FM, Gielen JL, Van Dyck P, Parizel PM (2008) Magnetic resonance imaging of variants of the knee. Singapore Med J 49(9):734–744

Swischuk LE (2002) Imaging of the cervical spine in children. Springer, Berlin

Van Hul E, Simons P, Malghem J, Parizel PM, Vanhoenacker F (2008) Une cause rare de pubalgie. Ortho-rhumato 6(4): 114–116

Vancauwenberghe T, Vanhoenacker FM, Van Den Abbeele K. (2009) Images in clinical radiology: painful os peroneum syndrome. JBR-BTR 92:232

Vandervliet EJ, Vanhoenacker FM, Snoeckx A, Gielen JL, Van Dyck P, Parizel PM (2007) Sports-related acute and chronic avulsion injuries in children and adolescents with special emphasis on tennis. Br J Sports Med 41(11): 827–831

Vanhoenacker F, Fabry K (2007) Heart-shaped sesamoid in multiple epiphyseal dysplasia. Pediatr Radiol 37(11): 1178

Vanhoenacker FM, Snoeckx A (2007) Bone marrow edema in sports: general concepts. Eur J Radiol 62(1):6–15

Vanhoenacker FM, Bernaerts A, Gielen J et al (2002a) Trauma of the pediatric ankle and foot. JBR-BTR 85(4):212–218

Vanhoenacker FM, Bernaerts A, Van de Perre S, De Schepper AM (2002b) MRI of painful bipartite patella. JBR-BTR 85:219

Williams H (2008) Normal anatomical variants and other mimics of skeletal trauma. In: Johnson KJ, Bache E (eds) Imaging of pediatric skeletal trauma. Springer, Berlin, pp 91–118

Zanetti M (2008) Founder's lecture of the ISS 2006: borderlands of normal and early pathological findings in MRI of the foot and ankle. Skeletal Radiol 37(10):875–884

Incidental Findings and Pseudotumours in Sports Injuries

A. Mark Davies, Suzanne E. Anderson-Sembach, and Steven L.J. James

Contents

A.M. Davies (✉) and S.L.J. James
Department of Radiology, Royal Orthopaedic Hospital,
Birmingham B31 2AP, UK
e-mail: wendy.Turner@roh.nhs.uk

S.E. Anderson-Sembach
Medical Imaging School, University of Notre Dame,
Sydney, Australia

Key Points

- Incidental abnormalities are a common finding on radiographs obtained for trauma in the child.
- Fractures in children following minor trauma may be due to pre-existing benign or malignant bone tumours.
- Congenital abnormalities in children revealed by imaging may be mistaken for tumours, e.g. anomalous muscles.
- Traumatic lesions in children revealed by imaging may be mistaken for tumours, e.g. stress fractures and avulsion injuries.

1 Introduction

Physical activity, sporting or otherwise, is required for the healthy development of the growing child into adulthood. Our underage society is polarising into those participating in moderate-to-excessive sports and those couch potatoes for whom recreation is largely confined to the playing of computer games. The growing skeleton in the former group is more susceptible to the effects of trauma than the healthy mature skeleton and can be exposed to forces well above that evolution intended or allowed for. All too often, because sport is so much a part of daily activity, both physicians and parents may fail to recognize the role of

A.H. Karantanas (ed.), *Sports Injuries in Children and Adolescents*,
Med Radiol Diagn Imaging, DOI: 10.1007/174_2010_51, © Springer-Verlag Berlin Heidelberg 2011

trauma when these children present with symptoms. The purpose of this chapter is to review the spectrum of trauma-related imaging abnormalities that may mimic a tumour (pseudotumours) and also those conditions that may be identified on imaging following injury either as an incidental finding or accompanying a traumatic lesion in the paediatric population. It is well recognized that the effects of skeletal trauma and occasionally tumours can be simulated by normal developmental variants, secondary ossification centres and radiographic artefacts. The prudent radiologist will regularly refer to one of the exhaustive treatises on normal variants when reporting radiographs of the immature skeleton (Keats and Anderson 2001; Köhler and Zimmer 1993). These diagnostic pitfalls are the subject matter of Chap. 2. Similarly, the radiologist needs to be aware of the normal variants seen in children in other forms of imaging such as focal areas of signal change on MR imaging of the feet in children mimicking marrow infiltration (Pal et al. 1999).

2 Incidental and Pre-Existing Bone Lesions

Previously undiagnosed lesions of bone may be identified following trauma in one of these two ways: First, as an incidental radiographic finding unrelated to the trauma or second, the pre-existing lesion may have weakened the bone, thereby pre-disposing to pathological fracture formation as the presenting complaint following a relatively minor injury. Benign bone lesions may present in either category. Malignant bone lesions will tend to present with either pain or a pathological fracture and not be first detected as an incidental finding. The caveat is that many children subsequently proven to have a bone malignancy will erroneously attribute the onset of symptoms to some episode of trauma. A study of 88 pathological fractures in paediatric patients showed that the commonest cause was simple bone cyst (SBC) (40%) followed by non-ossifying fibroma (19%), fibrous dysplasia (16%), osteosarcoma (15%) and aneurysmal bone cyst (ABC) (10%) (Ortiz et al. 2005). It is important when reviewing the radiographs of a fracture in a child with a history of only minor trauma that signs of a pre-existing abnormality are looked for.

2.1 Benign

2.1.1 Simple Bone Cyst

SBC, also known as unicameral bone cyst, is a common non-neoplastic lesion of childhood with almost 95% cases occurring before the age of 20 years. Typical sites are the proximal humerus (50%) and the proximal femur (25%) (Docquier and Delloye 2004). Clinically, the majority of SBCs are painless until minor trauma results in a pathological fracture. Over 75% cases therefore present with a fracture. In cases identified as an incidental finding without a fracture, the fracture risk can be calculated using a scoring system (Kaelin and Macewen 1989; Ahn and Park 1994). The radiographic appearances are those of a central metaphyseal lytic lesion with cortical thinning and mild bony expansion. Septation/trabeculation is not a prominent feature. A typical feature seen in up to 20% cases of SBC, but not pathognomonic, is the "fallen fragment sign" where a piece of the fractured cortex is seen to migrate to the dependent portion of the cyst (Fig. 1)

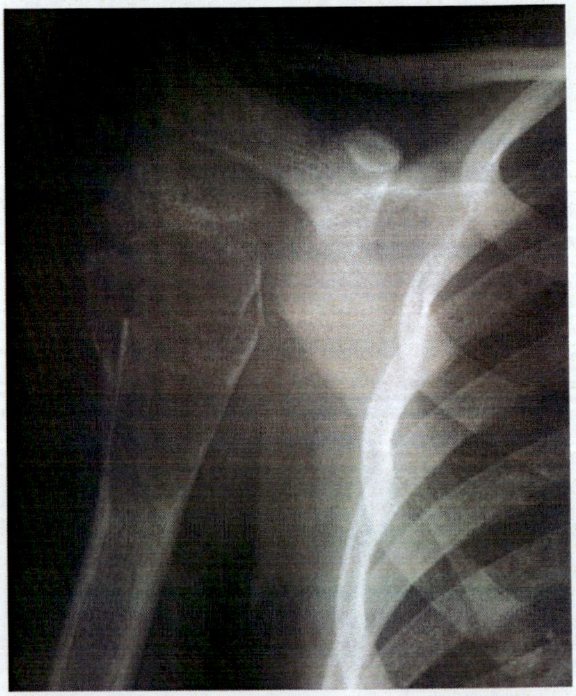

Fig. 1 Simple bone cyst. AP radiograph at presentation showing a pathological fracture and the "fallen fragment"

(Reynolds 1969). On MRI, the cyst contents appear mildly hypointense on T1-w and hyperintense on T2-w and STIR images. The thin cyst wall lining will show some minor enhancement with intravenous gadolinium. A fluid–fluid level may be seen in the presence of a recent fracture due to haemorrhage into the cyst. In time, the SBC will grow away from the growth plate and, depending on the extent of healing, may mimic other lesions such as fibrous dysplasia. Complications include repeated fracture, healing with deformity and growth arrest of the adjacent physis resulting in limb shortening (Violas et al. 2004). Over the years, numerous different treatments have been advocated for SBCs, including curettage and bone grafting, percutaneous steroid injection, autologous bone marrow injection, Ethibloc injection and intra-medullary nailing to mention only a few (Roposch et al. 2000). The wide variety of managements reflects the personal preference of the treating physician as well as the fact that no one procedure is convincingly more effective than any other. Internal fixation or intra-medullary nailing may be preferred for those fractures with a greater risk of displacement such as in the femur (Roposch et al. 2004; Vigler et al. 2006).

2.1.2 Aneurysmal Bone Cyst

ABC is another benign lesion of bone with 80% cases occurring in patients under the age of 20 years. ABC occurs as either a primary lesion (70% cases) or a secondary lesion in a pre-existing bone lesion (30% cases) (Cottalorda and Bourelle 2007). For a long time, it has been considered a non-neoplastic lesion with numerous different theories as to its pathogenesis. Interestingly, recent genetic and immunohistochemical studies are suggesting that primary ABC is after all a true neoplasm and not a reactive lesion (Leithner et al. 2004; Oliveira et al. 2004). Lesions predominate in the long bones (50% cases) and the spine, particularly the posterior elements (20% cases). The radiographic appearances have been described as a progression through four stages (Kransdorf and Sweet 1995). First, an initial phase when the lysis can mimic other benign bone lesions such as SBC and fibrous dysplasia (Parman and Murphey 2000). Second, an active or growth phase with marked expansion to give a "blown-out" appearance – mostly present in this phase with pathological fractures in 20% cases often with a history of minor trauma (Fig. 2a). Third and fourth, respectively, are

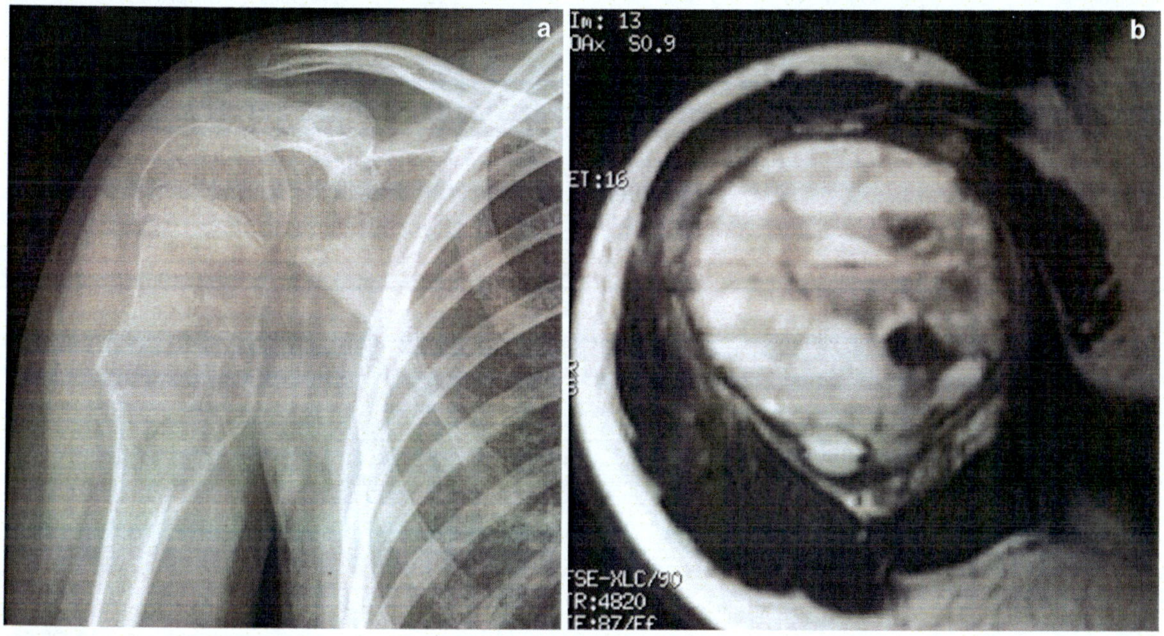

Fig. 2 Aneurysmal bone cyst. (**a**) AP radiograph showing a pathological fracture through the proximal humeral metaphysis. (**b**) Axial T2-w MR image showing multiple fluid–fluid levels

stabilization and healing phases with progressive thickening of the peripheral shell of the tumour. Eighty-five percent cases arise within medullary bone and 15% in a cortical or subperiosteal location (Maiya et al. 2002). Histologically, ABCs comprise multiple blood-filled cysts with intervening septae. Fluid–fluid levels due to the layering out of blood products within the cysts can be identified on CT and MRI (Fig. 2b). Fluid–fluid levels within bone and soft tissue lesions are a non-specific sign (Van Dyck et al. 2006). However, the commonest cause of a bone lesion in a child showing multiple fluid–fluid levels is an ABC (Davies et al. 1992), and lesions comprising a proportion greater than 2/3 fluid–fluid levels are more likely to be primary or secondary ABC than a malignancy (O'Donnell and Saifuddin 2004).

2.1.3 Non-Ossifying Fibroma

The commonest fibrous lesion of bone is the fibrous cortical defect and the histologically identical but larger non-ossifying fibroma. Both lesions are seen in childhood and adolescence, slightly more common in boys, with a predilection for the long bones around the knee. Fibrous cortical defects are seen in up to 30% of the normal population under the age of 15 years and are too small to present with a pathological fracture. They are, therefore, one of the commonest incidental bone lesions identified on radiographs of the knees in the paediatric population (Fig. 3). The radiographic appearances are those of a well-defined lytic lesion arising eccentrically within the metaphysis of a long bone. Larger non-ossifying fibromas can present with a pathological fracture following minor trauma (Fig. 4) (Drennan et al. 1974; Hase and Miki 2000). Arata et al. reported that if a non-ossifying fibroma involves more than 50% of the transverse diameter of the bone or measures greater than 33 mm in length, there is an increased risk of pathological fracture (Arata et al. 1981). A more recent series, however, showed that 59% cases of non-ossifying fibromas exceeded these threshold measurements without fracturing (Easley and Kneisl 1997). Common sense would suggest that the larger the non-ossifying fibroma the lesser the trauma that would be required to produce a pathological fracture.

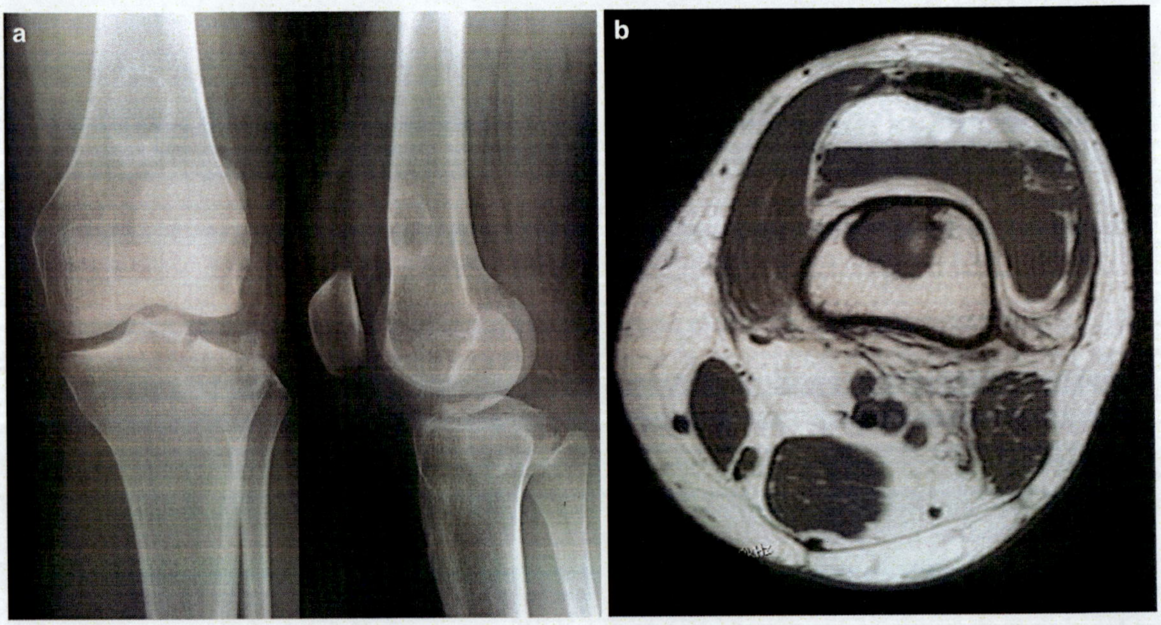

Fig. 3 Non-ossifying fibroma. (**a**) AP and lateral radiographs in a teenage girl presenting with a depressed fracture of the lateral tibial plateau following trauma. The non-ossifying fibroma in the distal femur was an incidental finding, which initiated more concern than the original fracture. (**b**) Axial T1-w MR image showing a lipohaemarthrosis in the suprapatellar pouch and the low signal intensity non-ossifying fibroma in the femur

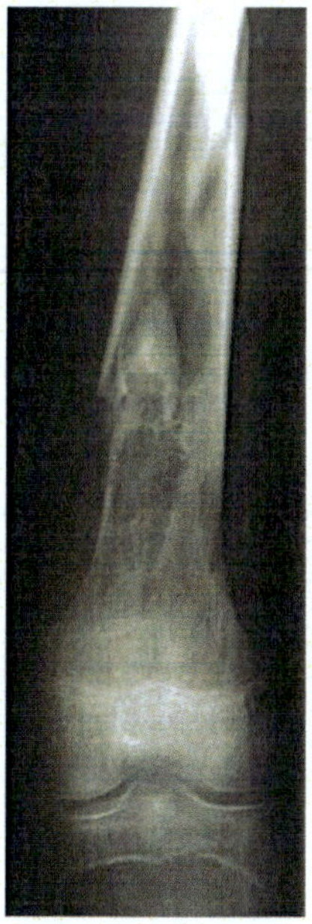

Fig. 4 Non-ossifying fibroma. AP radiograph following minor trauma showing a pathological fracture propagating proximally from the non-ossifying fibroma

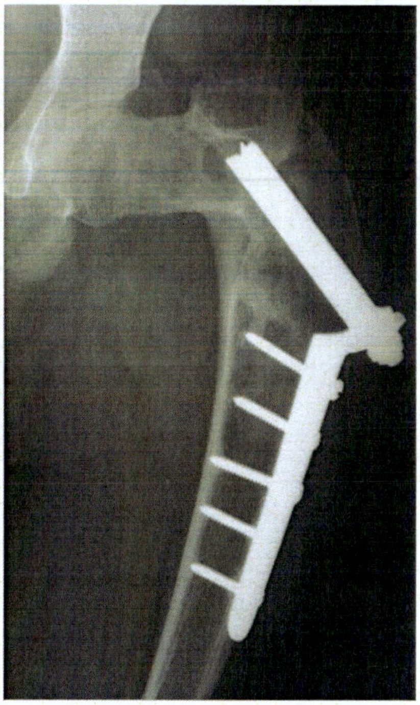

Fig. 5 Fibrous dysplasia. AP radiograph showing the typical shepherd's crook deformity of the proximal femur due to a combination of bone softening and repeated fractures with malunion. The internal fixation has failed to prevent the deformity progressing

2.1.4 Fibrous Dysplasia

Fibrous dysplasia is a developmental anomaly of bone in which the normal medullary space is replaced by fibroosseous tissue (Smith and Kransdorf 2000). It may affect a single bone (monostotic – 75% cases) or multiple bones (polyostotic – 25% cases). Small foci of monostotic fibrous dysplasia are not an uncommon incidental finding on radiographs. A variety of endocrinopathies can be associated with polystotic fibrous dysplasia. The classic example seen in up to one-third of females with polystotic disease is McCune–Albright syndrome in which there is fibrous dysplasia (frequently mono or hemimelic), café-au-lait spots and endocrine dysfunction notably precocious puberty. The radiographic appearances are those of a benign lytic or groundglass lesion in bone with mild-to-moderate expansion and endosteal thinning. This may result in small cortical fractures or, following minor trauma, complete fracture of the bone. Callus formation at the fracture site is dysplastic, and patients are therefore prone to a cycle of repeated fractures resulting in deformity (Kumta et al. 2000). A typical feature of involvement of the proximal femur is an increasing varus deformity (shepherd's crook deformity) resulting from malunion following fracture or progressive bone modelling due to abnormal biomechanics (Fig. 5) (Jung et al. 2006).

2.1.5 Enchondroma

Enchondroma is the second commonest benign tumour of bone after osteochondroma and is composed of mature hyaline cartilage arising within medullary bone. It comprises approximately 10% of all benign bone tumours and is the commonest tumour of the tubular bones of the hands and feet. Many cases are an incidental finding on radiographs obtained for unrelated reasons or present with a pathological fracture following minor trauma (Fig. 6). The main lesions appear lytic with minor expansion and varying degrees of cartilage mineralization described as flocculent, ring-and-arc or popcorn in appearance. The hands and feet are also common sites of involvement with the multiple forms of the tumour, Ollier disease and Maffucci's syndrome. Pathological fracture formation in enchondroma is no greater a problem in children than adults as shown by the paucity of publications on this subject when conducting an electronic search of the paediatric literature. The most serious complication seen rarely in solitary enchondroma but more common in both Ollier disease and Maffucci's

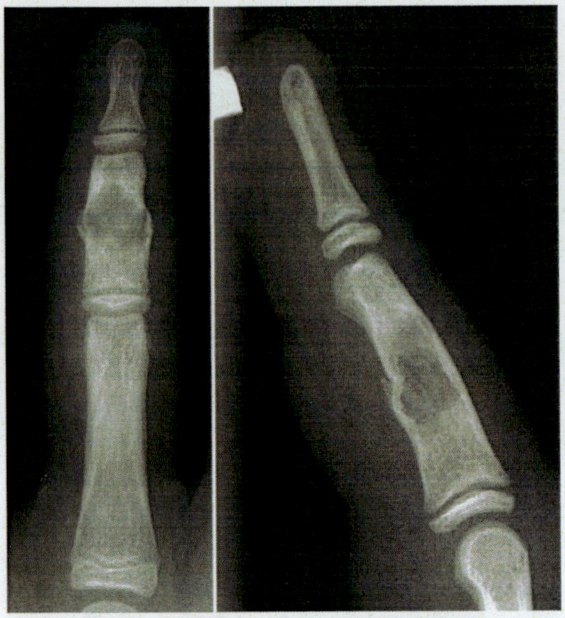

Fig. 6 Enchondroma. AP and lateral radiographs showing a pathological fracture through an enchondroma of the middle phalanx of the finger

syndrome is malignant transformation to a central chondrosarcoma that may present with a pathological fracture due to progressive bone destruction. Malignant change, however, is a complication really only seen in adults. Cellular atypia on histological examination, particularly in cartilage lesions in the hands and feet, should not be considered indicative of malignancy.

2.2 Malignant

Malignant lesions of bone in children do not as a rule present as an incidental finding on radiographs obtained following trauma or for other purposes. The marrow infiltration and subsequent cortical destruction will weaken the bone such that the presenting complaint is typically either pain or a pathological fracture. It is not unusual, however, for a child or his/her parents to attribute the gradual onset of symptoms due to malignancy to some episode of injury during sports.

2.2.1 Sarcoma

Pathological fracture through an osteosarcoma as the presenting complaint or during preoperative treatment is seen in 5–10% cases (Jaffe et al. 1987). They occur either spontaneously or as a result of minor trauma (Fig. 7). There is an increased risk in telangiectatic osteosarcoma as it is predominantly lytic (Huvos et al. 1982). It has been claimed that pathological fracture is associated with a poor outcome because of the dissemination of the tumour within the haematoma so that amputation is the preferred surgical treatment (Morris 1997; Scully et al. 2002). Some studies have suggested that limb-sparing surgery with adequate margins of excision can be achieved without compromising survival but may or may not have an increased risk of local recurrence (Abudu et al. 1996; Bacci et al. 2003; Natarajan et al. 2000). The risk of pathological fracture as the presenting complaint in Ewing sarcoma is similar to that in osteosarcoma (5–10% cases) (Fuchs et al. 2003). Two modes of presentation of pathological fracture of sarcoma in children merit special mention. First, there are the cases where the underlying tumour is so subtle as to be overlooked on the initial radiographs (De Santos and Edeiken 1985; Ramo et al. 2006). Second, where the tumour is mistaken for a benign bone tumour. In both situations, failure to recognize the underlying malignancy may lead to inappropriate internal fixation, thereby potentially disseminating the tumour along the whole length of the bone that in turn makes curative limb-salvage surgery problematic.

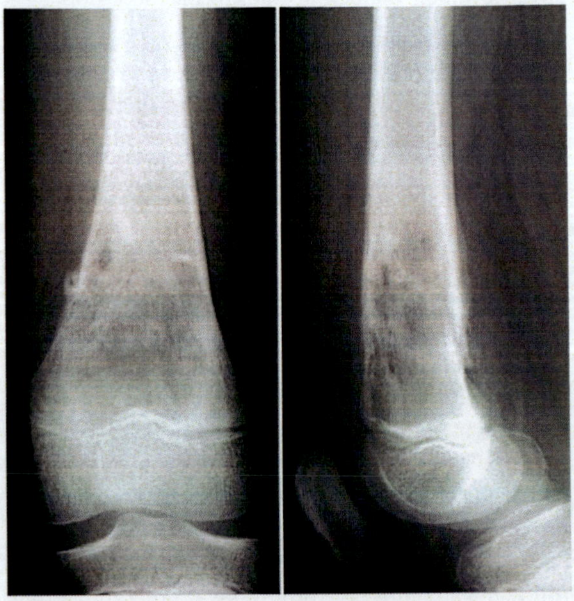

Fig. 7 Osteosarcoma. AP and lateral radiographs showing a pathological fracture developing through an osteosarcoma of the distal femur

2.2.2 Leukaemia

The leukaemias represent a group of diffuse malignancies of the bone marrow that frequently produce bony changes. The commonest form in children, particularly under 5 years of age, is acute lymphoblastic leukaemia (ALL). It would be extremely unlikely for leukaemia to be discovered as an incidental finding on imaging obtained following trauma. It is possible, however, that the leukaemic infiltration of the marrow might weaken the bone sufficient for the child to present with a pathological fracture following minor sports injury such as with vertebral body fractures producing wedging and/or collapse. The radiographic features seen in up to three quarters of patients include diffuse osteopenia, radiolucent and radiodense metaphyseal bands, osteolytic lesions and periosteal new bone formation. Observation of unexplained generalized osteopenia in a child should prompt urgent investigation to confirm/exclude ALL. MRI will reveal diffuse signal change, reduced on T1-w and raised on T2-w and STIR images, throughout the marrow (Thomsen et al. 1987).

3 Pre-Existing and Incidental Soft Tissue Lesions

3.1 *Accessory Muscles*

There are numerous accessory muscles described both at cadaveric dissection and on imaging, particularly using ultrasound and MRI. In children and adolescent athletes, these are most frequently incidental and identified on imaging for alternative indications; however, in some cases, the accessory muscle may be a cause of clinical symptoms. Accessory muscles may present as a consequence of local compression of neurovascular structures in confined anatomic spaces or rarely as a discrete mass lesion.

In the upper limb, accessory heads of biceps brachii, an accessory brachialis and an accessory head of flexor pollicis longus muscle have been described as potential causes of median nerve compression (Nakatani et al. 1998; Loukas et al. 2006; al-Qattan 1996). The anconeus epitrochlearis, which has an estimated prevalence of 11%, has been associated with ulnar nerve compression in the cubital tunnel in childhood (Boero and Sénès 2009). Anatomic variations in the hand and wrist are particularly common and include accessory abductor digiti minimi, extensor digitorum brevis manus, proximal origins of the lumbricals, palmaris longus inversus (Fig. 8), flexor digitorum superficialis indicis, flexor carpi radialis brevis vel profundus and accessory extensor carpi radialis (Timins 1999; Sookur et al. 2008). These typically present as pseudo mass lesions or are identified incidentally though there are reports describing compressive neuropathies of both the median and ulnar nerves (Timins 1999).

Lower limb accessory muscles become more common in the distal leg and ankle. There are sporadic reports of adolescent athletes presenting with peroneal nerve compression and foot drop from an anomalous biceps femoris muscle (Kaplan et al. 2008). Anatomic variations, including accessory slips of the medial and lateral heads of gastrocnemius, are reported as a cause

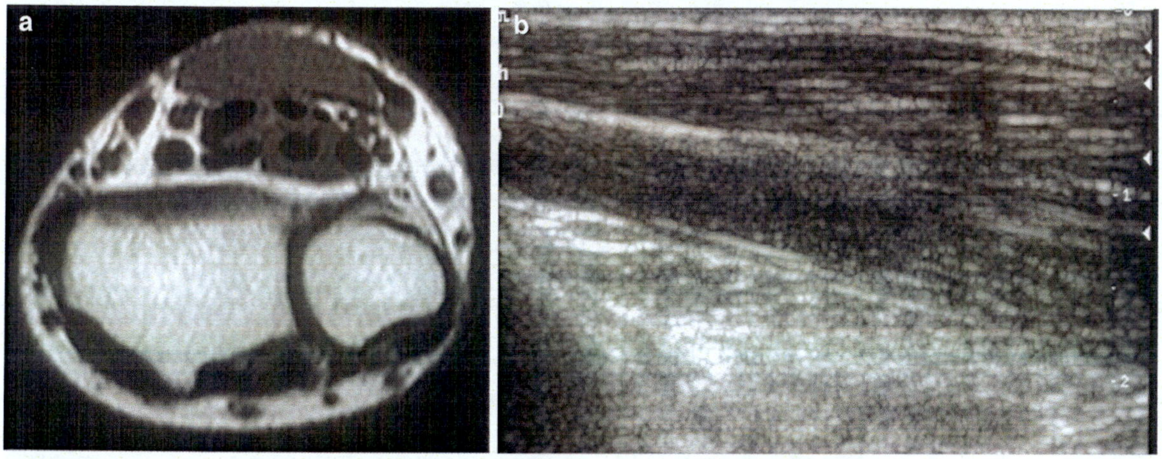

Fig. 8 Palmaris longus inversus muscle. (**a**) Axial T1-w MR image showing the anomalous muscle belly lying superficially in the palmar aspect of the wrist at the level of Lister's tubercle. (**b**) Longitudinal ultrasound at the same level shows normal echotexture from the anomalous muscle

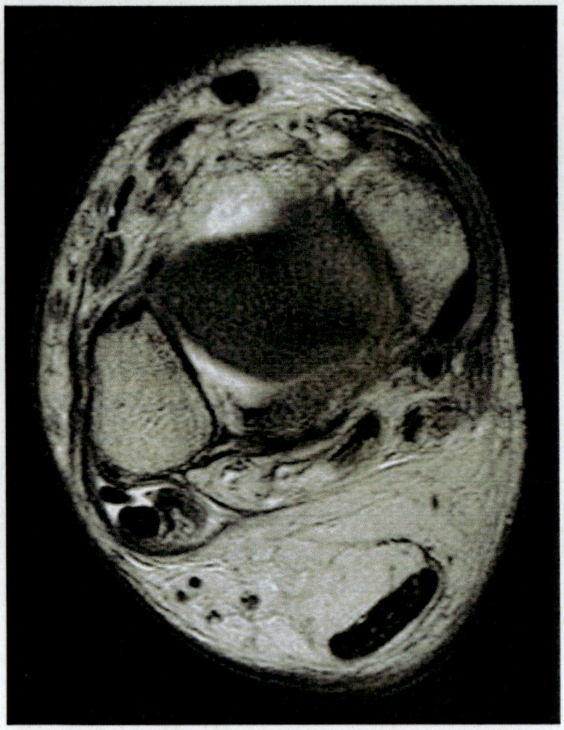

Fig. 9 Peroneus quartus muscle. Axial PD-w MR image showing the anomalous muscle immediately medial to the peroneus longus tendon and behind the lateral malleolus. This should not be confused with pathological processes of the peroneal tendons

for popliteal artery entrapment syndrome (PAES) which may present rarely in adolescents as intermittent claudication following exercise (Sookur et al. 2008). Six types of PAES have been described according to the relationship of the popliteal artery with the medial/lateral heads of gastrocnemius and their anomalous origins (Sookur et al. 2008). Further accessory muscles are reported in the popliteal region including tensor fasciae suralis and an accessory popliteus but have not been described as symptomatic variants in childhood/adolescence.

As with the hand, multiple accessory muscles occur in the foot and ankle region. These include peroneus tertius, peroneus quartus, peroneus accessorius, peroneocalcaneus externum, peroneocalcaneus internum and peroneus digiti minimi (Fig. 9) (Sookur et al. 2008). These will typically be identified incidentally and should be recognized to avoid misinterpretation as a longitudinal split within the peroneal tendons. On the medial side of the ankle, tarsal tunnel syndrome has been reported in childhood secondary to an accessory flexor digitorum longus muscle (Kinoshita et al. 2003). The accessory soleus has been described as a cause of exertion-related ankle and calf pain in association with a posteromedial mass in young athletes (Fig. 10) (Rossi et al. 2009; Christodoulou et al. 2004). Five variations in the accessory soleus have been reported based on their sites of insertion (Sookur et al. 2008).

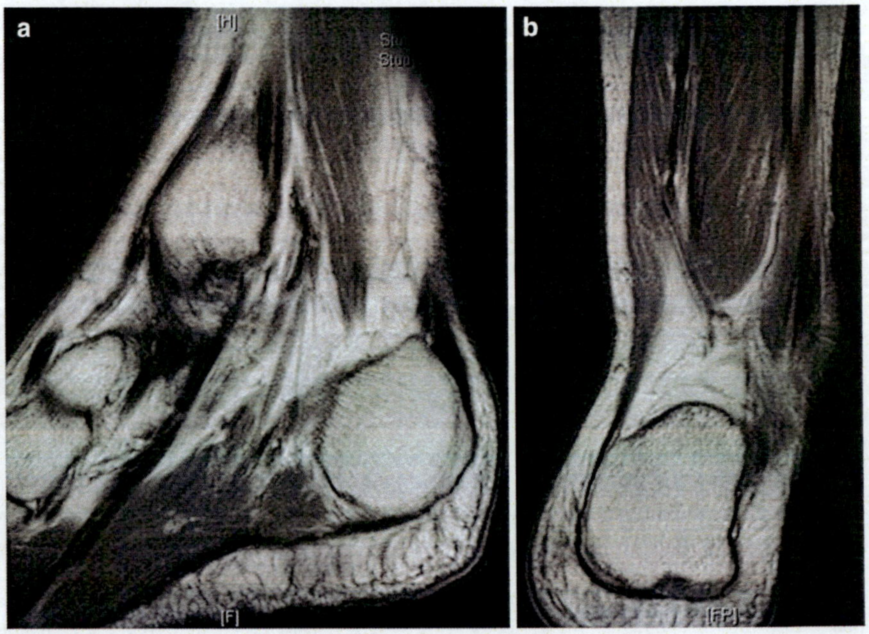

Fig. 10 Accessory soleus muscle. (**a**) Sagittal and (**b**) Coronal PD-w MR images showing the anomalous muscle deep to the Achilles tendon with a tendinous insertion to the superomedial aspect of the calcaneus. This is also known as the tibiocalcaneus internus muscle

4 Pseudotumours of Bone

4.1 Stress Fractures and Reactions

Fatigue-type stress fractures occur due to abnormal loading on normal bone. In the immature individual, if there is no history of recent increased activity, fatigue-type stress fractures are frequently mistaken for a primary sarcoma of bone (Levin et al. 1967; Provost and Morris 1969; Solomon 1974; Daffner et al. 1982; Burks and Sutherland 1984; Arrivé et al. 1988; Davies et al. 1989). The posteromedial aspect of the proximal tibia is the most common site for fatigue fractures in the child and is also the most common site to be misinterpreted on imaging as a sarcoma of bone (Davies et al. 1988). All too often, the periosteal new bone formation identified as ill-defined sclerosis en face and as a continuous lamella perpendicularly is interpreted as the early sign of an Ewing sarcoma or osteomyelitis (Fig. 11a) (Davies et al 1988). If the correct diagnosis of a stress fracture is not considered at this stage,

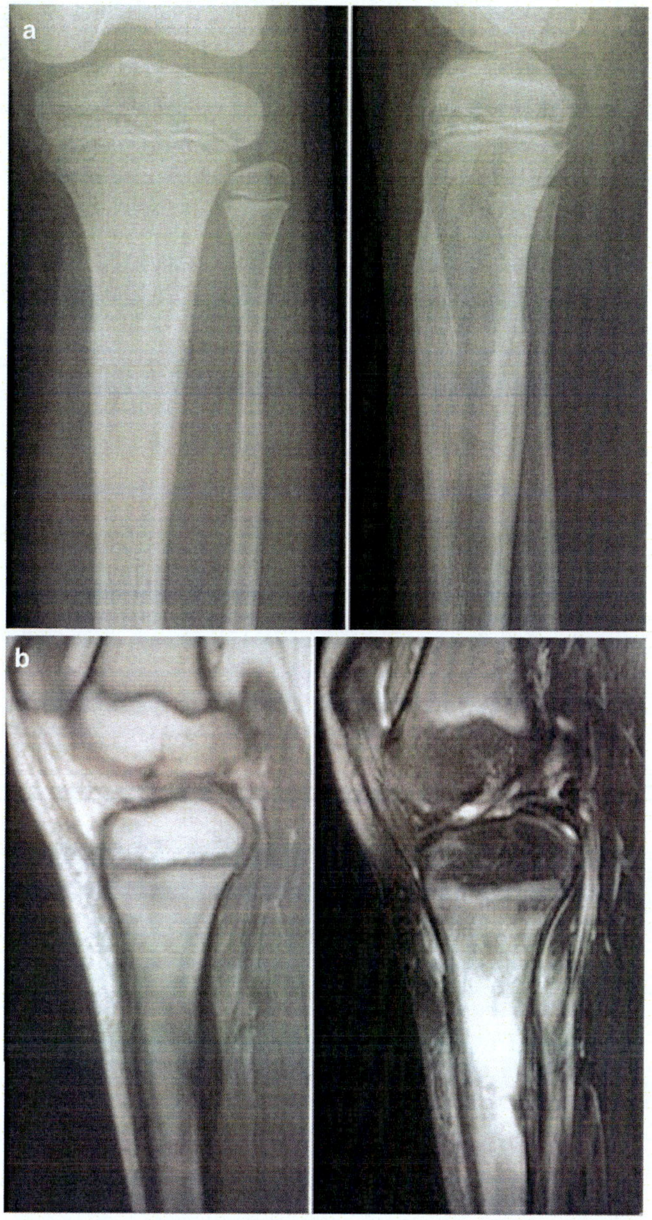

Fig. 11 Stress fracture. (**a**) AP and lateral radiographs showing a lamellar periosteal reaction along the proximal tibial diaphysis all too frequently mistaken for a sarcoma. (**b**) Sagittal T1-w and STIR MR images showing periosteal new bone formation with marrow and juxtacortical oedema/haemorrhage

further imaging with MRI may confuse the unwary radiologist as oedema and haemorrhage can be readily mistaken for marrow infiltration and extraosseous tumour spread (Fig. 11b) (Tyrrell and Davies 1994. Lee et al. 2005). Some authors have stressed the value of a multimodality imaging approach to the distinction of a stress fracture from a pathological fracture (Fayad et al. 2004, 2005) that does assume that the former has been included in the reporting radiologist's original differential diagnosis. In many cases, it is possible on both CT and MRI to identify the fracture as a focal cortical radiolucency/low signal intensity line traversing the cortex within the area of periosteal new bone formation. Fatigue fractures are just one end of the spectrum of bone response to abnormal loading. MRI can be utilized to differentiate stress fractures from shin splints (Aoki et al. 2004). MRI is also sufficiently sensitive to reveal subtle areas of marrow and juxtacortical oedema even when symptoms are absent or minimal (Bergman et al. 2004). These non-specific MRI changes are called stress reactions or stress phenomena and may be an incidental finding in children. They will typically resolve over a few weeks provided the source of the stress is removed. If signs persist or show progression, then an early sarcoma should be considered. It is not unusual with both fatigue fractures and stress reactions to see similar, if somewhat less pronounced, changes in the controlateral limb. This would be most unusual for a sarcoma unless it was multifocal, and then again it would be unlikely for the tumour to be symmetrically distributed.

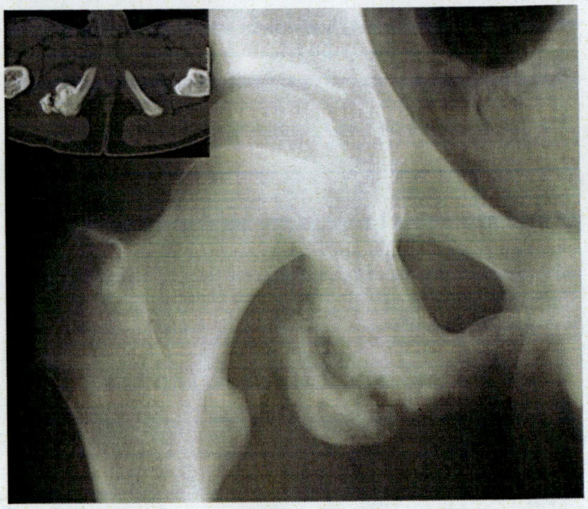

Fig. 12 Ischial avulsion injury. AP radiograph and axial-computed tomography (inset) showing a chronic avulsion of the ischial apophysis

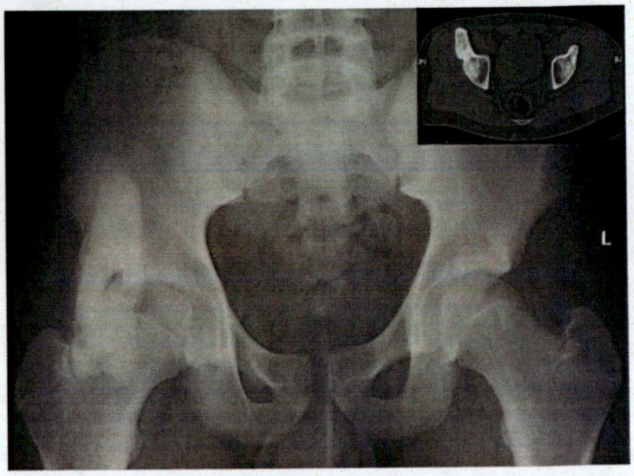

Fig. 13 Old anterior superior iliac apophyseal injury. AP radiograph and CT (inset) showing a bony exostosis at the site of the old avulsion injury

4.2 Avulsion Injuries

Avulsion injuries are common in the adolescent age group because the growth plate attachments of the apophyses to the underlying bone are relatively weak. Injuries may be acute or chronic in the latter due to repetitive microtrauma and overuse (Tehranzadeh 1987; El-Khoury et al. 1997; Donnelly et al. 1999; Stevens et al. 1999). The commonest site is the pelvis with over 50% cases involving the ischial apophysis, the origin of the hamstring muscles (Fig. 12) (Rossi and Dragoni 2001). Other typical sites in the pelvis include the anterior superior iliac spine (the origin of the sartorius muscle) and the anterior inferior iliac spine (the origin of the rectus femoris muscle) (Fig. 13). There is usually no diagnostic problem in acute injuries with the sudden onset of pain during an easily identified episode of physical activity/sport. However, if there is a delay in obtaining radiographs, the immature amorphous callus may mimic a surface tumour of bone. The MRI features of acute-on-chronic injuries can be pronounced with oedema and haemorrhage surrounding new bone formation in the juxta-apophyseal soft tissues and reactive oedema in the underlying bone marrow. If the blood supply to the ischial apophysis remains intact at the time of the acute avulsion, it may continue to grow and present in adulthood as a mature bony mass in the soft tissues of the buttock. Chronic muscle avulsive injuries can occur less commonly at other sites in the lower limb (Donnelly et al. 1999). One entity that merits mention in children if only because it can also mimic a sarcoma is femoral diaphyseal periostitis due to chronic stress at the insertion site of the adductor musculature (Anderson et al. 2001).

4.3 Periosteal Desmoid

The periosteal desmoid is an innocuous, incidental radiographic finding that frequently causes diagnostic problems following trauma in children. Understanding of this condition is not helped by the multiplicity of different names in the literature including cortical desmoid, avulsive cortical irregularity and cortical irregularity syndrome. It arises on the posteromedial ridge of the distal femoral metaphysis in adolescents, more common in boys, and is frequently bilateral. On radiographs, there is erosion or saucerization of the outer cortex with minor spiculated periosteal new bone formation (Fig. 14a). In the past, it has been attributed to mechanical stresses applied to the insertion of the adductor magnus muscle or the origin of the medial head of the gastrocnemius muscle (Bufkin 1971; Barnes and Gwinn 1974; Resnick and Greenway 1982; Pennes et al. 1984). Bone scintigraphy tends to show normal skeletal activity that is somewhat atypical for a trauma-related abnormality of bone (Dunham et al. 1980; Burrows et al. 1982; Craigen et al. 1994). Interestingly, MR imaging may show some oedema on the outer surface of the cortex and to a lesser extent in the underlying medulla that might tend to support a traumatic aetiology (Fig. 14b) (Posch and Puckett 1998). Whatever the pathogenesis, the important thing to note is that the process is self-limiting and of no immediate clinical consequence. Biopsy should be avoided.

4.4 Post-Traumatic Bone Cysts

Post-traumatic bone cysts are rare. One example recognized in the paediatric population arises in the distal radius following greenstick and torus fractures (Papadimitriou et al. 2005). It has been suggested that the cortical lucency is due to the release of intra-medullary fat through a breach in the cortex beneath an intact periosteum (Dürr et al. 1997). In time, the subperiosteal

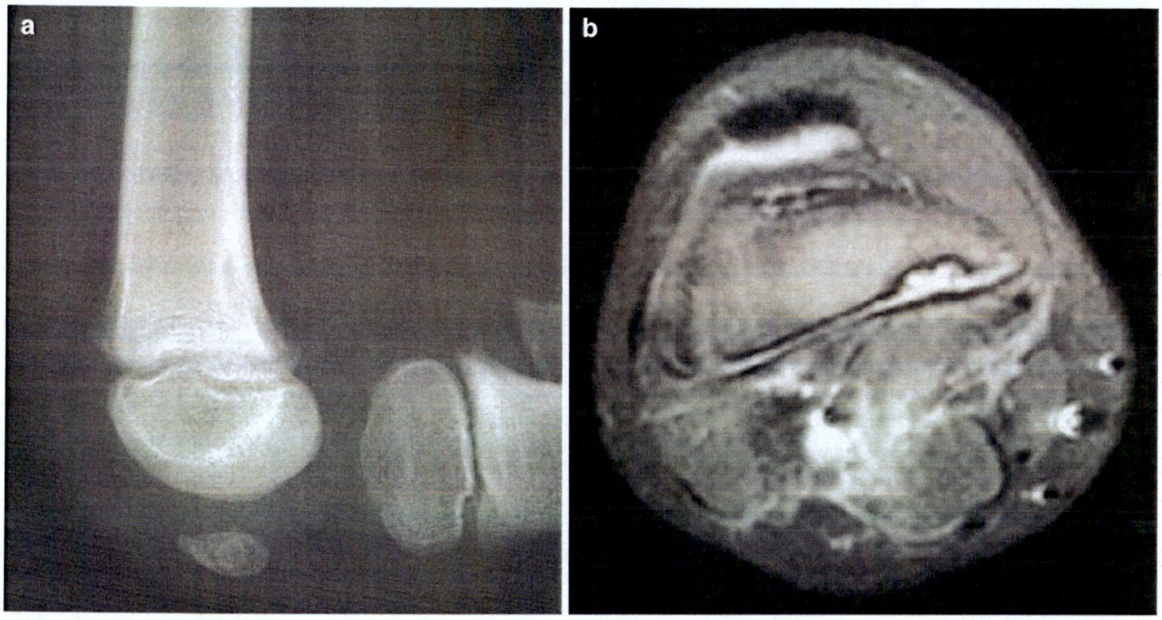

Fig. 14 Periosteal desmoid. (**a**) Lateral radiograph showing saucerization of the posteromedial cortex of the distal femoral metaphysis. (**b**) Axial fat-suppressed PD-w MR image showing the posteromedial metaphyseal defect with minor hyperintense oedema

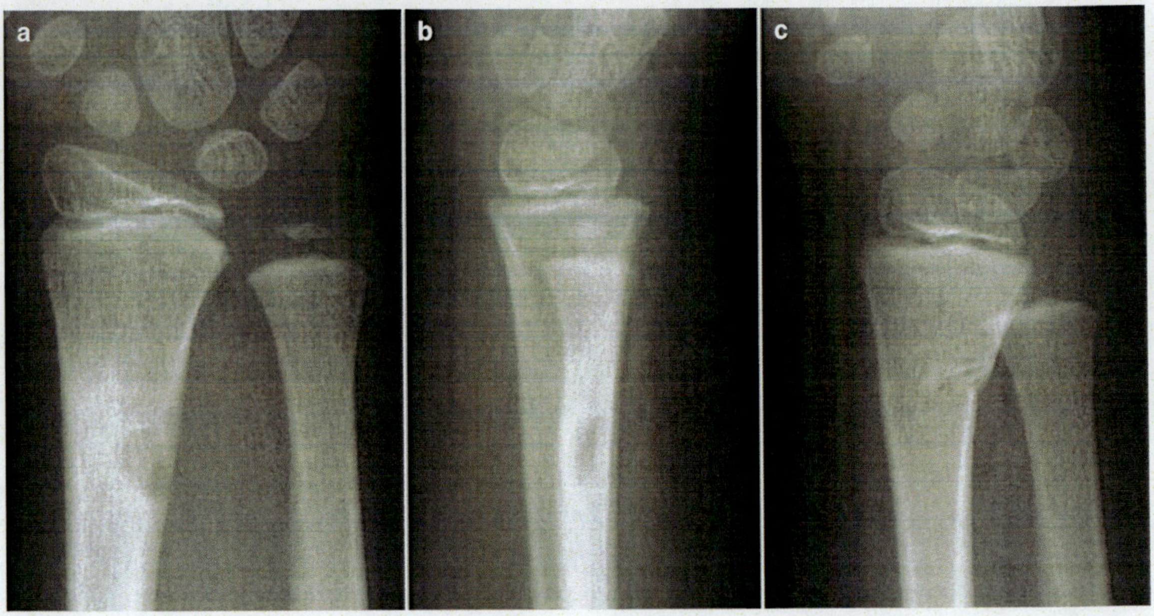

Fig. 15 Post-traumatic bone cyst. (**a–c**) PA and Lateral radiographs showing a cortically based lucency in the distal radius. PA radiograph obtained 6 months earlier shows the causative distal radial greenstick fracture

haematoma ossifies leaving the collection of fat as a cortically based lucency that may mimic a Brodie abscess or Langerhans cell histiocytosis (Fig. 15).

5 Pseudotumours of Soft Tissue

5.1 Haematoma

Haematoma may occur as a consequence of a direct impact of injury or secondary to an underlying muscle tear. In childhood, growth plate injury and avulsion fractures are more common than muscle injuries; however, muscle contusions and strains become more frequent in adolescence. Haematoma more commonly occurs as an inter-muscular location tracking between the fascial planes than as a true intra-muscular lesion; however, it is this latter entity that can occasionally present as a "pseudotumour" (Fig. 16). The differentiation of a soft tissue sarcoma with extensive intra-tumoral haemorrhage and a post-traumatic haematoma can be challenging. Correlation with the clinical history and presentation is required to assess whether the degree of abnormality on imaging can be explained by the severity and mechanism of injury (Kontogeorgakos et al. 2009).

The most common sites are the hamstring and quadriceps compartments though upper limb and abdominal wall (rectus sheath) haematomas are reported in adolescent athletes. There is usually a clear history of a significant muscle strain/tear though the time of presentation following the initial event is variable. The imaging appearances will vary with time depending on whether the patient is assessed in the acute, subacute or chronic phase. Both ultrasound and MRI are useful modalities in assessing for the presence of haematoma.

5.2 Penetrating Injuries

Penetrating injuries can lead to retained foreign bodies with numerous materials being implicated including wood, metal, grit and glass. Often an appropriate history can be sought from the patient or their immediate relatives. In sport, soft tissue injuries are common; however, puncture wounds with retained foreign bodies are rare in athletes. Occasionally, the history of an injury may not be forthcoming if the presentation is delayed from the initial event. Retained foreign bodies may cause a localized inflammatory reaction with the subsequent development of a foreign body granuloma. There are a number of reports of a foreign body

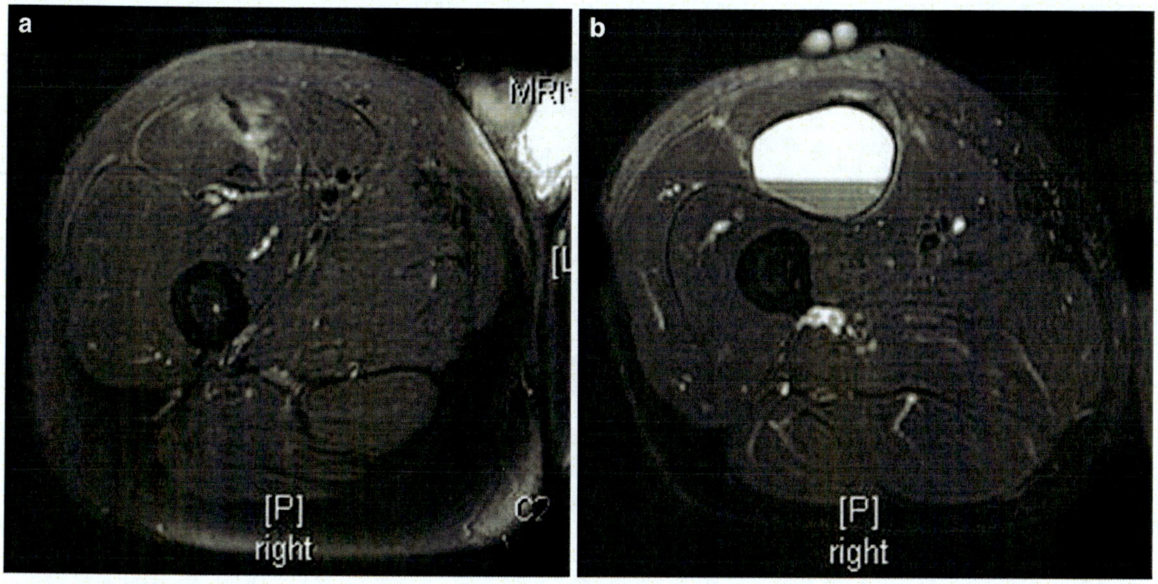

Fig. 16 Rectus femoris muscle haematoma. Axial fat-suppressed PD-w MR images. (**a**) The proximal image shows a thickened myotendinous junction with surrounding oedema. (**b**) The distal image shows a chronic intra-muscular haematoma containing a fluid–fluid level and a low signal intensity rim

granuloma mimicking soft tissue malignancy (Ando et al. 2009; Nakamura et al. 2008). Alternatively, a localized soft tissue infection may occur in the form of either cellulitis or local abscess formation, though this diagnosis is usually clinically more apparent.

Radiographs can be utilized to identify a radio-opaque material including metal and glass, but ultrasound is being used increasingly as the first line method of evaluating patients with retained foreign bodies (Peterson et al. 2002). This allows radiolucent lesions to be identified, and its high spatial resolution confers significant advantages over other cross-sectional modalities. It is also being utilized for percutaneous removal of the foreign body obviating the need for surgical exploration (Callegari et al. 2009). If a foreign body granuloma or abscess is suspected, then MRI will allow the local extent of this complication to be evaluated.

5.3 *Myositis Ossificans*

Myositis ossificans is the development of heterotopic ossification within the soft tissues, typically intramuscular. Some patients (<50%) give a history of prior trauma, but a significant number, particularly children, will not recall a pre-disposing acute injury. It is this latter group presenting with a painful soft tissue mass that can be mistaken clinically and on imaging for a sarcoma (Boutin et al. 2002). Myositis ossificans can also develop in association with paraplegia and extensive burns. While the latter category tends to occur around the hips and lumbar spine, 80% of the former arise in the large muscles of the extremities. Clinically, the lesion presents with pain, swelling and localized inflammation. Radiographs at presentation can be normal, but over a period of 4–6 weeks after injury or onset of symptoms, there is progressive peripheral mineralization (Fig. 17a). Identification of this peripheral distribution (zoning phenomenon) is an important diagnostic feature as it is not seen in soft tissue sarcomas. Serial radiographs or CT will show maturation of the lesion with increasing ossification extending from the periphery into the centre of the lesion (Fig. 17b) (Mccarthy and Sundaram 2005). If the lesion arises adjacent to bone, it may stimulate a periosteal reaction. At this location, it is sometimes called periostitis ossificans. The MRI appearances reflect the phase of development of the myositis ossificans. In the early phase before ossification, the lesion is usually isointense to muscle on T1-w with marked central hyperintensity on T2-w images (De Smet et al. 1992) with florid surrounding soft tissue oedema (Fig. 17c). The prominent oedema is another useful diagnostic feature as it reflects the inflammatory response, which would be most unusual around a soft

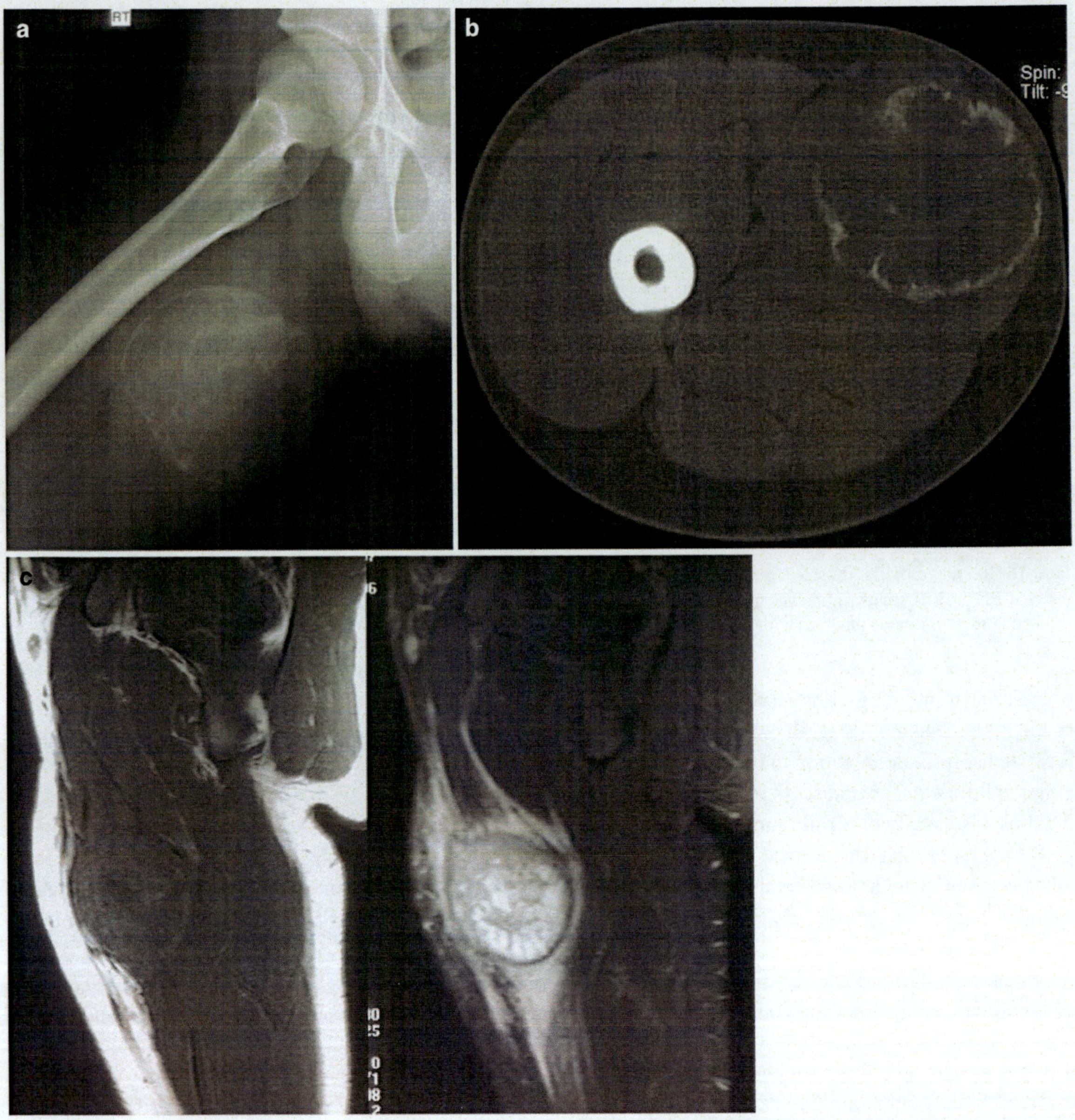

Fig. 17 Myositis ossificans. (**a**) Lateral radiograph showing an ossifying mass in the soft tissues of the upper thigh. (**b**) Computed tomography shows the zoning phenomenon with peripheral mineralization typical of myositis ossificans. (**c**) Sagittal T1-w and STIR MR images confirming the soft tissue mass. The low signal intensity rim is due to the mineralization, and there is peri-lesional oedema on the STIR image due to the florid inflammatory response

tissue sarcoma unless there has been recent biopsy or intra-tumoural haemorrhage (Jelinek and Kransdorf 1995). Correlation with radiographs is helpful as the subtle low signal intensity rim representing the early peripheral calcification may be easily overlooked. The variant arising on bone, periostitis ossificans, may stimulate some reactive marrow oedema in the underlying bone. Occasionally, fluid–fluid levels may be identified within the lesion. Caution should be exercised when interpreting a dynamic contrast-enhanced MR study in myositis ossificans as the time-intensity curve will typically show a slope similar to that of a high grade sarcoma (Verstraete et al. 1994). Over time, the soft tissue oedema around myositis ossificans subsides, the peripheral calcification thickens and the central portion ossifies eventually exhibiting signal characteristics similar to that of fatty marrow (Parikh et al. 2002). Biopsy should be avoided as the florid osteoblastic activity may be mistaken for an osteosarcoma.

References

Abudu A, Sferopoulos NK, Tillman RM, Carter SR, Grimer RJ (1996) The surgical treatment and outcome of pathological fractures in localised osteosarcoma. J Bone Joint Surg Br 78B:694–698

Ando A, Hatori M, Hagiwara Y, Isefuku S, Itoi E (2009) Imaging features of foreign body granuloma in the lower extremities mimicking a soft tissue neoplasm. Ups J Med Sci 114(1):46–51

Ahn JI, Park JS (1994) Pathological fractures secondary to unicameral bone cysts. Int Orthop 18:20–22

Anderson SE, Johnston JO, O'Donnell R, Steinbach LS (2001) MR imaging of sports-related pseudotumor in children: mid-femoral diaphyseal periostitis at insertion site of adductor musculature. Am J Roentgenol 176: 1227–1231

Aoki Y, Yasuda K, Tohyama H, Ito H, Minami A (2004) MR imaging in stress fractures and shin splints. Clin Orth Rel Res 421:260–267

Arata MA, Peterson HA, Dahlin DC (1981) Pathological fractures through nonossifying fibromas. J Bone Joint Surg Am 63A:980–988

Arrivé L, Selier N, Khalifa G, Seringer R (1988) Difficultés diagnostiques des appositions périostées unilamellaires symptomatiques isolées. J Radiol 69:351–356

Bacci G, Ferrari S, Longhi A, Donati D, Manfrini M, Giacomini S, Briccoli A, Forni C, Galletti S (2003) Nonmetastatic osteosarcoma of the extremity with pathologic fracture at presentation. Acta Orthop Scan 74:449–454

Barnes GR Jr, Gwinn JL (1974) Distal irregularities of the femur simulating malignancy. Am J Roentgenol 122:180–185

Bergman AG, Fredericson M, Ho C, Matheson GO (2004) Asymptomatic tibial stress reactions: MRI detection and clinical follow-up in distance runners. Am J Roentgenol 183:635–638

Boero S, Sénès FM (2009) Catena N (2009) Pediatric cubital tunnel syndrome by anconeus epitrochlearis: a case report. J Shoulder Elbow Surg 18(2):e21–e23

Boutin RD, Fritz RC, Steinbach LS (2002) MRI of muscle injury. Radiol Clin N Am 40:333–362

Bufkin WJ (1971) The avulsive cortical irregularity. Am J Roentgenol 112:487–492

Burks RT, Sutherland DH (1984) Stress fractures of the femoral shaft in children. Report of 2 cases and discussion. J Ped Orthop 4:614–616

Burrows PE, Greenberg ID, Reed MH (1982) The distal femoral defect: technetium-99 m pyrophosphate bone scan results. J Can Assoc Radiol 33:91–93

Callegari L, Leonardi A, Bini A, Sabato C, Nicotera P, Spano' E, Mariani D, Genovese EA, Fugazzola C (2009) Ultrasound-guided removal of foreign bodies: personal experience. Eur Radiol 19(5):1273–1279

Christodoulou A, Terzidis I, Natsis K et al (2004) Soleus accessories, an anomalous muscle in a young athlete: case report and analysis of the literature. Br J Sports Med 38(6):e38

Cottalorda J, Bourelle S (2007) Modern concepts of primary aneurysmal bone cyst. Arch Orthop Trauma Surg 127:105–114

Craigen MAC, Bennet GC, MacKenzie JR et al (1994) Symptomatic cortical irregularities of the distal femur simulating malignancy. J Bone Joint Surg Br 76B:814–817

Daffner RH, Martinez S, Gehweiler JA Jr, Harrelson JM (1982) Stress fractures of the proximal tibia in runners. Radiology 142:63–65

Davies AM, Evans N, Grimer RJ (1988) Fatigue fractures of the proximal tibia simulating malignancy. Br J Radiol 61:903–908

Davies AM, Carter SR, Grimer RJ, Sneath RS (1989) Fatigue fractures of the femoral diaphysis in the skeletally immature simulating malignancy. Br J Radiol 62:893–896

Davies AM, Cassar-Pullicino VN, Grimer RJ (1992) The incidence and significance of fluid-fluid levels on computed tomography of osseous lesions. Br J Radiol 65:193–198

De Smet AA, Noris MA, Fisher DR (1992) MR imaging of myositis ossificans: analysis of seven cases. Skeletal Radiol 21:503–507

Docquier PL, Delloye C (2004) Autologous bone marrow injection in the management of simple bone cysts in children. Acta Orthop Belg 70:204–213

Donnelly LF, Bisset GS, Helms CA, Squire DL (1999) Chronic avulsive injuries of childhood. Skeletal Radiol 28:138–144

Drennan DB, Maylahn DJ, Fahey JJ (1974) Fractures through large nonossifying fibromas. Clin Orthop 103:82–88

Dunham WK, Marcus NW, Enneking WF et al (1980) Developmental defects of the distal femoral metaphysis. J Bone Joint Surg Am 62A:801–806

Dürr LA, Stäbler A et al (1997) MRI of posttraumatic cyst-like lesions of bone after greenstick fracture. Eur Radiol 7: 1218–1220

Easley ME, Kneisl JS (1997) Pathologic fractures through nonossifying fibromas: is prophylactic treatment warranted. J Pediatr Orthop 17:808–813

El-Khoury GY, Daniel WW et al (1997) Acute and chronic avulsive injuries. Radiol Clin North Am 35:747–766

Fayad LM, Kawamoto S, Kamel IR et al (2004) Distinction of long bone stress fractures from pathological fractures on cross-sectional imaging: how successful are we? Am J Roentgenol 185:915–924

Fayad LM, Kamel IR, Kawamoto S et al (2005) Distinguishing stress fractures from pathologic fractures: a multimodality approach. Skeletal Radiol 34:245–259

Fuchs B, Valenzuela RG, Sim FH (2003) Pathologic fracture as a complication in the treatment of Ewing's sarcoma. Clin Orthop 415:25–30

Hase T, Miki T (2000) Autogenous bone marrow graft to nonossifying fibroma with a pathologic fracture. Arch Orthop Trauma Surg 120:458–459

Huvos AG, Rosen G, Bretsky SS, Butler A (1982) Telangiectatic osteogenic sarcoma: a clinicopathologic study of 124 patients. Cancer 49:1679–1689

Jaffe N, Spears R, Eftekhari F et al (1987) Pathologic fracture in osteosarcoma: impact of chemotherapy on primary tumor and survival. Cancer 59:701–709

Jelinek J, Kransdorf MJ (1995) MR imaging of soft tissue masses. Mass-like lesions that simulate neoplasms. Magn Reson Imaging Clin N Am 4:727–741

Jung ST, Chung JY, Seo HY, Bae BH, Lim KY (2006) Multiple osteotomies and intramedullary nailing with neck cross-pinning for shepherd's crook deformity in polystotic fibrous dysplasia. Acta Orthop Scand 77:469–473

Kaelin AJ, MacEwen GD (1989) Unicameral bone cysts: natural history and the risk of fracture. Int Orthop 13:275–282

Kaplan KM, Patel A, Stein DA (2008) Peroneal nerve compression secondary to an anomalous biceps femoris muscle in an adolescent athlete. Am J Orthop 37:268–271

Keats TE, Anderson MW (2001) Atlas of normal roentgen variants that may simulate disease, 7th edn. Mosby, St Louis

Kinoshita M, Okuda R, Morikawa J, Abe M (2003) Tarsal tunnel syndrome associated with an accessory muscle. Foot Ankle Int 24:132–136

Köhler A, Zimmer EA (1993) Borderlands of normal and early pathologic findings in skeletal radiography, 4th edn. Thieme Verlag, Stuttgart

Kontogeorgakos VA, Martinez S, Dodd L, Brigman BE (2009) Extremity soft tissue sarcomas presented as hematomas. Arch Orthop Trauma Surg [PMID 19838719]

Kransdorf MJ, Sweet DE (1995) Aneurysmal bone cyst: concept, controversy, clinical presentation, and imaging. AJR Am J Roentgenol 164:573–580

Kumta SM, Leung PC, Griffith JF, Chow LTC (2000) Vascularised bone grafting for fibrous dysplasia of the upper limb. J Bone Joint Surg (Br) 82B:409–412

Lee SH, Baek JR, Han SB, Sw P (2005) Stress fractures of the femoral diaphysis in children. J Pediatr Orthop 25:734–738

Leithner A, Machacek F, Haas OA, Lang S, Ritschl P, Radl R, Windhager R (2004) Aneurysmal bone cyst: a hereditary disease? J Pediatr Orthop 13B:214–217

Levin D, Blazina ME, Levine E (1967) Fatigue fractures of the shaft of the femur: simulation of malignant tumour. Radiology 88:883–885

Loukas M, Louis RG Jr, South G et al (2006) A case of an accessory brachialis muscle. Clin Anat 19:550–553

McCarthy EF, Sundaram M (2005) Heterotopic ossification: a review. Skeletal Radiol 34:609–619

Nakatani T, Tanaka S, Mizukami S (1998) Bilateral four-headed biceps brachii muscles: the median nerve and brachial artery passing through a tunnel formed by a muscle slip from the accessory head. Clin Anat 11:209–212

Maiya S, Davies AM, Evans N, Grimer RJ (2002) Surface aneurysmal bone cysts: a pictorial review. Eur Radiol 12:99–108

Morris HG (1997) Pathological fractures in bone sarcomas. Acta Orthop Scand 273S:106–107

Nakamura T, Kusuzaki K, Matsubara T, Matsumine A (2008) Uchida A (2008) Foreign-body granulomas in the trunk and extremities may simulate malignant soft-tissue tumors: report of three cases. Acta Radiol 49:80–83

Natarajan MV, Govardhan RH, Williams S, Gopal TSR (2000) Limb salvage surgery for pathological fractures in osteosarcoma. Int Orthop 24:170–172

O'Donnell P, Saifuddin A (2004) The prevalence and diagnostic significance of fluid-fluid levels in focal lesions of bone. Skeletal Radiol 33:330–336

Oliveira AM, Perez-Atayde AR, Inwards CY, Medeiros F, Derr V, His BL, Gebhardt MC, Rosenberg AE, Fletcher JA (2004) USP6 and CDH11 oncogenes identify the neoplastic cell in primary aneurysmal bone cysts and are absent on so-called secondary aneurysmal bone cysts. Am J Pathol 165:1773–1780

Ortiz EJ, Isler MH, Navia JE, Canosa R (2005) Pathologic fractures in children. Clin Orthop 432:116–126

Pal CR, Tasker AD, Ostlere SJ, Watson MS (1999) Heterogeneous signal in bone marrow on MRI of children's feet: a normal finding? Skeletal Radiol 28:274–278

Papadimitriou NG, Christophorides J, Beslikas TA et al (2005) Posttraumatic cystic lesion following fracture of the radius. Skeletal Radiol 34:411–414

Parikh J, Hyare H, Saifuddin A (2002) The imaging features of post-traumatic myositis ossificans, with emphasis on MRI. Clin Radiol 57:1058–1066

Parman LM, Murphey MD (2000) Alphabet soup: cystic lesions of bone. Semin Muscul Radiol 4:89–101

Pennes DR, Braunstein EM, Glazer GM (1984) Computed tomography of cortical desmoid. Skeletal Radiol 12: 40–42

Peterson JJ, Bancroft LW, Kransdorf MJ (2002) Wooden foreign bodies: imaging appearance. AJR Am J Roentgenol 178:557–562

Posch TJ, Puckett ML (1998) Marrow MR signal abnormality associated with bilateral avulsive cortical irregularities in a gymnast. Skeletal Radiol 27:511–514

Provost RA, Morris JM (1969) Fatigue fractures of the femoral shaft. J Bone Joint Surg (Am) 51A:487–488

al-Qattan MM (1996) Gantzer's muscle: an anatomical study of the accessory head of the flexor pollicis longus muscle. J Hand Surg [Br] 21:269–270

Ramo BA, Kyriakos M, McDonald DJ (2006) Osteosarcoma without radiographic evidence of tumor: case report. Clin Orthop 442:267–272

Resnick D, Greenway G (1982) Distal femoral cortical defects, irregularities and excavations: a critical review of the literature with the addition of histologic and paleopathologic data. Radiology 143:345–354

Reynolds J (1969) The "fallen fragment sign" in the diagnosis of unicameral bone cyst. Radiology 92:949–953

Roposch A, Saraph V, Linhart WE (2000) Flexible intramedullary nailing for the treatment of unicameral bone cysts in long bones. J Bone Joint Surg Am 82A:1447–1453

Roposch A, Saraph V, Linharty WE (2004) Treatment of femoral neck and trochanteric simple bone cysts. Arch Orthop Trauma Surg 124:437–442

Rossi F, Dragoni S (2001) Acute avulsion fractures of the pelvis in adolescent competitive athletes: prevalence, location and sports distribution of 203 cases collected. Skeletal Radiol 30:127–131

Rossi R, Bonasia DE, Tron A et al (2009) Accessory soleus in the athletes: literature review and case report of a massive muscel in a soccer player. Knee Surg Sports Traumatol Arthrosc 17(8):990–995

De Santos LA, Edeiken BS (1985) Subtle early osteosarcoma. Skeletal Radiol 13:44–48

Scully SP, Ghert MA, Zurakowski D, Thompson RC, Gebhardt MC (2002) Pathologic fracture in osteosarcoma: prognostic importance and treatment implications. J Bone Joint Surg Am 84A:49–57

Smith SE, Kransdorf MJ (2000) Primary musculoskeletal tumors of fibrous origin. Semin Musculoskelet Radiol 4: 73–88

Solomon L (1974) Stress fractures of the femur and tibia simulating malignant bone tumours. S Afr J Surg 12:19–25

Sookur PA, Naraghi AM, Bleakney RR et al (2008) Accessory muscles: anatomy, symptoms, and radiologic evaluation. Radiographics 28:481–499

Stevens MA, El-Khoury GY et al (1999) Imaging features of avulsion injuries. Radiographics 19:655–672

Tehranzadeh J (1987) The spectrum of avulsion and avulsion-like injuries of the musculoskeletal system. Radiographics 7:945–974

Thomsen C, Sorensen PG, Karle H et al (1987) Prolonged bone marrow T1-relaxation in acute leukaemia. Magn Reson Imaging 5:251–257

Timins ME (1999) Muscular anatomic variants of the wrist and hand: findings on MR imaging. AJR Am J Roentgenol 172:1397–1401

Tyrrell PNM, Davies AM (1994) Magnetic resonance imaging appearances of fatigue fractures of the long bones of the lower limb. Br J Radiol 67:332–338

Van Dyck P, Vanhoenacker FM, Vogel J, Venstermans C, Kroon HM, Gielen J, Parizel PM, Bloem JL, De Schepper AMA (2006) Prevalence, extension and characteristics of fluid-fluid levels in bone and soft tissue tumous. Eur Radiol 16:2644–2651

Verstraete KL, De Deene Y, Roels H, Dierick A, Uyttendaele D, Kunnen M (1994) Benign and malignant musculoskeletal lesions: dynamic contrast-enhanced MR imaging – parametric "First-Pass" images depict tissue vascularization and perfusion. Radiology 192:835–843

Vigler M, Weigl D, Schwarz M, Ben-Itzhak I, Salai M, Bar-On E (2006) Subtrochanteric femoral fractures due to simple bone cysts in children. J Pediatric Orthop 15B:439–442

Violas P, Salmeron F, Chapuis M, de Gauzy JS, Bracq H, Cahuzac JP (2004) Simple bone cysts of the proximal humerus complicated with growth arrest. Acta Orthop Belg 70:166–170

Current Role for Ultrasonography

Gina Allen and David Wilson

Contents

Key Points

- Ultrasound does not use radiation and does not need sedation, and so is the best way of imaging children when practical.
- Ultrasound has superb line pair resolution and therefore can look at the soft tissues in great detail and assess tendon muscle and ligament injury.
- Ultrasound has a long learning curve and the operator must be familiar with children and both normal and abnormal ultrasound appearances.
- The operator of the ultrasound should understand the problems that are specific to sport in children.

1 Introduction

Ultrasound is becoming the primary imaging technique of choice in sporting injury due to its easy availability and safety. It is possible to purchase portable high resolution ultrasound scanners which are affordable to the clinicians. Many machines are being purchased by sports physicians, physiotherapists and other medical professionals. This method of imaging is no longer reserved for radiologists.

The introduction of ultrasound as part of the core curriculum for the training of sports physicians and rheumatologists has confirmed and reinforced its value in sports medicine practice. Ultrasound examination is used as an adjunct to the clinical examination, which allows the imaging to be directed to the site of pain and abnormality. The additional benefits are that the young patient

G. Allen (✉)
Green Templeton College, University of Oxford, Oxford, UK
e-mail: georgina.allen@gtc.ox.ac.uk

D. Wilson
University of Oxford, Oxford, UK

A.H. Karantanas (ed.), *Sports Injuries in Children and Adolescents*,
Med Radiol Diagn Imaging, DOI: 10.1007/174_2010_11, © Springer-Verlag Berlin Heidelberg 2011

does not need sedation to have an ultrasound performed, the normal side can easily be examined for comparison and dynamic assessment of the movement of the affected area can be performed (Allen et al 2005).

Ultrasound is of greatest benefit when examining the soft tissues but can also detect bony abnormality when the lesion is superficial and peripheral joint effusions or synovitis.

Perhaps the most important element of training required of the sonographer is a detailed knowledge of anatomy beyond that normally taught in medical schools and different to that taught in surgical education (Bellah 2001; Sofka 2004; Wilson 2005; Allen and Wilson 2007).

2 Soft Tissue Injury

2.1 Muscle

The muscle-tendon-bone unit is different in children because the tendon does not insert directly into the bone but has an indirect insertion via the apophysis. This is the weak link in the muscle-tendon-apophysis-bone chain. In adults the musculotendinous junction is the weakest and tears occur in this location (Abalo et al. 2008; Sanders and Zlatkin 2008; McKinney et al. 2009).

Muscle has a multipennate structure and therefore has a characteristic appearance. Different muscle groups have different echogenicity and different stripped patterns on the sonogram related to the varied amount of fat and fibrofatty tissue. This pattern alters with the type of exercise the child is undertaking, as different sports use different muscle groups. Aerobic and anaerobic patterns of exercise also change the distribution of fat and muscle fibre. The dominant side of the patient will often have an increased muscle bulk, therefore asymmetry can be normal.

Muscular injury is well demonstrated using ultrasound, but is an uncommon injury in childhood, in part due to the plasticity of the tendon, bone and apophysis and in part due to the relative resilience of muscle in youth. Where muscular injury does occur however, it is usually due to direct contusion when the patient suffers a blow during contact sports. In late adolescence traction or overload injuries of muscle become more common.

Ultrasound examination of muscle in the first few hours after the injury may be misleading. The signs of an injury are alteration in the pennate pattern, disruption of fibres, abnormal bunching on dynamic motion and haemorrhage. Local oedema and neovascularity may be observed. In the early period after injury these signs may not be present. Paradoxically, MR is more sensitive at this stage. However, within 12–24 h the ultrasound features become clearer whilst diffuse oedema masks many of the signs using MR and makes interpretation difficult. This means that pitch or track side ultrasound examination may be misleadingly normal. Therefore, use MR for early diagnosis and ultrasound examination after 24 h. After one week both techniques are accurate.

If a muscular injury does not recover appropriately then the possibility of a retear or another diagnosis such as a tumour or myositis ossificans should be considered (Fig. 1). Ultrasound examination is particularly useful as it is more precise than MR in detecting calcification in muscle. It will detect mass lesions with sensitivity and precision whilst measuring abnormal blood flow without the need for intravenous injection of contrast agents (Micheli et al. 2009).

Experienced sonographers will not overlook soft tissue tumours and can readily discriminate solid mass lesions from relatively innocent cysts or ganglia (Fig. 2).

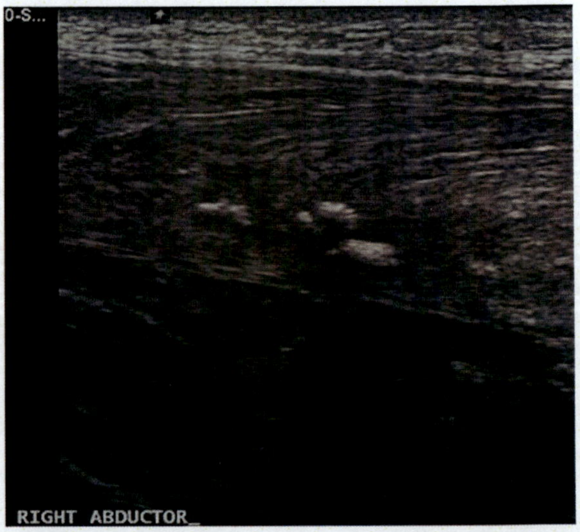

Fig. 1 An ultrasound image of myositis ossificans of the adductor longus muscle

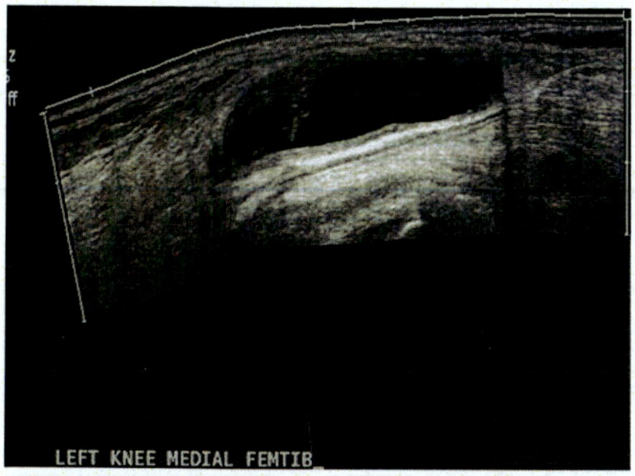

Fig. 2 An ultrasound image of a popliteal cyst which shows some internal echoes from a recent rupture

2.2 Tendons

Tendon injuries are uncommon in children, especially at the site commonly affected in adults – the musculotendinous junction. Most injuries occur at the apophysis where the tendon joins the bone. This is a common disorder that in our experience is rarely diagnosed. We suspect that many cases are overlooked and this is a particular problem in the lower limb (McKinney et al. 2009). Proper management is to immobilise and rest, to allow rapid recovery. Early mobilisation may lead to poor healing, long term dysfunction and even a mass lesion due to bony overgrowth. Entheseal injuries most often occur at the following sites of tendon attachment – the anterior superior iliac spine (sartorius insertion), the anterior inferior iliac spine (rectus femoris insertion), the lesser trochanter (iliopsoas insertion), and the tibial tuberosity (patellar tendon insertion). If the diagnosis is not considered then a radiograph may be reported as normal as the initial findings are often subtle. Often, in retrospect, there is some widening of the apophysis, but ultrasound examination can identify this injury more specifically with liquefying haematoma at the injured site and neovascularisation around the area of irregularity within the bone. In a chronic injury the only clue may be some fragmentation of bone at the site of the apophysis which appears different to the other side (Figs. 3 and 4).

Ultrasound is also preferred for the knee in cases where the symptoms are confined to the patella tendon. Tears, tendinopathy and enthesiopathy are readily detected using ultrasound (Bianchi et al. 2006). Patellar tendinopathy may occur in sports where there is excess loading, for example jumping sports such as basket ball or volley ball (Fig. 5). Here the presence of neovascularisation within the tendon can be used to detect disease and help guide the treatment. Follow up with Doppler ultrasound examination will show resolution of the neovascularity in response to treatment (Alfredson and Ohberg 2005).

Similarly ultrasound examination is accurate in assessing the iliotibial tract (especially for overuse pain and snapping syndromes).

2.3 Ligaments

Ligamentous injuries do occur in children, especially related to the ankle, but other problems within this age group also occur. Subluxation of the peroneal tendons is a much more common injury in young age groups. This may be due to the slow development of the fibro osseous tunnels and the fluctuating hormones in children in adolescence and can easily be identified on ultrasound using dynamic assessment looking for subluxation of the peroneal tendons.

Anterior cruciate ligament (ACL) injuries are more common in female adolescents compared to males. This was thought to be due to hormonal factors but there is also likely to be a genetic predisposition (Renstrom et al. 2008; Posthumus et al. 2009). MRI is still the gold standard for assessing knee problems, such as internal derangement (Prince et al. 2005). The superficial knee ligaments such as the medial and lateral collaterals can be assessed by ultrasound (Fig. 6). However, there are associated injuries often, and therefore, it is prudent to image with MRI. The internal knee ligaments are much better assessed by MRI.

Ligament anatomy is complex and as the abnormality that is sought is absence of a small structure, considerable skill and experience is required on the part of the examiner to detect ligament rupture. Having said this, with such knowledge, the addition of dynamic stress means that ultrasound examination may be more accurate than an MR examination.

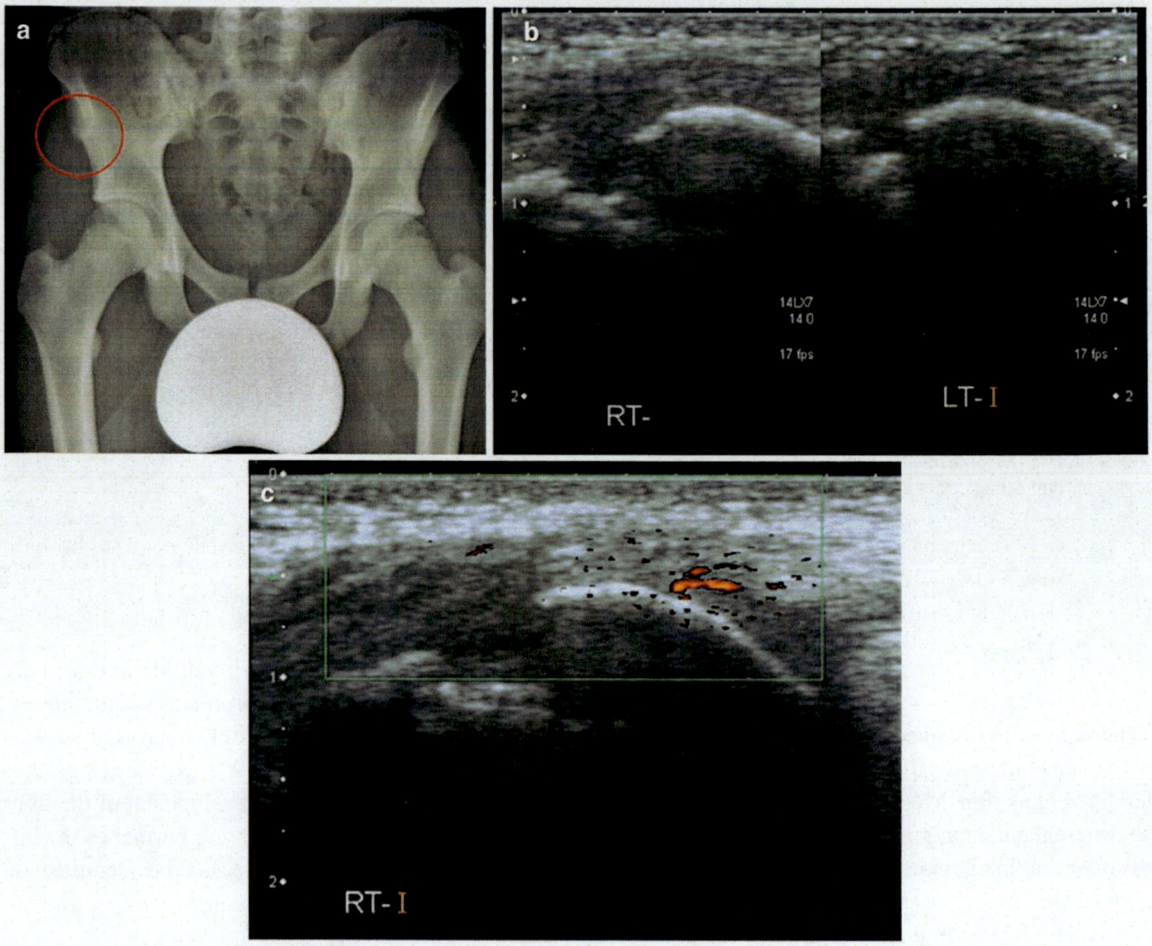

Fig. 3 Whilst the conventional radiograph (**a**) shows minor irregularity (circle), the ultrasound of the anterior inferior iliac spine shows widening (**b**) and increased vascularity on colour Doppler (**c**) compared to the normal side

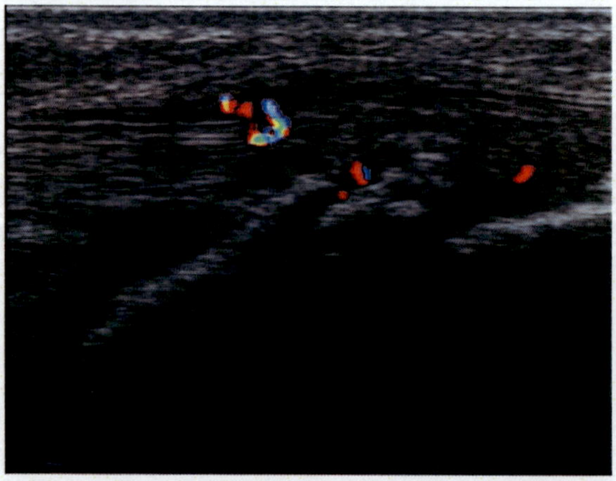

Fig. 4 Osgood–Schlatter's disease with a distal patellar tendinopathy shown by the reduced echogenicity and the neovascularisation on colour Doppler

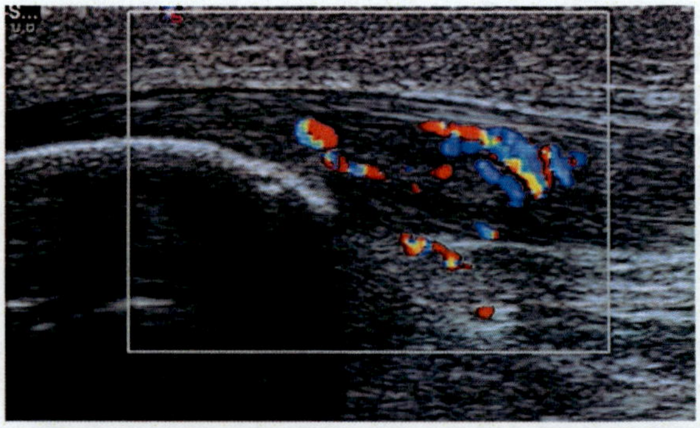

Fig. 5 Proximal patellar tendinopathy with neovascularisation on colour Doppler ultrasound

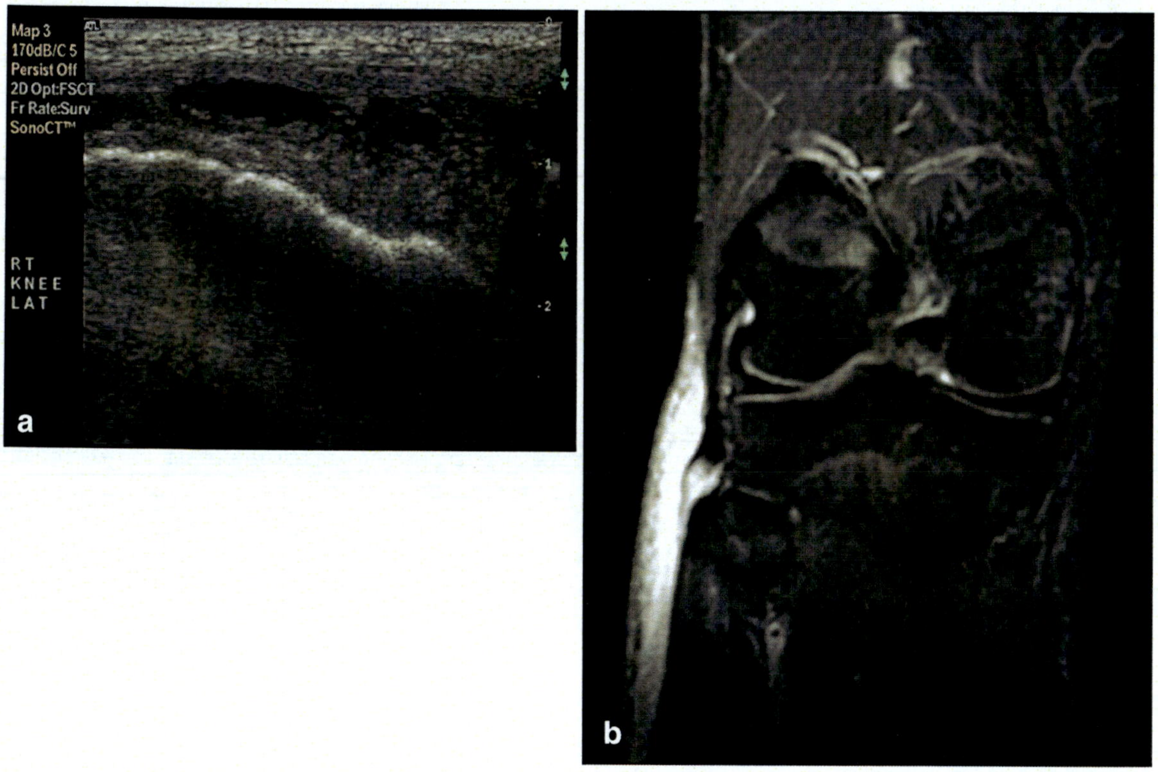

Fig. 6 A tear of the distal aspect of the lateral collateral ligament with liquefying haematoma in the centre on ultrasound (**a**) and an MRI of the same patient showing distal LCL disruption (**b**)

3 Joint Injury

Ultrasound can identify effusions within joints which may signal the presence of an occult fracture missed on plain radiography. Or indeed can assess the presence of an arthropathy with synovitis and neovascularisation. For these purposes the utility of ultrasound examination far exceeds the performance of other methods and is the technique of choice (Allen and Wilson 2007; Babyn and Doria 2005).

Hip pain in the child can have a number of causes and may be thought to be sport related. However in the 4 to 8 year old age group Perthes disease should be considered. In this disease 50% of patients will have an effusion. Irregularity of the epiphysis due to fragmentation may be detected with ultrasound in comparison to the other hip, but an MRI is the gold standard in the assessment of this disease, especially in the early stages where there may be necrosis of the femoral head, oedema and enlargement of the articular cartilage in comparison to the normal hip (Wirth et al. 1992; Terjesen 1993). Ultrasound may overlook the bone oedema that is an early sign, and any child with hip pain that cannot be explained by ultrasound examination should be considered for an MR study.

In the adolescent a slipped upper femoral epiphysis should be considered, especially in children between 12 and 16. It is safe to say that this condition does not occur under the age of 8. An effusion may be seen in approximately 70% of patients. Ultrasound may detect a slip of the epiphysis in comparison to the normal side, but a frog lateral radiograph is the preferred imaging (Terjesen 1992; Castriota-Scanderbeg and Orsi 1993). On occasion, MRI of the hip may be needed to confirm more subtle or early cases. This has significant impact on the patient whether sporting or not. In fact approximately 60% will have bilateral slipped upper femoral epiphysis and therefore imaging of the other side is recommended.

In unexplained hip pain apophyseal traction injuries should also be considered as discussed above. Osteomyelitis, tumours and pelvic disease may mimic hip symptoms. The serious diseases may be reasonably excluded by a normal MR examination (Jaramillo et al. 1995; Lang et al. 1998).

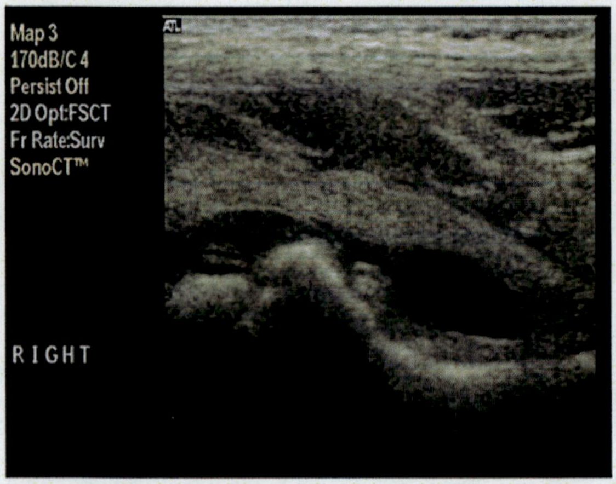

Fig. 7 An effusion and irregularity of the epiphysis in a case of Perthes disease

The majority of patients who develop painful hips in childhood have a transient synovitis which causes an effusion (Fig. 7). Ultrasound will detect this and can be used to guide an aspiration of this effusion (Fink et al. 1995; Berman et al. 1995). This can give immediate relief of pain and stop the effect of tamponade on the femoral vessels which has been cited as a potential cause of necrosis of the femoral head. More importantly however, aspiration of the hip can exclude the rare occurrence of a septic arthritis which may not be detected by any other means. It is not uncommon for the patient with septic arthritis to have normal laboratory signs in the early stages of infection, for example the ESR, CRP and white cell count are often normal.

Ultrasound examination should therefore be considered as the best screening test in the child with hip pain and can safely be used as the first-line imaging in the under 8 year olds when there is no significant history of trauma. When an injury occurs, a combination of ultrasound examination and conventional radiographs are important. Over the age of 8 a frog lateral view is important. If the symptoms cannot be explained by these examinations, then MR is an important next step (Alexander et al 1989). MR arthrography should be reserved for the very rare occasions when a labral tear is considered (Kocher and Tucker 2006).

Ultrasound can be used to look for an effusion within the knee but will not detect ACL, posterior cruciate ligament, articular surface or meniscal lesions adequately. Ultrasound is useful in the assessment of soft tissue lumps around the knee. It will determine whether the lesion is cystic or solid and can locate the origin of some masses around the knee, for example popliteal cysts or parameniscal cysts which can occur within this age group (Handy 2001). Ultrasound is the best way of imaging the rotator cuff in childhood.

Subdeltoid-subacromial bursitis and rotator cuff tears have been identified due to repetitive sporting activity, such as tennis players or overhead racket players. However as the unstable shoulder is potentially due to glenoid labrum or bone lesions, MR arthrography is the preferred way of imaging those with symptoms of apprehension on movement or recurrent dislocation.

4 Bone Injury

4.1 Spine

Ultrasound is not useful in injuries or the overuse syndrome of the spine. For back pain MRI is the preferred way of imaging. The most common lesions in children are pars interarticularis defects. Early detection of bone oedema, i.e. before the defect occurs, will allow appropriate reduction of athletic activity and healing. This is a particular problem in young gymnasts or adolescent fast bowlers (cricket) (Fig. 8).

Adolescent disc prolapse is rare but a disorder that is very often overlooked. It can be associated with a ring apophyseal fracture (Chang et al. 2008). The prolapse will generate severe local spasm and scoliosis. Flexibility of the spine in children allows the back to curve and avoid nerve compression. Back pain is very rare in children and all cases merit examination by an MRI (Fig. 9).

4.2 Entheses

If the patient presents with knee pain then clinical assessment is important in directing the correct imaging.

A diagnosis of Osgood Schlatter's disease or Sinding–Larsen–Johansson can be made clinically but

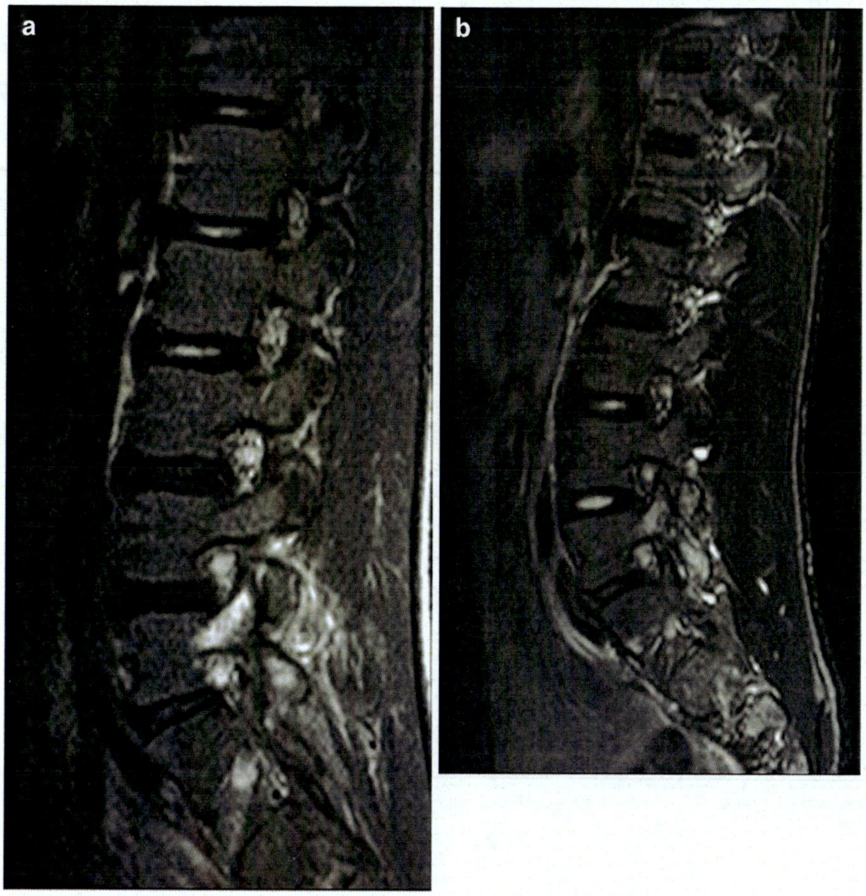

Fig. 8 An MRI showing oedema within the pars interarticularis in an adolescent gymnast (**a**). Six months later, a defect in the pars has occurred because the gymnast continued activity (**b**)

ultrasound can help the diagnosis without the use of radiation and may ascertain the presence of an associated patellar tendinopathy. These diagnoses show fragmentation of the bone at the site of these avulsion injuries of the developing secondary ossification centres, at the tibial tuberosity or the inferior pole of the patella (Abalo et al. 2008) (Fig. 10).

Sometimes pain in one area may be referred from other areas, so pain within the knee may be referred from the spine or the hip (Fig. 11). Clinical examination of the more proximal structures is often indicated.

4.3 Stress Injury

Stress fractures should also be considered especially in the adolescent female who may be anorexic due to their sport and excess training or have been using sport as a method of losing weight. Stress fractures in the peripheral skeleton can be identified with ultrasound. For example a stress fracture of the metatarsal can be detected by the periosteal reaction and the neovascularisation along the bone with a slight break in the cortex. The advantage of an ultrasound examination is that the patient can be assessed at the precise site of pain and symptoms may easily be correlated with the findings (Fig. 12).

Stress fractures seem to be more commonplace in Association football (soccer) and Rugby football even in children. This is thought to be due to boot design (Low et al. 2004).This is most common in the fifth metatarsal, but an apophysitis at the insertion of the peroneus brevis tendon at the base of the fifth metatarsal may produce similar symptoms. Opening of the epiphysis when compared to the normal side may be the only finding. Ultrasound examination is especially useful as in the growing skeleton all these sites have

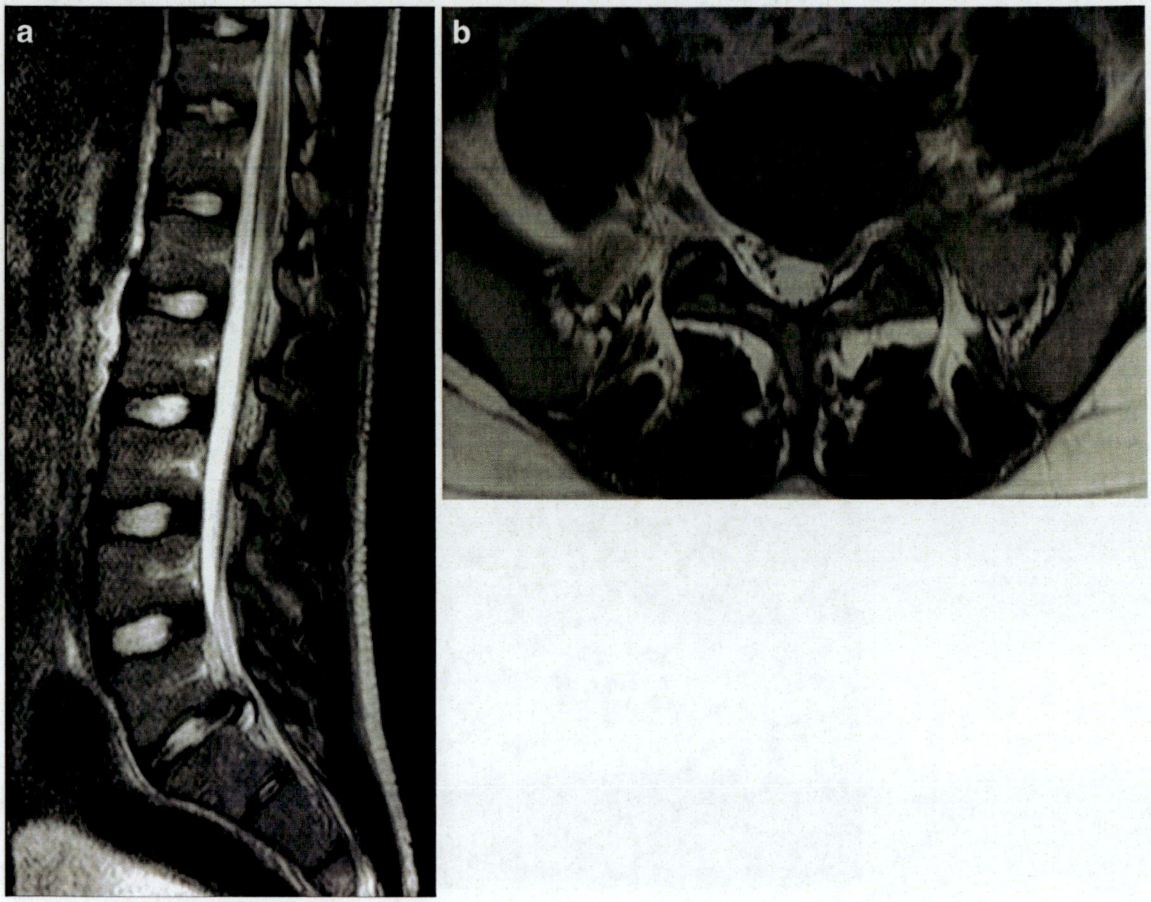

Fig. 9 An MRI showing a disc hernia in a 12-year-old child

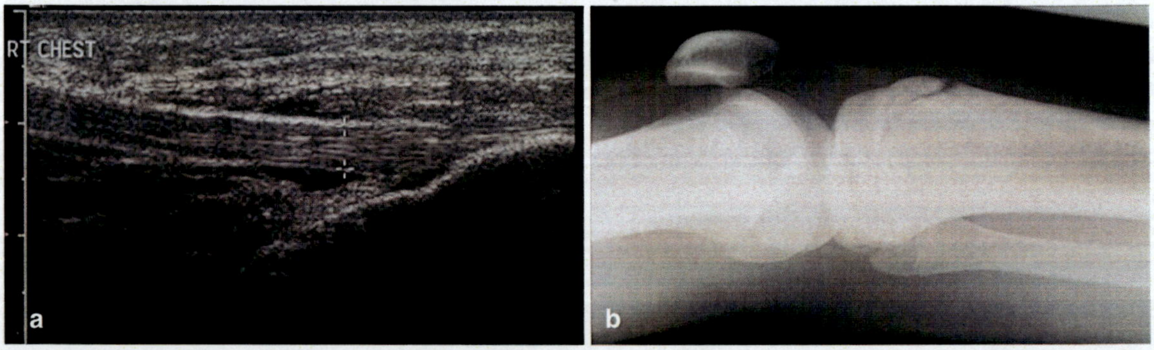

Fig. 10 An acute injury of the tibial tuberosity in a 13-year-old male. Note the fluid surrounding the distal patella tendon on ultrasound (**a**) and the swelling adjacent to the anterior tibial cortex on a radiograph (**b**)

high signal on T2-w MR images and MR often does not cover the opposite side. Arguably ultrasound is the best way to look for entheseal or epiphyseal separation (Pisacano and Miller 2003).

4.4 Fractures

Fractures can be seen using ultrasound. When the diagnosis has not been considered at the time of the

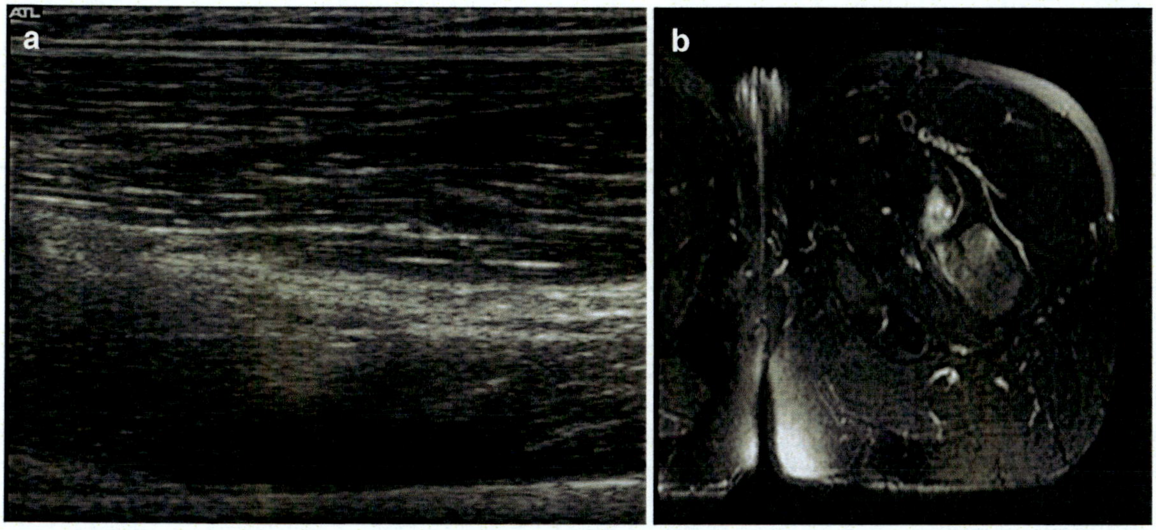

Fig. 11 Traumatic avulsion of the lesser trochanter in a gymnast. Ultrasound examination shows irregularity and local haematoma (**a**) and MR demonstrates both soft tissue and bone oedema (**b**). The bone element of the avulsion is hard to identify using MRI

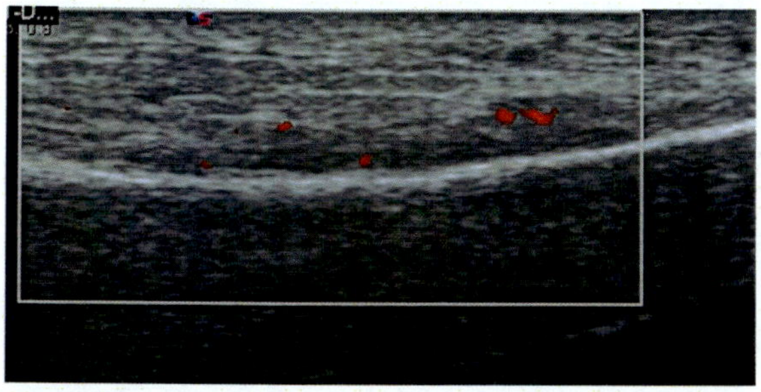

Fig. 12 A stress fracture of the fibula in a young marathon runner. Note the periosteal reaction and hematoma (low echoes paralleling the bone) and the neovascularisation

sporting injury, fractures may be overlooked clinically and they are sometimes first detected using ultrasound. Small avulsion fractures around the hand and wrist in particular can be identified when they were overlooked using conventional radiographs.

5 Mass Lesions

In this young age group other abnormalities can be identified with ultrasound such as painful fingers due to osteochondromas, neuromas of the ulnar nerve, or aneurysms of the ulnar arteries that occur in the squash racket or other racket players (Hammer hamate syndrome) (Muller et al. 1996) (Fig. 9). Ganglions are common even in children and popliteal cysts may also be detected. Both of these entities are fluid, and therefore, easy to distinguish with confidence with ultrasound (Wilson 2005; Allen 2008) (Fig. 13).

6 Conclusion

In our experience the greatest advantage of ultrasound is that it can often allow an imager the chance to talk to the patient in more depth, directing the examination to the point of swelling or pain. We are all guilty of labelling patients with a diagnosis, and sometimes, a negative ultrasound excluding our first diagnosis can be powerful in directing further thoughts. This is just as important in the athlete, as we will give the patient a diagnosis that supports their athletic pursuit and the problem may be unrelated.

Examples of this are a patient referred with peroneal tendinopathy who had normal peroneal tendons and whose pain was identified as related to the mid foot when he was examined by ultrasound. The ultrasound proposed that the diagnosis was a tarsal coalition which was confirmed using MRI.

Another athlete developed knee pain and her knee radiograph was reported as normal. Ultrasound examination was unremarkable, but concerns over the areas

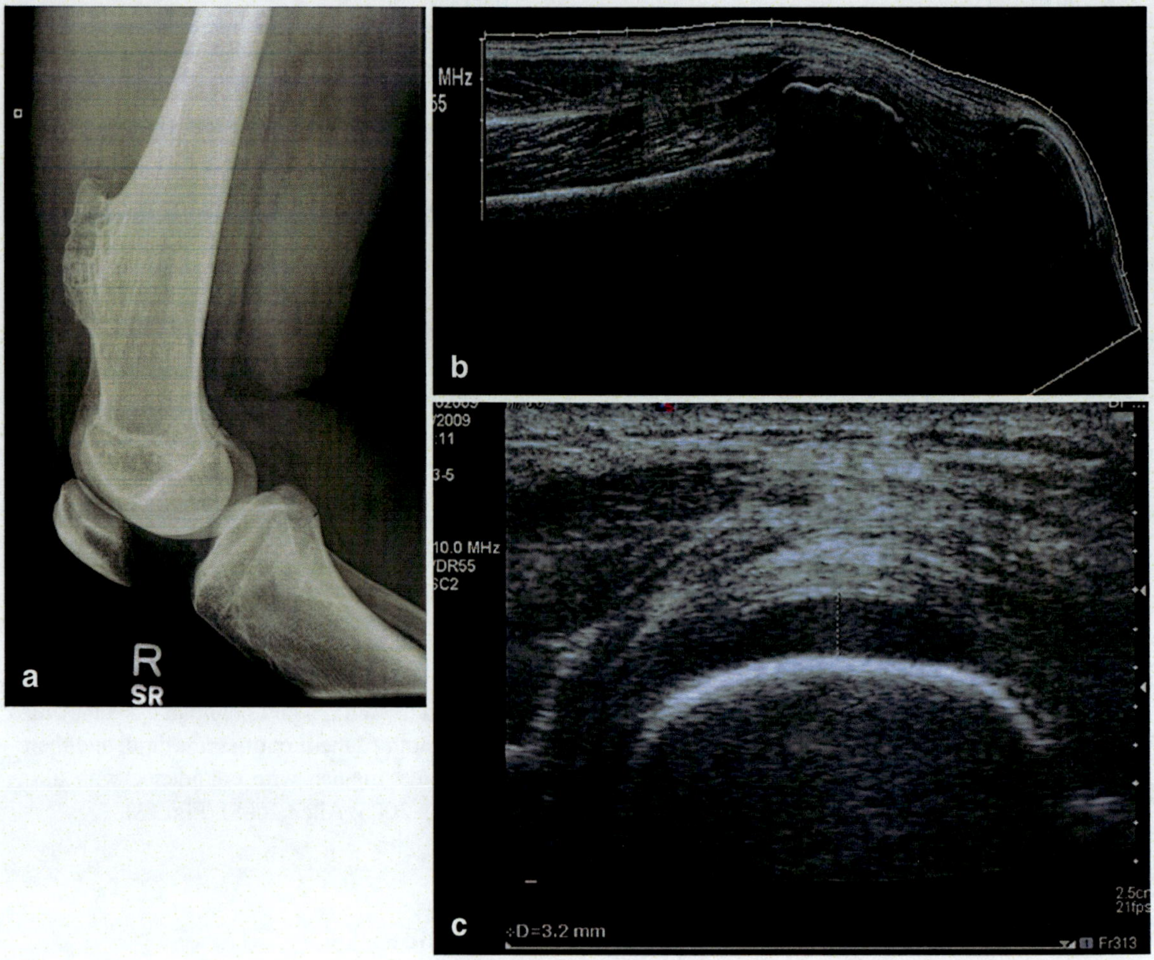

Fig. 13 A large osteochondroma arising from the anterior femur causing pain in a 15-year-old boy on running. Radiograph (**a**), extended field of view ultrasound (**b**) and transverse view showing a cartilage cap of only 3 mm supporting a benign lesion (**c**)

in the knee that cannot be assessed by ultrasound led to referral for an MRI. This showed a primary bone tumour of the proximal tibia.

Ultrasound is an important tool in the management of sporting injuries in children. There will be occasions when it is the only method of imaging required, times when it is an adjunct to other imaging and of course occasions where it is not a useful method (Alfredson and Ohberg 2005). To apply this form of imaging the clinical imager must understand the process of injury, the different nature of the developing musculoskeletal system, anatomy in detail, strengths and weaknesses of other imaging methods and above all have a broad clinical knowledge.

References

Abalo A, Akakpo-numado KG, Dossim A, Walla A, Gnassingbe K, Tekou AH (2008) Avulsion fractures of the tibial tubercle. J Orthop Surg (Hong Kong) 16:308–311

Alexander JE, Seibert JJ, Glasier CM et al (1989) High-resolution hip ultrasound in the limping child. J Clin Ultrasound 17:19–24

Alfredson H, Ohberg L (2005) Neovascularisation in chronic painful patellar tendinosis–promising results after sclerosing neovessels outside the tendon challenge the need for surgery. Knee Surg Sports Traumatol Arthrosc 13:74–80

Allen G (2008) The patient with a soft tissue lump. In: Wilson PBBM (ed) Imaging of the musculoskeletal system. Expert Radiology, Saunders, Elsevier, pp 1670–1678

Allen GM, Wilson DJ (2007) Ultrasound in sports medicine–a critical evaluation. Eur J Radiol 62:79–85

Allen G, Wilson D, Graham R, Jacob D (2005) Paediatric musculoskeletal ultrasound. J Radiol 86:1924–1930
Babyn P, Doria AS (2005) Radiologic investigation of rheumatic diseases. Pediatr Clin North Am 52:373–411, vi
Bellah R (2001) Ultrasound in pediatric musculoskeletal disease: techniques and applications. Radiol Clin North Am 39:597–618, ix
Berman L, Fink AM, Wilson D, McNally E (1995) Technical note: identifying and aspirating hip effusions. Br J Radiol 68:306–310
Bianchi S, Poletti PA, Martinoli C, Abdelwahab IF (2006) Ultrasound appearance of tendon tears. Part 2: lower extremity and myotendinous tears. Skeletal Radiol 35:63–77
Castriota-Scanderbeg A, Orsi E (1993) Slipped capital femoral epiphysis: ultrasonographic findings. Skeletal Radiol 22: 191–193
Chang CH, Lee ZL, Chen WJ, Tan CF, Chen LH (2008) Clinical significance of ring apophysis fracture in adolescent lumbar disc herniation. Spine (Phila Pa 1976) 33:1750–1754
Fink AM, Berman L, Edwards D, Jacobson SK (1995) The irritable hip: immediate ultrasound guided aspiration and prevention of hospital admission. Arch Dis Child 72:110–113, discussion 113–114
Handy JR (2001) Popliteal cysts in adults: a review. Semin Arthritis Rheum 31:108–118
Jaramillo D, Treves ST, Kasser JR, Harper M, Sundel R, Laor T (1995) Osteomyelitis and septic arthritis in children: appropriate use of imaging to guide treatment. AJR Am J Roentgenol 165:399–403
Kocher MS, Tucker R (2006) Pediatric athlete hip disorders. Clin Sports Med 25:241–253, viii
Lang P, Johnston JO, Arenal-Romero F, Gooding CA (1998) Advances in MR imaging of pediatric musculoskeletal neoplasms. Magn Reson Imaging Clin N Am 6:579–604
Low K, Noblin JD, Browne JE, Barnthouse CD, Scott AR (2004) Jones fractures in the elite football player. J Surg Orthop Adv 13:156–160
McKinney BI, Nelson C, Carrion W (2009) Apophyseal avulsion fractures of the hip and pelvis. Orthopedics 32:42
Micheli A, Trapani S, Brizzi I, Campanacci D, Resti M, de Martino M (2009) Myositis ossificans circumscripta: a paediatric case and review of the literature. Eur J Pediatr 168: 523–529
Muller LP, Rudig L, Kreitner KF, Degreif J (1996) Hypothenar hammer syndrome in sports. Knee Surg Sports Traumatol Arthrosc 4:167–170
Pisacano RM, Miller TT (2003) Comparing sonography with MR imaging of apophyseal injuries of the pelvis in four boys. AJR Am J Roentgenol 181:223–230
Posthumus M, September AV, O'Cuinneagain D, van der Merwe W, Schwellnus MP, Collins M (2009) The COL5A1 gene is associated with increased risk of anterior cruciate ligament ruptures in female participants. Am J Sports Med 37:2234–2240
Prince JS, Laor T, Bean JA (2005) MRI of anterior cruciate ligament injuries and associated findings in the pediatric knee: changes with skeletal maturation. AJR Am J Roentgenol 185:756–762
Renstrom P, Ljungqvist A, Arendt E et al (2008) Non-contact ACL injuries in female athletes: an International Olympic Committee current concepts statement. Br J Sports Med 42:394–412
Sanders TG, Zlatkin MB (2008) Avulsion injuries of the pelvis. Semin Musculoskelet Radiol 12:42–53
Sofka CM (2004) Ultrasound in sports medicine. Semin Musculoskelet Radiol 8:17–27
Terjesen T (1992) Ultrasonography for diagnosis of slipped capital femoral epiphysis. Comparison with radiography in 9 cases. Acta Orthop Scand 63:653–657
Terjesen T (1993) Ultrasonography in the primary evaluation of patients with Perthes disease. J Pediatr Orthop 13:437–443
Wilson D (2005) Paediatric musculoskeletal disease with an emphasis on ultrasound. Springer, Berlin
Wirth T, LeQuesne GW, Paterson DC (1992) Ultrasonography in Legg-Calve-Perthes disease. Pediatr Radiol 22:498–504

Shoulder: Sports-Related Injuries in Children and Adolescents

Amy Liebeskind, Varand Ghazikhanian, Shobi Zaidi, Usha Chundru, and Javier Beltran

Contents

A. Liebeskind (✉), V. Ghazikhanian, S. Zaidi, and J. Beltran
Department of Radiology, Maimonides Medical Center,
4802 Tenth Avenue, Brooklyn, NY 11219, USA
e-mail: amyliebeskind@yahoo.com

U. Chundru
San Francisco Magnetic Resonance Center, 1180 Post Street,
San Francisco, CA 94109, USA

A.H. Karantanas (ed.), *Sports Injuries in Children and Adolescents*,
Med Radiol Diagn Imaging, DOI: 10.1007/174_2010_12, © Springer-Verlag Berlin Heidelberg 2011

Key Points

- Pediatric shoulder sports injuries may be due to acute *macrotrauma* or *repetitive microtrauma*.
- *Anterior glenohumeral* joint dislocations as well as associated *Hill-Sachs, Bankart and multiple Bankart variant* lesions such as *Perthes, GLAD and ALPSA* may occur acutely.
- *Posterior glenohumeral* joint dislocations, as well as associated *reverse Hill-Sachs, reverse Bankart and POLPSA* may also occur.
- Skeletally immature individuals may sustain fracture injuries to the open physes (*Salter–Harris fractures*) of the humeral head, glenoid, coracoid and acromion.
- Children also sustain *clavicle fractures, acromioclavicular joint separations*, and less likely, *osteolysis of the distal clavicle and sternoclavicular joint separations.*
- *Myotendinous and myofascial strains,* as well as *soft tissue hematomas* also occur in children and adolescents. Chronic overuse injuries include *proximal humeral epiphysiolysis* (little league shoulder), *rotator cuff tendinopathy and impingement* as well as *rotator cuff tears.*
- *Anterior, posterior and multidirectional instability* may also occur.

Abbreviations

AC	Acromioclavicular
ALPSA	Anterior labroligamentous periosteal sleeve avulsion
CC	Coracoclavicular

GLAD	Glenolabral articular disruption
MRI	Magnetic resonance imaging
POLPSA	Posterior labroscapular periosteal sleeve avulsion
SC	Sternoclavicular
SH	Salter–Harris

1 Introduction

Sports injuries of the shoulder in children and adolescents differ from athletic injuries in adults due to anatomic differences in the growing skeleton. A thorough understanding of the anatomy and biomechanics of the shoulder in skeletally immature individuals is necessary to understand the pathophysiology, and imaging characteristics of the pediatric shoulder sports injuries.

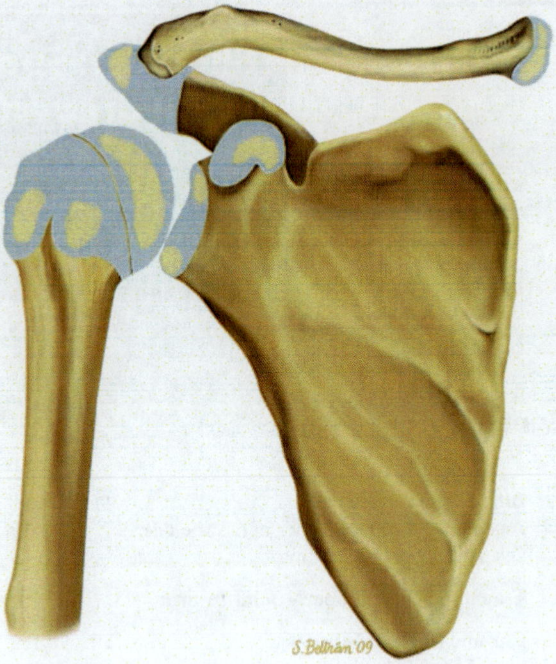

Fig. 1 Primary ossification centers of the proximal humerus, greater tuberosity and lesser tuberosity, which unite between the ages of 5–7 to form the proximal humeral epiphysis. Ossification centers of the acromion, coracoid, and glenoid are also illustrated

1.1 Anatomy and Biomechanics of the Shoulder

The humeral head originates from the primary ossification centers of the proximal humerus, greater tuberosity and lesser tuberosity, which unite between the ages of 5–7 to form the proximal humeral epiphysis. The physis between the proximal humeral epiphysis and metaphysis fuses between the ages of 14 and 17 in females and 16 and 18 in males (Fig. 1) (Chen and Diaz 2005; Webb and Mooney 2003).

The glenohumeral joint lacks the osseous stabilizing structures present in other joints and instead is stabilized by the muscles and ligaments attaching to the humerus, providing superior mobility while sacrificing stability (Herring 2008; Chen and Diaz 2005; Paterson and Waters 2000). There are static and dynamic stabilizers of the glenohumeral joint. The capsule, glenohumeral ligaments, and labrum provide static stability, while the deltoid, rotator cuff, long head of the biceps, and scapulothoracic muscles provide dynamic stability (Herring 2008; Chen and Diaz 2005; Paterson and Waters 2000; Jobe et al. 1998). Static stabilizers provide support during the extremes of motion, while dynamic stabilizers provide support during midrange of motion (Chen and Diaz 2005; Jobe et al. 1998).

The labrum deepens the socket circumferentially, and is the attachment point for the capsuloligamentous structures as well as the long head of the biceps tendon. Inferior and posterior translation of the humeral head in the adducted arm is prevented by the anterosuperior capsule and the rotator cuff interval structures (Chen and Diaz 2005; Jobe et al. 1998; O'Brien et al. 1990). Anteroposterior translation during abduction is prevented by the middle glenohumeral ligament during the midrange of external rotation, while the inferior glenohumeral ligament provides the same role (as well as preventing inferior translation) during abduction and maximal external rotation (Chen and Diaz 2005; O'Brien et al. 1990). The posterior capsule prevents posterior translation in the adducted, internally rotated and forward flexed arm (Chen and Diaz 2005).

The supraspinatus muscle abducts the humerus, while the infraspinatus and teres minor muscles externally rotate and flex the humerus, providing posterior dynamic glenohumeral stability. The subscapularis muscle internally rotates the humerus and provides anterior dynamic stability. The deltoid and scapulothoracic muscles position the scapula and provide stability at the glenohumeral articulation (Chen and Diaz 2005; Jobe et al. 1998; DiGiovine et al. 1992).

1.2 Overhead Throwing Motion

Overhead throwing techniques vary in different sports, but are fundamentally similar. The most studied throwing technique is the baseball pitch, which is divided into five phases (Fig. 2) (Chen and Diaz 2005; DiGiovine et al. 1992; Meister 2000).

Phase one is the windup portion in which the shoulder is in slight internal rotation with minimal muscle activity. Phase two is the early cocking stage, which begins when the ball leaves the nondominant hand and ends when the forward foot contacts the ground. The shoulder begins to abduct and rotate externally (Chen and Diaz 2005; Jobe et al. 1998; DiGiovine et al. 1992; Meister 2000). The deltoid is activated followed by the supraspinatus, infraspinatus, and teres minor (Chen and Diaz 2005; Jobe et al. 1998; DiGiovine et al. 1992; Meister 2000). In the late cocking phase (third stage) there is further abduction and maximal external rotation of the shoulder. The activity levels of the supraspinatus, infraspinatus, and teres minor peak during the late cocking phase, and the activity of the subscapularis and periscapularis muscles also increases. The increased activity levels of the rotator cuff muscles generate significant shearing forces across the anterior shoulder (Chen and Diaz 2005; Jobe et al. 1998; DiGiovine et al. 1992; Meister 2000). The long head of the biceps and the subscapularis help stabilize the

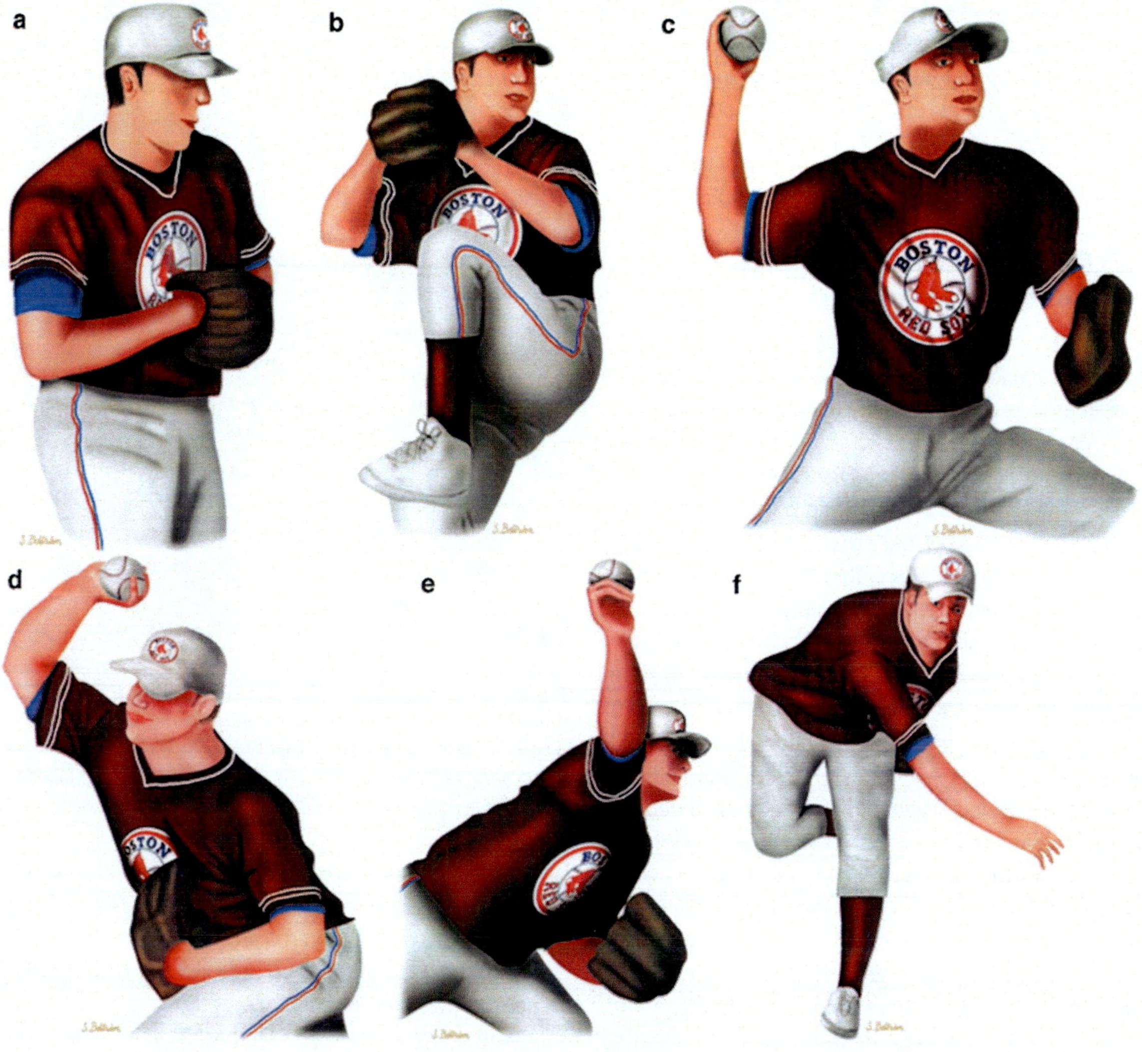

Fig. 2 The fundamental phases of the overhand throwing motion: (**a**) at rest. (**b**) Phase 1: the windup phase. (**c**) Phase 2: the early cocking phase. (**d**) Phase 3: the late cocking phase. (**e**) Phase 4: the acceleration phase. (**f**) Phase 5: the follow-through phase

glenohumeral joint in the late cocking phase (Chen and Diaz 2005; Jobe et al. 1998; DiGiovine et al. 1992; Itoi et al. 1993; Meister 2000). The fourth stage is the acceleration phase, where significant forward force is generated on the extremity, which results in internal rotation and adduction of the humerus. The activity levels of the periscapularis and subscapularis muscles peak in the acceleration phase (Chen and Diaz 2005; Jobe et al. 1998; Meister 2000; Pappas et al. 1985). The final phase is the follow-through phase, where the upper extremity decelerates and ends with completion of movement with the shoulder in maximal internal rotation. The posterior rotator cuff muscles as well as the deltoid, latissimus dorsi and subscapularis muscles stabilize the glenohumeral joint and prevent subluxation during the deceleration phase (Chen and Diaz 2005; DiGiovine et al. 1992; Itoi et al. 1993). A significant amount of torque is generated across the glenohumeral joint as the arm decelerates (Chen and Diaz 2005; Pappas et al. 1985).

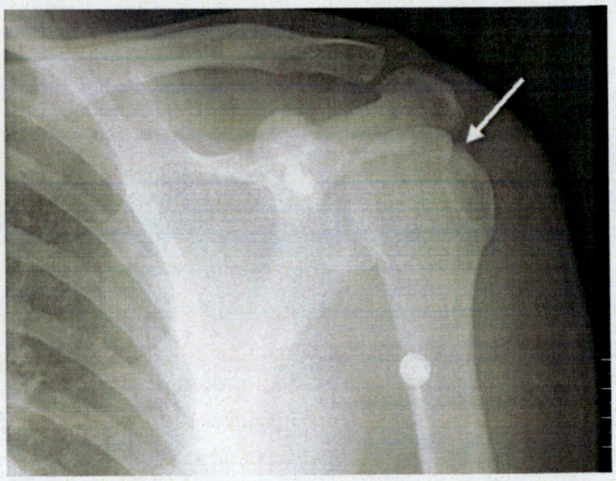

Fig. 3 Hill-Sachs fracture. AP radiograph of the shoulder reveals a fracture deformity of the superior posterolateral humeral head (*arrow*), after an anteroinferior glenohumeral dislocation

2 Traumatic Glenohumeral Joint Injuries

Traumatic glenohumeral joint dislocation is more common in adolescents who play contact sports and rare in younger children (Herring 2008; Gomez 2002; Marans and Angel 1992; Chen and Diaz 2005; Paterson and Waters 2000). Children with open physes are more likely to sustain a fracture of the proximal humerus during a traumatic dislocation. More than 90% of glenohumeral joint dislocations are anterior. Anterior dislocations are almost always caused by indirect force to an arm in the abducted, extended and externally rotated position. Other mechanisms include a fall on the outstretched arm or a blow to the posterior shoulder (Herring 2008; Gomez 2002; Marans and Angel 1992; Chen and Diaz 2005; Paterson and Waters 2000). Anterior dislocation is usually diagnosed on anteroposterior radiographs and can be confirmed on scapular Y and axillary views. During an anterior dislocation, the humeral head may strike the anteroinferior glenoid rim, and can produce a fracture of the superior posterolateral humeral head (Hill-Sachs fracture) (Fig. 3) (Greenspan 2004).

Hill-Sachs deformities are best visualized on an AP view with the arm in internal rotation, and can be confirmed on CT or MRI. On MRI, Hill-Sachs deformities are best seen on coronal oblique or axial images. Fracture of the anterior inferior osseous glenoid may also occur (osseous Bankart lesion) (Fig. 4) (Greenspan 2004), best visualized on AP radiographs with the arm in neutral position (Fig. 5).

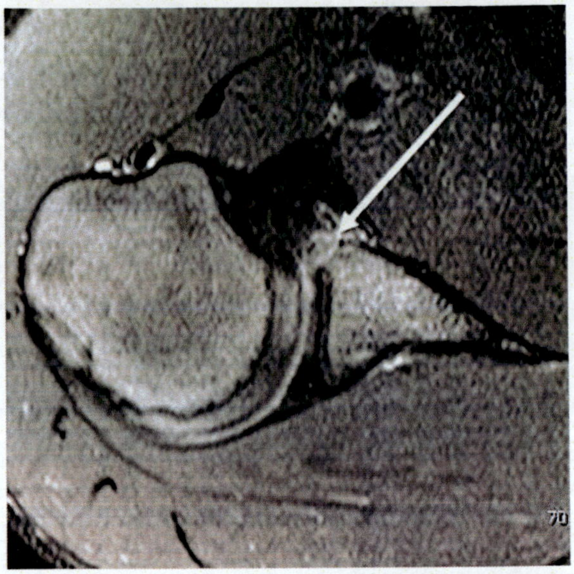

Fig. 4 Osseous Bankart lesion in a 16-year-old male after an anterior glenohumeral dislocation injury during a football game. The axial fat-saturated PD-w MR image of the shoulder reveals a fracture deformity of the anterior inferior osseous glenoid (*arrow*)

Cartilaginous Bankart lesions occur when the anteroinferior labrum is torn in the absence of osseous injury, and are detectable on MRI. A true Bankart lesion

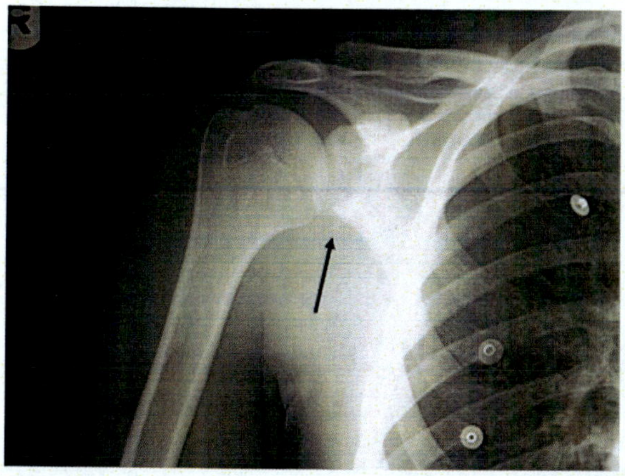

Fig. 5 Osseous Bankart lesion. AP radiograph of the shoulder reveals a fracture of the anterior inferior osseous glenoid with adjacent osseous fragment (*arrow*)

involves separation of the anteroinferior labrum from the underlying glenoid with periosteal disruption. Bankart variant lesions such as Perthes and anterior labroligamentous periosteal sleeve avulsion (ALPSA), as well as glenolabral articular disruption (GLAD) lesions are also best visualized on MRI. The Perthes lesion occurs when the scapular periosteum remains intact but is stripped medially, and the anterior labrum is avulsed from the glenoid but remains partially attached to the scapula by the intact periosteum, and the labrum may assume a normal position.

In ALPSA, there is an avulsion of the anterior labrum from the anteroinferior glenoid with an intact anterior scapular periosteum that has been stripped from the bone, but is still attached to the labrum. The anterior labroligamentous complex displaces medially and rotates inferiorly on the scapular neck (Helms et al. 2001). Finally, a GLAD may occur, which is a tear of the anterior inferior labrum with a glenoid chondral defect (Fig. 6).

Posterior glenohumeral joint dislocation is much more rare, and is usually due to direct force to the anterior shoulder, or indirect force applied to the arm with adduction, flexion and internal rotation (Herring 2008). Posterior dislocation may occur in patients sustaining electrical shock or seizure. During a posterior glenohumeral dislocation, the humeral head translates posterior to the glenoid fossa and often impacts the posteroinferior rim of the glenoid. This type of dislocation is more difficult to diagnose clinically and radiographically, due to the fact that the overlapping humeral head and glenoid fossa may appear to articulate

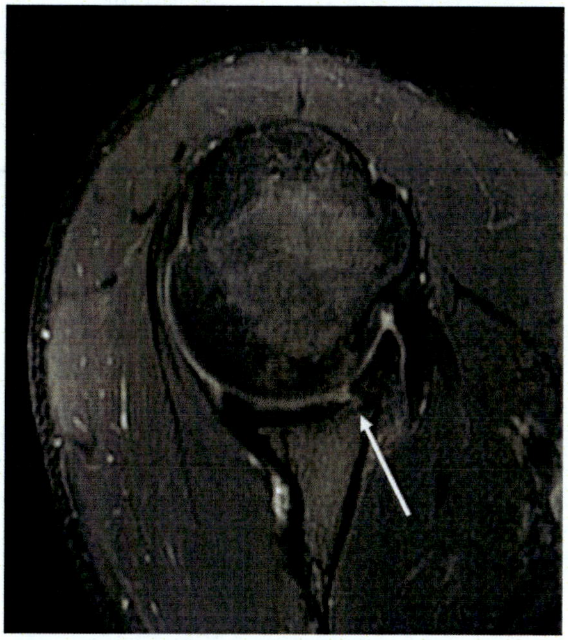

Fig. 6 Glenolabral articular disruption in a 16-year-old male after a football injury. The axial fat-saturated T2-w MR image reveals a tear of the anterior inferior labrum with a glenoid chondral defect (GLAD) (*arrow*), a Bankart variant lesion

normally on the AP view (Greenspan 2004). To increase sensitivity for posterior dislocation, the glenoid fossa is imaged in profile by rotating the patient 40° toward the affected side (Greenspan 2004), which will reveal obliteration of the normal glenohumeral joint space in patients with posterior dislocation (Fig. 7).

The axillary view can also be useful in patients with posterior dislocation but is difficult to obtain due to limited abduction of the arm (Greenspan 2004). The impaction of the humeral head on the posterior glenoid may cause fracture of the anteromedial aspect of the humeral head, (reverse Hill-Sachs) producing a "trough line," as well as a fracture of the posterior aspect of the glenoid (reverse Bankart), best seen on AP view with external rotation or the axillary view (Greenspan 2004). CT may directly show the reverse Bankart lesion (Fig. 8).

Posterior dislocation can also result in a posterior labroscapular periosteal sleeve avulsion (POLPSA), instead of a reverse Bankart fracture. POLPSA differs from a reverse Bankart fracture because the periosteum, although stripped, remains intact (Fig. 9).

The most common complication of traumatic dislocation of the glenohumeral joint is recurrent shoulder instability, which may manifest as repetitive episodes of fixed dislocation or symptoms such as a vague sense of

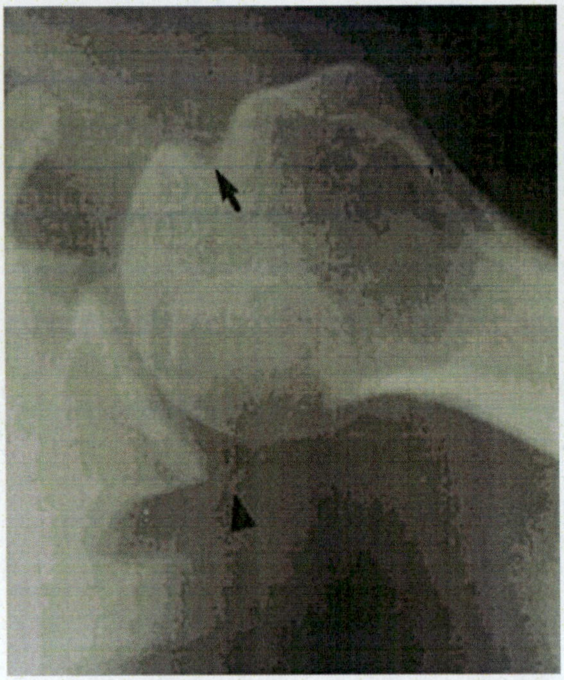

Fig. 7 Reverse Hill-Sachs fracture. An axillary view radiograph of the shoulder (status postreduction of a posterior glenohumeral dislocation) reveals a fracture deformity in the anteromedial aspect of the humeral head (*arrow*), caused by impact with the posterior glenoid (*arrowhead*)

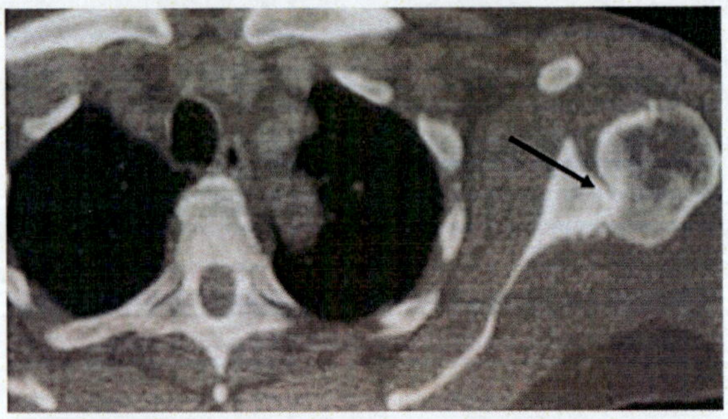

Fig. 8 Posterior dislocation. Axial CT image of the shoulder reveals a posterior glenohumeral dislocation with a fracture deformity in the anteromedial aspect of the humeral head (*arrow*), a reverse Hill-Sachs fracture

shoulder dysfunction or pain (Herring 2008). Recurrent shoulder instability may occur in 20–90% of adolescents and up to 100% in younger children with open physes (Herring 2008; Chen and Diaz 2005; Wagner and Lyne 1983; Greenspan 2004; Marans and Angel 1992; Paterson and Waters 2000), most often reflecting lack of complete healing of an anteroinferior labral avulsion as well as capsular laxity and incompetence

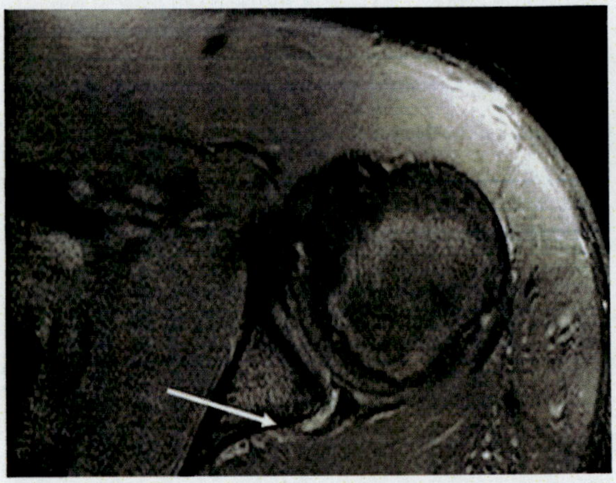

Fig. 9 Posterior labroscapular periosteal sleeve avulsion (POLPSA) in a 17-year-old male with shoulder instability. The oblique axial fat-saturated PD-w MR image reveals stripping of the posterior labroscapular periosteum. Unlike a reverse Bankart injury, the periosteum is still intact (*arrow*)

(Herring 2008; Paterson and Waters 2000; Krabak and Alexander 2008). Other complications include neurovascular injuries, most commonly involving the axillary nerve, and osteonecrosis of the humeral head (Herring 2008; Greenspan 2004).

3 Chronic Overuse Injuries

The most common overuse injuries of the shoulder in children are proximal humeral epiphysiolysis, rotator cuff tendinopathy and impingement, rotator cuff tears, anterior glenohumeral instability, posterior glenohumeral instability and multidirectional shoulder instability.

3.1 Little League Shoulder

Proximal humeral epiphysiolysis, also known as Little League shoulder, osteochondrosis of the proximal humerus and traction apophysitis of the proximal humerus is due to repetitive microtrauma in overhead athletes, most commonly in baseball pitchers (Herring 2008; Cassas and Cassettari-Wayhs 2006; Chen and Diaz 2005; Paterson and Waters 2000). It usually presents as nonspecific shoulder pain after throwing. It occurs in excessive throwing, especially after regimen changes, as well as in athletes with poor technique and muscle-tendon imbalance (Herring 2008; Cassas and Cassettari-Wayhs 2006; Chen and Diaz 2005).

On physical examination, patients usually present with point tenderness along the proximal humeral physis and anterolateral shoulder swelling with weakness on resisted abduction and internal rotation. Patients may also develop external rotation contractures with decreased internal rotation (Herring 2008; Cassas and Cassettari-Wayhs 2006; Chen and Diaz 2005).

AP radiographs with external rotation reveal proximal physeal widening. In more severe cases, stress fractures with metaphyseal demineralization and fragmentation as well as physeal irregularity and periosteal reaction can be seen (Herring 2008; Chen and Diaz 2005). These findings are believed to result from rotary torque generated during the cocking and acceleration phases throwing or from deceleration distraction forces during follow-through (Herring 2008). MRI demonstrates focal physeal widening, better seen on coronal and sagittal either fat-suppressed PD/T2-w or T2-w gradient echo sequences. Abnormal high signal on fat-suppressed images is also visualized in the metaphysis adjacent to the focal physeal widening (Figs. 10 and 11)

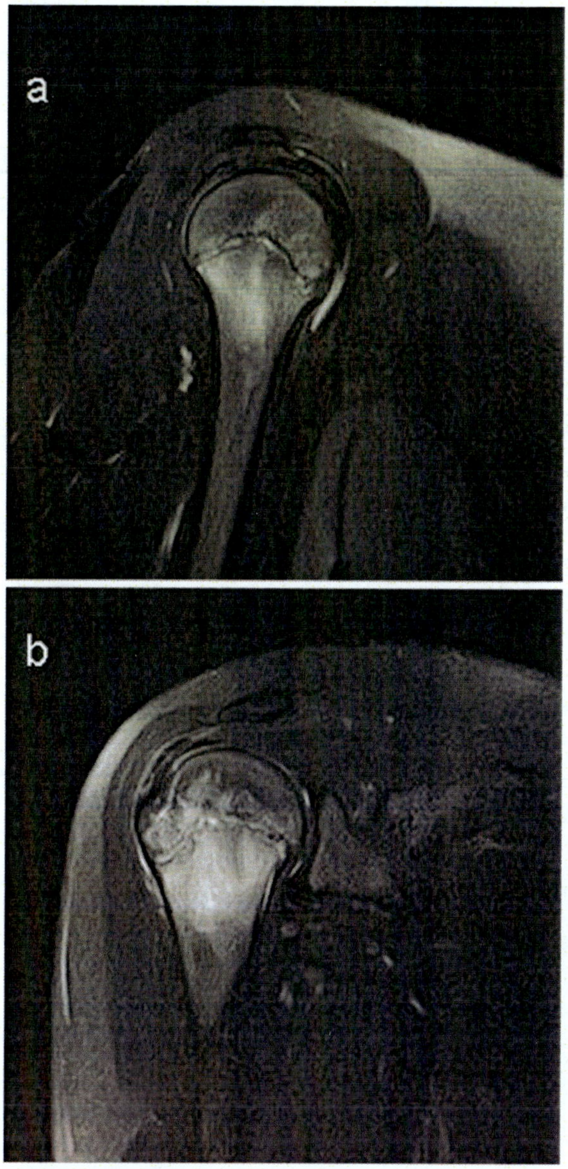

Fig. 10 Proximal humeral epiphysiolysis. (**a**) Sagittal, and (**b**) coronal fat-saturated T2-w MR images of the shoulder reveal focal physeal widening with extension of physeal high signal intensity into the metaphysis

3.2 Rotator Cuff Pathology

Adolescent athletes involved with overhead sports may suffer a variety of rotator cuff overuse injuries, including tendinopathy, myotendinous strains, and in extreme cases, rotator cuff tears. These injuries may result from cumulative tensile overload, outlet impingement, and instability associated with internal impingement (Chen and Diaz 2005). True outlet impingement is uncommon in adolescents (Gomez 2002; Chen and Diaz 2005). More commonly secondary or internal impingement occurs due to multidirectional instability. During abduction in patients with multidirectional instability, the pull of the deltoid muscle causes the humeral head to translate superiorly, trapping the supraspinatus tendon between the humeral head and acromion. This, in turn, causes inflammation or degenerative changes of the supraspinatus tendon, which produces clinical symptoms and signs similar to rotator cuff tendinopathy (Gomez 2002). Differentiating true impingement from underlying instability is essential as the treatments differ (Chen and Diaz 2005).

Patients usually complain of shoulder pain that worsens with activity, as well as possible stiffness and weakness (Chen and Diaz 2005). AP, outlet and axillary X-rays are usually negative. MRI reveals increased signal within the tendon on T2-w images, often with edema in the subacromial space (Chen and Diaz 2005).

Rotator cuff tears are rare in adolescents, making up less than 1% of all rotator cuff tears, but may be missed if not suspected (Gomez 2002; Tarkin and

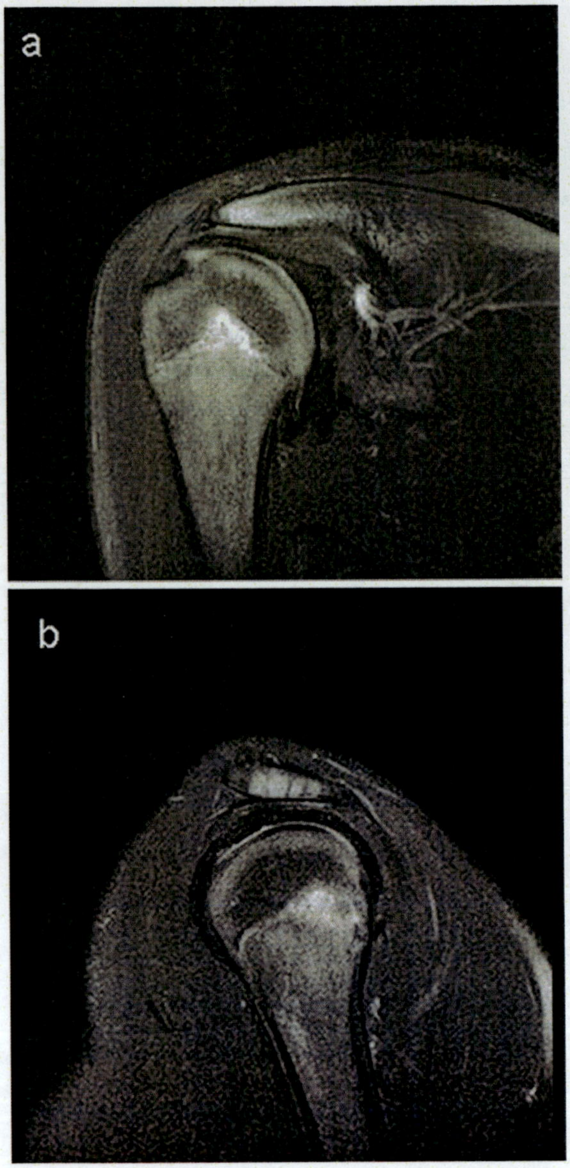

Fig. 11 Proximal humeral epiphysiolysis in a different patient. (**a**) Coronal, and (**b**) sagittal fat-saturated T2-w MR images of the shoulder again reveal focal physeal widening with extension of physeal high signal intensity into the metaphysis

Morganti 2005; Chen and Diaz 2005). In adolescents, significant trauma to the upper extremity must usually be sustained in order to tear the rotator cuff (Chen and Diaz 2005). Rotator cuff tears may also occur in adolescent athletes who perform chronic overhead throwing (Tarkin and Morganti 2005). Many rotator cuff tears in young athletes are due to an avulsion fracture

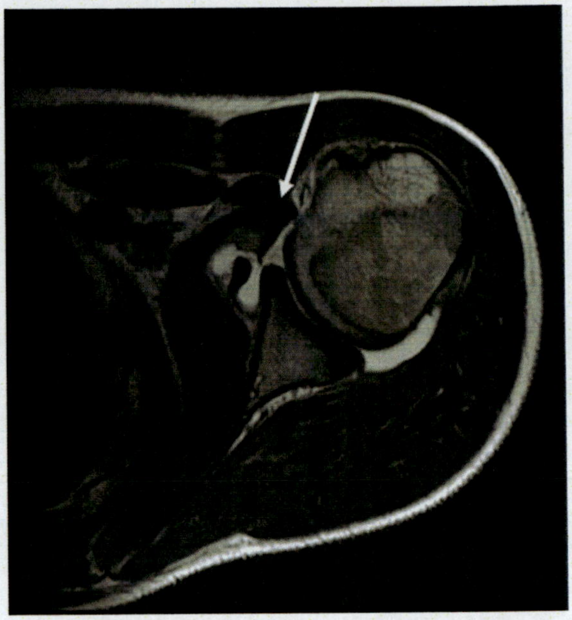

Fig. 12 The axial T2-w MR image of the shoulder reveals an avulsion fracture of the lesser tuberosity apophysis at the site of the subscapularis insertion (*arrow*)

of the lesser tuberosity apophysis with disruption of the subscapularis insertion, due to the relative weakness of the apophyseal physis compared to the myotendinous junction in children and adolescents (Figs. 12 and 13). Supraspinatus and infraspinatus tendon tears are less common but also occur (Levine and Pereira 2005; Tarkin and Morganti 2005).

Plain radiographs are usually normal, unless there is avulsion of the lesser tuberosity, which is best seen in the AP view (Tarkin and Morganti 2005). Occasionally, calcification may be identified adjacent to the affected tendon (Tarkin and Morganti 2005). On MRI, partial or less frequently full thickness tears are manifested by fluid signal defects within the tendon as seen in adult patients (Tarkin and Morganti 2005).

3.3 Anterior Glenohumeral Instability

Anterior glenohumeral instability is also associated with chronic overuse injuries in overhead sports. Usually, excessive and repetitive external rotation during overhead motion causes stress on the anterior

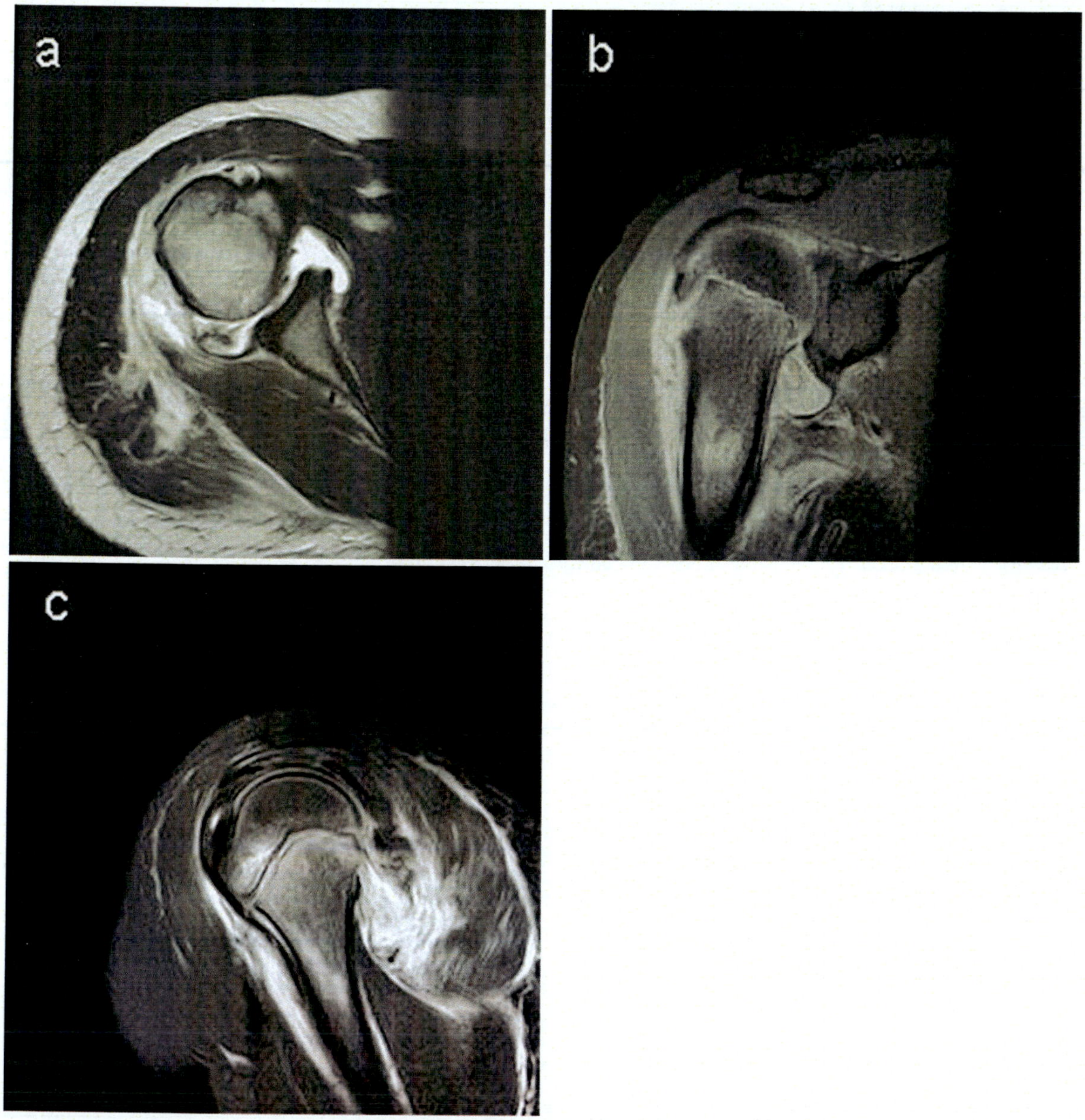

Fig. 13 The axial T2-w (**a**), and fat suppressed oblique coronal (**b**) and sagittal (**c**) MR images of the shoulder reveal avulsion injuries at the teres minor and latissimus dorsi insertions

capsule and ligamentous structures, which causes microtrauma leading to laxity of the ligaments (Chen and Diaz 2005). In the early phase, the dynamic stabilizers compensate for ligamentous laxity. As the muscles fatigue, there is anterior glenohumeral translation, which leads to instability (Chen and Diaz 2005). This may develop into secondary impingement of the rotator cuff anterosuperiorly against the coracoacromial arch during forward flexion, which may cause tendinits or undersurface tears (Chen and Diaz 2005; Ireland and Andrews 1988). Internal impingement of the rotator cuff may also occur as the humeral head translates anteriorly with the shoulder in abduction and external rotation (Chen and Diaz 2005; Jobe et al. 1989). As the static stabilizers become lax and the surrounding muscles begin to fatigue, increased anterior glenohumeral translation with the arm in the apprehension position pinches the cuff against the posterosuperior glenoid rim, causing internal impingement (Chen and Diaz 2005).

Patients usually complain of "dead arm" (lack of strength in the upper arm when it is abducted and externally rotated), or pain in the late cocking and early acceleration phases.

Plain radiographs are usually negative. MRI may show increased signal in the posterior cuff, or show redundancy of the anterior capsule (Chen and Diaz 2005).

3.4 Posterior Glenohumeral Instability

Posterior glenohumeral instability is rare compared to anterior glenohumeral instability, but its incidence has been rising due to chronic microtrauma to the posterior structures in repetitive overhead sports (Chen and Diaz 2005). Rarely, a single traumatic episode may result in posterior capsule injury and subluxation (Chen and Diaz 2005). The mechanism of injury is repetitive eccentric contraction during the deceleration and follow-through phases of throwing, which stretches the posterior capsule and causes microtears in the posterior rotator cuff (Chen and Diaz 2005; Fronek et al. 1989). In the absence of subluxation or posterior labral tears, X-rays and MRI are usually negative (Chen and Diaz 2005).

3.5 Multidirectional Shoulder Instability

Multidirectional shoulder instability is defined as subluxation in more than one direction, in the absence of a major traumatic event (Chen and Diaz 2005; Ireland and Andrews 1988). It usually occurs in athletes with repetitive shoulder abduction and external rotation, such as in gymnastics and swimming (Chen and Diaz 2005). Most of these athletes have underlying physiologic glenohumeral laxity that is exacerbated by microtrauma or by a traumatic insult, causing inability to maintain dynamic stability. These may lead to secondary rotator cuff tears. Patients usually present with vague symptoms such as "dead arm." They may also report a sensation of dislocation and spontaneous reduction.

Unless there is dislocation, X-rays are usually negative. MRI arthrography may reveal a redundant or patulous capsule with increased capsular volume (Chen and Diaz 2005).

4 Soft Tissue Injuries

Common sports-related soft tissue injuries in children and adolescents include soft tissue hematomas and myotendinous strains.

4.1 Soft Tissue Hematomas

Soft tissue injuries such as hematomas, which usually occur after an acute traumatic event, are best evaluated with MRI. MRI characteristics of hematomas vary depending on the temporal stage of the hematoma and the physical state of the hemoglobin in the collection. In the acute phase, up to the first 4 days, deoxyhemoglobin is the dominant molecule type and appears as low T1 and low T2 signal. In the early subacute phase, up to the first week, where methemoglobin is the dominant molecule, there is high T1 and low T2 signal, and in the late subacute phase, up to the first 3 weeks, there is high T1 and T2 signal. Finally, in the chronic phase, where there is hemosiderin, bilirubin and ferritin, there is low T1 and T2 signal with a low signal surrounding ring. After administration of IV contrast, hematomas typically demonstrate peripheral enhancement (Resnick 2002a).

4.2 Myotendinous and Myofascial Strains

In adolescents, myotendinous and myofascial strains occur as they do in adults. Myotendinous and myofascial strains are graded according to severity. In grade I strain, there is microscopic injury to the muscle, tendon or both, without significant loss of strength. On MRI, there is edema or hemorrhage, often at the myotendinous junction, best visualized as high signal on T2-w or STIR sequences. Perifascial fluid may be present (Resnick 2002b). In grade II strain, there is

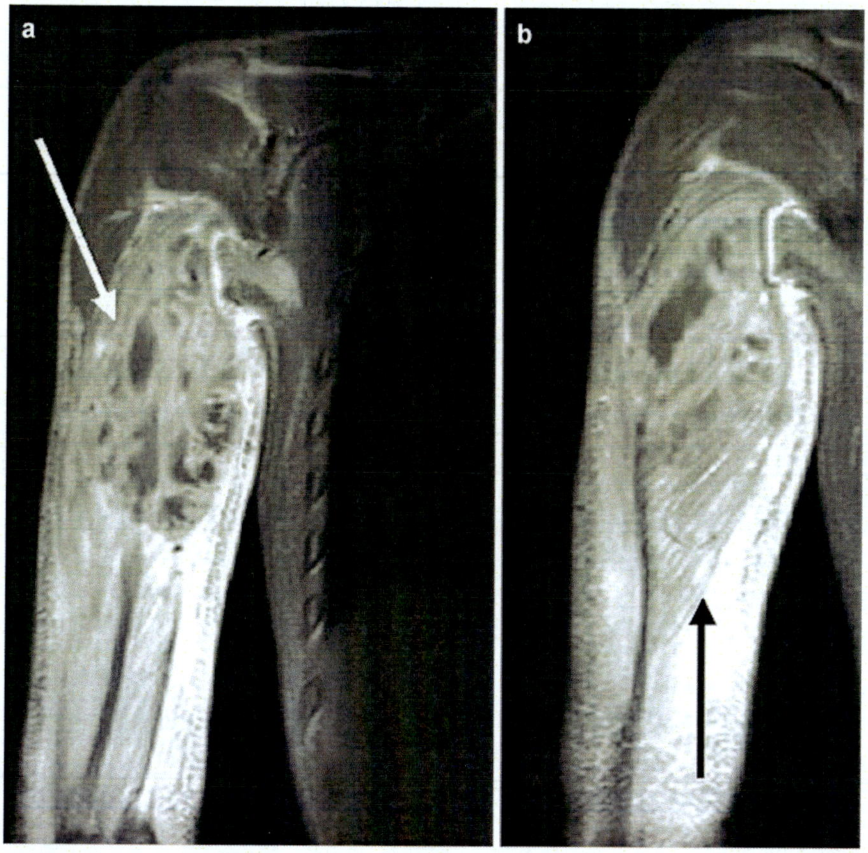

Fig. 14 (**a**) Post-contrast fat-saturated T1-w oblique coronal MR image of an adolescent following a lacrosse injury demonstrates a complex loculated fluid collection with peripheral and internal enhancement (*arrow*), compatible with a hematoma, which is subsequently resolved. (**b**) Also noted is perifascicular enhancement compatible with intramuscular (triceps) edema (*arrow*), creating a feathery appearance consistent with triceps muscular strain

partial thickness tearing of muscle fibers with associated loss of strength. On MRI, there is high T2-w or STIR signal, due to edema and hemorrhage, with disruption of some muscle fibers. There is often hematoma formation at the myotendinous junction as well as perifascial fluid (Resnick 2002b). In grade III strain, there is complete disruption of fibers with or without retraction, with significant associated loss of strength. On MRI there is complete disruption of fibers with fiber laxity. There may be a focal fluid collection within the resultant tendon fiber gap (Resnick 2002b) (Fig. 14).

5 Proximal Humerus Salter–Harris Fractures

The Salter–Harris (SH) classification is used to describe physeal fractures in pediatric patients for the purposes of both management and assessment of possible long-term complications (Rogers and Poznanski 1994). The types of SH fractures include (Fig. 15):

Type I – Transverse fracture through the hypertrophic zone of the physis.

Type II – Fracture extending from the physis into the metaphysis.

Type III – Fracture extending from the physis into the epiphysis.

Type IV – Fracture extending through the epiphysis, physis, and metaphysis.

Type V – Crush injury of the physeal plate.

Older children and adolescents commonly suffer type II SH fractures, whereas infants and small children more frequently sustain SH type I fractures. These two types of fractures account for the majority of physeal injuries. Type I–III fractures do not often damage the growth potential of the physis because they do not interrupt its critical blood supply. Additionally, these fractures rarely result in significant deformity due to the remodeling potential of the glenohumeral joint and

Fig. 15 Coronal section color illustration demonstrating the different Salter–Harris five (SH) physeal fractures

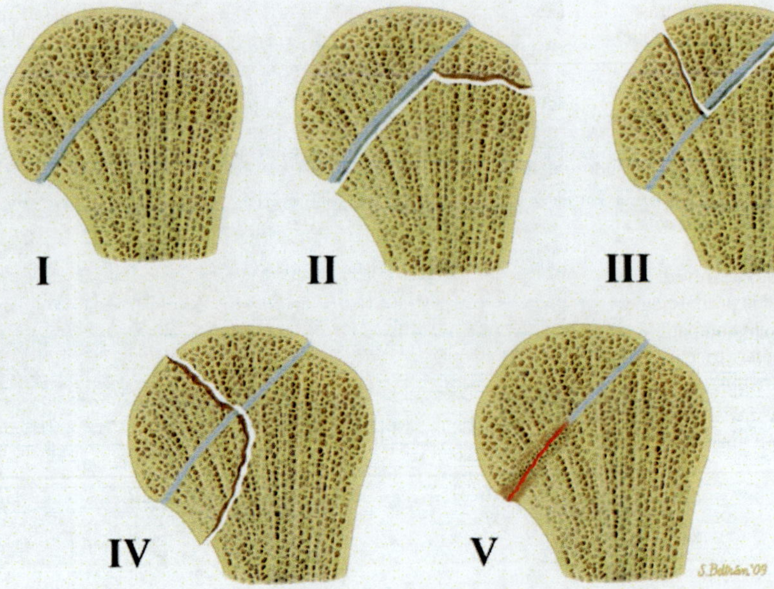

the universal motion of the joint itself (Herring 2008). Fractures that either cross the joint or result in spatial misalignment of portions of the physis (type IV and V) have the worst prognosis but are also the rarest types.

The vast majority of SH fractures are diagnosed with plain film radiography alone. In type I fractures, initial radiographs may only hint at a physeal separation. Follow-up X-rays may be needed to help establish the diagnosis. Type II fractures demonstrate a fracture line in the metaphysis extending to the growth plate. Type III fractures demonstrate a fracture line extending from the physis, through the epiphysis and to the articular surface. Type IV fractures appear as a combination of type II and type III fractures with a fracture line extending from the metaphysis, through the physis and epiphysis, to the articular surface. Type V fracture, similar to type I fractures, may not show a fracture line on initial images. Occasionally, additional imaging is required to guide management and for appropriate surgical planning. In these cases, CT with multiplanar reconstruction and MRI (Figs. 16 and 17) may be useful.

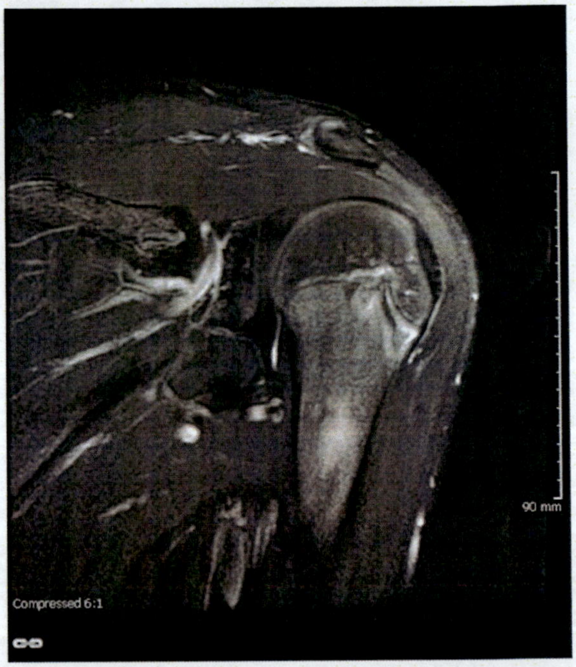

Fig. 16 SH type I fracture. An oblique coronal fat-saturated T2-w MR image of the shoulder demonstrates widening of the physis without an associated fracture of the metaphysis or epiphysis

6 Clavicle

The clavicle represents the only osseous connection between the upper extremity and the thorax and is therefore subjected to all forces exerted upon the arm. It is the first bone in the body to ossify and the medial epiphysis is the last to close. The clavicle has a double curved shape, with the juncture of the two curves at the midportion of the bone being the weakest point.

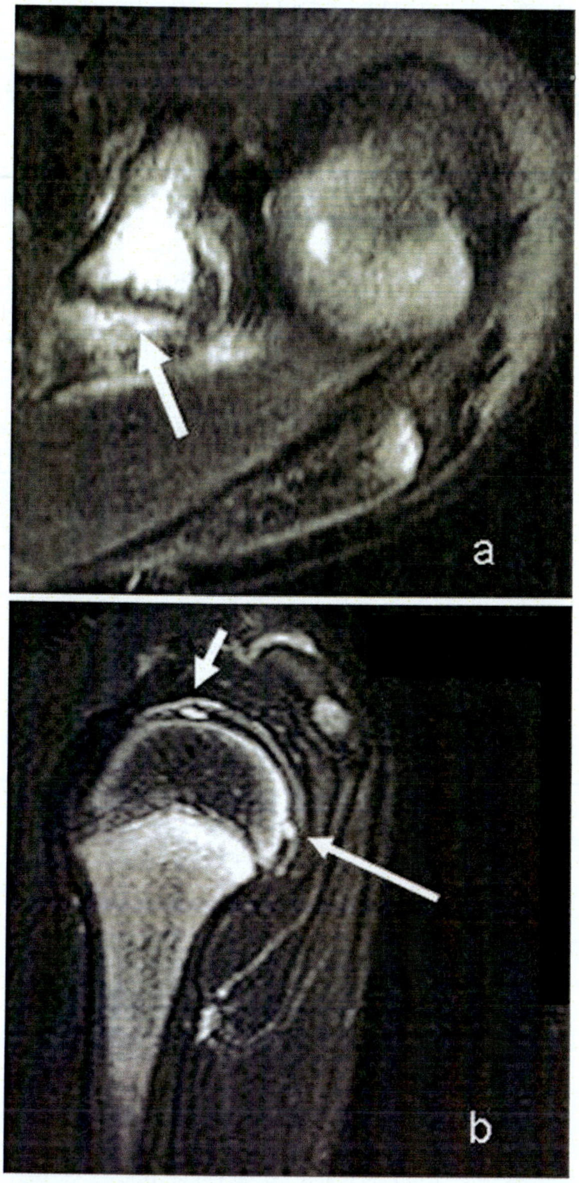

Fig. 17 (**a**) Axial T2-w fat-saturated MR image of a 10-year-old boy after a wrestling injury reveals a SH type I fracture of the coracoid process (*arrow*). (**b**) Incidentally noted, on oblique sagittal fat-suppressed T2-w MR image, also were two small focal areas of abnormal signal in the deep layers of the articular cartilage with intact overlying cartilage (concealed lesion) (*arrows*)

6.1 Clavicular Fractures

Due to its superficial location, the clavicle is frequently fractured (Kumar et al. 1989). In fact, the clavicle is the most commonly fractured bone in the pediatric population and represents 10–16% of all fractures in this age group. These fractures most often occur at two distinct times, the newborn period and in childhood. In the newborn, clavicular fractures are related to birth trauma, whereas in childhood they occur in the setting of a mobile child. The typical mechanism of injury results from a fall on outstretched hands or onto the lateral aspect of the shoulder (Paterson and Waters 2000). Stress or "academic" fractures may also be seen in students who carry heavy loads of books on their shoulders. Seventy-five to eighty percent of fractures involve the midportion, followed by the proximal portion (15–20%) and distal portion (5%). Fractures at the proximal and distal end of the clavicle are more likely to be epiphyseal disruptions due to the relatively stronger ligamentous attachments of the clavicle to the sternum and acromion, respectively. Most low-energy fractures that occur in sports result in a minimally displaced oblique fracture at the mid shaft. As the energy of the lateral force is increased, the fracture tends to be comminuted with a butterfly fragment and shortened.

Plain film radiography is the preferred method for evaluation of fractures to the midportion and distal clavicle (Fig. 18).

Due to the upward pull of the sternocleidomastoid muscle, a standard AP projection will show elevation of the proximal fracture fragment. The coracoclavicular (CC) ligament causes a downward pull of the distal fragment. A 30° cephalic view may be required in cases where a fracture is not seen on an AP projection in a patient with a high clinical suspicion for fracture. Fractures to the medial portion of the clavicle may be difficult to evaluate by radiograph alone and often

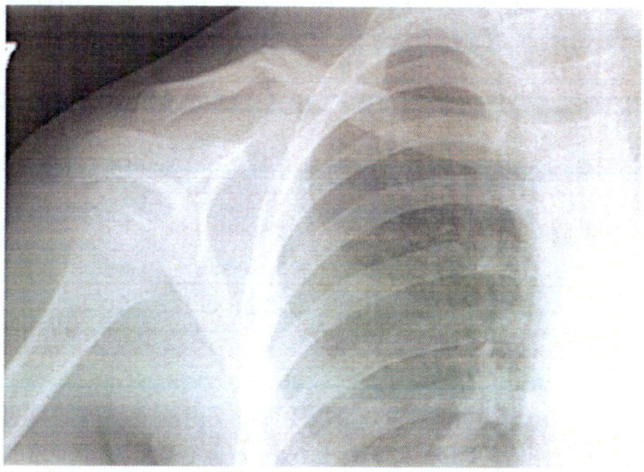

Fig. 18 Clavicle fracture. AP projection of the shoulder demonstrates a distal clavicle fracture. Typical of these fractures, there is superior retraction of the proximal fracture fragment

require a CT or MRI, especially in cases where the sternoclavicular (SC) joint may be involved. MRI provides more information regarding bone marrow abnormalities, disk or cartilaginous injury, and joint effusions.

6.2 Acromioclavicular Joint Separation

In addition to the articular surfaces or the distal clavicle and the acromion, the components of the acromioclavicular (AC) joint include, the AC ligament and the two processes of the CC ligament (trapezoid and conoid). The AC ligament is itself composed of four sets of ligaments, the stronger superior and inferior ligaments, and the weaker anterior and posterior ligaments. The AC ligament provides stability in the AP direction, while the CC ligament provides vertical stability. Prior to the age of 13, true AC dislocations are rare and account for only 10% of all clavicular injuries in children. The pediatric clavicle is surrounded by a periosteal sheath which contains the CC ligament, while the AC ligament remains exterior to the periosteal sheath. This anatomical relationship explains why the CC ligament often remains intact as a result of direct trauma, as opposed to the AC ligament, which is frequently injured.

The severity and therefore grading of AC separation is dependent upon both the degree of injury to the AC and/or CC ligament and displacement of the clavicle relative to the acromion. These injuries are graded according to the pediatric Rockwood classification (Fig. 19):

Type I – Radiographically normal joint without evidence of clavicular instability.

Type II – AC ligament disruption with mobility of the distal clavicle due to a partial tear of the periosteal tube.

Type III – Complete superior displacement of the distal clavicle through the periosteal tube.

Type IV–VI – Larger tear through the periosteal tube with more pronounced displacement of the clavicle posteriorly into the trapezius (IV), superiorly into the skin (V), or inferiorly under the coracoid process (VI). The CC ligament remains attached to the periosteal tube in type IV–VI separations.

Standard shoulder series radiographs are usually adequate to confirm a diagnosis of AC joint separation. A radiograph of the entire upper thorax may be helpful for comparison to the unaffected shoulder. Type I injuries may demonstrate mild soft tissue swelling, but appear otherwise unremarkable as compared to the opposite side. Type II separations may require stress radiographs to help distinguish them from a type I separation. As compared to type II separation, type III injuries will show increased subluxation of the AC joint space. Radiographs of type IV–VI will demonstrate their associated posterior, superior, and inferior clavicle dislocations, respectively. In certain cases an MRI may be required to definitively differentiate between a type II and III separation. In addition, it may also be useful if surgery is considered to identify additional disease. Ligamentous disruption is best seen on fat-suppressed PD-w or T2-w images when associated with surrounding blood or fluid (Alyas et al. 2008).

6.3 Osteolysis of the Distal Clavicle

Osteolysis of the distal clavicle can result from two distinct etiologies. It can occur as sequelae to direct trauma at the distal clavicle or the AC joint, with onset occurring anywhere from several weeks to several years after the traumatic event. Less frequently, it can occur as an overuse injury resulting from repetitive microtrauma, most commonly seen in weightlifting athletes. In either case, the clinical and radiographic natural history of the process is similar. Initially, patients complain of pain over the AC joint and limited range of motion at the shoulder. Early imaging demonstrates osteopenia at the distal clavicle and overlying soft tissue swelling. This is followed by erosion of 0.5–3.0 cm clavicle beginning at the subarticular cortex at the distal clavicle. Following this lytic phase, a reparative phase ensues, lasting 4–6 months (Levine et al. 1976). During this reparative phase, the distal clavicle can either undergo complete or partial reformation with resultant permanent widening of the AC joint. The pathogenesis of distal clavicular osteolysis, of either etiology is unclear. Theories include vascular compromise, autonomic nervous system dysfunction, reactive hyperemia, stress fractures, ischemic necrosis and a reactive synovitis (Kaplan and Resnick 1986).

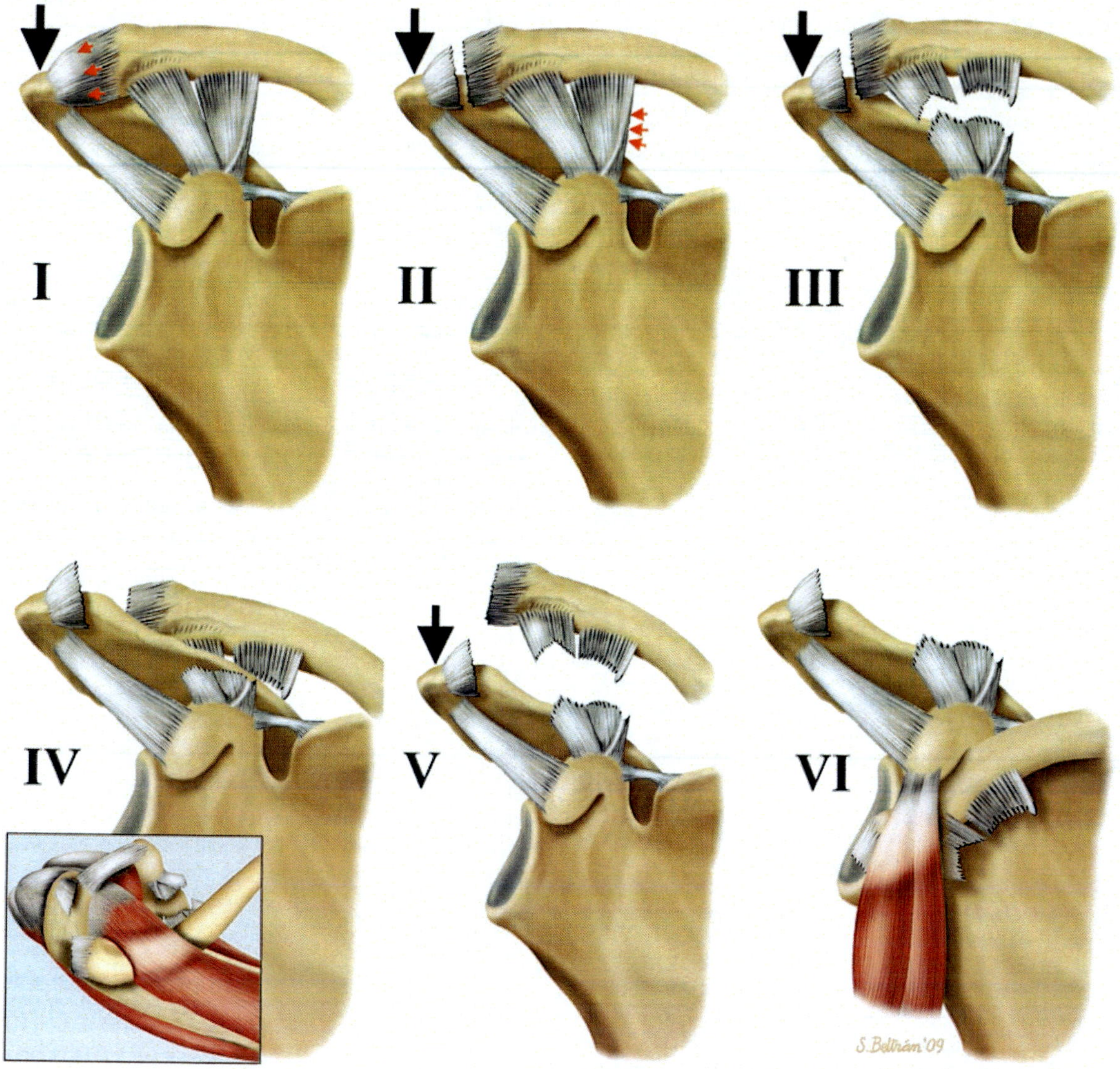

Fig. 19 Coronal section color illustration depicting the six types of acromioclavicular dislocations according to the pediatric Rockwood classification

6.4 Sternoclavicular Joint Separations

As opposed to true SC dislocations in adults, injuries to the medial clavicle in the skeletally immature often represent a medial physeal separation (pseudodislocation) as a result of a SH I or II fracture (Herring 2008). The shaft of the clavicle is displaced posteriorly or anteriorly while the medial epiphysis remains attached to the strong SC ligaments. These injuries occur as a result of traumatic forces on the shoulder being transmitted through the clavicle. Anterior displacements of the medial clavicle result from a posteriorly directed force being applied on the shoulder, while posterior displacements occur as a result of anteriorly directed forces on the shoulder. Severe posterior displacements may constitute a medical emergency as impingement of vital mediastinal structures may occur, including the great vessels, trachea, and esophagus.

A serendipity view radiograph, a tangential directed beam taken at 40° cephalad, may be needed for diagnosis as the SC joint may be obscured by the spinal, thoracic, and mediastinal structures on standard AP views (Kocher et al. 2000). Any equivocal radiographs should be supplemented with a CT examination of bilateral SC joints for definitive diagnosis and to rule-out a potential complicated posterior dislocation.

References

Alyas F, Curtis M, Speed C, Saifuddin A, Connell D (2008) MR imaging appearances of acromioclavicular joint dislocation. Radiographics 28(2):463–479, quiz 619

Cassas KJ, Cassettari-Wayhs A (2006) Childhood and adolescent sports-related overuse injuries. Am Fam Physician 73(6):1014–1022

Chen FS, Diaz VA (2005) Shoulder and elbow injuries in the skeletally immature athlete. J Am Acad Orthop Surg 13(3): 172–185

DiGiovine NM, Jobe FW, Pink M, Perry J (1992) An electromyographic analysis of the upper extremity in pitching. J Shoulder Elbow Surg 1:15–25

Fronek J, Warren RF, Bowen M (1989) Posterior subluxation of the glenohumeral joint. J Bone Joint Surg Am 71:205–216

Greenspan A (2004) Orthopedic imaging: a practical approach, 4th edn. Lippincott Williams & Wilkins, Philadelphia, pp 93–133

Gomez JE (2002) Upper extremity injuries in youth sports. Pediatr Clin N Am 49:593–626

Helms CA, Major NM, Anderson MW, Kaplan P, Dussault R (2001) Musculoskeletal MRI. Saunders, Philadelphia, pp 169–223

Herring JA (2008) Tachdjian's pediatric orthopaedics from the Texas Scottish Rite Hospital for Children, vol 3, 4th edn. Saunders, Canada, pp 2423–2451

Ireland ML, Andrews JR (1988) Shoulder and elbow injuries in the young athlete. Clin Sports Med 7:473–494

Itoi E, Kuechle DK, Newman SR, Morrey BF, An KN (1993) Stabilising function of the biceps in stable and unstable shoulders. J Bone Joint Surg Br 75:546–550

Jobe FW, Kvitne RS, Giangarra CE (1989) Shoulder pain in the overhand or throwing athlete: The relationship of anterior instability and rotator cuff impingement. Orthop Rev 18:963–975

Jobe FW, Tibone JE, Pink MM et al (1998) The shoulder in sports. In: Rockwood CA, Matsen FA III (eds) The shoulder, 2nd edn. Saunders, Philadelphia, pp 1214–1238

Kaplan PA, Resnick D (1986) Stress-induced osteolysis of the clavicle. Radiology 158(1):139–140

Kocher MS, Waters PM, Micheli LJ (2000) Upper extremity injuries in the paediatric athlete. Sports Med 30(2):117–135

Krabak BJ, Alexander E (2008) Shoulder and elbow injuries in the adolescent athlete. Phys Med Rehabil Clin N Am 19(2):271–285

Kumar R, Madewell JE, Swischuk LE, Lindell MM, David R (1989) The clavicle: normal and abnormal. Radiographics 9(4):677–706

Levine AH, Pais MJ, Schwartz EE (1976) Post-traumatic osteolysis of the distal clavicle with emphasis on early radiologic changes. AJR Am J Roentgenol 127:781–784

Levine B, Pereira D (2005) Avulsion fractures of the lesser tuberosity of the humerus in adolescents: review of the literature and case report. J Orthop Trauma 19(5):349–352

Marans HJ, Angel KR (1992) The fate of traumatic anterior dislocation of the shoulder in children. J Bone Joint Surg Am 74(8):1242–1244

Meister K (2000) Injuries to the shoulder in the throwing athlete: I. Biomechanics/pathophysiology/classification of injury. Am J Sports Med 28:265–275

O'Brien SJ, Neves MC, Arnoczky SP et al (1990) The anatomy and histology of the inferior glenohumeral ligament complex of the shoulder. Am J Sports Med 18:449–456

Pappas AM, Zawacki RM, Sullivan TJ (1985) Biomechanics of baseball pitching: a preliminary report. Am J Sports Med 13:216–222

Paterson PD, Waters PM (2000) Shoulder injuries in the childhood athlete. Clin Sports Med 19(4):681–692

Resnick D (2002a) Diagnosis of bone and joint disorders, vol 4, 4th edn. Saunders, Philadelphia, pp 4129–4273

Resnick D (2002b) Diagnosis of bone and joint disorders, vol 5, 4th edn. Saunders, Philadelphia, pp 4696–4768

Rogers LF, Poznanski AK (1994) Imaging of epiphyseal injuries. Radiology 191:297–308

Tarkin IS, Morganti CM (2005) Rotator cuff tears in adolescent athletes. Am J sports Med 33(4):596–601

Wagner KT, Lyne ED (1983) Adolescent traumatic dislocations of the shoulder with open epiphyses. J Pediatr Orthop 3(1): 61–62

Webb LX, Mooney JF (2003) Fractures and dislocations about the shoulder. In: Green NE, Swiontkowski MF (eds) Skeletal trauma in children, 3rd edn. Saunders, Philadelphia, pp 322–343

Elbow

Simon Porter and Eugene McNally

Contents

Key Points

- Supracondylar fractures are the most common in children.
- A visible posterior fat pad is the best clue to their presence. Significant displacement is associated with neurovascular complications.
- Lateral mass fractures are not common but are easily overlooked with devastating consequences.
- Medial avulsion injuries can be subtle if displaced into the joint. The mnemonic CRITOL tells us that if we see an apparent trochlear before a medial epicondyle ossification centre it is probably a displaced medial epicondyle.
- OCD of the capitellum is an important misuse injury in children. Careful scrutiny of the plain radiograph is needed to detect the injury.

1 Anatomy and Biomechanics

The elbow is a complex joint which has been described as one of the most congruous in the body. It is in effect three individual joints; the ulnohumeral and radiocapitellar which facilitate flexion/extension and the proximal radioulnar which facilitates pronation and supination. The normal range of flexion is from slight hyperextension to about 150°, and the range of pronation and supination is 75 and 85° respectively (Hutchinson and Wynn 2004).

The elbow capsule envelops all three articulations and has medial and lateral thickenings, the ulnar and lateral collateral ligament complexes. The ulnar collateral

S. Porter
Consultant Radiologist Craigavon Area
Hospital Lurgan Road, Portadown BT63 5QQ
e-mail: simonporter@doctors.org.uk

E. McNally (✉)
Consultant Musculoskeletal Radiologist Nuffield
Orthopaedic Centre & University of Oxford Old Road
Headington, Oxford OX37LD UK
e-mail: eugene.mcnally@gmail.com

A.H. Karantanas (ed.), *Sports Injuries in Children and Adolescents*,
Med Radiol Diagn Imaging, DOI: 10.1007/174_2010_13, © Springer-Verlag Berlin Heidelberg 2011

ligament (UCL) has a thick anterior band which is responsible for most of the stability at the elbow joint. It is the most easily identified component on MRI. The lateral ligament complex is less discrete and more difficult to visualize.

An understanding of the ossification process of the developing elbow is crucial in order to properly assess the radiographic anatomy and identify subtle pathology. Skeletal growth occurs at six ossification centres which have a predictable sequence of ossification and fusion. The mnemonic CRITOL is often used as an aide-memoire; the capitellum is the first to ossify at approximately 1 year, the radial head at 3 years, the internal (medial) epicondyle at 5 years, the trochlea at 7 years, the olecranon at 9 years and the lateral epicondyle at 10–11 years (Ouellette et al. 2008).

Acute injuries in young athletes predominantly take the form of fractures (Adirim and Cheng 2003). This is common in the upper extremity as children tend to protect themselves during a fall with an outstretched hand. Chronic elbow injuries usually occur in the throwing athlete and these are often grouped together under the term "little league elbow". The biomechanics of throwing is complex in an adult but this complexity is increased in an immature athlete because of the dynamic changes seen during normal development (Emery 2003; Kerssemakers et al. 2009).

2 Acute Injuries

2.1 Supracondylar Fractures

Elbow fractures are common in children between the ages of 5 and 7, accounting for 15% of all paediatric fractures (Omid et al. 2008). Supracondylar humeral fractures are the most common type, comprising between 50 and 70% (Alburger et al. 1992). Two thirds of all children admitted to hospital with an elbow injury have a supracondylar fracture.

The mechanism of injury is generally, a fall unto an outstretched hand with the elbow in full extension. The olecranon engages in it's fossa, acting as a fulcrum and resulting in fracture of the weakest point of the distal humerus, the thin cortex which connects the medial and lateral columns. As the fracture displaces, the anterior periosteum tears, leaving the posterior periosteum to act as a hinge. If the posterior periosteum is disrupted the elbow becomes unstable in both flexion and extension. The direction of fracture displacement indicates whether the medial or lateral periosteum is torn. The most common injury is a posteromedial displacement which usually has an intact medial periosteum.

The commonly used Gartland classification has low inter/intraobserver variability. Grade 1 injuries are undisplaced with an intact anterior humeral line. The fat pad sign may be the only evidence of a fracture. Grade 2 injuries are displaced with an intact posterior cortex but no translocation. Rotational deformity is not often seen. Grade 3 injuries have circumferential cortical disruption, usually with a rotational component.

Grade 3 injuries have a high incidence of neurovascular complications (Culp et al. 1990). If the distal metaphyseal spike projects medially, the median nerve and brachial artery can be compromised and if the spike projects laterally, the radial nerve may be compromised.

Proper radiographic evaluation requires AP and true lateral projections. The anterior humeral line is a line drawn along the anterior cortex of the distal shaft and in a normal study it should intersect with the middle third of the capitellum (Fig. 1). Baumann's angle is the angle between the long axis of the humeral shaft and the capitellar physis. The normal range is between 74–81° and is the same in both elbows. A reduction in Baumann's angle indicates rotation and varus tilt.

2.2 Physeal Fractures

2.2.1 Lateral Condyle Fracture

Fracture of the lateral condyle (lateral mass) is the second most common elbow fracture in children and is normally seen between 6–10 years of age (Shrader 2008). The mechanism of injury is either a valgus compression force from the radial head against the capitellum ("push off" type), caused by a fall on an outstretched hand with a flexed elbow, or a varus tensile force of the extensor muscles ("pull-off" type), caused by adducting the forearm with the elbow supinated.

Classification is on the basis of anatomic location or displacement. The Milch classification divides the fractures into two groups. Type 1 fractures traverse the capitellar ossification centre and extend to the articular surface lateral to the trochlear groove. This is a Salter–Harris IV injury. The more common type 2 fracture

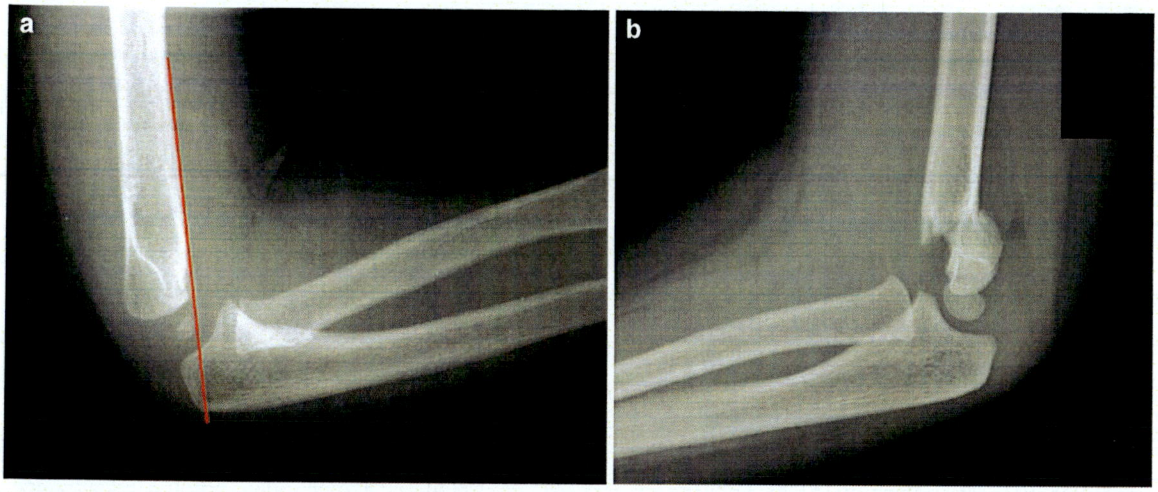

Fig. 1 (**a**, **b**) Grade 1 and 2 supracondylar fractures with disruption of the anterior humeral line

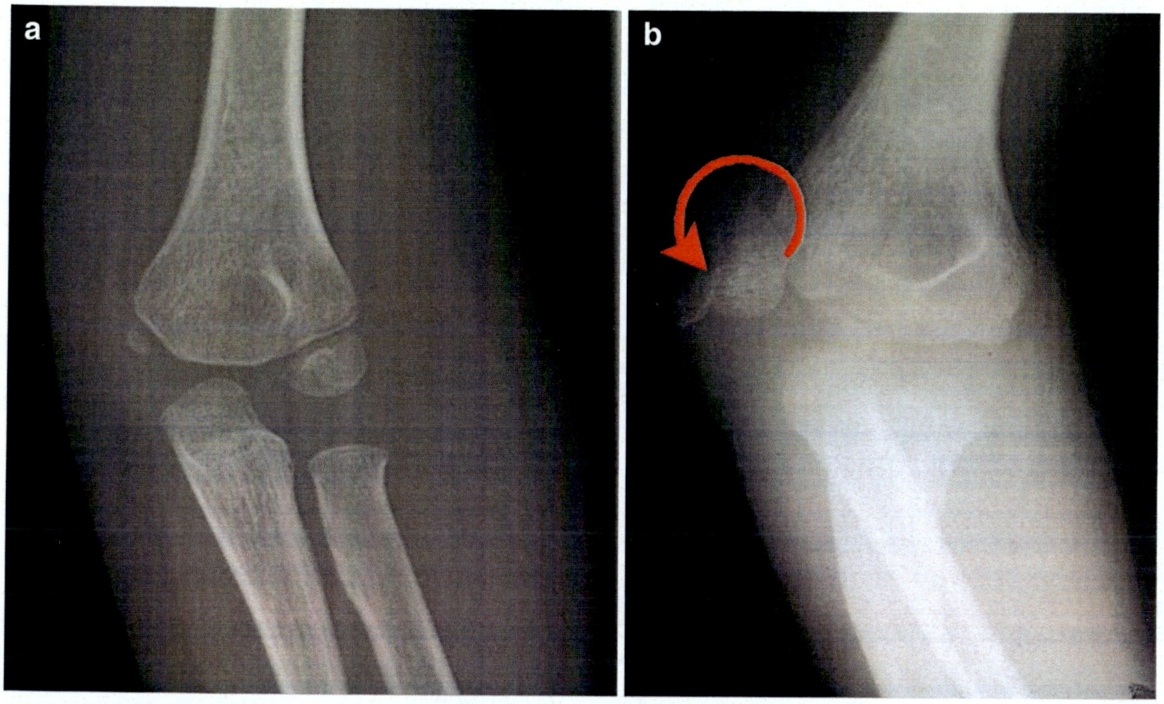

Fig. 2 Lateral condyle fractures with (**a**) subtle metaphyseal flake and (**b**) displacement and rotation

extends medial to the trochlear groove and results in an unstable injury.

The assessment of lateral condylar fractures is difficult and often only a small metaphyseal flake is appreciated. The degree of displacement is often better assessed on the lateral radiograph. An internal oblique radiograph has been shown to demonstrate both the amount of displacement, and the fracture morphology more clearly (Song et al. 2007). Classification should be based on the greatest displacement seen on at least three views (Fig. 2).

Differentiating between a lateral condylar injury and an entire physeal fracture can be difficult given the lack of ossification. With an entire physeal fracture, the radius and ulna are displaced *posteromedially* but with a lateral condyle fracture, stability afforded by the lateral crista is lost and the radius and olecranon can be displaced *posterolaterally*.

The problem with the Milch anatomic classification is that the fragments are primarily cartilaginous and the fracture line is not seen on plain films. Treatment can be based on the amount of displacement of the visible metaphyseal fragment; if there is more than 2 mm of displacement then there is an increased risk of complications, and open reduction with internal fixation is recommended (Song et al. 2008). When the amount of displacement is less than 2 mm it may be impossible to determine radiographically whether or not the fracture line extends to involve the articular surface. Historically, the recommendation in this case has been to undertake an open reduction and establish articular congruity. MRI can accurately evaluate the physis and potentially prevent unnecessary open reductions (Beltran et al. 1994; Griffith et al. 2001). Another way of evaluating articular involvement is by intraoperative arthrography.

2.2.2 Medial Epicondyle Fracture

Fractures of the medial epicondyle account for approximately 10% of all paediatric elbow fractures. They tend to occur later, the typical range is between 9–14 years, after the ossification centre has appeared. The mechanism of injury may involve a direct blow, valgus stress producing an avulsion-type injury, and dislocation. There is a strong association with elbow dislocation and it is reported that as many as 50% of these injuries occur concurrently.

With an undisplaced fracture the initial radiograph characteristically demonstrates loss of the medial soft tissue planes. Loss of the smooth physeal border of the epiphysis is strongly suggestive of an avulsion. An avulsed fragment is usually displaced inferiorly by the forearm flexors and with significant displacement the long axis of the fragment rotates medially. There may be an associated metaphyseal flake which is diagnostic of an avulsion.

The fracture fragment may become incarcerated within the joint space, usually between the trochlea and the semi-lunar notch of the ulna; this must be assumed when the fragment lies at the level of the joint line on any projection (Fig. 3). Because of the attachment of the UCL to the medial epicondyle and the ulna, posterolateral dislocation is frequently associated with avulsion. It is important to determine position of the medial epicondyle before and after reduction as incarceration does not occur until after the elbow is relocated. Comparison films may be helpful in these cases.

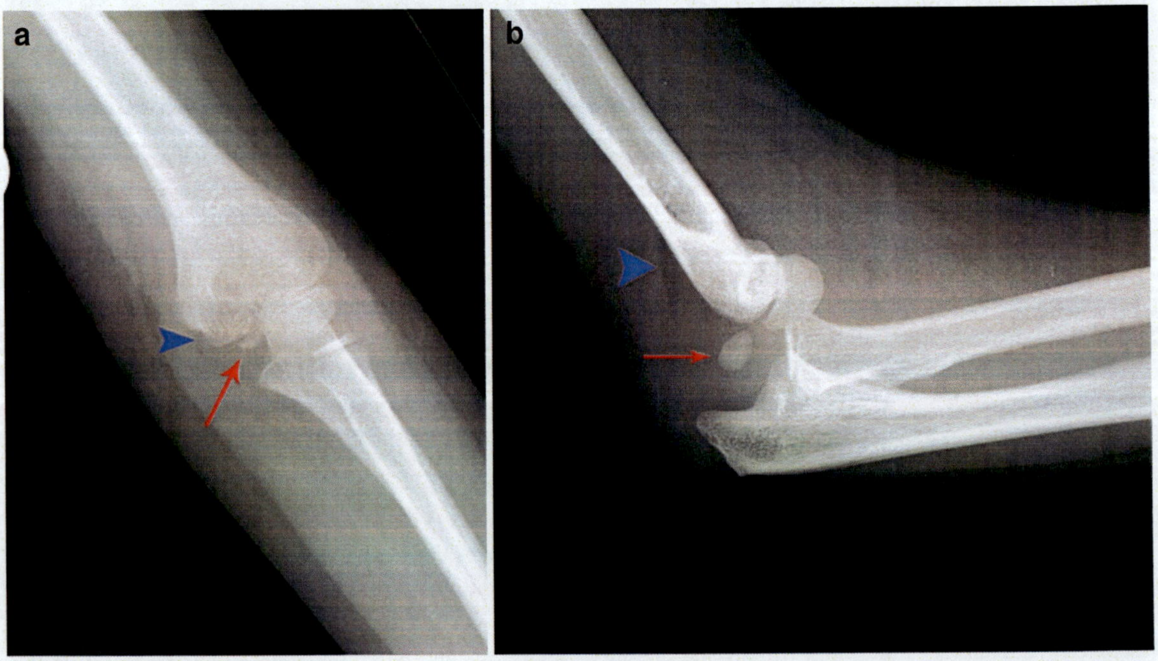

Fig. 3 (**a**) Incarcerated medial epicondyle (*red arrow*) and (**b**) dislocated elbow demonstrating an avulsed medial epicondyle (*red arrow*) and a posterior fat pad sign (*blue arrowhead*)

The incarcerated medial epicondyle is the raison d'être of CRITOL. It is easy to mistake the intra-articular ossification centre seen on the AP radiograph for the trochlea if the sequence of ossification is not properly appreciated (Silberstein et al. 1981). The authors therefore recommend using this mnemonic routinely when reviewing paediatric elbows, especially in the context of trauma.

Treatment is determined by the amount of fragment displacement; most surgeons will treat minimally displaced fractures (less than 5 mm) conservatively. Treatment of a displaced fracture, incarcerated within the joint always requires surgery.

3 Chronic Injuries

3.1 Medial Side Injuries

In 1960 Brogden et al. used the phrase "little league elbow" to describe a medial epicondyle fracture in an adolescent baseball pitcher. Unfortunately, today the nomenclature is confusing and the term is often used as an "umbrella", encompassing a number of conditions caused by repeated micro-trauma to vulnerable, developing areas of the paediatric elbow (Hang et al. 2004). The spectrum of injuries is considered for the purpose of this chapter in anatomical regions.

It has been well described that the aetiology of "little league elbow" relates to the valgus stress placed upon the elbow during early and late cocking phases of throwing (Klingele and Kocher 2002). The greatest force is applied to the epicondylar region and this produces an age-dependant pattern of injury.

3.1.1 Medial Epicondyle Apophysis

Medial epicondyle apophysitis is the typical overuse syndrome seen in young adults who have an immature elbow and expose themselves to abnormal and excessive forces. Although most commonly seen in baseball pitchers, the throwing action is not unique to baseball and the condition is also seen in tennis and gymnastics.

The radiographic findings associated with this condition are subtle and not uniform. Some patients with clinical findings have normal radiographs. When present the findings include fragmentation, irregularity, mild separation and enlargement. These findings are more readily appreciated when compared with the contralateral elbow.

In cases where conventional radiography is negative, an ultrasound may be particularly useful as it can be used to evaluate injury to the non-ossified cartilagenous growth centre.

MRI may be necessary to establish the diagnosis in the absence of radiographic findings. Typically, it demonstrates bone oedema on fat suppessed T2-w images with oedema also present in the surrounding soft tissue.

3.1.2 Ulnar Collateral Ligament Injury

As the adolescent thrower develops, the medial epicondyle begins to fuse and the maximum valgus stress is then preferentially transmitted across the UCL. This changes the pattern of injury from physeal to ligamentous.

The UCL is composed of anterior, posterior and transverse bands. The anterior band is the most important stabilizer. It originates on the inferior aspect of the medial epicondyle and inserts on the medial aspect of the coronoid process (the sublime tubercle). Because it is not well visualized at arthroscopy, it makes diagnosis at imaging even more important.

Stress radiographs can be undertaken for indirect evidence of ligamentous trauma. Distraction of the medial joint space by more than 1 mm, with respect to the normal side, is very suggestive of UCL injury. Heterotopic ossification of the ligament indicates a chronic tear (Mulligan et al. 2000).

Sonographically full thickness UCL tears are manifested as non-visualization of the ligament or alteration of the normal morphology (Fig. 4) (Miller et al. 2004). Using the same premise as radiography, joint distraction under valgus stress is also in keeping with a tear (De Smet et al. 2002). It has been reported that there was greater laxity in the medial joint space of collegiate baseball pitchers and that this correlated with medial joint symptoms. This would suggest that repetitive throwing causes medial joint laxity (Sasaki et al. 2002).

MRI has a valuable role in the diagnosis of UCL trauma (Mirowitz and London 1992). However, it is important to realize that the imaging characteristics of a developing UCL differ from those of an adult. A study by Sugimoto et al showed that the ulnar periosteum is a continuation of the UCL in the immature elbow, while in the mature elbow it appears to insert

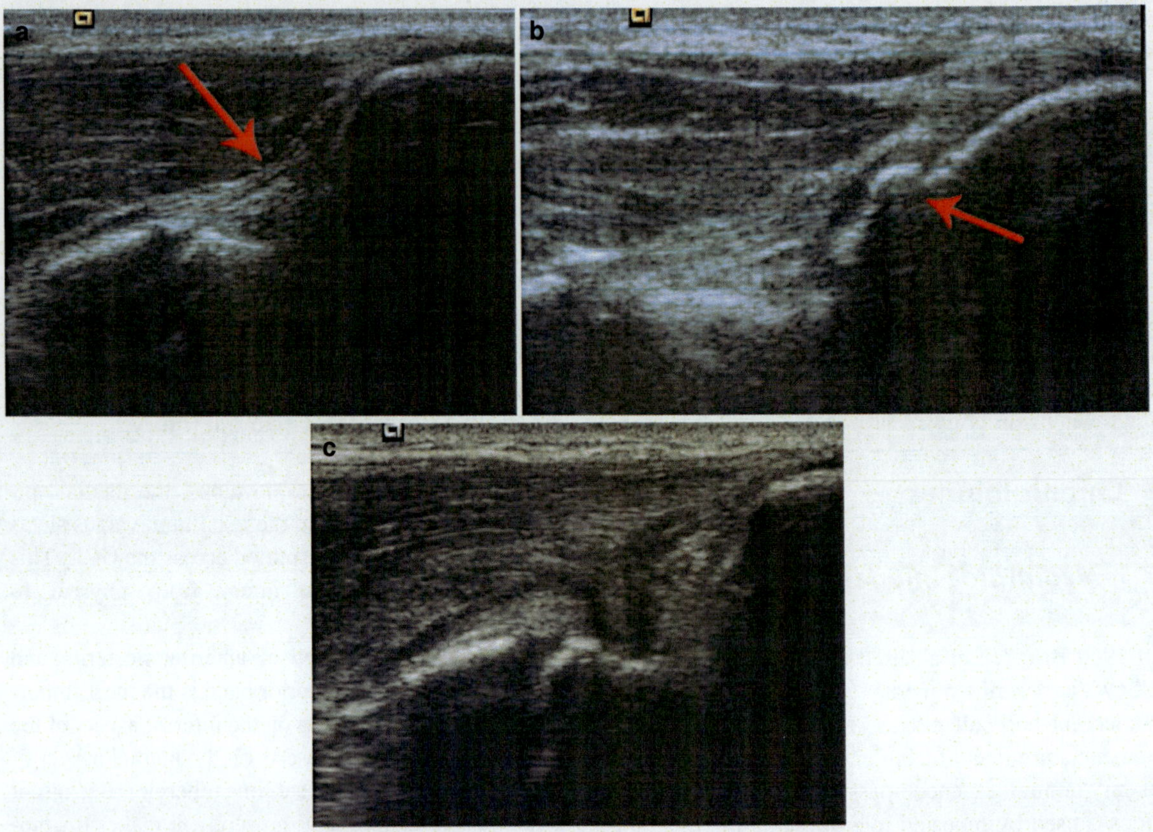

Fig. 4 US images of the UCL demonstrating (**a**) a normal ligament (*red arrow*) (**b**) avulsed bone fragment (*red arrow*) and (**c**) complete rupture

directly onto the cortex (Sugimoto and Ohsawa 1994). Also the proximal enthesis exhibits high T2 signal which can easily be mistaken for pathology.

MR arthrography has a high sensitivity and specificity for partial tears (Munshi et al. 2004). If there is complete tearing then ligament disruption and extracapsular leakage of contrast can occur. The appearance of distal extravasation of contrast at the expected site of coronoid insertion has been likened to a "T" shape.

3.1.3 Trochlear Osteochondral Lesions

Although much has been written regarding lateral osteochondral injuries in the context of "little league elbow" there is a paucity of literature relating to the paediatric trochlea. The trochlea represents only a small proportion of the total number of cases of osteochondral injuries of the elbow, with the capitellum accounting for the vast majority (Marshall et al. 2009). The exact incidence is difficult to determine given the small number of published studies.

The disparity in incidence may relate to the difference in axial loading forces, the trochlea takes only 40% of the overall load. It has also been suggested that the incidence and pattern may be accounted by for the vascular anatomy. There are two separate consistent vascular supplies to the trochlea. The lateral vessels cross the physis and supply the trochlear apex and lateral aspect, and the medial vessels enter through the non-articular surface to supply the medial aspect. Because there is a non-overlapping blood supply, there is a "watershed" area in the posteroinferior trochlea which is vulnerable to avascular necrosis. Two patterns of osteonecrosis have been described; type A "fishtail deformity" and type B "malignant varus deformity" (Beaty and Kasser 2006). Type A injuries are most often seen in the context of a Milch type 2 fracture of the lateral condyle which traverses the central trochlear groove and disrupts the lateral vessels. It may also be seen after a very distal supracondylar fracture. The outcome is a defect at the apex of the trochlear groove with the capitellum and the residual medial trochlea forming the lobes of a heterocercal fishtail. This pattern of injury does not often progress to deformity. However, when both medial and lateral vessels are disrupted, the pattern of injury is much more severe with involvement of the whole trochlea and subsequent angular deformities.

Early radiographic findings are subtle and although the lesion is uncommon, medial sided elbow pain in the clinical context of a previous injury should prompt consideration of further imaging with MRI.

MRI findings are variable and reflect the underlying pathology; there may be a well circumscribed area of hypointensity on T1-w imaging, eccentrically located in the lateral trochlea.

3.2 *Lateral Side Injuries*

During the late cocking and early acceleration phases of throwing the lateral elbow is subjected to compressive forces. There may also be shear forces exerted during the follow through phase. The repetitive injury caused by the compressive forces is probably the cause of lateral osteochondral injuries. There are two conditions of the humeral capitellum which have similar radiographic findings but differing clinical presentation and prognosis; osteochondritis dessicans (OCD) and Panner's disease.

3.2.1 Panner's Disease

Panner's disease is an osteochondrosis of the capitellum which usually presents between 4–8 years of age. It is the most common cause of lateral elbow pain in a young athlete and is almost exclusively seen in baseball pitchers. It is thought to represent avascular necrosis of the capitellar ossification centre secondary to trauma. The entire ossific nucleus is involved but the clinical course is benign and self-limiting. The treatment is conservative and the condition tends to resolve in most patients with restoration of the normal capitellar size and contour. There are rarely long term sequelae.

The radiographic findings are often diagnostic. They include a joint effusion, sclerosis, capitellar flattening and articular irregularity (Fig. 5a, b).

MRI findings are similar to those seen in Perthes disease of the hip with fragmentation and decreased signal on the T1-w images (Fig. 5c). The articular surface normally remains intact. Loose bodies are not typically a feature of Panner's disease.

3.2.2 Capitellar Osteochondritis Dessicans

The aetiology of capitellar OCD is unknown but repeated valgus compression and a tenuous blood supply has been proposed to explain the frequency of presentation in this area. It presents in an older age group than in Panner's disease, typically athletes between 11–16 years. As with Panner's disease, it is normally seen in the dominant arm of a throwing athlete.

Early radiographic findings are subtle and diagnosis may be facilitated by undertaking the AP radiograph with 45° flexion. The earliest signs are slight flattening and sclerosis of the superior aspect of the capitellum (Fig. 6). Articular surface collapse and loose body formation are not seen until a more advanced stage. The radiographic classification is as follows: grade 1, translucent shadow in the central or lateral capitellum; grade 2, separation between subchondral bone and the lesion; grade 3, loose bodies.

If the radiographs are normal and there is still a high index of suspicion then an MRI is indicated. The earliest MRI finding is reduced T1 signal in the superficial aspect of the capitellum; patients with this finding may have a better prognosis following conservative management (Fig. 6). As the disease process evolves, the capitellum develops increased T2 signal (Kijowski and De Smet 2005). Subsequently, the subchondral bone collapses and the overlying cartilage becomes unstable. Circumferential fluid surrounding the osteochondral fragment is indicative of instability. Ultimately, a loose body develops and occasionally concomitant radial head involvement is seen.

An important MR imaging pitfall to be aware of is the capitellar pseudodefect (Rosenberg et al. 1994). This occurs at the junction of the smooth articular surface of the capitellum with the non-articular surface. The junction is abrupt and accentuated by "troughlike undermining". Where the lateral capitellar margin overhangs the trough there is an apparent defect on both coronal and sagittal images. Care should be taken not to interpret this as an OCD or an impaction fracture.

Sonography has also been shown to be a reliable method for detection of unstable osteochondral lesions.

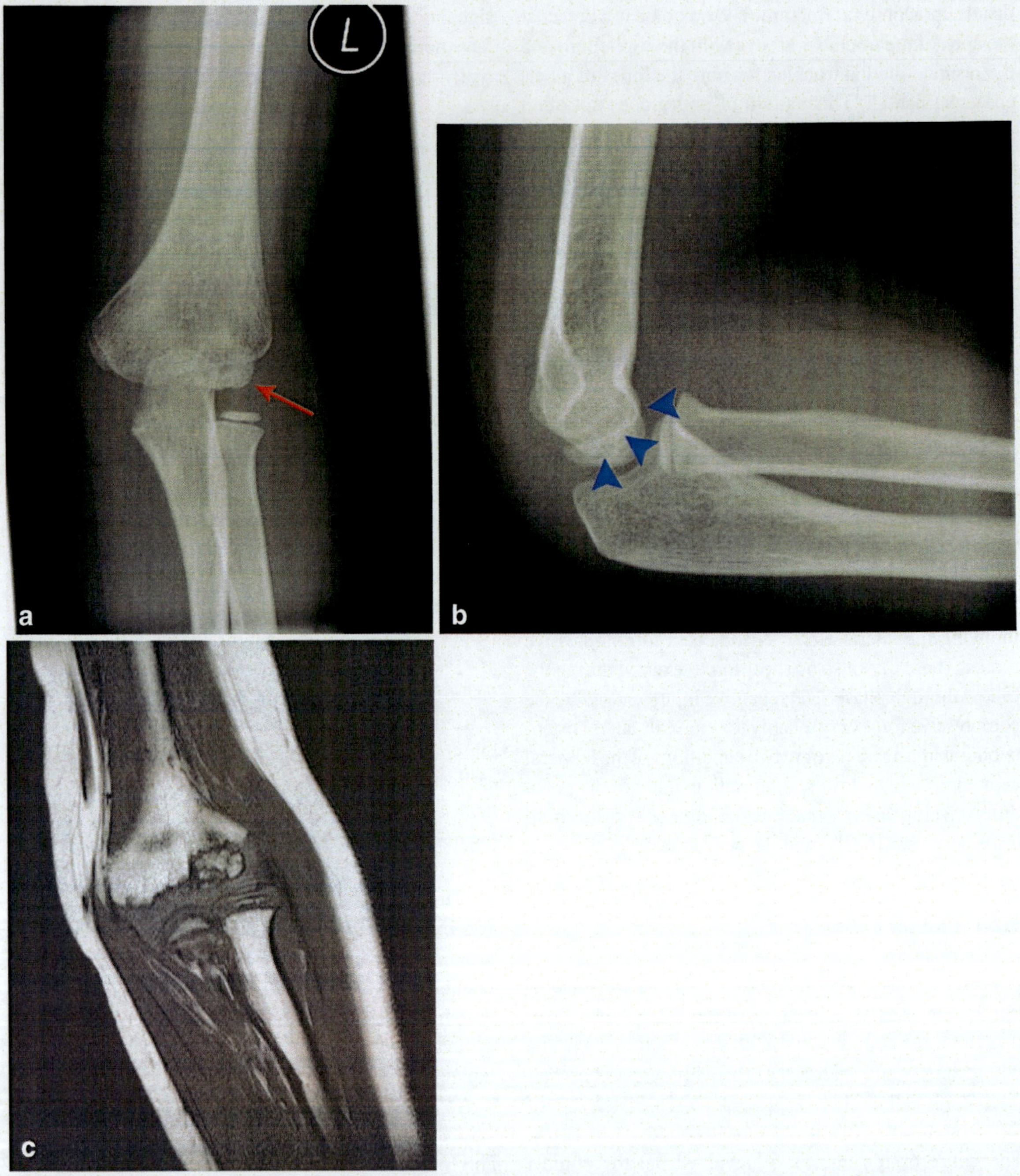

Fig. 5 The plain radiographs (**a**, **b**) demonstrate capitellar flattening with sclerosis (*red arrow* and *blue arrowheads*). MR (**c**) shows reduced T1 signal

3.3 Posterior Injuries

3.3.1 Olecranon Apophysitis

During pitching there are significant distracting forces generated by contraction of the triceps muscle. These forces are most prevalent during the acceleration phase. It has been hypothesized that the mechanism of injury of olecranon apophysitis is similar to that of Osgood–Schlatter's disease.

Radiographs may demonstrate soft tissue swelling with physeal widening, sclerosis and fragmentation.

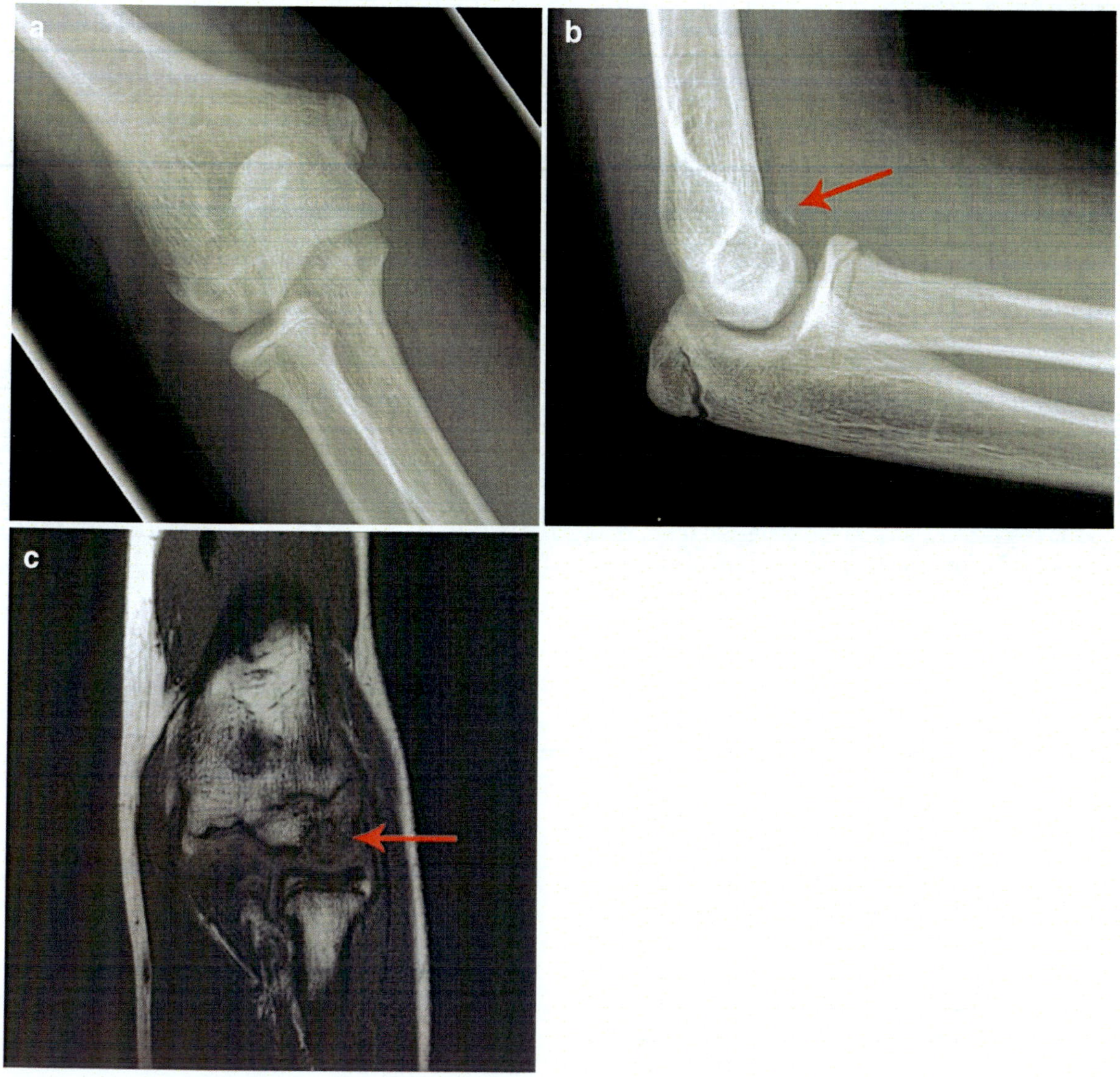

Fig. 6 Radiographs (**a**, **b**) demonstrate lucency of the subchondral bone and a loose body (*red arrow*) (**c**) The coronal T1-w MR image shows focal area of reduced signal (*red arrow*)

In subtle cases, the findings are more apparent when compared to the asymptomatic side. Normal radiographs do not exclude the diagnosis and further imaging with an MRI may be required in the correct clinical setting.

Once there has been an epiphyseal injury/distraction, continued stressful activity may prevent normal closure and result in a chronic non union. If conservative management fails in these patients then surgical fixation is indicated.

In the older adolescent athlete with a more mature, but still unfused apophysis, the same forces can cause a transverse fracture through the physis. The stress fractures seen in skeletally mature patients, through the olecranon tip and obliquely through the mid portion of the olecranon are seen much less commonly in children.

Also in the older adolescent athlete, posteromedial osteophytes may form and give rise to an impingement syndrome (Rosenberg et al. 2008).

The posterior joint is the location to look for effusion and synovial thickening. Ultrasound is particularly efficient in children and Doppler activity can indicate actively inflamed synovium. Involvement of several joints is indicative of juvenile idiopathic arthropathy.

3.4 Anterior Injuries

Anterior elbow injuries in the young athlete are uncommon. The distal biceps brachii is more commonly torn by an older athlete in the context of chronic injury. When present in a younger patient it is usually secondary to acute trauma. Ultrasound is the investigation of choice in the first instance. The most useful position is to examine distal tendon using a medially positioned probe in long axis, taking advantage of the acoustic window provided by pronator teres. The "cobra position" (Giuffre and Lisle 2005) is also employed to visualize the most distal part of the tendon. It is a posterior approach with the forearm pronated which reduces the anisotropic effect that frequently makes assessment difficult.

The brachialis tendon is susceptible to injury with overuse of the forearm in a pronated, semi-flexed position. This pattern is most commonly seem in extreme rock climbers, the so called "climbers elbow".

4 Conclusion

Sports injuries in the paediatric elbow encompass a broad spectrum of pathology. Musculoskeletal and neurological development result in age-dependant patterns of injury. This makes investigation more challenging and a multi-modality approach may be required to ensure an accurate diagnosis. In difficult cases it is possible to undertake dynamic assessment and compare with the normal side. Conventional radiography and ultrasound remain the first line investigations, with MR and CT reserved for more complex cases.

References

Adirim TA, Cheng TL (2003) Overview of injuries in the young athlete. Sports Med 33(1):75–81

Alburger PD, Weidner PL, Betz RR (1992) Supracondylar fractures of the humerus in children. J Pediatr Orthop 12(1): 16–19

Beaty JH, Kasser JR (2006) Rockwood and Wilkins fractures in children, 6th edn. Lippincott Williams & Wilkins, Philadelphia

Beltran J, Rosenberg ZS, Kawelblum M, Montes L, Bergman AG, Strongwater A (1994) Pediatric elbow fractures: MRI evaluation. Skeletal Radiol 23(4):277–281

Culp RW, Osterman AL, Davidson RS, Skirven T, Bora FW (1990) Neural injuries associated with supracondylar fractures of the humerus in children. J Bone Joint Surg Am 72(8):1211–1215

De Smet A, Winter T, Best T, Bernhardt D (2002) Dynamic sonography with valgus stress to assess elbow ulnar collateral ligament injury in baseball pitchers. Skeletal Radiol 31(11):671–676

Emery CA (2003) Risk factors for injury in child and adolescent sport: a systematic review of the literature. Clin J Sports Med 13(4):256–268

Emery KH (2006) Imaging of sports injuries of the upper extremity in children. Clin Sports Med 25(3)

Giuffre BM, Lisle DA (2005) Tear of the distal biceps branchii tendon: a new method of ultrasound evaluation. Australas Radiol 49(5):404–406

Gómez JE (2002) Upper extremity injuries in youth sports. Pediatr Clin North Am 49(3)

Griffith JF, Roebuck DJ, Cheng JC, Chan YL, Rainer TH, Ng BK, Metreweli C (2001) Acute elbow trauma in children: spectrum of injury revealed by MR imaging not apparent on radiographs. AJR Am J Roentgenol 176(1):53–60

Hang DW, Chao CM, Hang YS (2004) A clinical and roentgenographic study of little league elbow. Am J Sports Med 32(1): 79–84

Hutchinson MR, Wynn S (2004) Biomechanics and development of the elbow in the young throwing athlete. Clin Sports Med 23(4):531–544

Kerssemakers S, Fotiadou A, de Jonge M, Karantanas A, Maas M (2009) Sport injuries in the paediatric and adolescent patient: a growing problem. Pediatr Radiol 39(5): 471–484

Kijowski R, De Smet AA (2005) MRI findings of osteochondritis dissecans of the capitellum with surgical correlation. AJR Am J Roentgenol 185(6):1453–1459

Klingele KE, Kocher MS (2002) Little league elbow: valgus overload injury in the paediatric athlete. Sports Med 32(15): 1005–1015

Kocher MS, Waters PM, Micheli LJ (2000) Upper extremity injuries in the paediatric athlete. Sports Med 30(2): 117–135

Marshall KW, Marshall DL, Busch MT, Williams JP (2009) Osteochondral lesions of the humeral trochlea in the young athlete. Skeletal Radiol 38:479–491

Miller TT, Adler RS, Friedman L (2004) Sonography of injury of the ulnar collateral ligament of the elbow, initial experience. Skeletal Radiol 33(7):386–391

Mirowitz SA, London SL (1992) Ulnar collateral ligament injury in baseball pitchers: MR imaging evaluation. Radiology 185(2):573–576

Mulligan SA, Schwartz ML, Broussard MF, Andrews JR (2000) Heterotopic calcification and tears of the ulnar collateral ligament: radiographic and MR imaging findings. AJR Am J Roentgenol 175(4):1099–1102

Munshi M, Pretterklieber ML, Chung CB, Haghighi P, Cho J-H, Trudell DJ, Resnick D (2004) Anterior bundle of ulnar collateral ligament: evaluation of anatomic relationships by using MR imaging, MR arthrography, and gross anatomic and histologic analysis. Radiology 231(3):797–803

Omid R, Choi PD, Skaggs DL (2008) Supracondylar humeral fractures in children. J Bone Joint Surg Am 90(5):1121–1132

Ouellette H, Bredella M, Labis J, Palmer W, Torriani M (2008) MR imaging of the elbow in baseball pitchers. Skeletal Radiol 37(2):115–121

Rosenberg ZS, Beltran J, Cheung YY (1994) Pseudodefect of the capitellum: potential MR imaging pitfall. Radiology 191(3):821–833

Rosenberg ZS, Blutreich SI, Schweitzer ME, Zember JS, Fillmore K (2008) MRI features of posterior capitellar impaction injuries. AJR Am J Roentgenol 190(2):435–441

Rudzki JR, Paletta GA (2004) Juvenile and adolescent elbow injuries in sports. Clin Sports Med 23(4):581–608

Sasaki J, Takahara M, Ogino T, Kashiwa H, Ishigaki D, Kanauchi Y (2002) Ultrasonographic assessment of the ulnar collateral ligament and medial elbow laxity in college baseball players. J Bone Joint Surg Am 84-A(4): 525–531

Shrader MW (2008) Pediatric supracondylar fractures and pediatric physeal elbow fractures. Orthop Clin North Am 39(2):163–171

Silberstein MJ, Brodeur AE, Graviss ER, Luisiri A (1981) Some vagaries of the medial epicondyle. J Bone Joint Surg Am 63(4):524–528

Sofka C, Potter HG (2002) Imaging of elbow injuries in the child and adult athlete. Radiol Clin North Am 40:251–265

Song KS, Kang CH, Min BW, Bae KC, Cho CH (2007) Internal oblique radiographs for diagnosis of nondisplaced or minimally displaced lateral condylar fractures of the humerus in children. J Bone Joint Surg Am 89(1):58–63

Song KS, Kang CH, Min BW, Bae KC, Cho CH, Lee JH (2008) Closed reduction and internal fixation of displaced unstable lateral condylar fractures of the humerus in children. J Bone Joint Surgery Am 90(12):2673–2681

Sugimoto H, Ohsawa T (1994) Ulnar collateral ligament in the growing elbow: MR imaging of normal development and throwing injuries. Radiology 192(2):417–422

Wrist and Hand

Ana Navas Canete, Milko C. de Jonge, Charlotte M. Nusman, Maaike P. Terra, and Mario Maas

Contents

Key Points

- Radiologists diagnosing overuse injuries in hand and wrist must have detailed knowledge of anatomy, sports specific biomechanics and sense of awareness of the sports specific pathology.
- Overuse injury in wrist and hand can occur in bones, tendons, ligaments, vessels and nerves.
- Plain film, with standardized PA and lateral films is the mainstay for initial imaging workup.
- MRI is extremely helpful, particularly when using a dedicated wrist coil and high field strength (1.5 or 3.0 T) MR scanners. Routinely there is no need for MR arthrography.

1 Introduction

The wrist is still thought a difficult joint to evaluate, both by treating clinicians and radiologists. Since the wrist is a complex joint that biomechanically transmits forces generated at the hand through to the forearm, wrist pain often occurs in high performing athletes. Thus both sport physicians and radiologists will frequently encounter this pathology.

Plain radiography, performed in a standardized manner with true PA and lateral views still remains the mainstay of initial imaging workup. In specific cases, these standard projections have to be completed with additional projections depending on the suspected lesion and clinical presentation (Demondion et al. 2008). The use of high frequency ultrasound (US), with dedicated probe, is currently accepted as a powerful tool for analysing superficial tendon, nerve and other soft tissue pathology.

A. Navas Canete, M.C. de Jonge, C.M. Nusman, M.P. Terra, and M. Maas (✉)
Department of Radiology, Academic Medical Center, Meibergdreef 9, Amsterdam 1105 AZ, The Netherlands
e-mail: m.maas@amc.uva.nl

A.H. Karantanas (ed.), *Sports Injuries in Children and Adolescents*,
Med Radiol Diagn Imaging, DOI: 10.1007/174_2010_14, © Springer-Verlag Berlin Heidelberg 2011

MR imaging (MRI) is considered the imaging study of choice to evaluate chronic wrist pain, when plain film fails to provide the exact diagnosis. Since high field MRI has emerged, evaluation of small structures, such as triangular fibrocartilage complex (TFCC) and intercarpal ligaments is feasible. However we need to stress that a dedicated wrist coil is more important than the high field strength. Tailoring the imaging protocol is essential when dealing with high performing athletes.

Anatomy may serve as a guiding tool. Thus we have chosen to divide the pathology following anatomical landmarks focusing to most frequently encountered disorders and those that require increase in awareness amongst radiologists.

2 Radial Wrist Pain

2.1 Bones

2.1.1 Gymnast's Wrist and Distal Radial Stress Fracture

The radial side of the wrist carries 80% of the axial load and the ulnar side the remaining 20% (Palmer and Werner 1984). The incidence of wrist and hand pathology in the sporting population is approximately 25%. This tends to be higher in those sports using the hand and the wrist frequently, like in *gymnastics*. A unique aspect of gymnastics is the regular use of the upper extremities to support body weight. Events such as the pommel horse, balance beam and floor exercise include many elements that subject the wrist joint to recurrent loading with relatively large static and dynamic forces. Under these particular conditions, radial wrist pain is common among gymnasts of both sexes. Since gymnasts typically begin training at young ages, the growth plates of the wrist are a potential site of injury. Elite female and male gymnasts may initiate training as early as 6 and 9 years, respectively, with peak performance being 10 or more years away. During this period, the degree of difficulty of manoeuvres practiced and performed, and the volume and intensity of training increase dramatically (Caine and Nassar 2005).

In case of an adult gymnast, with closed physis, the repetitive stress on the radius provocates a radial stress fracture/stress response of the bone. In young athletes, growth plates that are non-fused are a well known site of injury. In experimental studies performed in an attempt to understand the physiopathology of the distal radial physeal injury (Gymnast's wrist), it was shown when shortening the ulna to produce an ulnar variance of −2.5 mm, the load born by the radius was increased to 96% (Palmer and Werner 1984). In children with open growth plates, the ulnar variance is typically negative, with a mean of approximately −2 mm (Hafner et al. 1989). Because of that, the loading of the distal radius in young gymnastics exceeds 80%. Nevertheless, recent studies have not confirmed a relationship between ulnar variance and wrist pain nor between ulnar variance and stress injury to the distal radial physis (DiFiori et al. 2002; Dobyns and Gabel 1990). The distal radial growth plate injury has been reported primarily on the basis of radiographic findings (Dobyns and Gabel 1990; Caine et al. 2003). The classical radiographic criteria include one or more of the following: widening of the growth plate, cystic changes of the metaphyseal aspect of the growth plate, a beaked effect of the distal aspect of the epiphysis, and haziness within the usually radiolucent area of the growth plate (Fig. 1). Although grading of radiographic findings of the distal radial physis has been proposed (DiFiori et al. 2002), no clear relationship with prognosis has been established. MRI can show the same radiological findings as the plain radiographs or subtle radiological findings such as bone marrow oedema adjacent to the physis in a young patient, confirming the diagnosis of a gymnast's wrist (Fig. 2).

In our clinical experience, gymnasts with imaging findings of physeal injury or stress fracture in the distal radius should refrain the compression loading of the wrist joint for 6 weeks. At that time, a reassessment should be performed before considering a gradual return to training. Repeat radiographs at regular intervals combined with clinical follow-up evaluation after skeletal maturity is needed to elucidate the long-term effect of gymnastics on the wrist (Dobyns and Gabel 1990).

2.1.2 Scaphoid Stress Fracture

Less common than lower-extremity stress fractures, upper-extremity stress fractures are becoming recognized more frequently. High clinical suspicion is required for diagnosis because the historical and physical features can be vague. Regarding the scaphoid stress fracture, the same biomechanical mechanism that was described

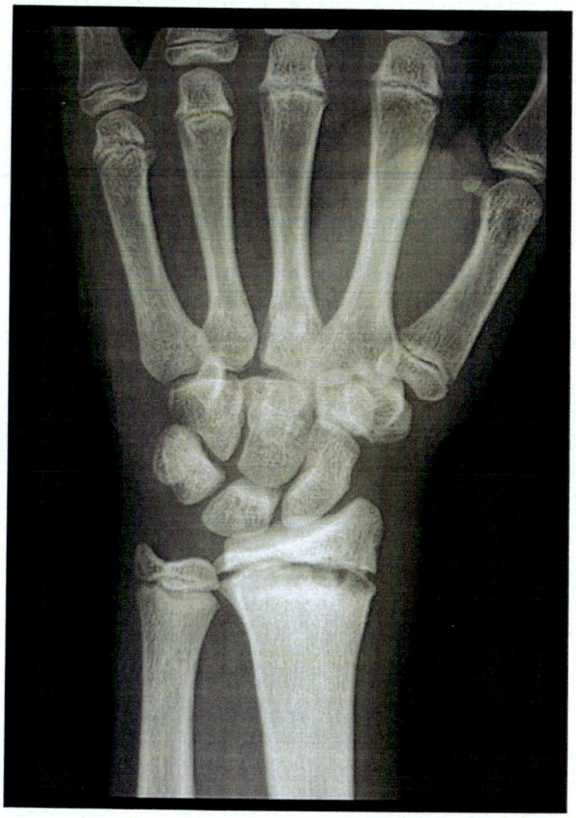

Fig. 1 Gymnast's wrist in a 12-year-old female gymnast. PA radiograph of the left wrist shows in the distal radius widening of the growth plate, beaked effect of the distal aspect of the epiphysis and haziness within the usually radiolucent area of the growth plate

before to explain the distal radial physeal injury is applied as well. Because of this, the association between a distal radius fracture/physeal injury and the stress fracture of the scaphoid is common and well known in the literature (Inagaki and Inoue 1997; Hernán-Prado and Laplaza 2001). The *gymnasts* are again especially predisposed to this kind of injury (Matzkin and Singer 2000; Engel and Feldner-Busztin 1991).

Loading of the distal radius during the exercises and abduction and dorsiflexion of the wrist in gymnastics are suggested as likely pathomechanisms of this injury. Besides, the scaphoid occupies a unique anatomical position in the wrist, bridging the proximal and distal carpal rows and acts as a connecting rod between the two rows. Because of this relation, the scaphoid may receive shearing and torsional forces by excessive and repetitive wrist movements, causing failure of the body structure at the level of the waist and subsequent the fracture of the bone.

Other sports have been related with the development of a stress fracture of the scaphoid: a *shot putter* (Mazione and Pizzutillo 1981) due to repetitive forced dorsiflexion of the wrist and *badminton players* (Brutus and Chahidi 2004) due to repeated shearing and torsion forces by excessive wrist movement from hitting a shuttle. Also an unusual case of a stress fracture of the scaphoid in a *competitive diver* has been observed (Hosey et al. 2006).

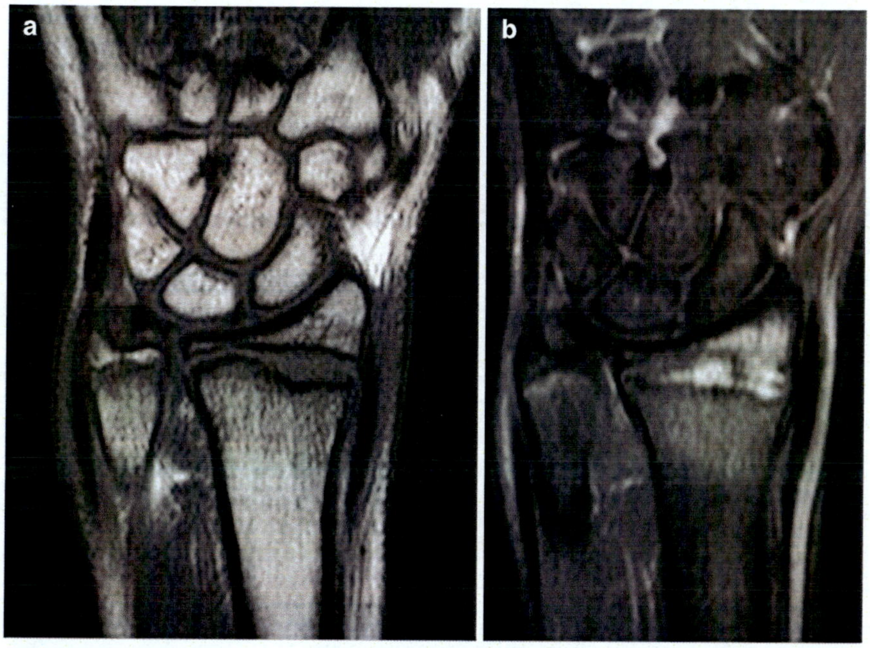

Fig. 2 Gymnast's wrist in a 12-year-old female gymnast. The coronal T1-w (**a**) and corresponding coronal STIR (**b**) MR images clearly depict widening of the growth plate, beaked effect of the distal aspect of the epiphysis and bone marrow oedema adjacent to the growth plate

Plain radiographs are often inconclusive, but MRI usually helps elucidate the diagnosis. Typical MRI findings include periostal reaction and marrow oedema, as well as fracture line. Multi detector computed tomography (MDCT) may be helpful if the fracture needs to be visualized, or to distinguish between a stress reaction (no fracture line visible) and a real stress fracture (Jones 2006; Brukner and Bennel 1997).

2.1.3 Scaphoid Impaction Syndrome

The scaphoid impaction syndrome (SIS) occurs usually as result of repetitive hyperextension stresses such as those occurring in floor exercises of *gymnasts* and when *weightlifters* rest the weight bar on their palms or from excessive push-ups (Webb and Rettig 2008; Stabler et al. 1997).

The symptoms are pain, weakness and tenderness at the dorsoradial aspect of the wrist usually aggravated by dorsiflexion. The SIS is caused by impingement of the scaphoid against the radius due to forced dorsiflexion, forming an osteophyte on the dorsoradial aspect of the scaphoid. Plain radiographs may show an osteophyte on the dorsoradial aspect of the scaphoid. On MDCT these osteophytes are more easily detected (Fig. 3). MRI may show associated soft tissue/bone marrow oedema as a consequence of the impingement.

2.2 Tendons

2.2.1 De Quervain's Syndrome

De Quervain's syndrome is a typical example of overuse tenosynovitis of the wrist. Athletes who practice sports such *golf, tennis* and other racquet sports, *volleyball* and *handball* may be affected by this condition (Rossi et al. 2005; Tagliafico et al. 2009). All these sports have in common the alteration of the normal kinematics of the tendons of the first extensor compartment of the wrist, abductor pollicis longus (APL) and extensor pollicis brevis (EPB), resulting in a chronic microtrauma of the tendons at the level of the radial styloid. Due to this, a thickening of the extensor retinaculum of the wrist and subsequent impingement of the tendons in the fibro-osseous canal result in the development De Quervain's tendinopathy.

Clinically, patients complain of pain and tenderness at the radial side of the wrist during pinch grasping or thumb or wrist movements. The pain may radiate to the thumb or up to the volar aspect of the wrist. Athletes may complain also of difficulty gripping and often rub over the radial styloid when describing the condition. A positive *Finkelstein test* provides further confirmation of the diagnosis. Plain radiographs are only helpful in ruling out bony pathology, such as severe carpometacarpal (CMC) osteoarthritis. Initial evaluation often is done with high resolution US. US findings include tendon thickening and synovial sheath thickening with

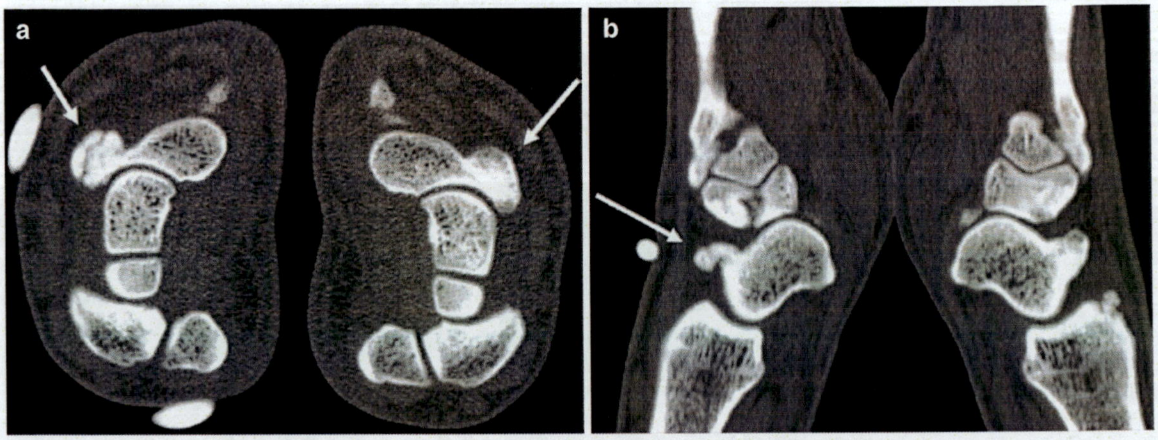

Fig. 3 Scaphoid impaction syndrome in a 21-year-old female former gymnast with dorsoradial wrist pain. MDCT with axial (**a**) and sagittal (**b**) MPR shows a prominent osteophyte on the dorsoradial aspect of the scaphoid bone on both sides (*arrows*)

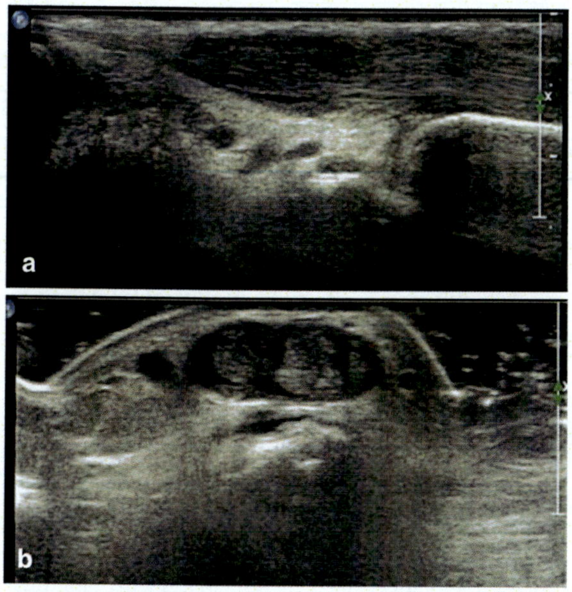

Fig. 4 De Quervain's syndrome in an 18-year-old male professional tennis player. The longitudinal (**a**) and axial (**b**) ultrasound (US) images, show thickening of tendons and tendon sheaths. In addition, peritendinous oedematous changes (hypoecoic halo) around the tendons of the first extensor compartment are shown

peritendinous oedematous changes resulting in a peritendinous hypoecoic halo in all patients (Fig. 4) (Diop et al. 2008).

Injection of corticosteroid into the sheath, with or without US guidance, reduces tendon thickening and inflammation. A dose of 0.5 mL of 1% of Lidocaine and 0.5% of a long-acting corticosteroid preparation can be injected either simultaneously or sequentially. Just one injection relieves the symptoms in approximately 50% of patients. A second injection given at least 1 month later relieves symptoms in another 40–45% of patients (Diop et al. 2008; Sawaizumi et al. 2007).

In our clinical experience MRI does not play an active role in the diagnosis of this disease.

2.3 Nerves

2.3.1 Wartenberg's Syndrome

The *Wartenberg's syndrome* is the isolated nerve entrapment of the cutaneus branch of the radial nerve causing significant pain in the lower one third of the forearm on the radial side (Lanzetta M, Foucher G. 1993) The cutaneus branch of the radial nerve emerges between the tendon of the brachioradialis and the extensor carpi radialis longus (ECRL) (Tryfonidis et al. 2005).

In athletes it is caused by the repetitive ulnar deviation and pronation causing compression between the tendons of the brachioradialis and the ECRL, especially in *weightlifters* with tight wrist bands.

The patients complain of pain and paresthesias with forearm pronated.

At the clinical exploration, typically forearm pronation worsens symptoms with paraesthesia in the distribution of the radial sensory nerve. The *Tinel's sign* (it is performed by lightly percussing over the nerve to elicit a sensation of tingling in the distribution of the nerve) may also be positive (Plate and Green 2000).

The association between the Wartenberg's syndrome and De Quervain's disease is well known in the literature (Lanzetta and Foucher 1995; Fragniere et al. 2001) and occasionally the clinical manifestation of a Wartenberg's syndrome may be confused with a Quervain's tendinopathy.

The diagnosis is based on electrodiagnostic studies and following a local anaesthetic block. High-resolution US examination may be able to depict subtle abnormalities of the superficial cutaneous branch of the radial nerve.

3 Ulnar Wrist Pain

The ulnar side of the wrist has been referred to as the "black box" of the wrist and its pathology has been compared with that of low back pain. This is due to the complexity of the structures that can potentially be injured on the ulnar aspect of the wrist and also due to the particular biomechanical properties of the ulnar side of the wrist. The ulnar-sided wrist pain can be disabling because of limitation of pronation-supination during sports such as tennis and golf, apart of others. The combination of an exquisite physical examination and a detailed history will contribute to the exact location of the problem which is helpful in terms of tailoring the appropriate radiological evaluation.

The pain can be located on the distal ulna (stress fracture of the distal ulna), on the ulnar border of the wrist (ulnocarpal impaction syndrome, extensor carpi ulnaris (ECU) subluxation/tendinopathy, distal radio-ulnar joint instability) or a bit distal from the border of the wrist joint (stress fractures of the hook of the hamate and piso-triquetal chondromalacia). In the athletes and due to repeated trauma on the hand palm, the ulnar nerve can also be compressed at the level of the wrist causing an ulnar neuropathy with a characteristic clinical manifestation (numbness in the medial side of the wrist/hand and in the little finger).

3.1 Bone

3.1.1 Stress Fractures of the Ulna

Stress fractures of the ulna are uncommon injuries but have been reported in athletes involved in various sports. The mechanisms involving ulnar stress fractures remain unclear. As we discussed at the beginning of this chapter, the radial side of the wrist is the important weight-bearing surface; meanwhile the role of the ulnar side of the wrist has more to do with movement. Postulated causes of stress fractures of the ulna include repetitive muscle tension, torsion forces, and compression forces. Ulnar stress fractures have been reported in athletes who exert substantial physical stresses on the ulna by repetitive excessive pronation during sports. These have been seen more frequently in *tennis players* who use double-handed backhand strokes (Fragniere et al. 2001; Young et al. 1995; Bollen et al. 1993) but also in *softball pitchers* (Tanabe et al. 1991), *table tennis players* (Dufek et al. 1999; Petschnig et al. 1997), *weightlifters* and *bodybuilders* who lift excessive weights (Hamilton 1984; Steunebrink et al. 2008) and *spinner bowlers* with repeated flexor profundus muscle contraction (Hsu et al. 2005). Other sports have been associated with stress fractures of the ulna such as *volleyball* and *golf* (Koskinen et al. 1997). Stress fracture of the ulnar styloid process has been reported in a *kendo player* (Japanese fencing) (Itadera et al. 2001). In this particular sport, the exercise of the kendo requires to flex the non-dominant wrist in an ulnar direction, causing the disorder.

Tennis is the sport most frequently involved in the development of a stress fracture of the ulna and are characteristically located in the non-dominant arm of athletes using a two-handed backhand stroke. The typical complaint is an insidious onset of pain during playing. Like in all overuse type of injuries, the athlete will not recall a recent history of trauma in this area. The pain subsides at rest, but symptoms return when the athlete resumes the original activity. The common findings on physical examination include tenderness or pain on palpation or percussion on the ulna. Erythema or oedema can also be present. Radiologic investigation should always start with plain radiographs, but the stress fracture may not be evident for the first 2–4 weeks after the onset of symptoms. An early accurate diagnosis is essential for avoiding both complications and prolonged delay of return to competition. MRI is the preferred test for diagnosis. The MRI findings of stress fractures typically follow one of two patterns.

The stress response or reaction does not show any fracture line or band; instead, the injury may have diffuse areas of hypointensity on T1-w images, with increased signal intensity on fat suppressed T2-w and short-tau inversion recovery (STIR) images (Lee and Yao 1988). In the second pattern if activity is not interrupted, the fracture line is demonstrated with a hypointense line on all pulse sequences, with surrounding bone marrow and soft tissue oedema.

3.1.2 Ulnocarpal Impaction Syndrome

The ulnocarpal impaction syndrome, also known as ulnar abutment or ulnocarpal loading, is a *degenerative condition* characterized by ulnar wrist pain, swelling and limitation of the motion related to excessive load bearing across the ulnar aspect of the wrist. The type of stroke and grip in racquet sports and more frequently in *tennis* can predispose to this injury. In racquet sports during the stroke the wrist is extended and pronated and the ECU tendon is relaxed. The movement of the head of the ulna is therefore not limited. Forced translation of the head of the ulna dorsally or a hyper-pronation or hyper-supination may cause a tear of the articular disc or of the peripheral attachment of the radio-ulnar ligaments. This can cause pain due to the torn cartilage interposing between highly congruent surfaces during motion or by causing micro or macro instability to the distal radio-ulnar complex. In the ulna-positive athlete, the chronic impaction between the ulnar head and the TFCC and the ulnar aspect of the carpus results in the spectrum of abnormalities that constitute the ulnocarpal impaction syndrome. Styloid magna and rarely negative ulnar variance may also be predisposing factors. Other sports that require repetitive wrist and hand motion such as *rowing*, *hockey*, *golf*, *baseball* and those inducing loading at the hand and wrist such as *gymnastics*, *shot put*, *cycling* and *weightlifting* have been associated with this syndrome. The ulnocarpal impaction syndrome can appear years after a fracture of the distal radius (with residual radial shortening and abnormal dorsal tilt and secondary ulna plus), premature physeal closure of the distal radius or after a previous radial head resection (Guha and Marynissen 2002).

The spectrum of radiological manifestations includes (Cerezal et al. 2002): degenerative tear of the TFCC; chondromalacia of the lunate bone, triquetral bone, and distal ulnar head; instability or tear of the lunotriquetral ligament; and finally osteoarthritis of the ulnocarpal and distal radioulnar joints (Fig. 5). The only radiological modality for diagnosing this syndrome is MRI. High resolution imaging, high field strength and the use of a dedicated wrist coil for the evaluation of the TFCC are mandatory (Magee 2009). The TFCC lesions associated with the ulnar impaction syndrome are degenerative on arthroscopy according to Palmer's classification (Palmer 1989). The differential diagnosis must include Kienböck disease, intraosseous ganglion and a true subchondral cyst formation.

3.1.3 Stress Fractures of the Hook of the Hamate

Normally the fracture of the hook of the hamate is due to an acute trauma or a sharp strike against the hamate hook while swinging in *golf*, *baseball*, *tennis* or *hockey*. In all these sports, during the swing, the stress of the impact is transmitted up the shaft to the hand, causing the fracture in the upper hand. The non-dominant hand is typically affected.

Nevertheless, some of these athletes due to repeated stress can develop also a stress fracture of the hook of the hamate. Just a few cases of stress fractures have been reported in the literature (Guha and Marynissen 2002; Ardèvol and Henriquez 2002; Bayer and Schweizer 2009). Like in other stress fractures, usually they have only a few symptoms and a high clinical suspicion is mandatory to find the correct diagnosis. These patients complain of gradual onset of pain on the ulnar aspect of the wrist and tenderness. Plain radiographs usually do not show any evidence of stress fractures and thus MRI is more effective for diagnosing unclear cases.

3.1.4 Pisotriquetal Chondromalacia

Chondromalatia of the pisotriquetal affects sports that require holding a club, handle or a bat; with powerful forces of the forearm such as *golf*, *baseball*, *tennis*, *hockey*, *squash* and *badminton* (Helal 1978a, b; Linscheid and Dobyns 1985). During the swing in these sports, the stress of the impact is transmitted from the forearm to the hand, causing chronic trauma between triquetrum and pisiforme resulting in pisotriquetal chondromalacia. In an attempt to understand the pathophysiology of

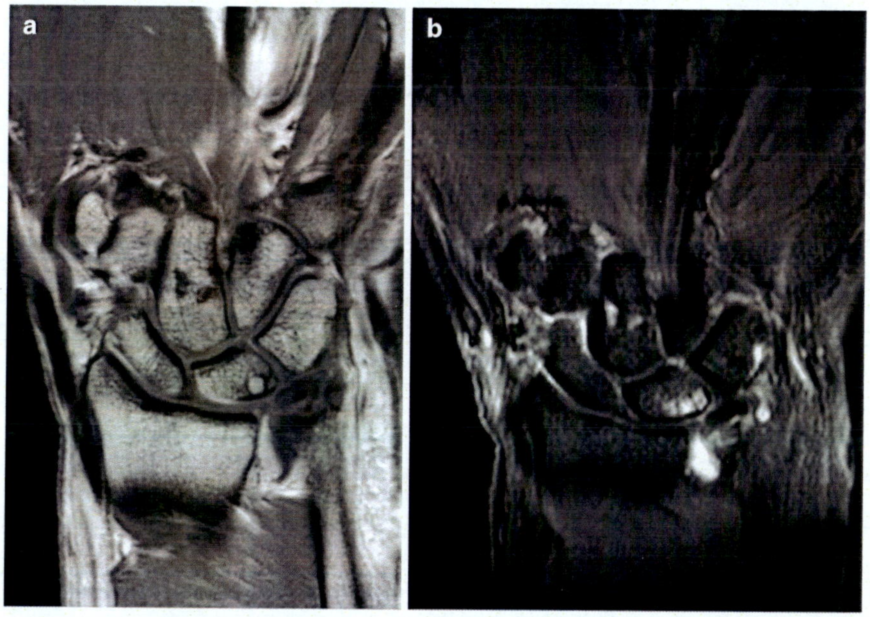

Fig. 5 Ulnocarpal impaction syndrome in a 26-year-old male amateur tennis player. The coronal T1-w (**a**) and STIR (**b**) MR images show the subchondral changes in keeping with chondromalacia of the lunate bone (ulnar side) with synovitis and a degenerative TFCC tear

the strain at the pisotriquetal joint, Beckers and Koebke (Beckers and Koebke 1998) investigated the distribution of forces to pisiform and pisotriquetal joint and the role of these structures in the transfer of forces within the carpus from the forearm. They concluded that the pisiform mechanically contributes to the stability of the ulnar column of the wrist. It has two main functions: it holds the triquetum in a correct position and prevents its subluxation even in extreme extension and it also acts as a fulcrum while transducing powerful forearm forces to the hand.

This injury, causing in athletes significant clinical symptoms and disability, is a commonly encountered abnormality in arthroscopy but rarely diagnosed by radiologists. Because of this, an athlete with chronic ulnar-sided wrist pain, in whom no other cause can be found, the pisotriquetal chondromalacia should be suspected.

The diagnosis may also be difficult to distinguish from other ulno-carpal problems from the radiological point of view. The plain radiographs are frequently negative. Additional views of the P-T joint can be helpful in detecting joint space narrowing and small osteophytes with sclerosis. Early degenerative diseases may be seen well on MRI as early alterations in cartilage contour morphology (fibrillation, surface irregularity) or changes in cartilage thickness. Advanced degenerative chondral lesions typically manifest on MRI as multiple areas of cartilage thinning of varying depth and size. Cartilage defects are typically demonstrated with obtuse margins and may be associated with corresponding subchondral regions of increased T2-w signal reflective subchondral oedema or cysts or low signal intensity reflective subchondral sclerosis (Recht et al. 2005). MDCT can detect the degenerative changes in the joints in a later phase (Fig. 6).

In the top athlete, early diagnosis (in most of the cases with MRI or even with arthroscopy) provides the best chance for successful treatment.

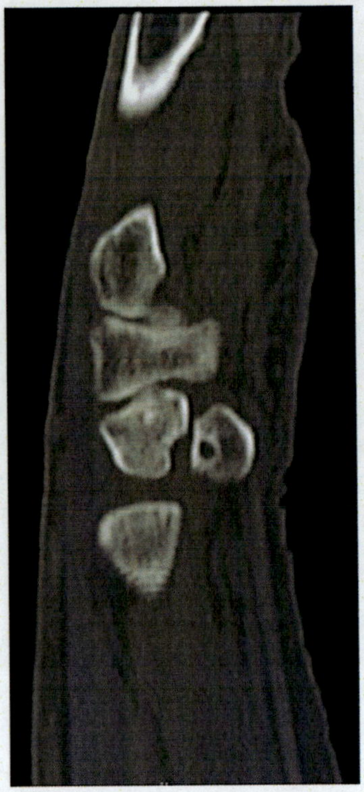

Fig. 6 Pisotriquetal chondromalacia in a 36-year-old male golf player. MDCT (MPR sagittal reconstruction) shows a late phase of a pisotriquetal chondromalacia with degenerative changes in the pisotriquetal joint

3.2 Tendon

3.2.1 Extensor Carpi Ulnaris tendinopathy

The origin of the ECU muscle is on the lateral epicondyle of the humerus and its insertion on the base of the fifth metacarpal (dorsal side). The distal tendon of the ECU muscle resides within its own subsheath, which is distinct from the extensor retinaculum and this, stabilizes the tendon within its groove along the distal ulna (Spinner and Kaplan 1970). The main actions of this muscle are the extension and the ulnar deviation (adduction) of the wrist.

The injury of the ECU tendon can be divided in two types: chronic tendinopathy and traumatic injury. The chronic overuse related tendinopathy of the ECU is a common sport overuse injury related normally to *racquet sports* with repetitive wrist motion such as *tennis, squash, badminton* and *racquetball* (Montalvan et al. 2006). The pain in the athletes with tendinopathy of the ECU tendon initially occurs when the player changes technique, equipment or surface. The pain is located around the ulnar side of the wrist, along and under the ulnar styloid. It is felt with the first strokes of the racquet, then gradually fades, and disappears after 5–10 min. It usually follows the same pattern the next day. At rest, the player is aware of minor discomfort under the ulnar styloid. Prompt diagnosis will allow for the appropriate treatment and will allow the player to get back to the court and prevent the development of chronic discomfort. As was commented previously, pinpointing the cause of dorsal ulnar-sided wrist pain is a diagnostic challenge even to the most experienced physicians, especially if the pain becomes chronic. The clinical findings are often non-specific and can mimic disorders of the distal radio-ulnar joint. Recently, in an effort to improve the diagnostic value of the physical examination in patient with ulnar-sided wrist pain and reduce imaging studies, the *ECU synergy test* has been introduced (Ruland and Hogan 2008). This test contributes to distinguish between intra-articular and extra-articular pathology in the athlete with ulnar-sided wrist pain. Acute tendinopathy of the ECU will cause swelling over the tendon sheath and possible crepitus. In players with chronic pain over the ECU tendon (tendinopathy) swelling may not be present. The diagnosis can be confirmed, and in dubious cases supported, by ultrasonography (preferably) or MRI. The ultrasonography can measure the tendon size, longitudinal splits, tendon sheath effusion and synovial hypertrophy (Fig. 7). The treatment is based on the injection in the tendon sheath of the ECU 3 mL of 1% lidocaine and 40 mg of a long-acting corticosteroid preparation.

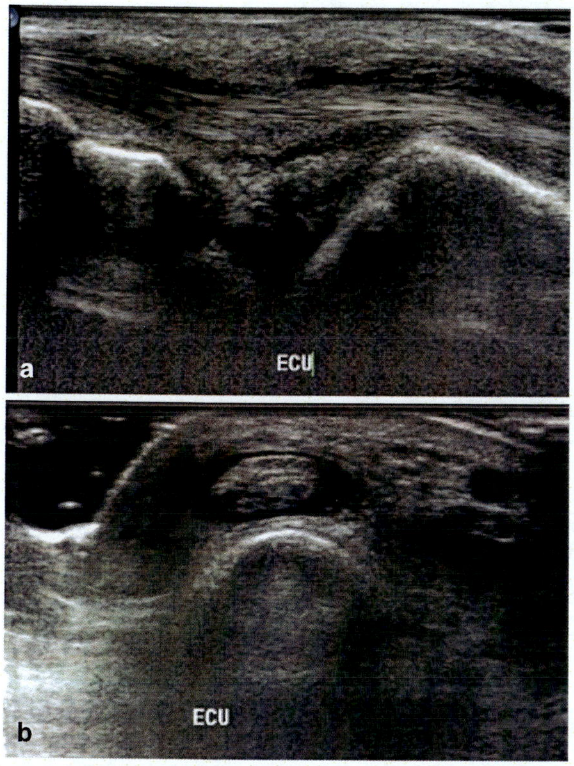

Fig. 7 Extensor carpi ulnaris (ECU) tendinopathy in a 27-year-old male professional tennis player with ulnar-sided wrist pain. US shows effusion and synovial hypertrophy around the ECU tendon in both the longitudinal (**a**) and axial (**b**) images

3.2.2 Subluxation of the ECU

In patients with chronic ulnar-sided pain (with a positive synergy test) in whom the diagnosis of a tendonitis/tenosynovitis of the ECU can not be established, other underlying causes of the pain should be considered: instability of the tendon with subluxation of the ECU and erosions on the floor of the sixth extensor compartment.

The instability of the tendon with its subluxation outside the groove can be assessed with the help of dynamic US. During the dynamic US a painful snapping of the ulnar wrist during supination and pronation can be detected (MacLennan et al. 2008).

The erosion of the sixth compartment floor has been given very little attention in the literature as a potential cause of chronic ulnar-sided wrist pain in athletes. In patients with persistent pain despite usual treatment, an erosion of the sixth compartment floor should be suspected (Fig. 8).

Patients often relate the onset of pain with a twisting motion during sports activities. A "pop" is felt and the ulnar-sided aspect of the wrist becomes painful. If the structures that give stability to the tendon (retinaculum, linea jugata) are partially ruptured, further instability of the tendon without true subluxation occurs. The presence of an unstable tendon will cause chronic inflammation, swelling and erosion of the floor of the sixth dorsal space causing chronic ulnar-sided wrist pain in these patients (Carneiro et al. 2005).

3.3 Nerves

3.3.1 Ulnar Tunnel Syndrome

The *ulnar tunnel syndrome* (UTS) or *Guyon's canal syndrome* is a compression neuropathy of the ulnar nerve when it crosses the Guyon's canal. The Guyon's canal is a tunnel formed medially by the pisiform bone and laterally by the hook of the hamate. In this tunnel the nerve passes deep to the palmar carpal ligament and superficial to the flexor retinaculum. Accompanying the nerve through this canal are the ulnar artery and vein. Once in the canal, the ulnar nerve divides into its terminal branches: the superficial (sensory) and the deep (motor) branches. Symptoms associated with Guyon's canal syndrome fall into three types depending on the level and type of compression involved (Gross and Gelberman 1984).

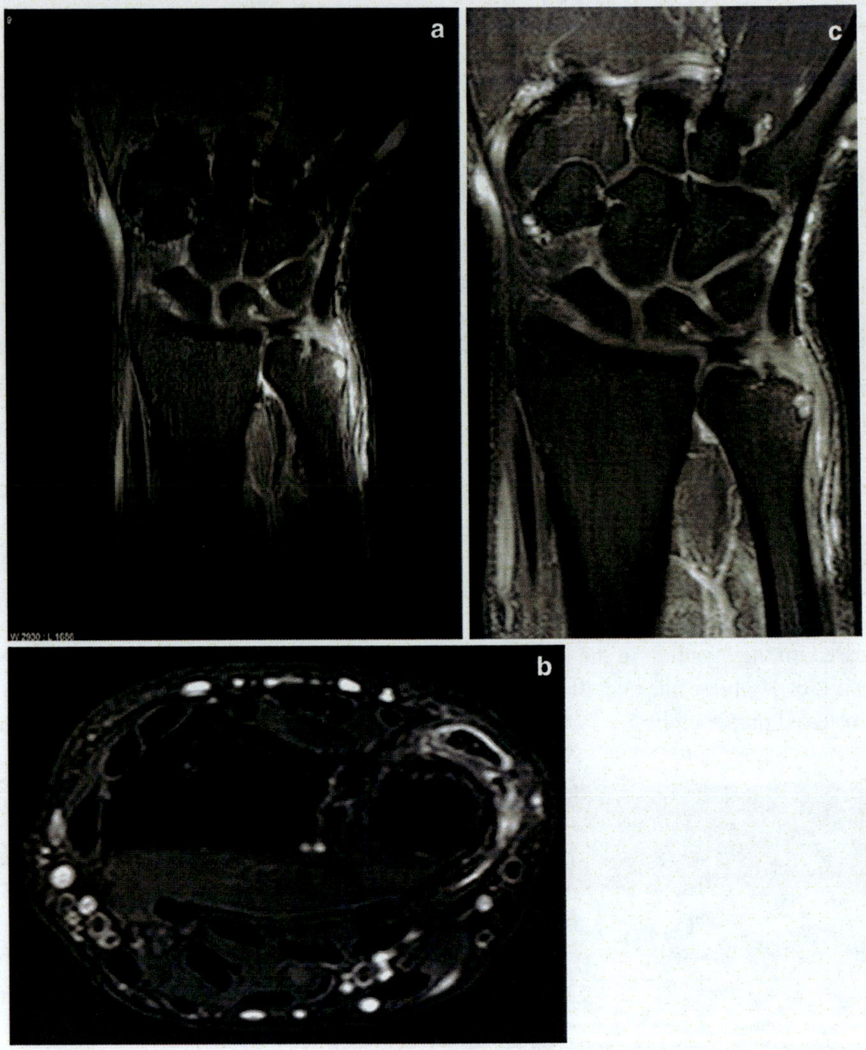

Fig. 8 Erosion of the sixth compartment floor in a 41-year-old male amateur tennis player. The coronal STIR (**a**) and fat suppressed axial T2-w (**b**) MR images, show erosion on the floor of the sixth compartment with concomitant inflammatory changes around the extensor capi ulnaris tendon. After intravenous contrast administration, marked enhancement is seen (**c**)

This syndrome can be caused by mass lesions (accessory muscles, arthritic changes, tumours, ganglia or vascular thrombosis) but in athletes, it is normally caused by chronic trauma. Symptoms of UTS are commonly experienced by *avid bicyclists* (Kalainov and Hartigan 2003; Maimaris and Zadeh 1990). Cyclists can experience this kind of neuropathy related to hand placement on the handlebars. The ulnar nerve is at risk due to the pressure and force applied though handlebars and brakes. Other sports have been associated, but less frequently, with UTS: *formula 1 driver* (Masmejean et al. 1999) and *wheelchair athletes* (Burnham and Steadward 1994).

The diagnosis is based on the clinical history and the electro-diagnostic studies. The ultrasonography can measure the nerve size and show mass lesions causing the syndrome but it plays a less important role than in other kind of neuropathies, due to difficulty in the evaluation of the ulna nerve in the Guyon's canal.

4 Dorsal Wrist Pain

4.1 Bone

4.1.1 Stress Injury of the Lunate

The stress injury of the lunate is a condition only vaguely described in the literature. Nevertheless, our experience is that this entity is not so rare, but its association with other conditions, obscure its proper diagnosis. Tennis and similar sports have been related to the development of this injury (Maquirriain and Ghisi 2007). It has been reported that the type of grip used, determines the development of this kind of injury (Maquirriain and Ghisi 2006). The patient complains of pain in the dorsal side of the wrist at the level of the proximal carpal row. The diagnosis is based on MRI which shows bone marrow oedema without any fracture line.

4.1.2 Capitate Avascular Necrosis

Avascular necrosis (AVN) of the capitate bone in athletes is an important, although rare, cause of spontaneous onset of wrist pain. This entity should be considered in athletes with dorsal wrist pain of unknown origin especially in sports such as *gymnastics* or *weight-lifting*. These two sports have in common the extreme loading of the wrist with axial compression and microtrauma combined with an inherent "weak" blood supply (Bürger et al. 2006). The association of these two conditions constitute the basis of the development of an AVN of the os capitate. Like the scaphoid, the proximal part of the capitate obtains its blood supply by means of diffusion or retrograde blood supply. This particular vascularisation pattern of the bone predisposes to the development of AVN.

The diagnosis of this entity should start with plain radiographs. These can be normal during the initial stages but later they can show sclerosis of the os capitate, progressive loss of height of the bone, fragmentation and at the late phase degenerative changes involving the surrounding joints. Our role as radiologists is the early detection of this entity to prevent the dramatic consequences of a premature osteoarthritis. Because of this, MRI, which is the method to early depict AVN, should be performed in those athletes with dorsal wrist pain of unknown origin when plain X-rays are negative. The radiological criteria and stages of the osteonecrosis are the same as in the case of the osteonecrosis of the lunate (Golimbu et al. 1995; Bartelmann et al. 2001). In our clinical experience, the use of paramagnetic contrast is also mandatory. The degree of vascular enhancement relates to the viability of the necrotic segment and this parameter is essential for the clinical management of the patient.

4.2 Tendon

4.2.1 Intersection Syndrome

Intersection syndrome is not a cause of strictly dorsal-sided wrist pain but rather affects the dorsal side of the distal forearm. This painful condition is mentioned herein since it exhibits clinical similarities with other disorders described previously such as DeQuervain's syndrome. This syndrome has a high incidence in *rowers* and *weight-lifters* (McNally et al. 2005). The intersection syndrome is an inflammatory process of the second extensor compartment tendons of the forearm, characterized by the presence of pain and swelling proximal to the Lister tubercle of the distal radius. Symptoms occur where the first extensor compartment tendons (APL and EPB) cross over the second extensor compartment tendons, extensor carpi radialis brevis (ECRB) and ECRL tendons. In sports such as *rowing* and *weight-lifting,* repetitive resisted extension is required and the friction of the tendons of the first extensor compartment against the second is constant, causing this overuse syndrome.

The diagnosis is based on a proper physical examination and most of the time no special tests are required. The main challenge is distinguishing intersection syndrome from a DeQuervain's syndrome. In unclear cases complementary studies are required. US and MRI may show peritendinous fluid/oedema concentrically surrounding the first and the second extensor compartments (Fig. 9).

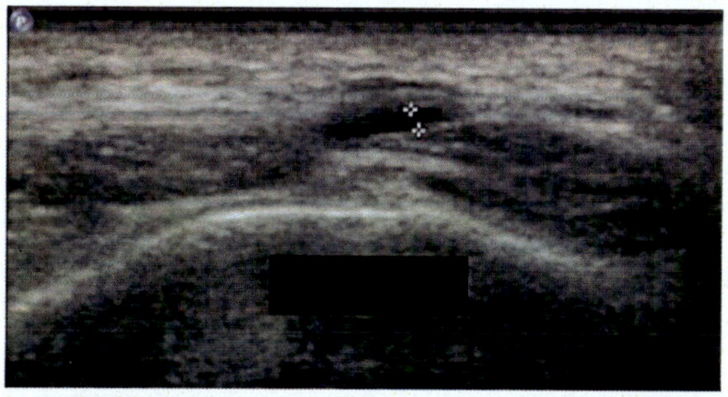

Fig. 9 Intersection syndrome in a 28-year-old professional rower. US (axial view) shows peritendinous fluid concentrically surrounding the first and the second extensor compartments

4.3 Soft Tissue

4.3.1 Dorsal Impingement Syndromes

The dorsal wrist impingement is a controversial syndrome. In the majority of cases, no specific radiological findings that could support the diagnosis exist whereas variable results have been reported to the standard treatment. Typically, this syndrome has been attributed to a pinching of the dorsal wrist capsule between the ECRB and the dorsal ridge of the scaphoid during specific manoeuvres. It occurs especially in recreational athletes with poor swing mechanics. There are no specific tests for dorsal wrist impingement. Its diagnosis is based on the patient's history and on how and when the pain started. The pain of this syndrome is not a generalized one, but a specific pain in a specific spot, usually brought on by certain hand and wrist movements. The diagnosis is also made by ruling out any other wrist problems that could be responsible (Henry 2008).

5 Palmar Wrist Pain

5.1 Tendon

5.1.1 Wrist Flexor Tendinopathy

The tendinopathy of the flexor tendons at the level of the wrist is also an overuse injury that occurs frequently in specific sports. The tendinopathy can occur in all tendons but it is most common in the flexor carpi ulnaris tendon (FCU), flexor carpi radialis tendon (FCR) and flexor digitorum tendon.

FCU tendinopathy is more often seen in *racquet sports* due to direct impact of the handle against the wrist as well as due to repetitive stretching that occurs as the wrist is forcefully whipped into extremes of position. The FCU tendon has a broad area of insertion into the pisiform and in the hypothenar fascia and patients with tendinopathy complain of vague pain anywhere from the forearm to the ulnar and palmar side of the hand. Sometimes the pain is well localized at the level of the pisiform making the diagnosis in this case easier.

FCR tendinopathy is also normally related with *racquet sports*. The FCR tendon passes through a groove in the trapezium and passes near the scaphotrapezial and metacarpotrapezial joints as it approaches its insertion onto the volar surface of the second metacarpal. A racquet sport athlete with pain in the course of the FCR tendon should be suspected of suffering such a tendinopathy (Osterman et al. 1988).

The flexor digitorum tendinopathy is more common in sports requiring repetitive pulling (e.g. climbers and rowers) or prolonged pressure on the palms (cycling) (Heuck et al. 1992). These tendons pass through the carpal tunnel and can both mimic and cause carpal tunnel syndrome (CTS), including median nerve compression.

Like in other tendinophaties described before, the diagnosis is based on the clinical exploration and just in unclear cases the US or MRI may be required.

5.2 Nerves

5.2.1 Carpal Tunnel Syndrome

The CTS is a wrist injury that causes damage to the median nerve, which radiates from the forearm into the hand. To be more precise, the CTS describes an irritation of the synovial membranes around the tendons in the carpal tunnel and this inflammation results in a compression of the median nerve. This syndrome can result from anything that irritates the tendons of the carpal tunnel and in turn causes pressure on the median nerve. In athletes, this syndrome is related to sports that involve repetitive and intense wrist motion such as *racquet sports*, *golf* and *bowling* (Osterman et al. 1988; White and Johnson 2003). This compression neuropathy has been also described in *wheelchair sports* (Vanlandewijck et al. 2001).There are a number of tests that can discriminate the CTS from other causes of tingling and loss of hand function. The *Tinel test* is performed with pressure being placed on the location of the median nerve, just above the wrist. If a tingling sensation is experienced in the thumb or fingers, the nerve is probably compressed. The *Phalen test* involves the person extending the arm and flexing the wrist inward; if tingling is experienced, CTS is a strong possibility. This syndrome can be confirmed preferably by abnormal electrophysiological tests. Depending on the degree of impact on daily functioning of the athlete the treatment for CTS may be conservative or surgical.

6 Overuse Athletic Injuries in Hand

6.1 Bone

In athletes most fractures in the hand are stable, since regularly they are caused by low energy injury (Rettig 2004). A stress fracture may develop as a result from overuse of the extremity during daily sports related activity. Plain radiographs including PA, lateral and oblique views with external rotation are advised (www.acr.org). There also is evidence that adding an internally rotated oblique view, the fracture conspicuity will increase (Street 1993).

6.1.1 Stress Fracture of the Metacarpal Bone

As previously commented, stress fractures are usually encountered in athletes but just a few cases involving the metacarpal bones have been reported in the literature. Metacarpal stress fractures have been described in different sports but mainly in *tennis players* (Bespalchuk et al. 2004; Muramatsu and Kuriyama 2005) and *softball players* (Jowett and Brukner 1997). Consequently, metacarpal stress fractures should be considered in athletes with persistent hand pain where repetitive grip function is used. For its diagnosis, MRI is the method of choice.

6.1.2 PIP Joint Injury

This is the most commonly injured joint in sports (Rettig 2004). Injuries include both bone and soft tissues, including fracture, fracture/dislocation, collateral ligaments injury and volar plate injury. Regarding ligaments, the radial collateral is the most frequently injured one, commonly seen in ball handling sports such as *basketball*, *American football*, *volleyball* and *baseball* (Rettig 2004). All PIP injuries should be radiologically assessed to prevent malunion of an intraarticular fracture, described as the *coach finger* (McCue and Cabrera 1992). Besides the three or four radiographic views, no additional imaging is required for diagnosis and treatment (Fig. 10). Radiologists need to be aware that when plain film shows a small volar calcification only, suggesting a small avulsion injury, this can very well be the tip of the iceberg, meaning a volar plate injury. In the case of a total rupture, Swan-neck deformity can occur and is thought a surgical emergency. Late complications of untreated volar plate rupture include recurrent instability of the joint and early osteoarthritis.

6.1.3 Thumb Injury

Thumb injuries are common in all sorts of sports. In assessing thumb injuries, additional radiographs are described in evaluating this complex joint (Carlsen and Moran 2009). Fractures that frequently occur at the base of the thumb are the Bennett's and the Rolando's (Carlsen and Moran 2009). *Bennet fracture* is an intraarticular fracture, caused by adduction force applied on a partially flexed thumb, separating the volar ulnar aspect of the metacarpal base. This fragment is hold in place by the anterior oblique ligament. In American football this is frequently described in the quarterback's throwing hand, impacted on a helm (Rettig 2004). This unstable fracture causes the metacarpal shaft to subluxate dorsally, proximally and radially. *The Rolando fracture* describes a comminuted fracture of the base of the thumb, especially the Y or T-pattern (Carlsen and Moran 2009). MDCT with multiplanar reconstructions enables delineation of the true extend of the injury, allowing adequate surgical management. There is no role for MRI in this kind of injuries.

6.2 Ligaments

6.2.1 Ligaments of the Thumb

The collateral ligaments of the thumb MP joint need some detailed attention. The *skier's* or *gamekeeper's thumb* caused by a radially directed force leading to a ulnar collateral ligament injury, often occurs in *ball handling sports* (e.g. volleyball, basketball), *contact collision sports* and *skiing*. Injury of the ulnar collateral ligament occur more frequently compared to the radial side. Displacement of the ligament proximal and superficial to the adductor pollicis aponeurosis, hampering healing of the rupture is called *Stener* lesion and is a complication of the UCL injury. Most often these injuries are described to occur in the absence of a significant osseous fragment. When a fragment is seen, proximal to the adductor hood, a *bony Stener* lesion is suggested (Carlsen and Moran 2009). MRI is considered the most accurate imaging technique to assess the extension of

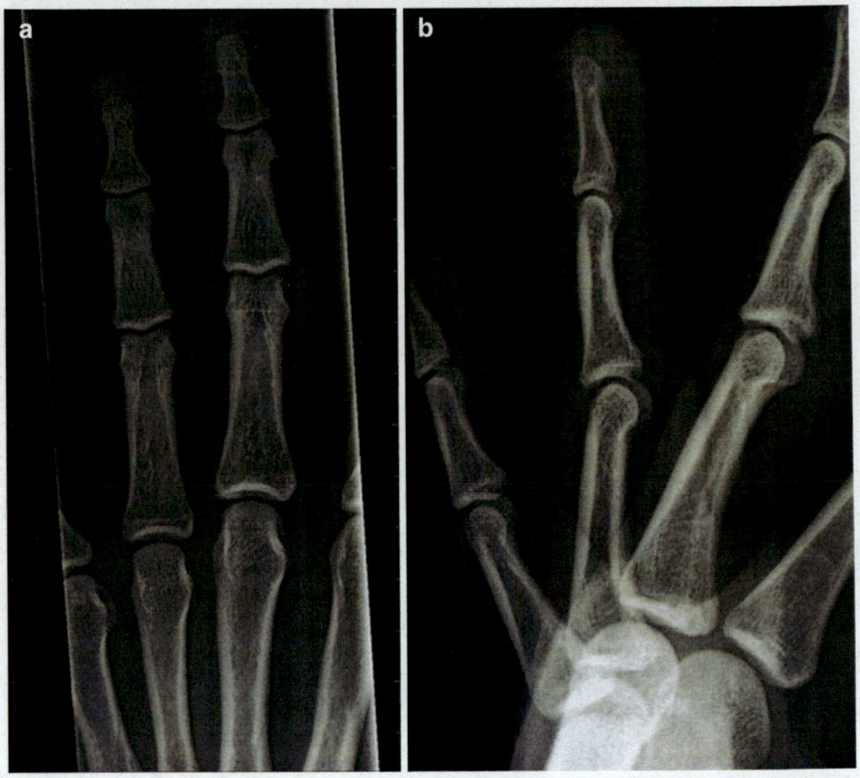

Fig. 10 Volar plate injury in a 20-year-old male basketball player: (**a**) the PA view is normal. (**b**) The lateral radiograph of the third right finger shows a small volar calcification in the PIP joint suggesting an avulsion injury of the volar plate

this lesion (Carlsen and Moran 2009; Plancher et al. 1999). The chronic type of the UCL injury is described as the "*gamekeeper's thumb*". The injury was originally described in Scottish gamekeepers, who used to break the necks of rabbits between thumb and index finger, leading to UCL overuse and thumb laxity (Carlsen and Moran 2009; Campbell 1955).

6.2.2 Mallet Finger

This is a disruption of the terminal extensor tendon at the distal insertion on the distal phalanx. This type of injury is known as *drop finger or baseball finger*, since it often occurs in baseball and softball, basketball or American football. No need for radiological assessment is described. When asked for, US is advised, yet not easily performed.

6.2.3 Boutonniere Deformity

This is the rupture of a central slip of the extensor mechanism at its insertion into the base of the middle phalanx. This injury needs no imaging for diagnosis.

6.2.4 Pulley Injury

An important overuse injury to the ligamentous pulley system structures of the fingers is found in rock climbers. This entity is known as the "*climber's finger*" (Yamaguchi and Ikuta 2007). With the increase in popularity of indoor climbing, this pathological entity has become frequently encountered outside areas where rock climbing is a very common sport. With the formation of a crimp hold, using mainly the middle and ring finger, a maximal load of 700 N can be placed on the pulley when climbing. As a result, the biological strength of the pulley system, especially the A2 and A4, can exceed its strength limit and closed pulley rupture may occur (Schöffl and Schöffl 2006; Klauser et al. 2002).

Characteristic symptoms include an acute onset of sharp pain and loss of tight grip combined with a loud popping noise. A tender palpable mass may be found volarly between PIP and MCP joints (Yamaguchi and Ikuta 2007; Schöffl and Schöffl 2006). When the A2 pulley is ruptured, an increased distance of the flexor tendon to the bone may be palpated. However clinically it is difficult to give an exact differentiation between pulley strain, partial or complete rupture (Yamaguchi and Ikuta 2007). In a recently proposed diagnostic-therapeutic algorithm, imaging work up starts with AP and lateral radiographs, for exclusion of fracture (acute or chronic stress fracture) or volar plate avulsion (Schöffl and Schöffl 2006). When no fracture is seen dynamic high resolution US is advised. Using high frequency technique with a stand off gel pad, the relation of the flexor tendon with the underlying bone can be depicted, once the learning curve is past (Klauser et al. 2002). The measurement in the longitudinal plane of the tendon-bone distance both in extension and active flexion is the important finding. Normally a distance of 0.14 cm during extension and 0.30 cm in active flexion is found: in injuries this can increase to 0.51 cm in forced flexion with a complete rupture (Schöffl and Schöffl 2006). The distance measured allows grading, with a grade 1 strain injury when <2 mm, and a single or multiple rupture when higher distances are measured. Grading will contribute to treatment planning (Klauser et al. 2002). US may show additional findings in climbers, such as tendon sheath cysts, tenosynovitis, PIP joint effusion, and fibrosis (Fig. 11) (Klauser et al. 1999). MRI also has proven highly accurate in detecting these pulley injuries.

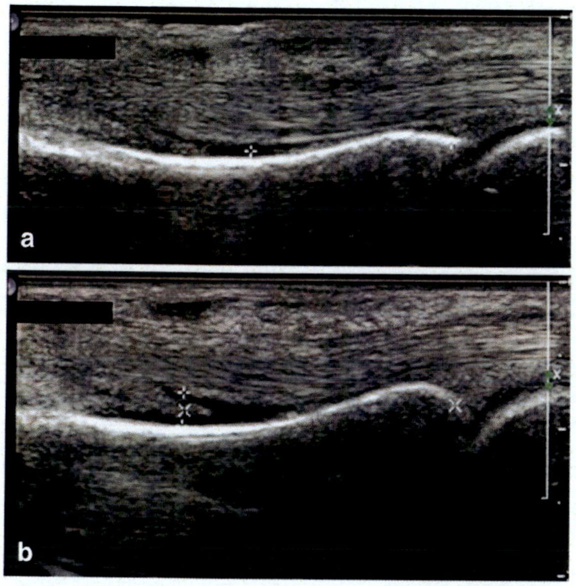

Fig. 11 Pulley injury in a 35-year-old rock climber with acute onset of pain and loss of tight grip in the third right finger during climbing. US (longitudinal view) of the third right finger (**a**) and left finger (**b**) shows an increased tendon-bone distance on the left side with effusion in PIP joint consisting with a pulley injury

6.3 Vascular

6.3.1 Traumatic Aneurysm of the Posterior Circumflex Humeral Artery

In our hospital we have had some experience with *volleyball players* with painful fingers. Reekers et al. (1993) were the first to describe this entity in three professional volleyball players who presented with progressive or intermittent painful often pale or cyanotic hand, with dysesthesia in the fingers. On angiography small microemboli in the digital arteries of the dominant right hand were found. In a second publication the underlying pathology was described as traumatic aneurysm of the posterior circumflex humeral artery (PCHA) in three and occlusion of the PCHA in another three volleyball players (Reekers and Koedam 1998). Pathophysiology was thought to be a recurrent blunt trauma of the vessel wall by smashing or blocking the ball, combining strong contractions of the pectoralis muscle and an anatomically vulnerable position of the PCHA (Reekers et al. 1993). This pathology was suggested as "a volleyball players" disease, and is underestimated due to non awareness of the treating clinicians (Reekers et al. 1993; Reekers and Koedam 1998). Failure to recognize a vascular injury in these highly trained athletes is expected as the symptoms often are subtle, starting with coolness of fingers and loss of endurance or strength. Increased level of suspicion is required in these athletes to promptly diagnose and accurately treat a potentially limb-threatening injury (Arko et al. 2001). Next to volleyball is *baseball pitching* and *tennis* thought to be sports at risk for developing this entity. For diagnosis, angiography or nowadays contrast enhanced MR angiography is the modality of choice (Fig. 12). Endovascular treatment is an effective alternative to the surgical management (Reekers et al. 1993; Reekers and Koedam 1998; Vlychou et al. 2001).

6.4 Hypothenar Hammer Syndrome

Another uncommon vascular overuse syndrome to be included in the differential diagnosis in patients, who present with hand and finger pain, is the *hypothenar hammer syndrome*. This well known pathology often is found in men with a mean age of 40 years in an

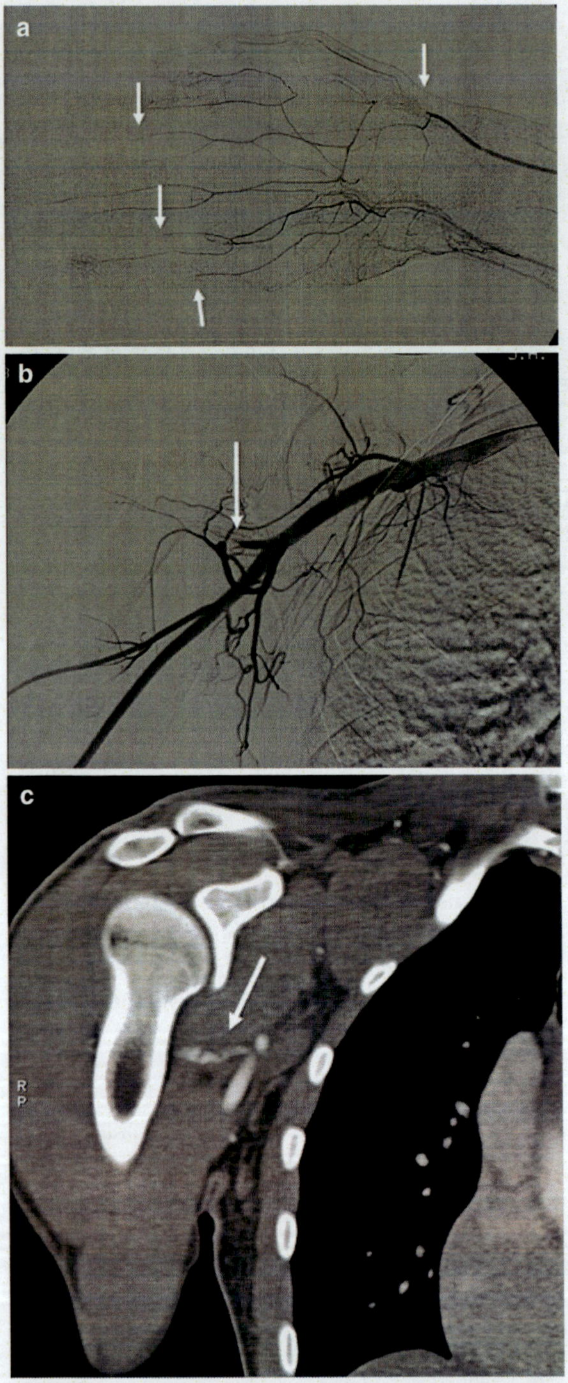

Fig. 12 Vascular injury to the fingers in a volleyball player. (**a**) DSA shows multiple areas of small emboli in small arteries of various fingers (*arrows*). (**b**) Shows an abrupt stop of the posterior circumflex humeral artery in another volleyball player, (**c**) CT angiography shows the injured vessel. (Courtesy Professor J.A. Reekers)

occupational setting, in which the worker uses the ulnar hypothenar side of the hand as a tool to hammer, or push hard objects (Ablett and Hackett 2008). Workers at risk are metal workers, auto mechanics and carpenters. However, this syndrome is also seen in athletes who experience trauma to the palm of the hand when striking: it is reported in sports such as *baseball, karate, badminton, golf, tennis, volleyball* and also in *break-dancing* (Ablett and Hackett 2008).

The injured structure is the superficial branch of the ulnar artery, distally from Guyon's canal, that is compressed against the hook of the hamate. With injury of the vessel wall, with potential aneurysm and periadventitial scarring, vascular narrowing occurs, resulting in microemboli that can occlude digital arteries. Angiography is thought the gold standard for diagnosis, showing tortuosity of the ulnar artery with corkscrew appearance, aneurysm formation and occluded ulnar located digital arteries (Ablett and Hackett 2008).

7 Final Remarks

In a world of increasing gaming amongst people of all ages, new overuse type of injuries occur. Prolonged use of electronic games cause serious problems (Osterman et al. 1987). Mandall described a 68 years old grandmother, gaming 3–4 h a day with her grandchildren, who presented with a volar plate rupture of the first MCPJ as overuse injury (Mandal et al. 2005). It is thought that gaming biomechanics with chronic hyperextension of the thumb is causing this lesion. The first thumb injury, due to playing Nintendo game, called "nintendinitis", was a tendinopathy of the extensor pollicis longus tendon (Brasington 1990). Pain syndromes as myofascial pain syndrome of the wrist and intrinsic muscles of the hand are described related to gaming (Zapata et al. 2006). The newer games, with the Nintendo "Wii", in which players make movements that simulate real sports activities are also known for their overuse related injuries (Bonis 2007; Nett et al. 2008).

References

Ablett CT, Hackett LA (2008) Hypothenar hammer syndrome: case reports and brief overview. Clin Med Res 6:3–8

American College of Radiology. Appropriateness criteria. www.acr.org
Ardèvol J, Henriquez A (2002) Hook of the hamate non-union: suspicion of stress-induced mechanism in a hockey player. Knee Surg Sports Traumatol Arthrosc 10:61–63
Arko FR, Harris EJ, Zarins CK, Olcott C IV (2001) Vascular complications in high-performing athletes. J Vasc Surg 33: 935–942
Bartelmann U, Kalb K, Schmitt R, Fröhner S (2001) Radiologic diagnosis of lunate necrosis. Handchir Mikrochir Plast Chir 33:365–378
Bayer T, Schweizer A (2009) Stress fracture of the hook of the hamate as a result of intensive climbing. J Hand Surg Eur 34:276–277
Beckers A, Koebke J (1998) Mechanical strain at the pisotriquetral joint. Clin Anat 11:320–326
Bespalchuk A, Okada K, Nishida J (2004) Stress fracture of the second metacarpal bone. Skeletal Radiol 33:537–540
Bollen SR, Robinson DG, Crichton KJ et al (1993) Stress fractures of the ulna in tennis players using a double-handed backhand stroke. Am J Sports Med 21:751–752
Bonis J. (2007) N Engl J Med 7;356(23):2431–2432
Brasington R (1990) Nintendinitis. New Engl J Med 322: 1473–1474
Brutus JP, Chahidi N (2004) Could this unusual scaphoid fracture occurring in a badminton player be a stress fracture? Chir Mai 23:52–54
Brukner P, Bennell K. (1997) Sports Med 24(6):419–29. Review
Bürger H, Müller EJ, Kälicke T (2006) Avascular necrosis of the capitate in athletes. Sportverletz Sportschaden 20: 91–95
Burnham RS, Steadward RD (1994) Upper extremity peripheral nerve entrapments among wheelchair athletes: prevalence, location, and risk factors. Arch Phys Med Rehabil 75: 519–524
Caine D, Nassar L (2005) Gymnastics injuries. Med Sport Sci 48:18–58
Caine D, Sands WA, Caine DJ, Borms J (2003) Scientific aspects of women's gymnastics 45:46–71
Campbell CS (1955) Gamekeepr's thumb. J Bone Joint Surg 37B:148–149
Carlsen BT, Moran SL (2009) Thumb trauma: Bennett fractures, Rolando fractures, and ulnar collateral ligament injuries. J Hand Surg 34A:945–952
Carneiro RS, Fontana R, Mazzer N (2005) Ulnar wrist pain in athletes caused by erosion of the floor of the sixth dorsal compartment. Am J Sports Med 33:1910–1913
Cerezal L, Del Piñal F, Abascal F et al (2002) Imaging findings in ulnar-sided wrist impaction syndromes. Radiographics 22:105–121
Demondion X, Boutry N, Khalil C et al (2008) Plain radiographs of the wrist and hand. J Radiol 89:640–651
DiFiori JP, Puffer JC, Aish B, Dorey F (2002) Wrist pain, distal radial physeal injury, and ulnar variance in young gymnasts: does a relationship exist? Am J Sports Med 30:879–885
Diop AN, Ba-Diop S, Sane JC et al (2008) Role of US in the management of the Quervain's tenosynovitis: review of 22 cases. J Radiol 89:1081–1084
Dobyns JH, Gabel GT (1990) Gymnast's wrist. Hand Clin 6:493–505
Dufek P, Ostendorf U, Thormählen F (1999) Stress fractures of the ulna in a table tennis player. Sportverletz Sportschade 13:62–4
Engel A, Feldner-Busztin H (1991) Bilateral stress fracture of the scaphoid. A case report. Arch Orthop Trauma Surg 110: 314–315
Fragniere B, Landry M, Siegrist O (2001) Stress fracture of the ulna in a professional tennis player using a double-handed backhand stroke. Knee Surg Sports Traumatol Arthrosc 9: 239–241
Golimbu CN, Firooznia H, Rafii M (1995) Avascular necrosis of carpal bones. Magn Reson Imaging Clin N Am 3:281–303
Gross MS, Gelberman RH (1984) The anatomy of the distal ulnar tunnel. Clin Orthop 196:238–247
Guha AR, Marynissen H (2002) Stress fracture of the hook of the hamate. Br J Sports Med 36:224–225
Hafner R, Poznanski AK, Donovan JM (1989) Ulnar variance in children: standard measurements for evaluation of ulnar shortening in juvenile rheumatoid arthritis, hereditary multiple exostosis and other bone or joint disorders in childhood. Skeletal Radiol 18:513–516
Hamilton HK (1984) Stress fracture of the diaphysis of the ulna in a body builder. Am J Sports Med 12:405–406
Helal B (1978a) Chronic overuse injuries of the piso-triquetal joint in racquet game palyers. Br J Sports Med 12:195–198
Helal B (1978b) Racquet player's pisiform. Hand 10:87–90
Henry M (2008) Arthroscopic management of dorsal wrist impingement. J Hand Surg 33:1201–1204
Hernán-Prado MA, Laplaza FJ (2001) Distal radius epiphysiolysis associated with scaphoid fractures in immadure patients: report of two cases and review of the literatura. J Orthop Trauma 15:73–77
Heuck A, Hochholzer T, Keinath C (1992) MRI of the hand and wrist of sports climbers. Imaging of injuries and consequences of stress overload. Radiologe 32:248–254
Hosey RG, Hauk JM, Boland MR (2006) Scaphoid stress fracture: an unusual cause of wrist pain in a competitive diver. Orthopedics 29:503–505
Hsu MC, Lue KH, Lin ZI (2005) Stress fracture at the junction of the middle and distal third of the ulnar diaphysis in a spinner bowler: a case report and a review of the literature. Knee Surg Sports Traumatol Arthrosc 13:499–504
Inagaki H, Inoue G (1997) Stress fracture of the scaphoid combined with the distal radial epiphysiolysis. Br J Sports Med 31:256–257
Itadera E, Ichikawa N, Hashizume H, Inoue H (2001) Stress fracture of the lunar styloid process in kendo player- a case report. Hand Surg 6:109–111
Jones GL (2006) Upper extremity stress fractures. Clin Sports Med 25:159–174
Jowett AD, Brukner PD (1997) Fifth metacarpal stress fracture in a female softball pitcher. Clin J Sport Med 7:220–221
Kalainov DM, Hartigan BJ (2003) Bicycling-induced ulnar tunnel syndrome. Am J Orthop 32:210–211
Klauser A, Bodner G, Frauscher F et al (1999) Finger injuries in extreme rock climbers, assessment of high resolution ultrasonography. Am J Sports Med 27:733–737
Klauser A, Frauscher F, Bodner G et al (2002) Finger pulley injuries in extreme rock climbers: depiction with dynamic US. Radiology 222:755–761

Koskinen SK, Mattila KT, Alanen AM, Aro HT (1997) Stress fracture of the ulnar diaphysis in a recreational golfer. Clin J Sports Med 7:63–65

Lanzetta M, Foucher G (1993) Entrapment of the superficial branch of the radial nerve (Wartenberg's syndrome). A report of 53 cases. Int Orthop 17:342–345

Lanzetta M, Foucher G (1995) Association of Wartenberg's syndrome and De Quervain's disease: a series of 26 cases. Plast Reconstr Surg 96:408–412

Lee JK, Yao L (1988) Stress fractures: MR imaging. Radiology 169:217–220

Linscheid RL, Dobyns JH (1985) Athletic injuries of the wrist. Clin Orthop Relat Res (198):141–151

MacLennan AJ, Nemechek NM, Waitayawinyu T, Trumble TE (2008) Diagnosis and anatomic reconstruction of extensor carpi ulnaris subluxation. J Hand Surg 33:1682–1683

Magee T (2009) Comparison of 3-T MRI and arthroscopy of intrinsic wrist ligament and TFCC tears. AJR Am J Roentgenol 192:80–85

Maimaris C, Zadeh HG (1990) Ulnar nerve compression in the cyclist's hand: two cases and review of the literature. Br J Sports Med 24:245–246

Mandal A, Imran D, Erdmann M (2005) Prolonged use of electronic games-a word of caution. Injury 36:218–219

Maquirriain J, Ghisi JP (2006) The incidence and distribution of stress fractures in elite tennis players. Br J Sports Med 40:454–4

Maquirriain J, Ghisi JP (2007) Stress injury of the lunate in tennis players: a case series and related biomechanical considerations. Br J Sports Med 41:812–815

Masmejean EH, Chavane H, Chantegret A et al (1999) The wrist of the formula 1 driver. Br J Sports Med 33:270–273

Matzkin E, Singer DI (2000) Scaphoid stress fracture in a 13-year-old gymnast: a case report. J Hand Surg [Am] 25: 710–713

Mazione M, Pizzutillo PD (1981) Stress fracture of the scaphoid waist. A case report. Am J Sports Med 9:268–269

McCue FC III, Cabrera JM (1992) Common athletic digital joint injuries of the hand. In: Strickland JW, Rettig AC (eds) Hand injuries in athletes. WB Saunders, Philadelphia, pp 49–94

McNally E, Wilson D, Seiler S (2005) Rowing injuries. Semin Musculoskelet Radiol 9:379–396

Montalvan B, Parier J, Brasseur JL et al (2006) Extensor carpi ulnaris injuries in tennis players: a study of 28 cases. Br J Sports Med 40:424–429

Muramatsu K, Kuriyama R (2005) Stress fracture at the base of second metacarpal in a soft tennis player. Clin J Sport Med 15:279–280

Nett MP, Collins MS, Sperling JW (2008) Magnetic resonance imaging of acute 'wiitis' of the upper extremity. Skeletal Radiol 37:481–483

Osterman AL, Weinberg P, Miller G (1987) Joystick digit. JAMA 257:782

Osterman AL, Moskow L, Low DW (1988) Soft-tissue injuries of the hand and wrist in racquet sports. Clin Sports Med 7:329–348

Palmer AK (1989) Triangular fibrocartilage complex lesions: a classification. J Hand Surg 14:594–606

Palmer AK, Werner FW (1984) Biomechanics of the distal radioulnar joint. Clin Orthop Relat Res 187:26–35

Petschnig R, Wurnig C, Rosen A, Baron R (1997) Stress fracture of the ulna in a female table tennis tournament player. J Sports Med Phys Fitness 37:225–227

Plancher KD, Ho CP, Cofield SS et al (1999) Role of MR imaging in the management of "skier's thumb". Magn Reson Imaging Clin N Am 7:73–84

Plate AM, Green SM (2000) Compressive radial neuropathies. Instr Course Lect 49:295–304

Recht MP, Goodwin DW, Winalski CS, White LM (2005) MRI of articular cartilage: revisiting current status and future directions. AJR Am J Roentgenol 185:899–914

Reekers JA, Koedam N (1998) Volleyball-related ischemia of the hand. Cardiovasc Intervent Radiol 21:261

Reekers JA, den Hartog BMG, Kuyper CF et al (1993) Traumatic aneurysm of the posterior circumflex humeral artery: a volleyball player's disease? J Vasc Interv Radiol 4:405–408

Rettig AC (2004) Athletic injuries of the wrist and hand: part II Overuse injuries of the wrist and traumatic injuries to the hand. Am J sports Med 32:262–273

Rossi C, Cellocco P, Margaritondo E, Bizzarri F, Costanzo G (2005) De Quervain disease in volleyball players. Am J Sports Med 33:424–427

Ruland RT, Hogan CJ (2008) The ECU synergy test: an aid to diagnose ECU tendonitis. J Hand Surg 33A:1777–1782

Sawaizumi T, Nanno M, Ito H (2007) De Quervain's disease: efficacy of intra-sheath triamcinolone injection. Int Orthop 31:265–268

Schöffl VR, Schöffl I (2006) Injuries to the finger flexor pulley system in rock climbers: current concepts. J Hand Surg Am 31A:647–654

Spinner M, Kaplan EB (1970) Extensor carpi ulnaris: its relationship to the stability of the distal radio-ulnar joint. Clin Orthop 68:124–129

Stabler A, Heuk A, Reiser M (1997) Imaging of the hand: degeneration, impingement and overuse. Eur J Radiol 25: 118–128

Steunebrink M, de Winter D, Tol JL (2008) Bilateral stress fracture of the ulna in an adult weightlifter: a case report. Acta Orthop Belg 74:851–855

Street JM (1993) Radiographs of phalangeal fractures: importance of the internally rotated oblique projection for diagnosis. AJR Am J Roentgenol 160:575–576

Tagliafico AS, Ameri P, Michaud J, Derchi LE, Sormani MP, Martinoli C (2009) Wrist injuries in nonprofessional tennis players: relationships with different grips. Am J Sports Med 37:760–767

Tanabe S, Nakahira J, Bando E et al (1991) Fatigue fracture of the ulna occurring in pitchers of fast-pitch softball. Am J Sports Med 19:317–321

Tryfonidis M, Jass GK, Charalambous CP et al (2005) Superficial branch of the radial nerve piercing the brachioradialis tendon to become subcutaneous: an anatomical variation with clinical relevance. Hand Surg 10:141

Vanlandewijck Y, Theisen D, Daly D (2001) Wheelchair propulsion biomechanics: implications for wheelchair sports. Sports Med 31:339–367

Vlychou M, Spanomichos G, Chatziioannou A et al (2001) Embolisation of a traumatic aneurysm of the posterior circumflex humeral artery in a volleyball player. Br J Sports Med 35:136–137

Webb BG, Rettig LA (2008) Gymnastic wrist injuries. Curr Sports Med Rep 7:289–295

White JC, Johnson RK (2003) Unusual entrapment neuropathy in a golf player. Neurology 60:885

Yamaguchi T, Ikuta Y (2007) Climber's finger. Hand Surg 12:59–65

Young CC, Raasch WG, Geiser C (1995) Ulnar stress fracture of the nondominant arm in a tennis player using a two-handed backhand. Clin J Sports Med 5:262–264

Zapata LG, Moraes AJ, Leone C et al (2006) Pain and musculoskeletal pain syndromes related to computer and video game use in adolescents. Eur J Pediatr 165:408–414

Contents

R.J. Robinson
The Mid Yorkshire Hospitals NHS Trust, Pinderfields Hospital, Wakefield, UK

P. Robinson (✉)
Chapel Allerton Musculoskeletal Imaging Department,
The Leeds Teaching Hospitals NHS Trust, Leeds, UK
e-mail: p.robinson@leedsth.nhs.uk

Key Points

- Athletic injury to the pelvis and groin is often difficult to accurately diagnose clinically due to the complex anatomy of the region and frequent coexisting pathology. Injury can occur in both acute and chronic settings with different imaging modalities suitable depending on the particular clinical question.
- Acute injury in this age group mainly involves apophyseal avulsion as this is the weakest point within the muscle bone interface.
- Chronic injury includes apophysitis, athletic pubalgia, tendinopathy, bursitis and stress fractures. Other rarer diagnoses such as groin hernias should also be considered as a potential source for patient symptoms.
- Imaging mainly involves the use of ultrasound and magnetic resonance imaging although plain radiography, computed tomography and nuclear medicine studies all have specific roles.

1 Introduction

The pelvis and groin is a complex anatomical region with a multitude of causes for activity and non-activity related symptoms. Clinical diagnosis can be difficult with potentially multiple co-existing injuries. Understanding the regional anatomy, pathologies and appropriate investigations is vital for diagnostic accuracy. This is especially pertinent in the paediatric and adolescent age groups due to unique physiological and anatomical changes that occur before skeletal

A.H. Karantanas (ed.), *Sports Injuries in Children and Adolescents*,
Med Radiol Diagn Imaging, DOI: 10.1007/174_2010_15,

maturity. Athletic pelvic injury occurs less frequently than injuries involving the extremities accounting for approximately 5–8% of injuries in high school athletes (Anderson et al. 2001). Sports which involve quick acceleration, rapid direction change and kicking such as soccer, ice hockey, American football, Australian rules football, fencing and baseball are particularly susceptible to injury. Acute childhood and adolescent sports injury mainly involves avulsion fractures and less commonly muscle and tendon tears. Overuse injuries include apophysitis, tendinopathy, bursitis, pubalgia and stress fractures. The majority of sporting injury occurs in males but there is increasing female participation in organized sport with high school girls representing the fastest growing group under 18 years of age. Consideration of differences between male and female pelvic anatomy is necessary to provide optimum injury assessment (Cheng et al. 2000; Loud and Micheli 2001).

This chapter will highlight the appropriate investigative methods in both acute and chronic injury to facilitate accurate diagnosis and influence management.

2 Groin Hernia

Groin hernias occur in up to 4.4% of children and 98% of these occur in children under 13 years old. Approximately 99% of childhood hernias are indirect, direct hernias account for less than 1% and femoral hernias occur even less frequently (Ein et al. 2006). A single strenuous event does not often cause herniation (Sanjay and Woodward 2007) although it may precipitate detection due to raised intrabdominal pressure. This is more likely to affect older adolescents in sports such as weight lifting (Diamond and Gregory 2007). Recognition of groin hernias may offer the athlete a potential cure for symptoms through surgical repair.

2.1 Inguinal Anatomy

The inguinal canal is composed of several muscle and fascial layers which allow passage of the spermatic cord (or round ligament), vessels, nerves and lymphatics from the abdomen to the external genitalia. The medial half of the inguinal ligament is formed by the external oblique aponeurosis and also comprises the inferior wall of the canal. This extends posteriorly forming a u shaped channel containing the spermatic cord (or round ligament) when viewed in cross section (Figs. 1 and 2). The superior boundary is formed by the internal oblique and transversus abdominis, which blend together to form the conjoined tendon medially which also forms the posterior wall. The deep ring is a deficiency in the posterior wall, through which the spermatic cord (round ligament) and other contents enter the canal. The superficial inguinal ring is a defect in the medial external oblique aponeurosis and marks the exit of the canal. The inguinal canal is obliquely orientated and extends medially and inferiorly from the deep ring towards the pubis and superficial ring. In children its orientation is less oblique than that seen in adults (Vergnes et al. 1985). In prepubescent children the deep inguinal ring lies medial to the midway point of the inguinal ligament (Parnis et al. 1997).

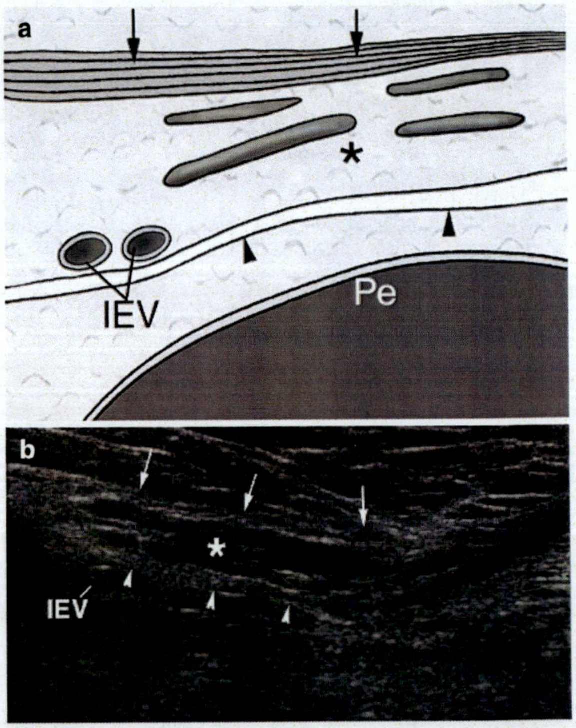

Fig. 1 Normal right inguinal canal anatomy long axis. (**a**) Diagram and (**b**) sonogram show inguinal ligament (*arrows*), inferior epigastric vessels (IEV), posterior wall (*arrowheads*), peritoneum (Pe) with vessels and fat in canal (*asterisk*)

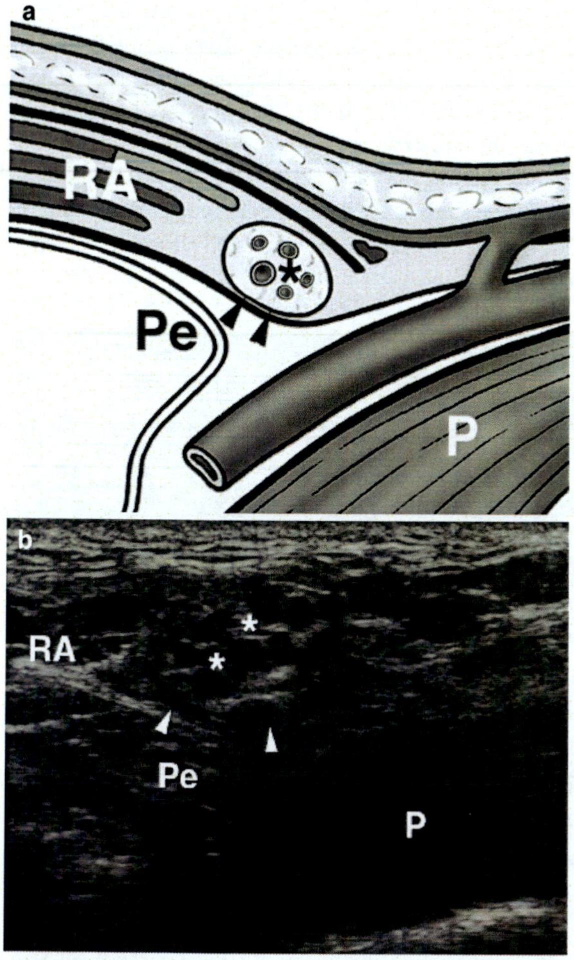

Fig. 2 Normal inguinal anatomy short axis. (**a**) Diagram and (**b**) sonogram show psoas (P), rectus abdominis (RA), posterior wall (*arrowheads*), peritoneum (Pe) with vessels and fat in canal (*asterisk*) (part a from Robinson et al. (2006))

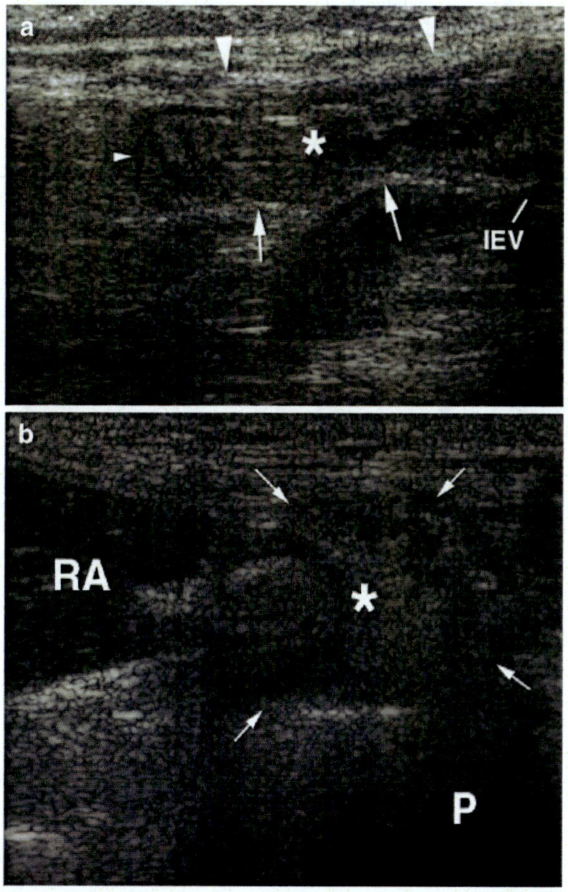

Fig. 3 Indirect hernia in two different athletes. (**a**) Transverse (long axis) sonogram shows inguinal ligament (*large arrowheads*), posterior wall (*arrows*) with a hernia of bowel (*asterisk*) within the canal arising lateral to the inferior epigastric vessels (IEV) and extending medially (*small arrowhead*). (**b**) Sagittal (short axis) sonogram shows psoas (P), rectus abdominis (RA) and canal expansion (*arrows*) by an indirect hernia of fat and bowel (*asterisk*) (compare to Fig. 2b)

2.2 Inguinal Pathology

The main potential area of weakness within the inguinal canal is the deep ring resulting in an indirect hernia due to persistent patent processus vaginalis and is considered a congenital abnormality (Figs. 3 and 4). Fluid can become encysted within a remnant of the processus vaginalis (or canal of Nuck) with communication with the peritoneal cavity or scrotum (Fig. 4).

The presence of an indirect hernia is not always significant as it can be found in many asymptomatic individuals (Ein et al. 2006). Direct inguinal hernias occur due to a posterior wall weakness and enter the canal medial to the inferior epigastric vessels (IEVs) and deep ring (Shadbolt et al. 2001; Jamadar et al. 2006).

2.3 Inguinal Canal Imaging

Ultrasound is the primary imaging method for detection of hernia in the paediatric and adolescent population and is more accurate than clinical examination. Technique accuracy is between 92 and 95% for indirect hernia detection (Erez et al. 1993; Kervancioglu et al. 2000; Hata et al. 2004). Disadvantages of ultrasound

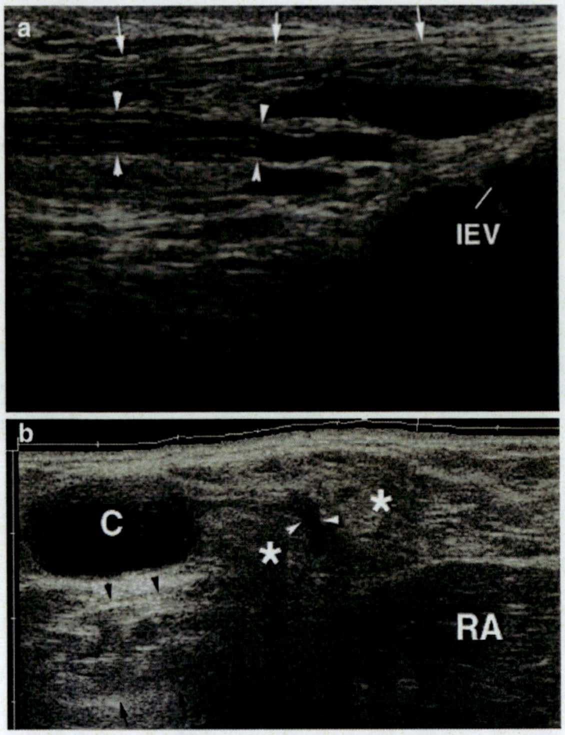

Fig. 4 (**a**) Asymptomatic male athlete with patent processus vaginalis (PPV). Transverse (long axis) sonogram shows left inguinal ligament (*arrows*) and fluid between to two layers of peritoneum (*arrowheads*) that communicated through the deep ring and moved on straining. (**b**) Symptomatic female athlete with canal of Nuck. Longitudinal eFOV sonogram shows right inguinal ligament (*black arrowheads*), posterior wall (*black arrows*) and cyst (C) with neck (*white arrowheads*) extruding from the medial inguinal canal into oedematous subcutaneous tissues (*asterisk*). Rectus abdominis (RA)

can relate to operator dependence. MRI can demonstrate inguinal canal anatomy at rest and dynamic techniques have been described. Little evidence currently exists regarding its accuracy for paediatric hernias. The inguinal region should however remain an important review area when using MRI for suspected pathology elsewhere in the pelvis.

2.3.1 Inguinal Hernia Sonographic Technique

Ultrasound should be performed using a high frequency linear transducer (above 10 MHz). The patient is initially imaged supine and asked to increase intraabdominal pressure (by performing the valsalva manoeuvre) at each stage of the examination. This is critical as many hernias reduce spontaneously. The examination can also be performed in a sitting or standing position, which along with the ability of examining the asymptomatic groin for comparison offers distinct advantages over other imaging techniques.

Scanning transversely (along the long axis of the canal) an indirect hernia arises lateral to the IEVs and extends along the long axis of the canal. Orientating the probe sagittally (along the short axis of the canal), the hernia will distend the canal and efface its contents (Figs 3–5).

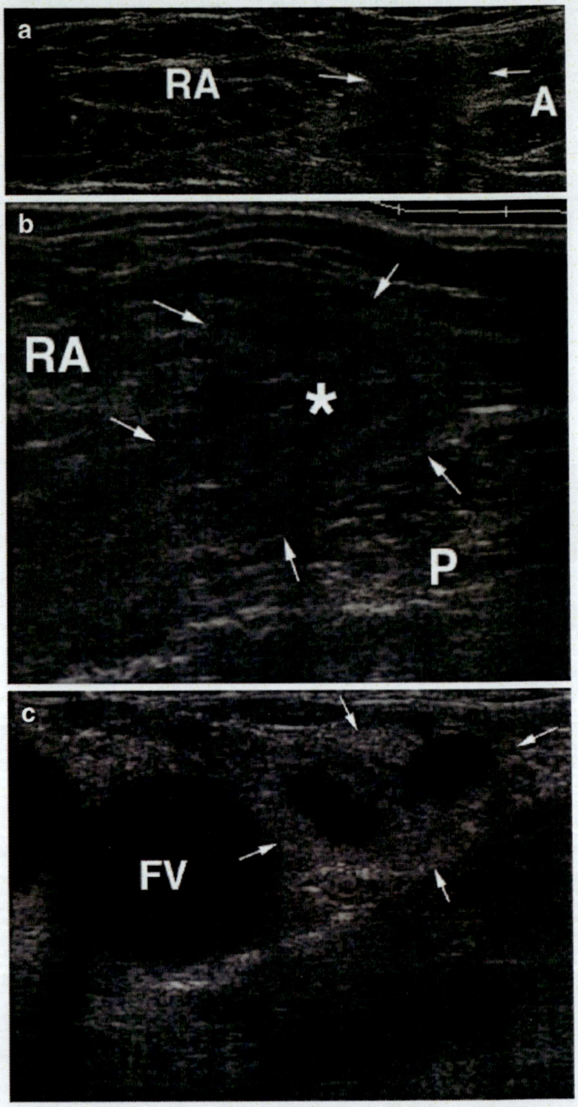

Fig. 5 Other hernias. (**a**) Transverse eFOV sonogram shows left Spigelian hernia (*arrows*) extending between the rectus abdominis (RA) and lateral abdominal muscles (A). (**b**) Sagittal (short axis) sonogram shows a direct hernia (*arrows*) entering and filling the inguinal canal through a posterior wall defect. Psoas (P), rectus abdominis (RA). (**c**) Transverse sonogram shows right femoral hernia with fat and fluid (*arrows*) filling the femoral canal medial to the femoral vein (FV)

Direct hernias originate medial to the IEVs and are usually more localized than indirect hernias. Scanning transversely the hernia will protrude through the posterior wall and when viewed in the sagittal plane will enter the canal from a posterior superior position (Fig. 5) (Robinson et al. 2006).

Hernias can consist of peritoneum, fat and bowel. Evaluation is made for reducibility and signs of incarceration, which include free fluid in the hernial sac, bowel wall thickening and fluid within the herniated bowel loop (Rettenbacher et al. 2001).

2.4 Femoral Hernia

Femoral hernias are uncommon in the paediatric age group accounting for less than 1% of groin hernias and are commonly mistaken for inguinal hernias clinically (Radcliffe and Stringer 1997). The femoral sheath contains the femoral artery, vein and femoral canal (lateral to medial). The femoral canal is located medial to the vein and is a space, which normally allows venous expansion in the absence of a hernia (Shadbolt et al. 2001).

2.4.1 Femoral Hernia Sonographic Technique

Ultrasound is an accurate technique for detection and is performed with the transducer located inferior to the inguinal ligament and medial to the femoral vessels. On performing the Valsalva manoeuvre the femoral vein (FV) normally dilates. In the presence of a hernia, the hernial sac causes femoral canal expansion, compressing or preventing the FV from completely expanding (Fig. 5) (Jamadar et al. 2006).

3 Athletic Pubalgia

Athletic pubalgia is a term which describes a number of pathological entities, which cause symptoms of exertional groin pain. Proposed pathologies occur in and around the pubic symphysis, sharing similar mechanisms of injury and symptoms. In a study of youth soccer players groin pain (athletic pubalgia) accounted for approximately 8% of injuries. Groin injuries are more likely in patients who mature early reflecting the higher incidence of overuse injury with increasing age (Volpi et al. 2003; Le Gall et al. 2007). Theories proposed for athletic pubalgia include sportsman's hernia, osteitis pubis, parasymphyseal enthesopathy and nerve entrapment syndromes (Akita et al. 1999).

In reality the close relationship of structures and their common biomechanical roles suggests injury to one of the structures in this region may predispose to injury elsewhere and synchronous injuries are common (Ekberg et al. 1988). The early detection of this condition enables appropriate management, which is usually conservative involving rest and anti-inflammatory medication.

3.1 Pubic Anatomy and Biomechanics

The pubic symphysis has many muscle and ligamentous attachments. The inguinal ligament attaches to the pubic tubercle positioned on the lateral aspect of the pubic crest. The pubic bodies have an anteromedial apophysis which fuses late on in adolescence or early adulthood (Fig. 6). This anteromedial position is also where there is capsular attachment and merging with the tendinous structures of the adductor group and rectus abdominis (RA) (Figs. 6 and 7).

These attachments are dynamic stabilizers of the anterior pelvis acting as relative antagonists during rotation and extension at the waist (Standring 2005; Robinson et al. 2007). Injury to one of these muscles can affect equilibrium leading to relative instability at the pubic symphysis, or peri-symphyseal soft tissues (Robinson et al. 2007; Omar et al. 2008). The interaction between the closely applied anatomic structures seen around the pubic symphysis suggests that alteration in structure of any of these elements may affect the normal balance of the region precipitating athletic pubalgia (Fig. 7). Proposed pathological entities for the cause of symptoms are discussed below.

3.2 Causes of Athletic Pubalgia

3.2.1 Sportsman's Hernia

Sportsman's hernia is a phrase that has evolved from its original description relating to chronic groin pain caused by posterior inguinal wall deficiency without

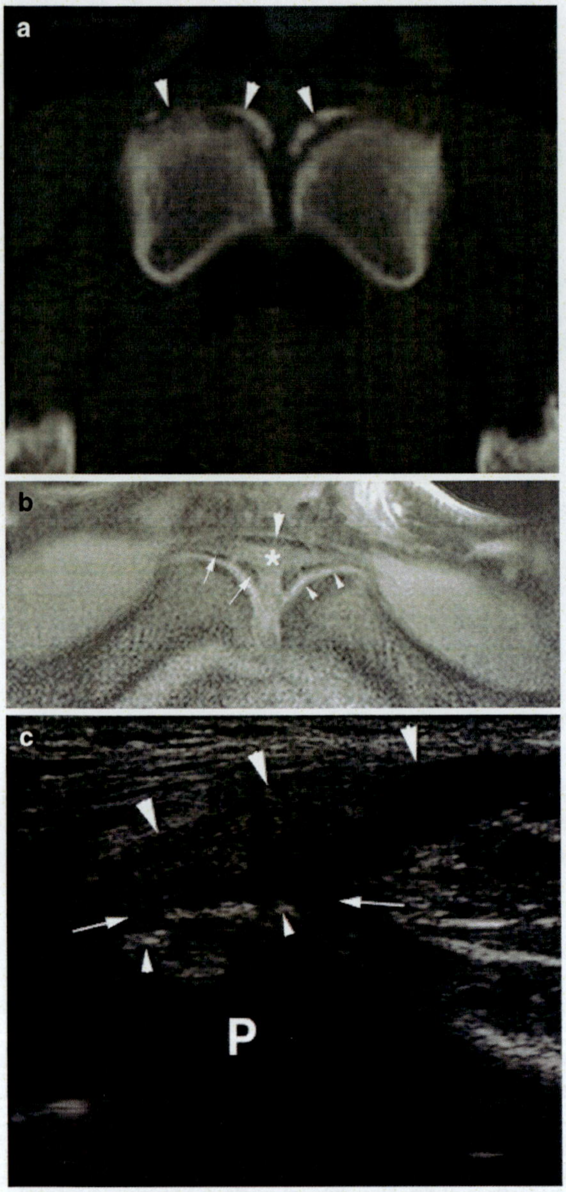

Fig. 6 Pubic apophysis. (**a**) Axial CT shows anteromedial apophyses (*arrowheads*). (**b**) Axial oblique fat suppressed T2-w MR image shows the anteromedial apophyses (*small arrows*), cartilage (*small arrowheads*), capsular tissues (*asterisk*) and merging rectus abdominis tendon anteriorly (*large arrowhead*). (**c**) Sagittal sonogram shows the normal irregular apophysis (*small arrowheads*) and cartilage with anterior capsular tissues (*arrows*) and merging adductor longus tendon (*large arrowheads*)

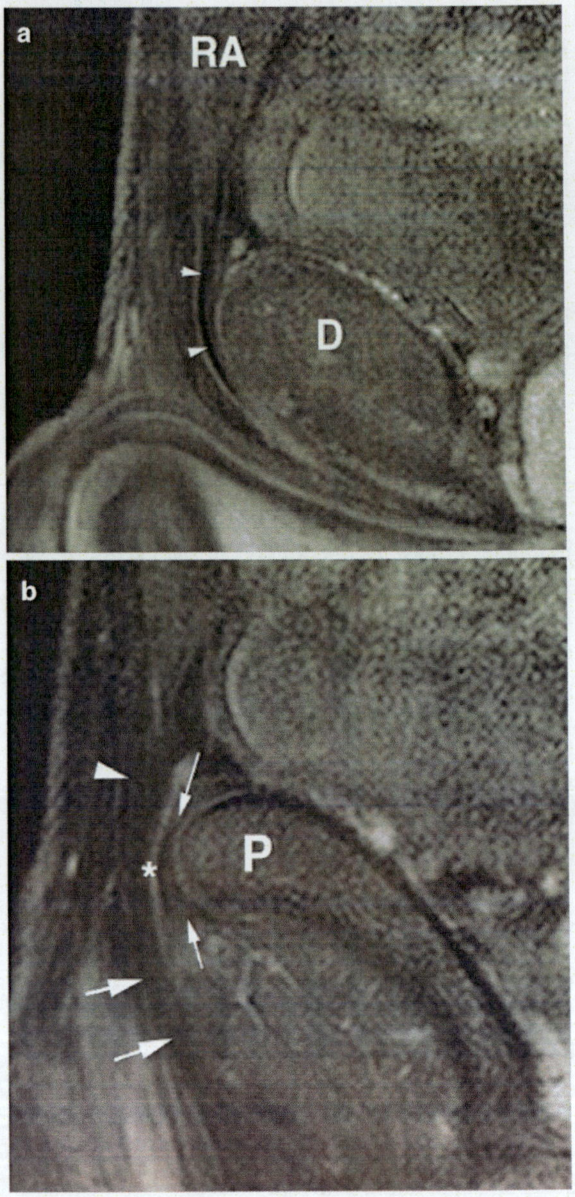

Fig. 7 Symphyseal anatomy. High resolution MR images from a volume acquisition show (**a**) Midline symphyseal disc (D) with distal rectus abdominis (RA) tendon wrapping around its anterior margin (*arrowheads*). (**b**) Para-sagittal apophysis (*small arrows*) and pubis (P) merging anteriorly with the capsule (*asterisk*), distal RA tendon (*arrowhead*) and proximal adductor longus tendon (*large arrows*) (part b from Robinson et al. (2007))

clinical evidence of hernia (Gilmore 1998). Since the inception of this theory many works have been published attributing chronic athletic related groin pain to multiple different pathologies in the groin region (Gilmore 1998; Irshad et al. 2001; Joesting 2002; Kumar et al. 2002; Zoga et al. 2008). The absence of a true hernia along with the pathophysiological and clinical ambiguity exhibited in this condition mean the term is confusing. No specific imaging features are seen (at ultrasound or MRI) and often an incipient hernia or aponeurotic injury cannot be diagnosed until operation.

3.2.2 Osteitis Pubis

Osteitis pubis is thought to be a biomechanical arthropathy caused by an imbalance in strength of the pelvic and abdominal musculature leading to relative symphysis instability. Chronic repetitive microtrauma due to shearing and distraction forces causes an oedematous response producing osteitis and periostitis leading to inappropriate osteoclastic activity and possible bone resorption (Omar et al. 2008). One study has suggested that osseous stress injury is the most significant contributor to symptoms rather than inflammation (Verrall et al. 2008). Osteitis pubis is described in sports involving rapid changes in direction such as soccer, Australian rules football and hockey. It also affects long distance runners (Verrall et al. 2005).

3.2.3 Pubic Enthesopathy

Another cause for chronic groin pain within the spectrum of athletic pubalgia is injury to the musculotendinous insertions of the adductor group and rectus sheath. Injury is thought to occur due to imbalance between the common tendinous attachments in this region (Robinson et al. 2004; Koulouris 2008) causing tendinopathy and enthesopathy at their soft tissue attachments and the adjacent pubic apophysis (Benjamin et al. 2006).

3.3 Imaging Athletic Pubalgia

3.3.1 General Principles

It is suggested that athletic pubalgia be utilized as a more accurate term for radiological use as it describes the clinical findings before surgical or imaging confirmation of the specific cause for symptoms.

3.3.2 Plain Radiographs and Bone Scintigraphy

Plain radiography in adolescents with athletic pubalgia is often normal and is only of value for excluding other injuries such as fracture or hip abnormality. Flamingo views may demonstrate pubic symphysis instability, by a difference of 2 mm in cranio-caudal height of the adjacent inferior pubic rami but are rarely positive. Bone scintigraphy may show increased pubic uptake but findings are often non-specific, may be seen in asymptomatic patients and has been superseded by MRI.

3.3.3 Ultrasound

Ultrasound is a valuable tool in imaging acute tendon injury (Kälebo et al. 1992) and groin tendinopathy (Koulouris 2008). Cortical irregularity is seen as part of the normal apophysis and asymptomatic tendinopathy (hypoechoic thickening) can occur in professional athletes before the age of 18 (Fig. 6c). Greater specificity can be obtained by applying direct pressure over areas of perceived abnormality to see if symptoms are provoked during real time imaging (Kälebo et al. 1992). However MRI is superior for detecting low level soft tissue change and bone oedema.

3.3.4 MRI Technique

MRI offers the most complete method for imaging of athletic pubalgia being both sensitive (98%) and specific (89–100%) for the detection of parasymphyseal abnormality (Brennan et al. 2005; Robinson et al. 2006; Zoga et al. 2008). A wide field of view is recommended for the initial sequences to enable review of the hip and inguinal regions as well as the pubis thus directing subsequent more focused, higher resolution sequences. The addition of an axial oblique sequence offers excellent visualization of the parasymphyseal musculotendinous insertions (Figs. 8–10). Fat-suppressed Gadolinium-enhanced sequences can increase detection of entheseal and subchondral changes (Fig. 9) (Robinson et al. 2004).

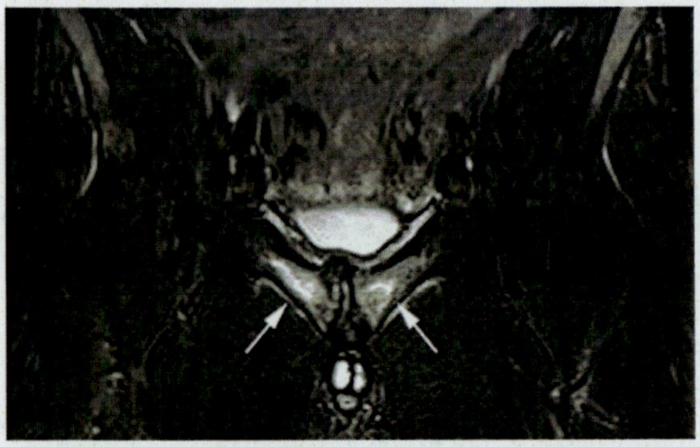

Fig. 8 Athlete with severe bilateral pubalgia. Coronal STIR MR image shows marked symmetrical pubic bone marrow oedema (*arrows*) extending into the soft tissues. This symmetrical pattern can be termed "osteitis pubis"

3.3.5 Imaging features of Sportsman's Hernia

Imaging has little role in making a positive diagnosis of incipient hernia or aponeurotic injuries described surgically. However it is useful to try and identify other causes of groin pain relating to structures found in this region. It has been claimed that posterior inguinal wall deficiency can be demonstrated by ultrasound as marked bulging of the posterior inguinal wall (Fig. 11) (Orchard et al. 1998). However, this finding is seen in many asymptomatic individuals (Steele et al. 2004) and a negative result does not exclude the diagnosis. In patients imaged with MRI for symptoms thought to represent sportsman's hernia or athletic pubalgia the commonest findings are injury to the RA (at or just proximal to its insertion),

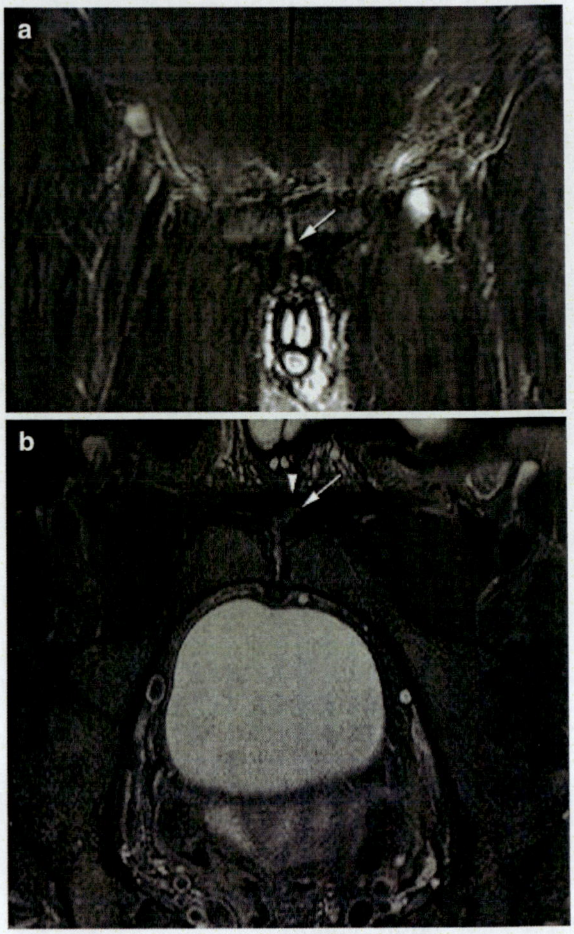

Fig. 10 Athlete with left sided pubalgia. (**a**) Coronal STIR MR image shows a left sided symphyseal cleft (*arrow*). (**b**) Axial oblique fat suppressed T2-w MR image shows the cleft (*arrow*) is due to disruption and oedema at the junction of the left adductor longus tendon (*arrowhead*) and the capsular tissues

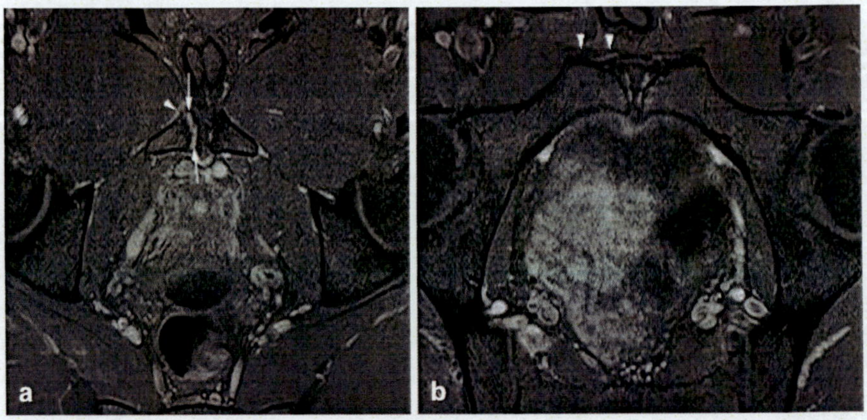

Fig. 9 Athlete with right sided pubalgia. (**a**) Axial oblique fat suppressed T1-w post IV gadolinium MR image shows marked enhancement of the right inferior pubic apophysis (*arrows*), capsular tissue and adductor brevis origin (*arrowhead*). (**b**) A more superior image shows normal appearances at the adductor longus origin (*arrowheads*)

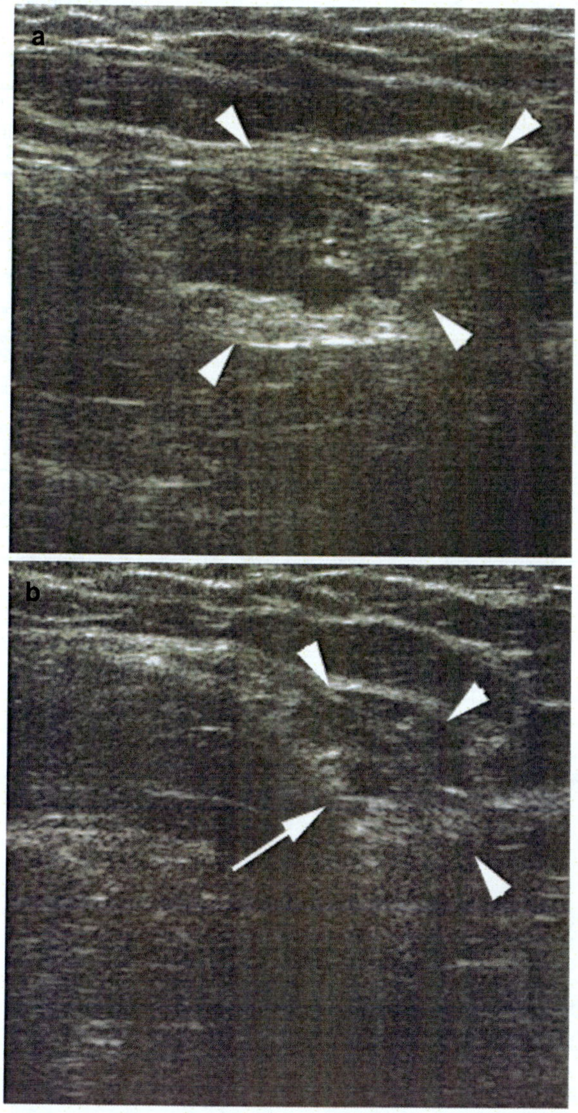

Fig. 11 Asymptomatic athlete. Sagittal (short axis) sonograms show (**a**) normal inguinal canal (*arrowheads*) at rest. (**b**) During valsava manoeuvre there is compression of the canal into a crescent shape (*arrowheads*) by marked posterior wall movement (*arrow*)

adductor origin and "osteitis pubis" (Omar et al. 2008; Zoga et al. 2008).

3.3.6 Imaging features of Osteitis Pubis

MRI can show bilateral florid pubic bone marrow and surrounding soft tissue oedema with fluid in the symphysis (Fig. 8). This classical appearance is less commonly seen with more subtle and asymmetrical appearances typically present in most athletes.

3.3.7 Imaging features of Parasymphyseal Enthesopathy

MRI typically shows asymmetrical entheseal based (soft tissue and pubic subchondral) oedema and is the commonest imaging finding in athletes with pubalgia (Verrall et al. 2001). This can occur in unilateral, bilateral, focal or diffuse patterns and correlates well with symptoms (Figs. 9 and 10) (Cunningham et al. 2007). In addition gadolinium enhancement of the adductor enthesis and anterior pubis also correlates well with patient symptoms (Robinson et al. 2004). Interpretive caution is required as bone oedema can be seen in asymptomatic athletes especially those undergoing heavy training (Paajanen et al. 2008). In the adolescent athlete moderate to severe bone oedema can be seen in asymptomatic patients related to bone maturation rather than injury (Lovell et al. 2006). The presence of a secondary symphyseal cleft has a high correlation with the side of reported pain although is not seen in all patients (Fig. 10) (O'Connell et al. 2002; Cunningham et al. 2007). The secondary cleft is not detected in asymptomatic populations suggesting its presence is a good evidence of symptomatic pathology and MRI has been shown to be 100% sensitive and specific for its detection (Brennan et al. 2005). Later changes such as articular surface irregularity, osteophyte formation, bony sclerosis, joint misalignment and subchondral cysts can also be demonstrated (Cunningham et al. 2007). Observation should be made for sacral or sacro-iliac joint abnormality as co-existing pathology, due to pelvic ring imbalance, however this rarely occurs in practice (Major and Helms 1997).

4 Apophyseal Injury

The pelvic apophyses are particularly susceptible to sporting injury due to the large forces generated by the pelvic musculature (Donnelly et al. 1999). Apophyseal injury is more commonly seen in adolescents as the physis is the weakest point of the musculotendinous osseous unit (Rossi and Dragoni 2001). There are three types of apophyseal injury; (1) Apophysitis (stress injury) caused by repetitive microtrauma, (2) Acute avulsion fracture caused by a single traumatic event and (3) Chronic non-union of an avulsion fracture. Clinical presentation and treatment options differ between the separate types of injury.

4.1 Pelvic Apophyseal Anatomy

Apophyseal injury can occur at any time during skeletal development up to 25 years dependent on the age of bony fusion. Injury occurs most often during adolescence with the average incidence around 14 years (Rossi and Dragoni 2001). Table 1 summarises the relevant pelvic muscle apophyseal attachments and their ages of appearance and fusion.

4.2 Acute Apophyseal Avulsion

Acute injury occurs due to a single episode of sudden, violent or unbalanced muscle contraction generating indirect forces which overwhelm the apophyseal attachment (Fig. 12) (Stevens et al. 1999; Kocher and Tucker 2006). Multiple injuries can occur concurrently as well as injuries of different ages and combinations of acute and chronic injury.

4.3 Apophysitis (Apophyseal Stress Injury)

Chronic apophyseal stress injury (apophystis) occurs due to overuse from repetitive sporting activity. Recurrent stresses result in physis microtrauma, where the

Table 1 Pelvic apophyseal muscle attachments and age of apophyseal fusion (Risser 1958; Eich et al. 1992; Standring 2005; Butler et al. 1999)

Apophysis	Muscle attachments	Age of appearance of apophysis (years)	Age of fusion of apophysis (years)
Ischial tuberosity	Semimembranosus, semitendinosus, biceps femoris	13–15	20–25
Anterior inferior Iliac Spine	Straight head rectus femoris	13–15	16–18
Anterior superior iliac spine	Sartorius, tensor fascia latae	13–15	20–25
Pubic symphysis	External oblique, internal oblique, transversus abdominus, rectus abdominus, pectineus, gracilis, adductor longus, adductor brevis, adductor magnus	18–20	20–25
Iliac crest	Internal and external oblique Transversus abdominus Gluteus medius Tensor fascia latae	13–15	21–25

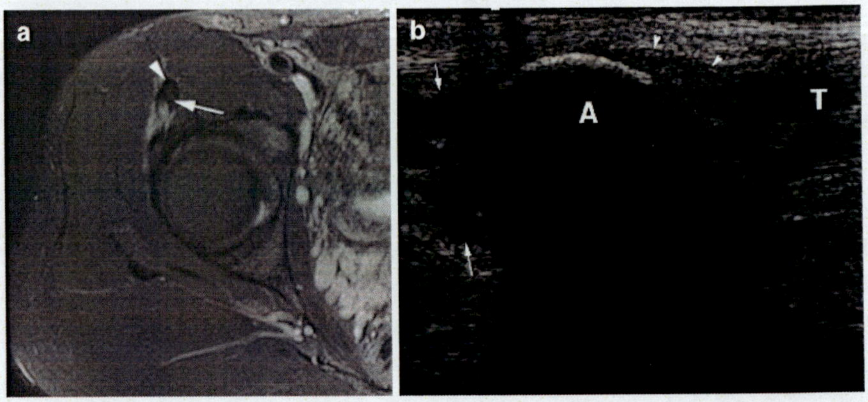

Fig. 12 Apophyseal fractures. (**a**) Axial fat suppressed T2-w MR image shows avulsion of the right inferior iliac spine (*arrow*) with intact tendon (*arrowhead*). (**b**) Sagittal sonogram shows the apophysis (A), intact fibrocartilage (*arrowheads*) and tendon (T). Note haematoma (*arrows*) at avulsion site

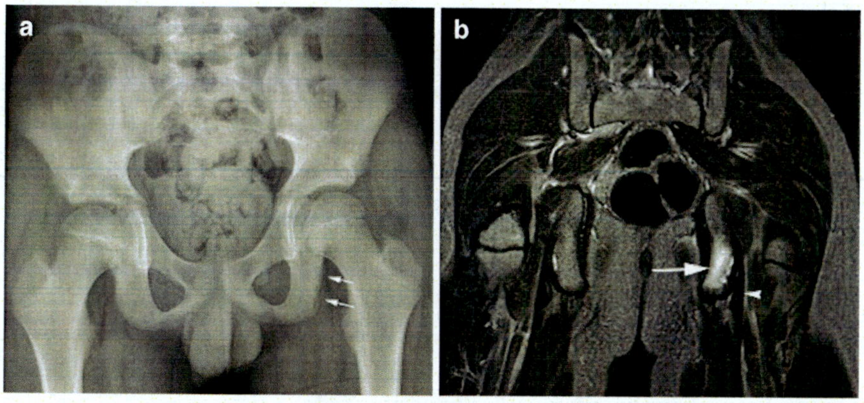

Fig. 13 Sprinter with ischial pain. (**a**) Pelvic radiograph shows left ischial osteopoenia (*arrows*). (**b**) Corresponding fat suppressed T2-w MR image shows normal hamstring tendons (*arrowhead*) with extensive apophyseal and ischial bone marrow oedema (*arrow*)

ability to repair itself is outpaced by the repetition of injury (Micheli and Fehlandt 1992). Pathologically it is thought that this causes chondrocyte hypertrophy leading to physeal widening along with adjacent bone microfractures (Fig. 13) (Hébert et al. 2008).

4.4 Imaging in Apophyseal Injury

The AP radiograph is the most appropriate initial investigation to demonstrate the acutely displaced apophysis without the need for further investigation. Radiographically occult injuries are seen in patients with unossified apophyses, fibrocartilage injury and can occur if the bony pelvis obscures the displaced fragment (Lazović et al. 1996).

Apophysitis can have complex imaging appearances ranging from minimal physeal widening to rarefaction, bone lysis, periosteal reaction, prominent callus formation and sclerosis in the healing phase (Fig. 13a). These appearances can be mistaken for aggressive processes such as infection or malignancy (Yamamoto et al. 2004). Similar findings occur when using CT for injury evaluation although its cross sectional capabilities may offer greater characterization of difficult cases. However it is rarely used in the paediatric population because of radiation dose (Stevens et al. 1999).

Ultrasound is more sensitive than plain radiography and is able to detect injury in those without ossification centres, fibrocartilage injury and has the ability for dynamic examination. Hypoechoic oedema or haemorrhage in the region of the apophysis and surrounding soft tissues may be seen (Fig. 12b). Widening of the normally hypoechoic physis and mobility of the apophysis during dynamic examination indicates an unstable avulsion (Lazović et al. 1996). Hyperaemia seen on power Doppler settings has been described in acute injuries. However its value in chronic injury is uncertain (Pisacano and Miller 2003). MRI in acute avulsion demonstrates increased signal on fat suppressed T2-w sequences at the avulsion site and local soft tissues representing haematoma and oedema (Figs. 12 and 14). Retraction of greater than 2 cm can lead to extended morbidity and poor healing, with surgical management often advocated in these patients (Kocher and Tucker 2006). Periosteal stripping at the tendon attachment sites along with retraction of the displaced bone or cartilage fragment and attached tendon can be seen (Fig. 14). Small cortical avulsion fragments that are marrow deficient may be easily missed with MRI and are better assessed by ultrasound.

In the healing phase imaging may show extensive hypertrophic ossification and deformity, which can mimic aggressive pathology if a history of trauma is not elucidated. Ultrasound and plain radiography are often useful in confirming a mature non aggressive process if MRI still shows oedematous change.

MRI is also useful in the healing phase to distinguish chronic non union from fibro-osseous union. In non union MRI reveals persistent high signal on fat suppressed T2-w and STIR sequences, between the displaced apophyseal fragment and the underlying bone (Vandervliet et al. 2007). Fibro-osseous union shows focal hypointense signal across the apophyseal growth-plate although fibrous or osseous distinction cannot always be made (Jaramillo et al. 1990).

Bone scintigraphy as well as MRI is sensitive in the early stages of apophysitis but MRI is the more specific technique of choice in this young population. MRI changes in apophysitis include mild apophyseal widening of 3–5 mm along with increased T2-w signal of the physis, adjacent muscle and bone marrow (Hébert et al. 2008). Surgical resection of hypertrophic

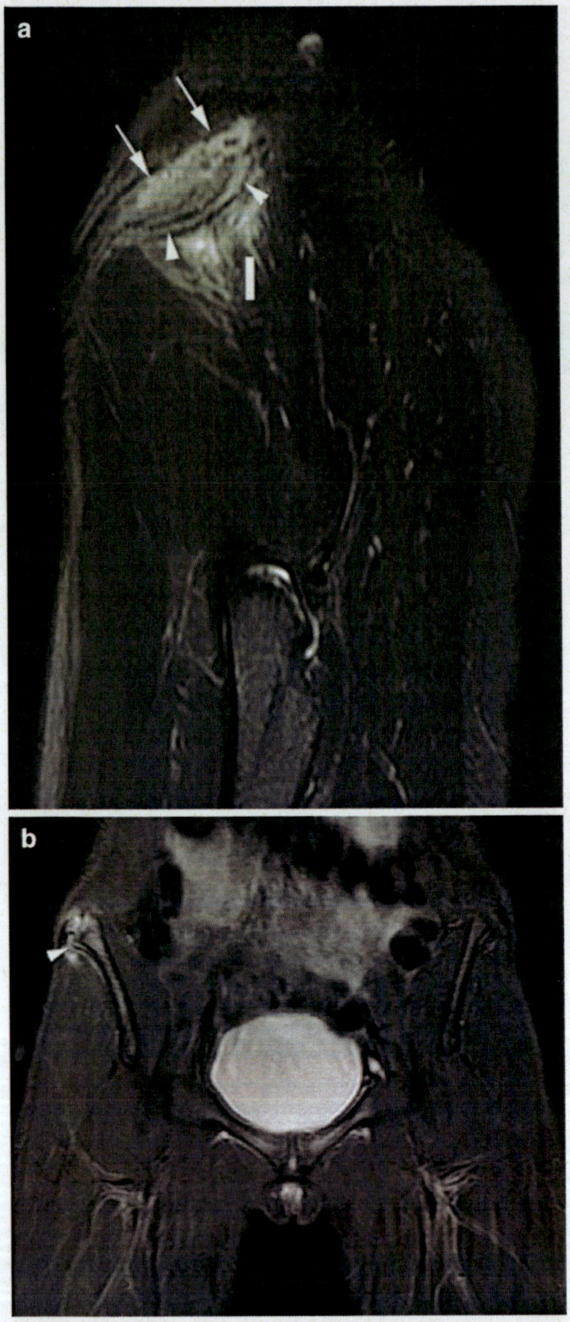

Fig. 14 Gymnast with acute severe left hip pain. (**a**) Sagittal and (**b**) coronal fat suppressed T2-w MR images shows apophyseal avulsion (*arrowheads*) from the right iliac crest (*arrows*) with oedema in iliacus (I) muscle

ossification can be performed in patients with continued symptoms or localized pressure effects such as sciatic nerve compression (Anderson et al. 2001).

5 Muscle Injury

In contrast to adults the paediatric athlete is less likely to suffer from muscle strain (due to the inherent apophyseal weakness discussed before). Muscle contusion remains common comprising up to 38% of paediatric injuries (Sorensen et al. 1996). Around the pelvis and groin muscular strain is most likely to occur in the biceps femoris or adductor longus, however muscle involvement is somewhat dependent on the sporting activity performed (Maffulli et al. 1996).

5.1 Imaging of Pelvic Muscle Injury

As in other regions of the body ultrasound and MRI are the primary modalities for detection of suspected muscle injury. Ultrasound is the preferred initial method for imaging muscle tears due to its accessibility and cost. However some institutions may use MRI as their primary modality especially if athletes have significant muscle bulk precluding easy ultrasound access or for detecting low grade injury (Fig. 15) (Järvinen et al. 2005).

5.2 Delayed Onset Muscle Soreness

Delayed onset muscle soreness describes pain occurring hours to days following exercise. It is particularly associated with eccentric muscle contraction and manifests with increases in plasma creatine kinase levels (Evans et al. 1998). Imaging changes on MRI are similar to low grade muscle strains with increased signal on fat suppressed T2-w and STIR sequences, indicating oedema. In severe cases, muscle necrosis can rarely occur (Armfield et al. 2006).

6 Tendinopathy

Tendon injury also occurs less frequently in the immature athlete due to the inherent weakness at the apophysis (Soprano and Fuchs 2007). In the groin dancers and runners in particular can experience iliopsoas tendinopathy as a consequence of the internal snapping hip syndrome (Winston et al. 2007).

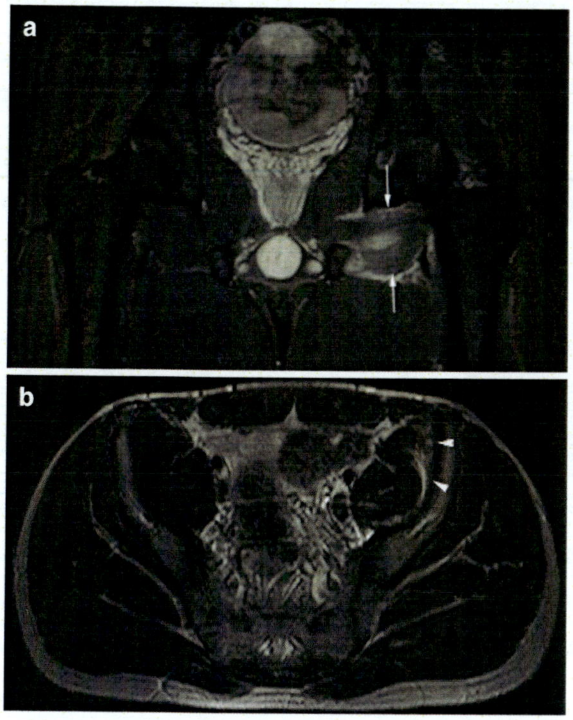

Fig. 15 Acute muscle injuries. (**a**) Coronal fat suppressed T2-w MR image shows intrasubstance oedema (*arrows*) consistent with grade 2 obturator externus tear. (**b**) Axial T2-w MR image shows left iliacus oedema (*arrowheads*) consistent with a grade 2 tear as more than 5% of the muscle volume is affected

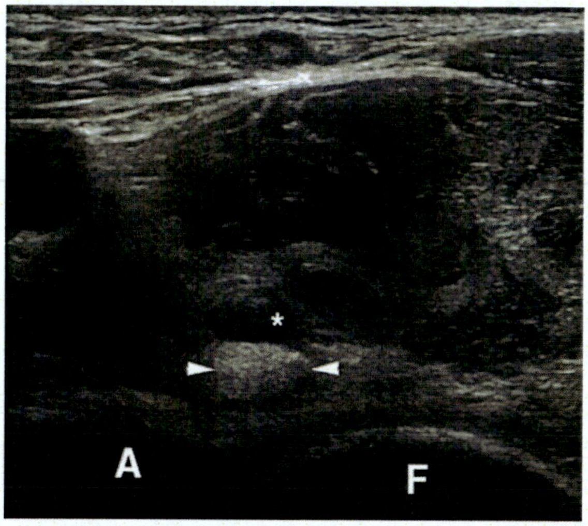

Fig. 16 Runner with snapping hip. Transverse sonogram shows femoral head (F), acetabulum (A) and iliopsoas tendon (*arrowheads*) with surrounding oedema (*asterisk*). Juddering translation was confirmed on hip flexion

6.1 Tendon Imaging

Plain radiographs have little role beyond the exclusion of other diagnoses or avulsion. Ultrasound and MRI are appropriate, however because of increased soft tissue bulk in the pelvis low grade tendinopathy detected by MRI can be missed by ultrasound (Campbell and Grainger 2001).

6.2 Internal Snapping Hip Syndrome

The internal snapping hip syndrome can cause severe anterior inguinal pain, which may coexist with an audible or palpable snap (Vaccaro et al. 1995). Snapping hip syndrome can be caused by intra and extra articular mechanisms. The internal (medial) syndrome is extra-articular involving flipping of the iliopsoas tendon over the iliacus or iliopectineal eminence (Deslandes et al. 2008). MRI offers greater anatomic coverage enabling assessment for intra-articular causes. However, the real time capabilities of ultrasound make it the preferred method for confirmation of this condition. Ultrasound technique involves a dynamic examination during hip flexion-abduction-external rotation revealing a jerky return to neutral position of the iliopsoas tendon producing the audible snap against the superior pubic ramus (Fig. 16). Bifid tendons and tendon impingement due to paralabral cysts or spurs have also been demonstrated (Deslandes et al. 2008). Treatment is generally conservative initially involving anti-inflammatory medication and biomechanical re-education.

7 Bursitis

Bursitis in the adolescent athlete is likely to be caused by overuse injury relating to repetitive irritation from overlying tendons. However, other causes such as infection should always be considered. The most commonly affected pelvic bursae are the trochanteric, iliopsoas and ischial. Iliopsoas bursitis is caused by friction from the overlying iliopsoas tendon (Fig. 17). Ischial and gluteal "bursitis" may occur as a complication of chronic tendon injury or direct injury. However free

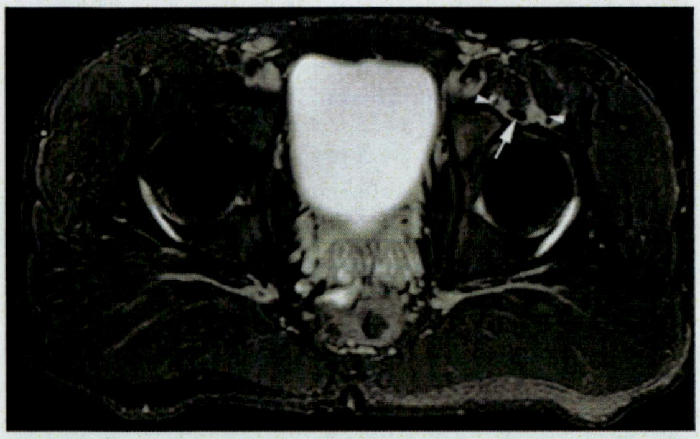

Fig. 17 Axial fat suppressed T2-w MR image shows left iliopsoas tenosynovitis (*arrowheads*) and normal tendon (*arrow*)

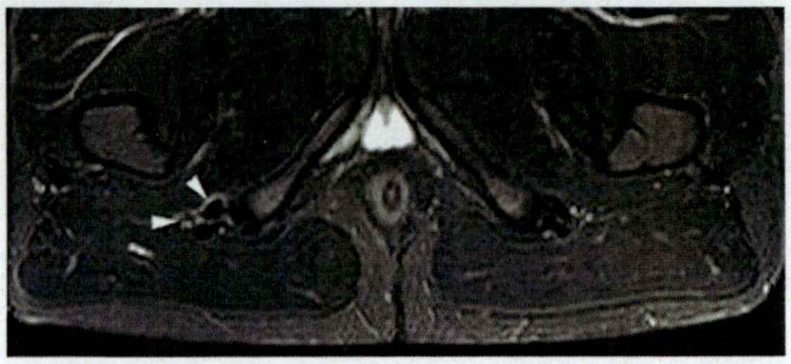

Fig. 18 Runner with chronic right hamstring pain. Axial fat suppressed T2-w MR image shows right paratenon oedema (*arrowheads*) with normal tendons

fluid is not typically seen (Bencardino and Palmer 2002) at ultrasound and MRI with paratenon oedema more common than bursitis (Fig. 18). Ultrasound also offers imaging guidance for injection into the oedema to aid diagnosis or treatment (Adler et al. 2005). Due to the anatomical communication between the hip joint and bursa in 15% of patients, the iliopsoas bursa can be distended due to a hip joint effusion rather than primary bursitis (Bencardino and Palmer 2002).

8 Osseous Injury

Acute pelvic fracture is unusual with only 3.5% of paediatric pelvic fractures resulting from athletic activity (Torode and Zieg 1985). Pelvic fractures are generally associated with high-speed collisions in activities such as cycling, skiing and skating (Cheng et al. 2000) although significant pelvic fractures have been reported with lower energy mechanisms (Stilger et al. 2000). These injuries are investigated and treated as any other significant non sports related trauma and are not covered in this chapter.

8.1 Pelvic Fatigue (Stress) Injury

In the paediatric and adolescent age groups fatigue fractures are becoming increasingly more prevalent especially with long distance running (Micheli and Curtis 2006). They are most commonly seen after an inappropriate increase in activity intensity or with vigorous newly undertaken exercise (Sofka 2006). Pelvic injury most often occurs in the proximal femur (90%) while injury to the pelvic ring mostly involves the inferior pubic ramus and sacrum (Kiuru et al. 2003).

8.2 Imaging of Pelvic Fatigue Fractures

Multiple imaging modalities can be used for the detection of fatigue fracture but MRI is the most sensitive and specific modality currently (Fig. 19).

Plain radiography is generally insensitive to early injury and changes lag behind clinical presentation. Injury to the pubic rami and femur are likely to be more visible than injury elsewhere in the pelvis but the sacrum is particularly poorly seen (Kiuru et al. 2003; Micheli and Curtis 2006). Early radiographic changes can rarely include faint cortical radiolucency but a negative plain radiograph cannot exclude a fatigue fracture. Periosteal new bone formation can be seen approximately 10 days after the initial injury pattern commences progressing to complete fracture if left untreated (Sofka 2006).

In cases with refractory symptoms or a high clinical suspicion further imaging is warranted. CT may allow fracture lines to be detected earlier especially in the sacrum or to differentiate between other causes of symptoms such as osteoid osteoma. CT is suggested as a problem solving tool if MRI is inconclusive.

Bone scintigraphy and MRI are extremely sensitive for early detection of stress remodelling and fracture. Bone scintigraphy contrast resolution may be improved by the use of single photon emission computed tomography (SPECT) (Bryant et al. 2008).

MRI currently is the gold standard in the investigation of stress fractures. Bone marrow oedema is

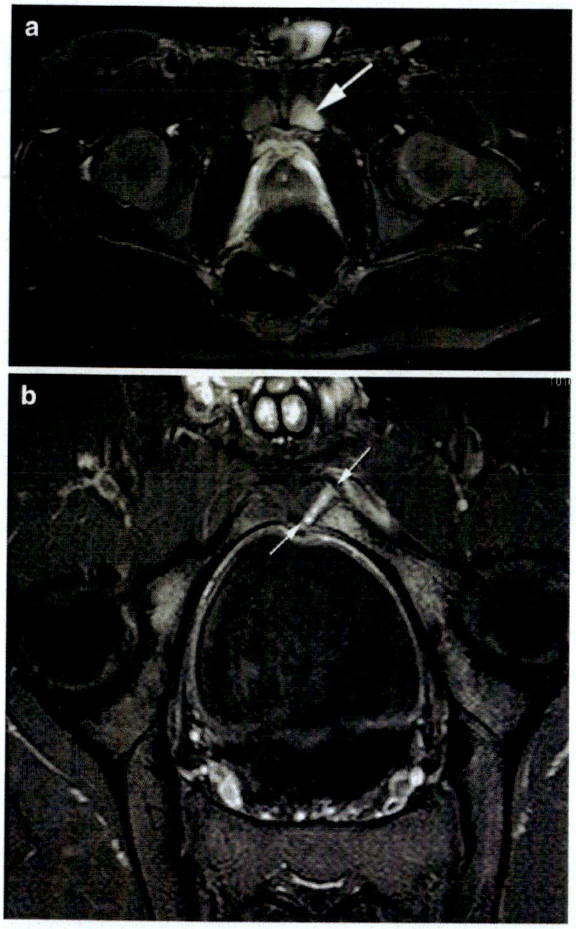

Fig. 19 Osseous stress injuries. (**a**) Axial fat suppressed T2-w MR image shows left pubic oedema (*arrow*) with no fracture. (**b**) Axial oblique fat suppressed T1-w post IV gadolinium MR image shows marked enhancement of a linear left pubic stress fracture (*arrows*). The patient presented with pubalgia

seen in areas of stress reaction (Fig. 19a) (Bryant et al. 2008). Linear signal voids may be seen on all sequences if there is an advanced stress injury or progression to fracture (Fig. 19b) (Ahovuo et al. 2004). Periosteal reaction and cortical thickening can also be demonstrated. Some caution is required when interpreting the presence of bone marrow oedema as it can be seen in asymptomatic physically active patients (Sofka 2006) and also may be a non specific finding relating to other pathology such as infection or tumour. In non specific or atypical findings correlation with other modalities such as CT may be necessary. Following onset of treatment fatty marrow conversion may be seen but imaging parameters should return to normal within 6 months (Ahovuo et al. 2004; Slocum et al. 1997).

9 Specific Considerations in the Female Athlete

Until puberty males and females are comparable in physical condition and essentially equal in all sports (Greydanus and Patel 2002). Female differences should remain at the back of the radiologists mind as symptoms may relate to gynaecological anatomy (Fig. 4b). Endometriosis, ovarian cysts and pelvic inflammatory disease are non athletic causes for symptoms which may be apparent on MRI performed for investigation of athletic pain (Loud and Micheli 2001). The female athlete triad of disordered eating, osteoporosis and amenorrhea increases the risk of stress fractures, which are more commonly seen around the pelvis in female than in male athletes.

10 Non-athletic Related Pelvic and Groin Pain

Non-athletic related pathologies (Table 2) can masquerade as sports injuries with similar symptoms but potentially devastating effects. In many instances a plain radiograph or ultrasound examination can lead to exclusion of tumour or infection. However, these pathologies should be considered if imaging for suspected athletic injury is negative or shows unusual findings (Fig. 20).

Table 2 Non-athletic causes of pelvic and groin pain

Developmental	Developmental dysplasia Legg–Calve Perthe's disease Slipped capital femoral epiphyses
Neoplasia	Primary bone malignacies E.g. Osteosarcoma, Ewing sarcoma, osteoid osteoma
Infectious causes	Septic Arthritis Osteomyelitis Pelvic inflammatory disease Epipydidymitis and orchitis
Inflammatory causes	Endometriosis Inflammatory bowel disease
Referred pain	Knee, spine, hip
Visceral abnormalities	Testicular torsion Gynaecological abnormalities Abdominal causes e.g. appendicitis, IBD Urinary tract infection

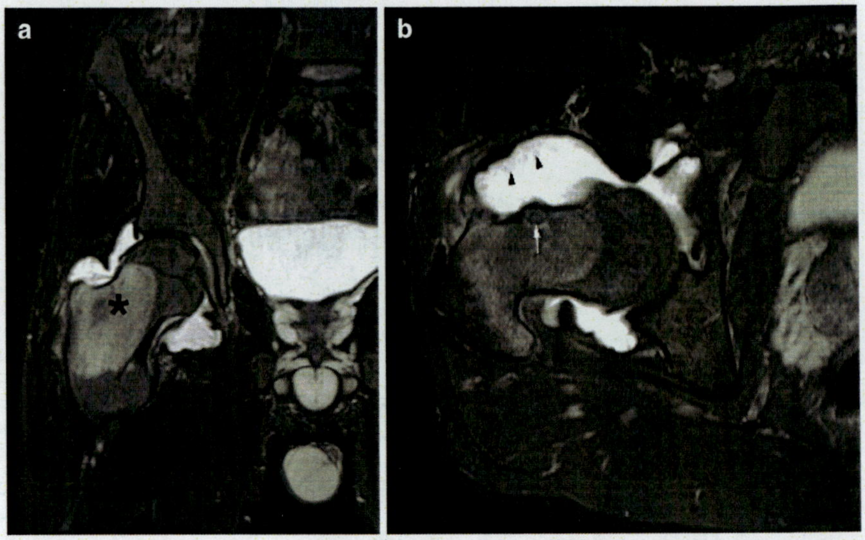

Fig. 20 Athlete with right hip pain. (**a**) Coronal and (**b**) axial fat suppressed T2-w MR images show a large hip effusion, synovitis (*arrowheads*) and femoral neck oedema (*asterisk*) not typical for stress injury. The axial images confirm an intra-capsular osteoid osteoma (*arrow*)

Acknowledgements The authors would like to thank Dr L.M. White and Dr M. Blacksin for their image contribution.

References

Adler RS, Buly R, Ambrose R, Sculco T (2005) Diagnostic and therapeutic use of sonography-guided iliopsoas peritendinous injections. AJR Am J Roentgenol 185:940–943

Ahovuo JA, Kiuru MJ, Visuri T (2004) Fatigue stress fractures of the sacrum: diagnosis with MR imaging. Eur Radiol 14:500–505

Akita K, Niga S, Yamato Y et al (1999) Anatomic basis of chronic groin pain with special reference to sports hernia. Surg Radiol Anat 21:1–5

Anderson K, Strickland SM, Warren R (2001) Hip and groin injuries in athletes. Am J Sports Med 29:521–533

Armfield DR, Kim DH, Towers JD et al (2006) Sports-related muscle injury in the lower extremity. Clin Sports Med 25:803–842

Bencardino JT, Palmer WE (2002) Imaging of hip disorders in athletes. Radiol Clin North Am 40:267–287

Benjamin M, Toumi H, Ralphs JR et al (2006) (2006)Where tendons and ligaments meet bone: attachment sites ('entheses') in relation to exercise and/or mechanical load. J Anat 208:471–490

Brennan D, O'Connell MJ, Ryan M et al (2005) Secondary cleft sign as a marker of injury in athletes with groin pain: MR image appearance and interpretation. Radiology 235:162–167

Bryant LR, Song WS, Banks KP et al (2008) Comparison of planar scintigraphy alone and with SPECT for the initial evaluation of femoral neck stress fracture. AJR Am J Roentgenol 191:1010–1015

Butler P, Mitchell AWM, Ellis H (1999) Applied radiological anatomy. Cambridge University Press, Cambridge, UK

Campbell RS, Grainger AJ (2001) Current concepts in imaging of tendinopathy. Clin Radiol 56:253–267

Cheng TL, Fields CB, Brenner RA et al (2000) Sports injuries: an important cause of morbidity in urban youth. Pediatrics 105:E32

Cunningham PM, Brennan D, O'Connell M et al (2007) Patterns of bone and soft-tissue injury at the symphysis pubis in soccer players: observations at MRI. AJR Am J Roentgenol 188:W291–W296

Deslandes M, Guillin R, Cardinal E et al (2008) The snapping iliopsoas tendon: new mechanisms using dynamic sonography. AJR Am J Roentgenol 190:576–581

Diamond A, Gregory A (2007) The male adolescent athlete: specific concerns. Pediatr Ann 36(730–731):735–737

Donnelly LF, Bisset GS, Helms CA, Squire DL (1999) Chronic avulsive injuries of childhood. Skeletal Radiol 28: 138–144

Eich GF, Babyn P, Giedion A (1992) Pediatric pelvis: radiographic appearance in various congenital disorders. Radiographics 12: 467–484

Ein SH, Njere I, Ein A (2006) Six thousand three hundred sixty-one pediatric inguinal hernias: a 35-year review. J Pediatr Surg 41:980–986

Ekberg O, Persson NH, Abrahamsson PA et al (1988) Longstanding groin pain in athletes. A multidisciplinary approach. Sports Med 6:56–61

Erez I, Kovalivker M, Schneider N, Glaser E, Lazar L, Motovic A (1993) Elective sonographic evaluation of inguinal hernia in children an effective alternative to routine contralateral exploration. Pediatr Surg Int 8:415–418

Evans GF, Haller RG, Wyrick PS et al (1998) Submaximal delayed-onset muscle soreness: correlations between MR imaging findings and clinical measures. Radiology 208: 815–820

Gilmore J (1998) Groin pain in the soccer athlete: fact, fiction and treatment. Clin Sports Med 17(4):787–793, vii

Gray H, Standring S (2005) Gray's Anatomy 39Ed: The anatomical basis of clinical practice. Elsevier Churchill Livingstone, Edinburgh.

Greydanus DE, Patel DR (2002) The female athlete. Before and beyond puberty. Pediatr Clin North Am 49:553–580, vi

Hata S, Takahashi Y, Nakamura T et al (2004) Preoperative sonographic evaluation is a useful method of detecting contralateral patent processus vaginalis in pediatric patients with unilateral inguinal hernia. J Pediatr Surg 39:1396–1399

Hébert KJ, Laor T, Divine JG et al (2008) MRI appearance of chronic stress injury of the iliac crest apophysis in adolescent athletes. AJR Am J Roentgenol 190:1487–1491

Irshad K, Feldman LS, Lavoie C et al (2001) Operative management of "hockey groin syndrome": 12 years of experience in National Hockey League players. Surgery 130:759–764, discussion 7646

Jamadar DA, Jacobson JA, Morag Y et al (2006) Sonography of inguinal region hernias. AJR Am J Roentgenol 187: 185–190

Jaramillo D, Hoffer FA, Shapiro F, Rand F (1990) MR imaging of fractures of the growth plate. AJR Am J Roentgenol 155:1261–1265

Järvinen TA, Järvinen TL, Kääriäinen M et al (2005) Muscle injuries: biology and treatment. Am J Sports Med 33:745–764

Joesting DR (2002) Diagnosis and treatment of sportsman's hernia. Curr Sports Med Rep 1:121–124

Kälebo P, Karlsson J, Swärd L, Peterson L (1992) Ultrasonography of chronic tendon injuries in the groin. Am J Sports Med 20:634–639

Kervancioglu R, Bayram MM, Ertaskin I, Ozkur A (2000) Ultrasonographic evaluation of bilateral groins in children with unilateral inguinal hernia. Acta Radiol 41:653–657

Kiuru MJ, Pihlajamaki HK, Ahovuo JA (2003) Fatigue stress injuries of the pelvic bones and proximal femur: evaluation with MR imaging. Eur Radiol 13:605–611

Kocher MS, Tucker R (2006) Pediatric athlete hip disorders. Clin Sports Med 25:241–253, viii

Koulouris G (2008) Imaging review of groin pain in elite athletes: an anatomic approach to imaging findings. AJR Am J Roentgenol 191:962–972

Kumar A, Doran J, Batt ME et al (2002) Results of inguinal canal repair in athletes with sports hernia. J R Coll Surg Edinb 47:561–565

Lazović D, Wegner U, Peters G, Gossé F (1996) Ultrasound for diagnosis of apophyseal injuries. Knee Surg Sports Traumatol Arthrosc 3:234–237

Le Gall F, Carling C, Reilly T (2007) Biological maturity and injury in elite youth football. Scand J Med Sci Sports 17:564–572

Loud KJ, Micheli LJ (2001) Common athletic injuries in adolescent girls. Curr Opin Pediatr 13:317–322

Lovell G, Galloway H, Hopkins W, Harvey A (2006) Osteitis pubis and assessment of bone marrow edema at the pubic symphysis with MRI in an elite junior male soccer squad. Clin J Sport Med 16:117–122

Maffulli N, So WS, Ahuja A, Chan KM (1996) Iliopsoas haematoma in an adolescent Taekwondo player. Knee Surg Sports Traumatol Arthrosc 3:230–233

Major NM, Helms CA (1997) Pelvic stress injuries: the relationship between osteitis pubis (symphysis pubis stress injury) and sacroiliac abnormalities in athletes. Skeletal Radiol 26:711–717

Micheli LJ, Curtis C (2006) Stress fractures in the spine and sacrum. Clin Sports Med 25:75–88, ix

Micheli LJ, Fehlandt AF (1992) Overuse injuries to tendons and apophyses in children and adolescents. Clin Sports Med 11:713–726

O'Connell MJ, Powell T, McCaffrey NM et al (2002) Symphyseal cleft Injection in the diagnosis and treatment of osteitis pubis in athletes. AJR Am J Roentgenol 179:955–959

Omar IM, Zoga AC, Kavanagh EC et al (2008) Athletic pubalgia and "sports hernia": optimal MR imaging technique and findings. Radiographics 28:1415–1438

Orchard JW, Read JW, Neophyton J, Garlick D (1998) Groin pain associated with ultrasound finding of inguinal canal posterior wall deficiency in Australian Rules footballers. Br J Sports Med 32:134–139

Paajanen H, Hermunen H, Karonen J (2008) Pubic magnetic resonance imaging findings in surgically and conservatively treated athletes with osteitis pubis compared to asymptomatic athletes during heavy training. Am J Sports Med 36: 117–121

Parnis SJ, Roberts JP, Hutson JM (1997) Anatomical landmarks of the inguinal canal in prepubescent children. Aust N Z J Surg 67:335–337

Pisacano RM, Miller TT (2003) Comparing sonography with MR imaging of apophyseal injuries of the pelvis in four boys. AJR Am J Roentgenol 181:223–230

Radcliffe G, Stringer MD (1997) Reappraisal of femoral hernia in children. Br J Surg 84:58–60

Rettenbacher T, Hollerweger A, Macheiner P et al (2001) Abdominal wall hernias: cross-sectional imaging signs of incarceration determined with sonography. AJR Am J Roentgenol 177:1061–1066

Risser JC (1958) The Iliac apophysis; an invaluable sign in the management of scoliosis. Clin Orthop 11:111–119

Robinson P, Barron DA, Parsons W et al (2004) Adductor-related groin pain in athletes: correlation of MR imaging with clinical findings. Skeletal Radiol 33:451–457

Robinson P, Hensor E, Lansdown MJ et al (2006) Inguinofemoral hernia: accuracy of sonography in patients with indeterminate clinical features. AJR Am J Roentgenol 187: 1168–1178

Robinson P, Salehi F, Grainger A et al (2007) Cadaveric and MRI study of the musculotendinous contributions to the capsule of the symphysis pubis. AJR Am J Roentgenol 188: W440–W445

Rossi F, Dragoni S (2001) Acute avulsion fractures of the pelvis in adolescent competitive athletes: prevalence, location and sports distribution of 203 cases collected. Skeletal Radiol 30:127–131

Sanjay P, Woodward A (2007) Single strenuous event: does it predispose to inguinal herniation? Hernia 11:493–496

Shadbolt CL, Heinze SB, Dietrich RB (2001) Imaging of groin masses: inguinal anatomy and pathologic conditions revisited. Radiographics 21:S261–S271

Slocum KA, Gorman JD, Puckett ML, Jones SB (1997) Resolution of abnormal MR signal intensity in patients with stress fractures of the femoral neck. AJR Am J Roentgenol 168:1295–1299

Sofka CM (2006) Imaging of stress fractures. Clin Sports Med 25:53–62, viii

Soprano JV, Fuchs SM (2007) Common overuse injuries in the pediatric and adolescent athlete. Clin Pediatc Emerg Med 8:7–14

Sorensen L, Larsen SE, Rock ND (1996) The epidemiology of sports injuries in school-aged children. Scand J Med Sci Sports 6:281–286

Steele P, Annear P, Grove JR (2004) Surgery for posterior inguinal wall deficiency in athletes. J Sci Med Sport 7:415–421, discussion 422–423

Stevens MA, El-Khoury GY, Kathol MH et al (1999) Imaging features of avulsion injuries. Radiographics 19:655–672

Stilger VG, Alt JM, Hubbard DF (2000) Traumatic acetabular fracture in an intercollegiate football player: a case report. J Athl Train 35:103–107

Torode I, Zieg D (1985) Pelvic fractures in children. J Pediatr Orthop 5:76–84

Vaccaro JP, Sauser DD, Beals RK (1995) Iliopsoas bursa imaging: efficacy in depicting abnormal iliopsoas tendon motion in patients with internal snapping hip syndrome. Radiology 197:853–856

Vandervliet EJ, Vanhoenacker FM, Snoeckx A et al (2007) Sports-related acute and chronic avulsion injuries in children and adolescents with special emphasis on tennis. Br J Sports Med 41:827–831

Vergnes P, Midy D, Bondonny JM, Cabanie H (1985) Anatomical basis of inguinal surgery in children. Anat Clin 7:257–265

Verrall GM, Slavotinek JP, Fon GT (2001) Incidence of pubic bone marrow oedema in Australian rules football players: relation to groin pain. Br J Sports Med 35:28–33

Verrall GM, Slavotinek JP, Barnes PG, Fon GT (2005) Description of pain provocation tests used for the diagnosis of sports-related chronic groin pain: relationship of tests to defined clinical (pain and tenderness) and MRI (pubic bone marrow oedema) criteria. Scand J Med Sci Sports 15: 36–42

Verrall GM, Henry L, Fazzalari NL et al (2008) Bone biopsy of the parasymphyseal pubic bone region in athletes with chronic groin injury demonstrates new woven bone formation consistent with a diagnosis of pubic bone stress injury. Am J Sports Med 36:2425–2431

Volpi P, Pozzoni R, Galli M (2003) The major traumas in youth football. Knee Surg Sports Traumatol Arthrosc 11:399–402

Winston P, Awan R, Cassidy JD, Bleakney RK (2007) Clinical examination and ultrasound of self-reported snapping hip syndrome in elite ballet dancers. Am J Sports Med 35: 118–126

Yamamoto T, Akisue T, Nakatani T et al (2004) Apophysitis of the ischial tuberosity mimicking a neoplasm on magnetic resonance imaging. Skeletal Radiol 33:737–740

Zoga AC, Kavanagh EC, Omar IM et al (2008) Athletic pubalgia and the "sports hernia": MR imaging findings. Radiology 247:797–807

Hip

Apostolos H. Karantanas

Contents

A.H. Karantanas
Department of Radiology, University Hospital, Stavrakia, GR 711 10, Heraklion, Greece
e-mail: akarantanas@gmail.com

Key Points

- Hip and groin injuries are usually seen with kicking, running and jumping athletic activities. Both recreational and elite young athletes can be involved.
- Plain X-rays are the initial examination although usually unremarkable.
- CT can be helpful in certain cases such as tiny avulsion injuries, intraarticular loose bodies and myositis ossificans.
- MR imaging of the hip depicts radiographically occult osseous abnormalities such as stress injuries, musculotendinous injuries and bursitis.
- US in children and adolescents may be used as an alternative to MR imaging method, for superficial injuries.

1 Introduction

The overall incidence of sports-related hip injuries in both recreational and elite athletes is low compared with other anatomical areas. Studies in high school athletes reported an incidence of hip area injuries of 5–9% (Delee and Farney 1992; Gomez et al. 1996). Adolescent athletes are able to describe both the symptoms and the mechanism of injury. On the other hand, children with hip injuries may present clinically in variable ways: hip pain, painless hip with radiating pain to the knee or distal thigh, refusal to bear weight, limp or abnormal gait, and restricted movement of the lower extremity. The lack of specificity of the clinical symptoms induces clinical dilemmas on the diagnosis

A.H. Karantanas (ed.), *Sports Injuries in Children and Adolescents*,
Med Radiol Diagn Imaging, DOI: 10.1007/174_2010_57, © Springer-Verlag Berlin Heidelberg 2011

and treatment. The anatomic variations in the growing skeleton such as soft structure of the thick articular cartilage, laxity of the ligaments and increased strength of the tendon insertions with regard to the underlying bone, underline the difficulties in arriving to a correct diagnosis. On the other hand, unique injury patterns can be seen in young athletes who have underlying pediatric hip disorders such as slipped capital femoral epiphysis, and Legg-Calve-Perthe's disease.

Hip injuries can result in increased rehabilitation time. The complex anatomical and biomechanical considerations along with the peculiarities of the immature skeleton further enhance the role of imaging for accurate diagnosis. The most common sports-related hip disorders include avulsions, stress injuries, labral and osteochondral injuries, and soft tissue disorders such as muscle strains and contusions, tendinopathies and iliopsoas bursitis. Conventional radiographs should be the initial examination. Ultrasonography (US) has an evolving role as a first line imaging study, mainly for superficial structures. Magnetic resonance (MR) imaging has proven efficient in demonstrating a wide spectrum of disorders originating in both bones and soft tissues. An optimized MR imaging protocol, should be constructed and tailored according to the clinical problem. Large field of view coronal T1-w and fat suppressed PD/T2-w or STIR images should be matched with focused unilateral high resolution ones depending upon the clinically suspected pathology. MR arthrography is reserved for the depiction and characterization of intra-articular lesions. Computed tomography (CT) can be useful in certain circumstances, such as for diagnosing non-displaced or chronic avulsion injuries, as well as in examining patients who are contraindicated to undergo MR imaging.

2 Osseous Injuries

2.1 Avulsion Injuries

Apophyseal injury is more commonly seen in adolescents as the physis is weaker than the musculotendinous insertion (Rossi and Dragoni 2001). The distinct types of apophyseal injury, the commonly involved apophyses with their expected age of fusion and the corresponding tendon insertions, have already been discussed in the previous chapter (see Table 8.1). Avulsion injuries around the hip area are rare and usually located at the lesser trochanter (Gamble and Kao 1997). Other avulsion fractures are located at the ischial tuberosity, anterior inferior iliac spine and the anterior superior iliac spine (Moeller 2003). The imaging findings of the various types of avulsion injuries have been already discussed in the previous chapter.

Most of the cases are *acute* avulsions which result from a forceful, unbalanced and eccentric muscular contraction (El-Khoury et al. 1997). Typically, there is a history of a single traumatic event and therefore the clinical and radiographic diagnosis is easy. Surgical intervention is required for fractures displaced more than 2 cm or in cases of failed conservative treatment (Kocher and Tucker 2006). In radiographically occult injuries without significant displacement, MR imaging will show the bone marrow and soft tissue edema close to the apophysis which is slightly widened (Figs. 1 and 2). This finding cannot be distinguished from that seen in *apophysitis* which results from repetitive microtrauma. Apophysitis might represent the earliest in the spectrum of apophyseal injuries, and if not recognized, acute avulsions, usually during kicking, will occur. Thus, apophysitis may pre-exist and predispose to an acute avulsion or may exist as a chronic process. Indeed, it is the history which will direct towards the correct diagnosis, yet not altering the treatment decisions.

Chronic avulsion injuries in terms of non-union of an avulsion fracture, may demonstrate clinical and radiographic findings which occasionally are confusing (Tehranzadeh 1987). Sprinters, cheerleaders and gymnasts as well as football, and track athletes are prone to these injuries (Brandser et al. 1985; Tehranzadeh 1987). Irritation of the sciatic nerve may occur either due to fragment impingement on the nerve or to callus formation during healing (Combs 1994). These injuries may lead to osteolysis and may be misinterpreted as infection or Ewing sarcoma (Tehranzadeh 1987). MR imaging and CT can be quite diagnostic in these cases (Figs. 3 and 4). Chronic avulsive changes can be recognized on fat suppressed images by the bright signal of the slight widening of the physis (Figs. 4 and 5) and/or the contiguous marrow reaction (Fig. 6).

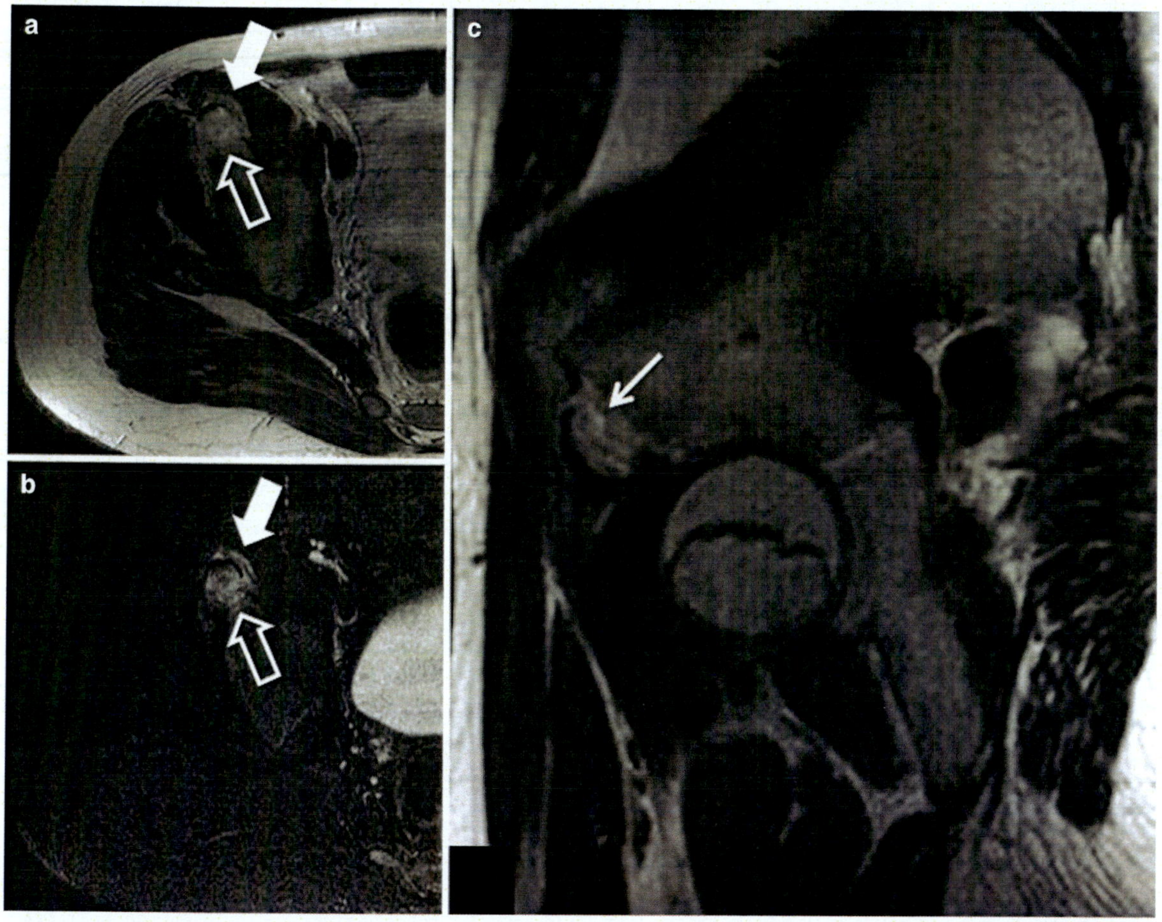

Fig. 1 Radiographically occult acute avulsion injury in a 14 year-old male wrestling athlete with a recent injury. The transverse T2-w MR images (**a**, **b** with fat suppression) and the sagittal T2-w MR image (**c**), show the minimal displacement (*thin arrow*), the bone marrow edema (*open arrows*) and the soft tissue edema (*arrows*) in the right anterior inferior iliac spine

2.2 Legg-Calve-Perthe's Disease

Legg-Calve-Perth's (LCP) disease (osteochondrosis), is an idiopathic self-limiting disorder, corresponding to avascular necrosis of the femoral head. It is seen in the first decade of life, mainly involving males. The younger a child at the onset of the disease, the greater the time she/he has for subsequent growth and remodeling. Although not directly related to sports activities, this disorder might impose diagnostic problems, in young athletes who report a history of repetitive microtrauma. Early MR imaging findings include subchondral femoral fracture, synovitis and joint effusion, bone marrow edema and epiphyseal fragmentation. Subchondral fractures in athletic patients might simulate stress injuries (Figs. 7 and 8). Early postocontrast images may show the lack of perfusion in the involved epiphysis, as opposed to the contralateral normal one. Members of the same family may be involved (Fig. 9). The goal of treatment for LCP in the young child is to maintain the proper congruity of the hip joint. As a complication of poorly treated LCP, the femoral head may be flattened and become incongruous with the acetabulum. This abnormal relationship may result to labral tears and chondral injury.

2.3 Slipped Capital Femoral Epiphysis

Slipped capital femoral epiphysis (SCFE) is a Salter Harris I fracture through the proximal femoral growth plate. SCFE is regarded as the most common hip

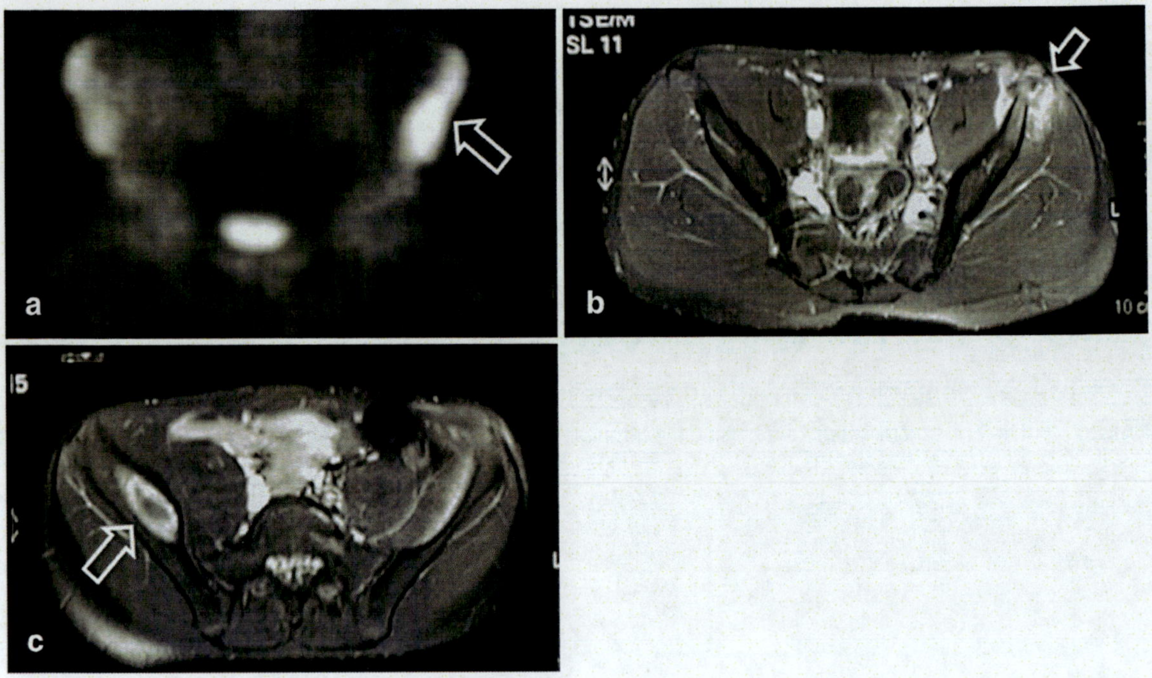

Fig. 2 Radiographically occult avulsion injury in a 16 year-old male track athlete with a recent injury during rapid acceleration and pain on both sides above the hip joints. (**a**) The bone scintigram shows uptake on the left side in keeping with an injury of the anterior superior iliac spine (*arrow*). The fat suppressed contrast enhanced T1-w MR images, confirm the avulsion injury with soft tissue and bone marrow enhancement on the left (*arrow* in **b**) and in addition depict a strain with peripheral enhancement of the right iliac muscle (*arrow* in **c**)

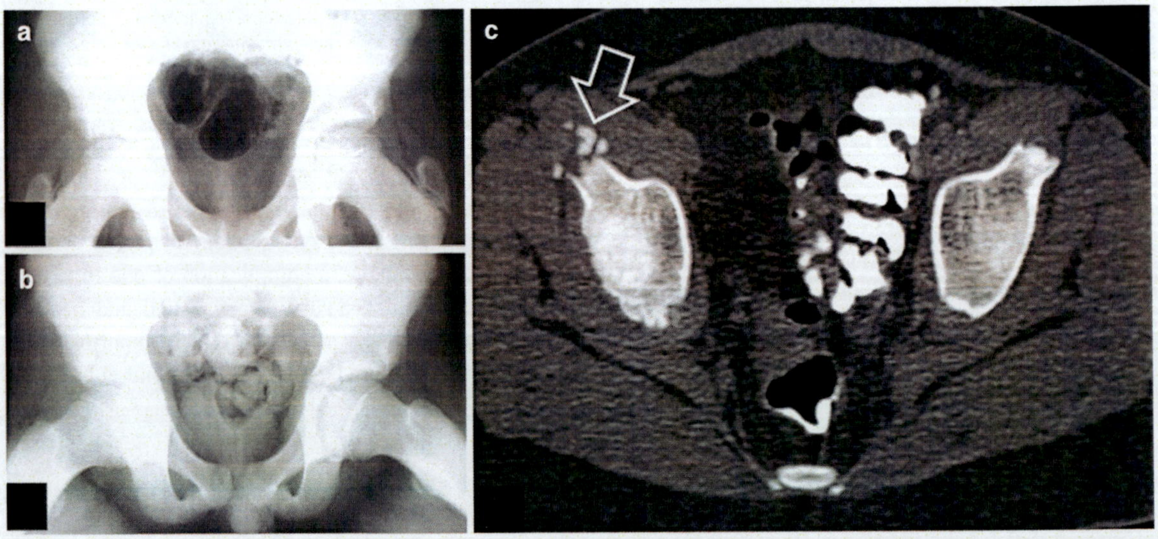

Fig. 3 Chronic avulsion injury of the anterior inferior iliac spine, in a 13 year-old male football player with a history of 2-month injury and pain above the right hip joint. The AP (**a**) and lateral (**b**) radiographs are unremarkable. (**c**) The axial CT image shows abnormal and amorphous calcifications within the insertion of the rectus femoris tendon (*arrow*). This appearance may be confused with more aggressive disorders

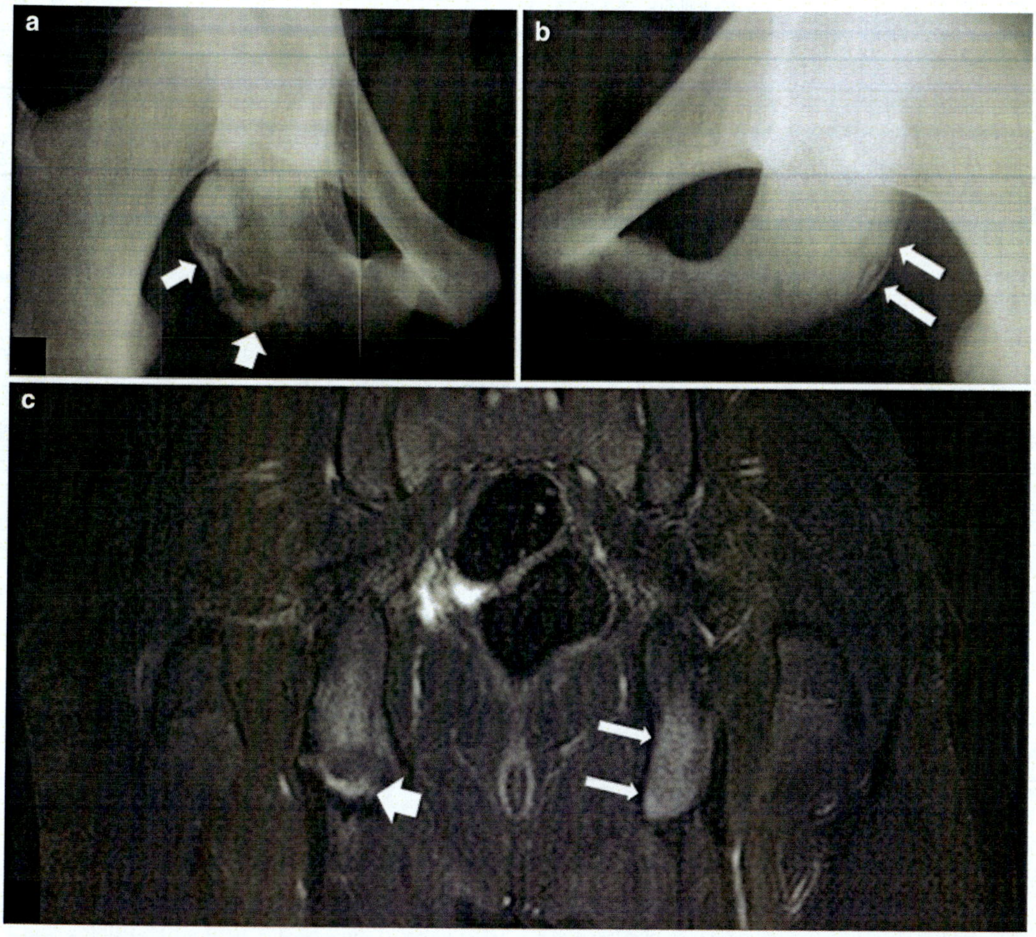

Fig. 4 Bilateral hip and gluteal pain in a 15 year-old male football player, with a history of injuries 6 months before imaging. (**a**) The plain AP radiograph shows on the right side irregular appearance of the ischial body and tuberosity, resulting from callus formation of an old avulsion fracture (*arrows*). (**b**) On the left side, a normal apophysis is seen (*arrows*). (**c**) The coronal STIR MR image, shows a bright signal in the right ischial tuberosity in keeping with chronic avulsion (*arrow*). On the left, reactive bone marrow edema (stress injury) is depicted (*thin arrows*)

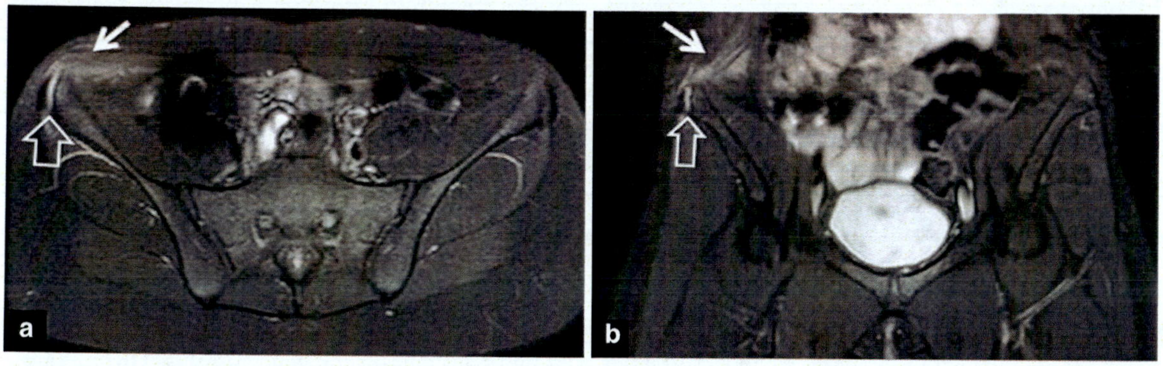

Fig. 5 A chronic avulsion injury in the right anterior superior iliac spine, in a 14 year-old female track athlete. The axial (**a**) and coronal (**b**) fat suppressed proton density MR images, show a bright signal within the apophysis (*open arrows*) and associated soft tissue edema (*white arrows*)

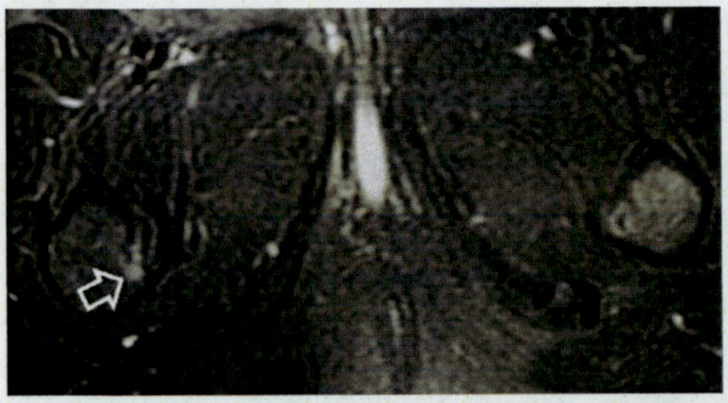

Fig. 6 Bone marrow edema (*arrow*) in an 11 year-old male football player with repetitive microtrauma and apophysitis at the insertion of the right iliopsoas tendon

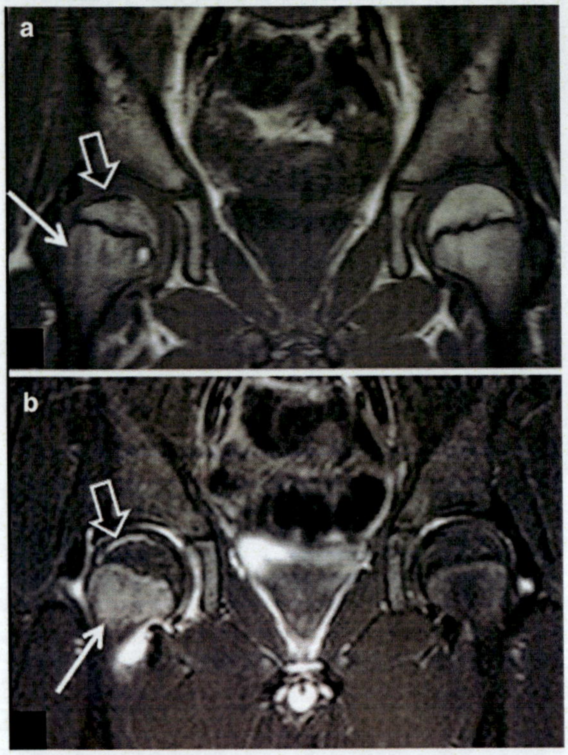

Fig. 7 Early Legg-Calve-Perthe's osteochondrosis of the right hip in a 10 year-old male football athlete. The coronal T1-w (**a**) and STIR (**b**) MR images show a subchondral fracture (*open arrow*), synovitis with joint effusion, and bone marrow edema (*thin arrow*). Note the asymmetric appearance in the bone marrow of the femoral heads, in keeping with deficient perfusion of the right

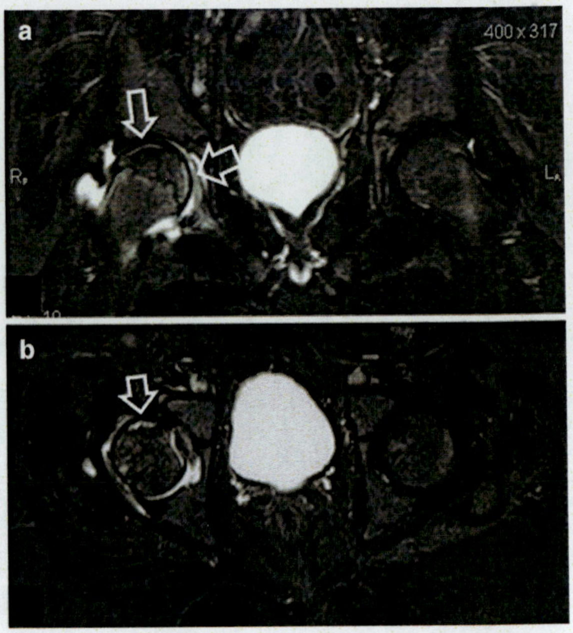

Fig. 8 Early Legg-Calve-Perthe's osteochondrosis of the right hip in a 9 year-old female tennis player. The coronal (**a**) and axial (**b**) fat suppressed T2-w MR images show subchondral fracture in the femoral head (*open arrows*) and synovitis with joint effusion

disorder of adolescence, with an increased prevalence among males, and with peak onset around 11 years of age. Increased body mass index is a significant risk factor for its development, with both biomechanical and endocrinological factors being also implicated. As with LCP disease, no direct relation seems to exist with sports activities. Thus, the main goal of imaging is to early depict SCFE in young athletes and to rule out irrelevant sports related injuries.

The earliest radiographic findings consist of widening of the growth plate and osteopenia of the head and neck. In more advanced cases, there is displacement of the neck with regard to head. This displacement ("olisthesis" in Greek) can be evaluated on the AP view by using a line drawn tangential to the lateral edge of the femoral neck. This should intersect the femoral head, with at least a small portion of the femoral head, typically the same on both sides, located lateral to the line. If not, SCFE should be suspected. SCFE is best appreciated on the frog-leg lateral view of the pelvis.

Accurate MR imaging diagnosis relies on depiction of the morphologic changes and the abnormal signal in the growth plate and the surrounding bone marrow. Coronal fat suppressed images are useful to demonstrate the increased growth plate, and comparison with the normal contralateral hip is useful (Dwek 2009). Multiplanar imaging is important for depicting the displacement of the femoral head (Fig. 10). MR imaging is useful to evaluate the vascular integrity of the

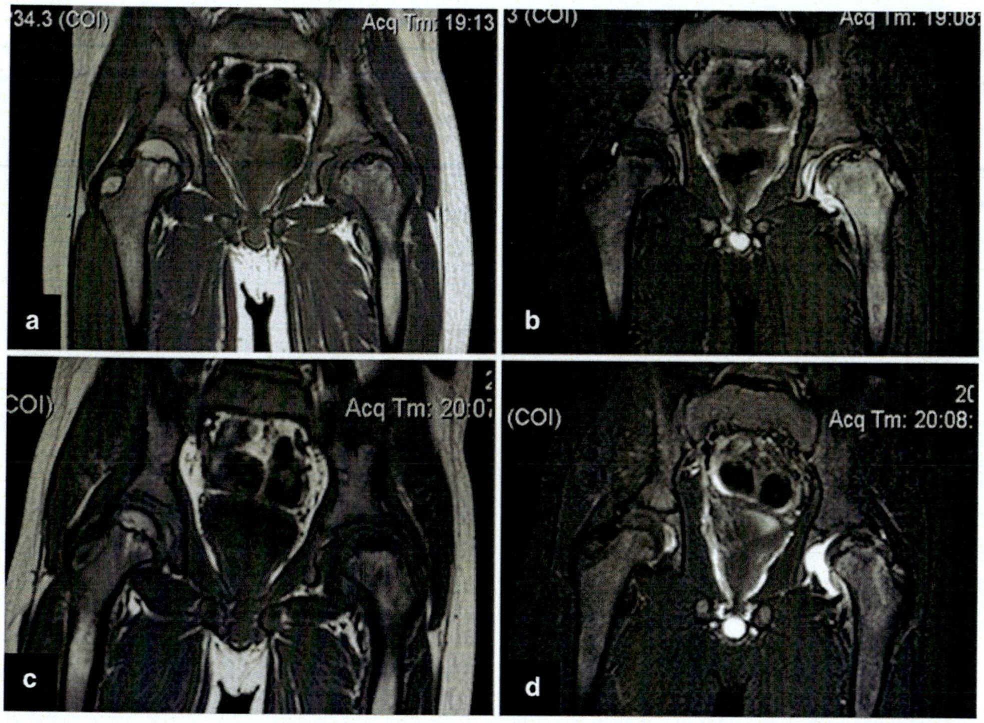

Fig. 9 Two male brothers, football players and Taekwondo athletes, 8 year old (**a** and **b**) and 9 year-old (**c** and **d**) with left hip joint pain, limp and limited joint function presenting simultaneously. The coronal T1-w (*left*) and fat suppressed T2-w (*right*) MR images, show fragmentation of the left femoral heads, synovitis and bone marrow edema, in keeping with Legg-Calve-Perthe's osteochondrosis

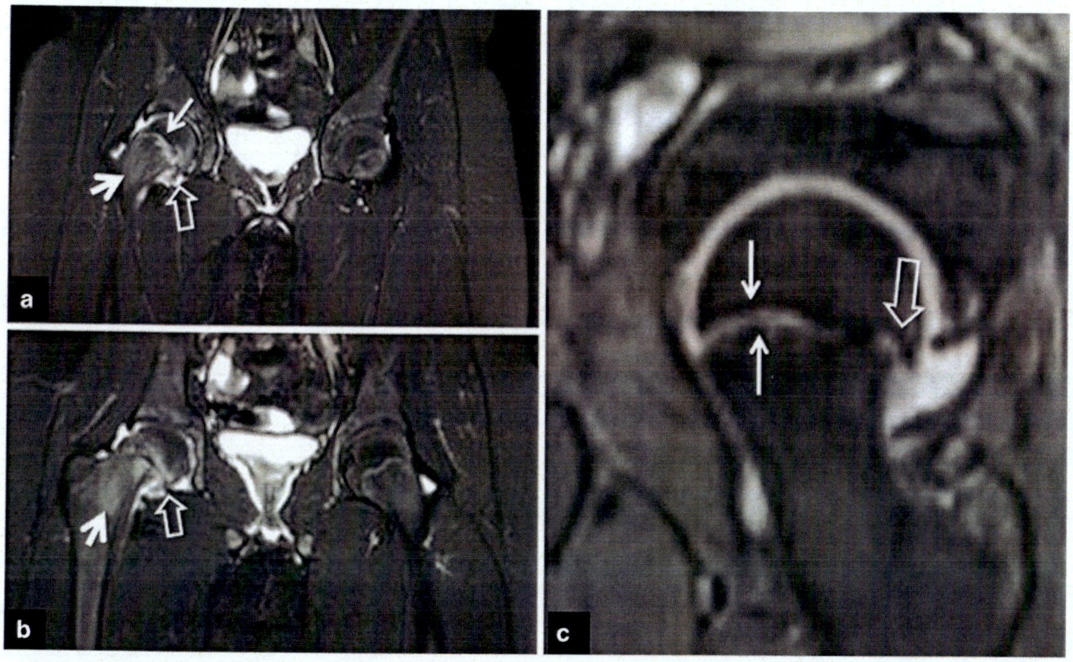

Fig. 10 A 15 year old male handball athlete, with right slipped femoral capital epiphysis. The coronal fat suppressed PD-w (**a**, **b**) and oblique axial T2* (**c**) MR images, show the epiphysiolysis (*thin arrows*), epiphysiolistheris (*open arrows*), bone marrow edema (*short arrows*) and the joint effusion

femoral head with the use of fat suppressed contrast enhanced T1-w images. A lack of enhancement suggests osteonecrosis.

2.4 Stress Injuries

Stress fractures and reactions, account for about 20% of all sports-related injuries. Stress injuries involving the growing skeleton are of "fatigue," type, resulting from normal bone being subjected to abnormal and repetitive forces (Anderson and Greenspan 1996). Children are rarely involved. These injuries are seen usually in adolescents as they require high impact of training before they are clinically and radiologically present. They occur more commonly in female athletes as they have reduced muscle bulk compared to males (Hodnett et al. 2009). Stress related injuries represent a wide spectrum ranging from stress reaction to overt fractures. The typical clinical symptoms are exercise-related pain with relief at rest. The persisting pain at rest usually indicates a more severe injury.

Sites of stress injuries with pain referred to the hip include the inferomedial femoral neck, superior and inferior pubic rami, acetabular roof, subcortical femoral head and very rarely the sacrum (Bogost et al. 1995). Stress injuries present with local pain during or after physical exercise. Femoral neck and inferior pubic ramus stress fractures occur in joggers and long distance runners. Plain X-rays should be used as the initial method for imaging the osseous structures involved. However, the initial plain X-rays can be negative in up to 65% of cases and follow-up films may demonstrate findings in 50% of the patients (Spitz and Newberg 2002). When the fractures are not seen in the initial films, they are called occult. Bone scintigraphy is very sensitive for detection of stress fractures but lacks spatial resolution, imposes radiation burden and shows a high false-positive rate (Shin et al. 1996). Overall it has a limited role for follow up as it can be positive for up to 10 months after injury (Rupini et al. 1985).

MR imaging is the method of choice for demonstrating stress injuries because of its high sensitivity for imaging the bone marrow and its high-contrast resolution (Deutsch et al. 1997).

Stress response or stress reaction is a pre-fracture condition characterized by low signal on T1-w and high signal on T2-w and STIR sequences, due to repetitive trauma to the bone marrow, without any fracture line (Figs. 11–13). Periosteal and parosteal soft tissue edema may be seen. This condition is differentiated from bone contusion only with history, by means of one single traumatic effect occurring in the latter. Bone bruise is rare in the hip and groin area both in the growing skeleton and adults. Although asymptomatic bone marrow edema has been reported to occur in the lower limbs in adult athletes, it is currently not known if this finding could also be seen in the hips of children and adolescents involved in sports.

Stress fractures are shown as hypointense areas on T1-w and hyperintense on fat suppressed T2-w because

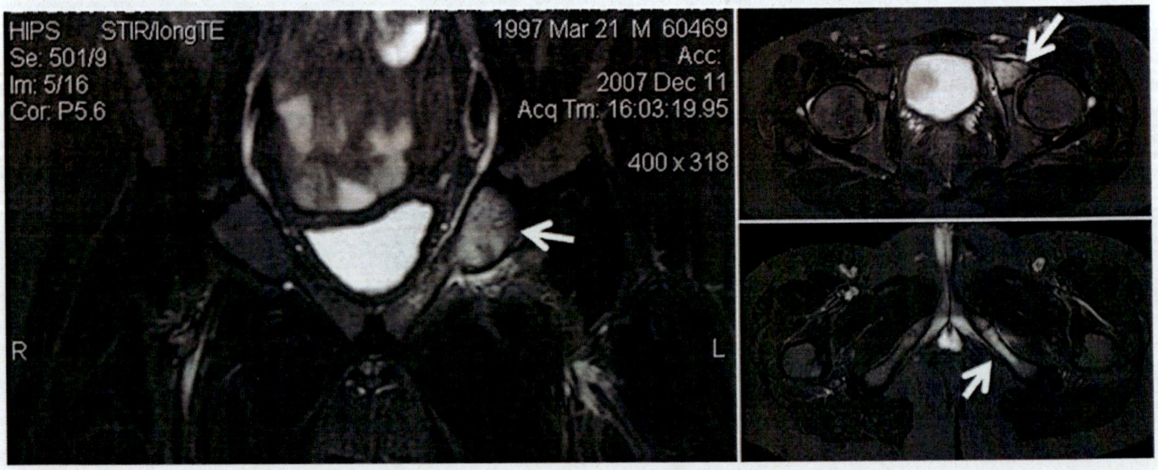

Fig. 11 Stress reaction in a 10 year-old male football player demonstrated with bone marrow edema on fat suppressed MR images within the ischiopubic rami (*arrows*). Parosteal soft tissue edema is also seen

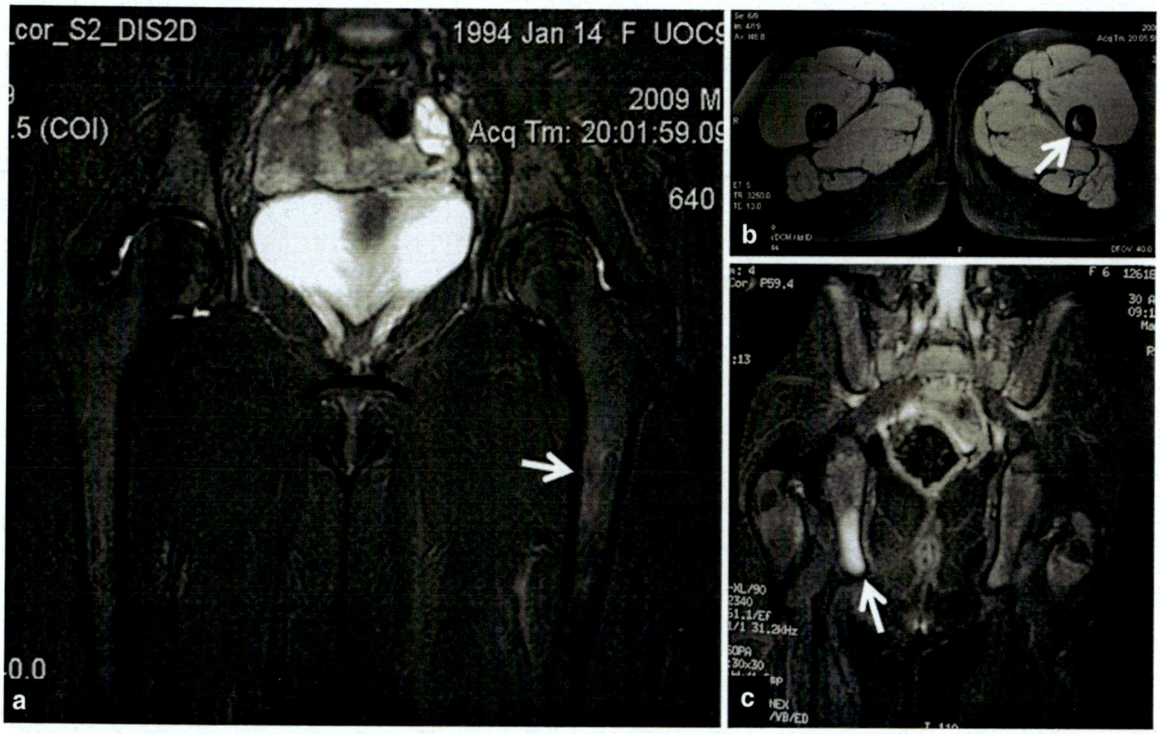

Fig. 12 Stress reaction without fracture in two athletes. The first patient is a 15-year-old female basketball player with a 2-month pain in the left thigh. The coronal STIR (**a**) and the axial fat suppressed PD-w (**b**) MR images, show a subtle area of bone marrow edema during the resolution phase of clinical symptoms (*arrows*). (**c**) The coronal STIR MR image shows bone marrow edema within the ischial bone (arrow) in a 6-year-old girl following intense trampoline playing during the last 2 weeks

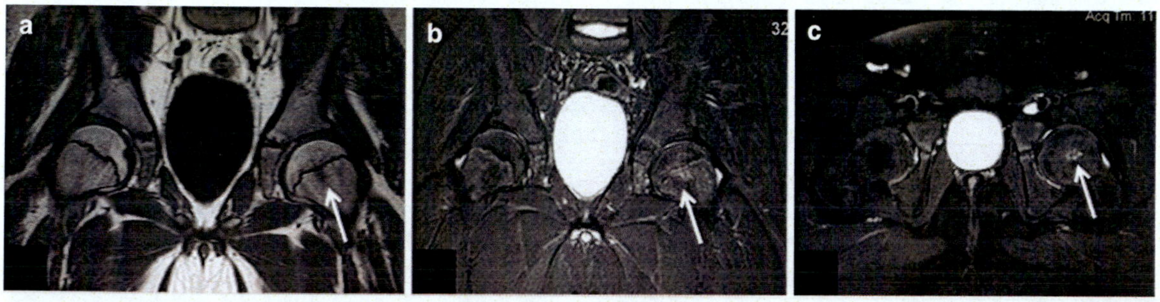

Fig. 13 Stress reaction in a 13-year-old male football player with increased body mass index. The coronal T1-w (**a**), coronal STIR (**b**) and axial fat suppressed T2 (**c**) MR images, show a focal abnormal signal intensity lesion (*arrows*). This finding is similar to Salter Harris type V lesions. Complete resolution of symptoms occurred within 6 weeks, with just weight bearing protection

of the bone marrow edema and hemorrhage. Within this abnormal area, a low signal intensity line crossing the edematous area up to the cortex can be seen on T2-w images (Figs. 14 and 15) (Deutsch et al. 1989). This low signal intensity fracture line may be obvious on T1-w images as well. MR imaging has been shown to be 100% accurate in differentiating stress fractures from other causes of sports-related disorders in the hip (Shin et al. 1996). MR imaging can be quite useful for the follow-up of elite athletes as it allows, by using fat-suppressed sequences, to assess the conversion of the bone marrow signal back to normal, in about 3 months (Slocum et al. 1997). The majority of stress fractures has a good prognosis and is healed in a few weeks with conservative treatment. Stress fracture displacement, non-union or associated osteonecrosis may occur in

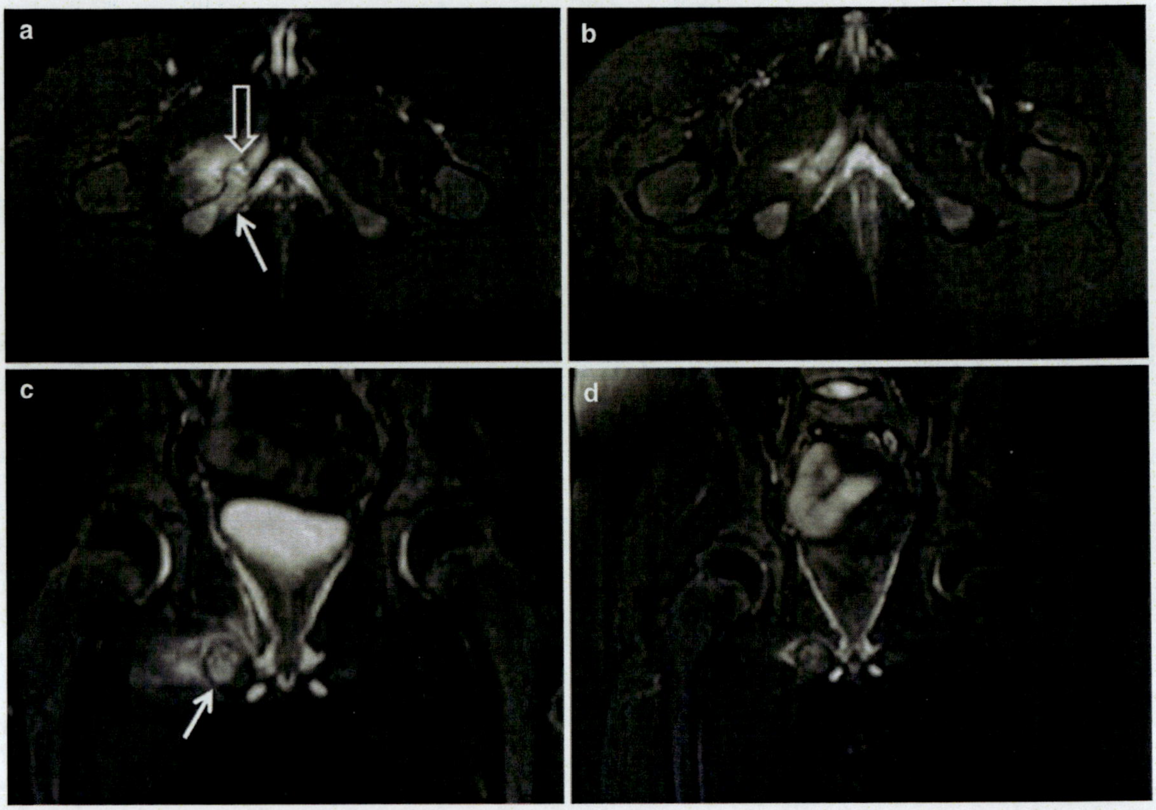

Fig. 14 A stress fracture of the pubic bone in a 14 year-old male jogger. Fat suppressed MR images in the axial (**a**) and coronal (**b**) planes show the bone marrow edema (*arrows*), the low signal intensity fracture line (*open arrow*) and the soft tissue changes. The low signal intensity line posterior to the fracture represents the normal synchondrosis. The corresponding MR images 1 month following rest, show reduction of the findings, in keeping with the clinical improvement

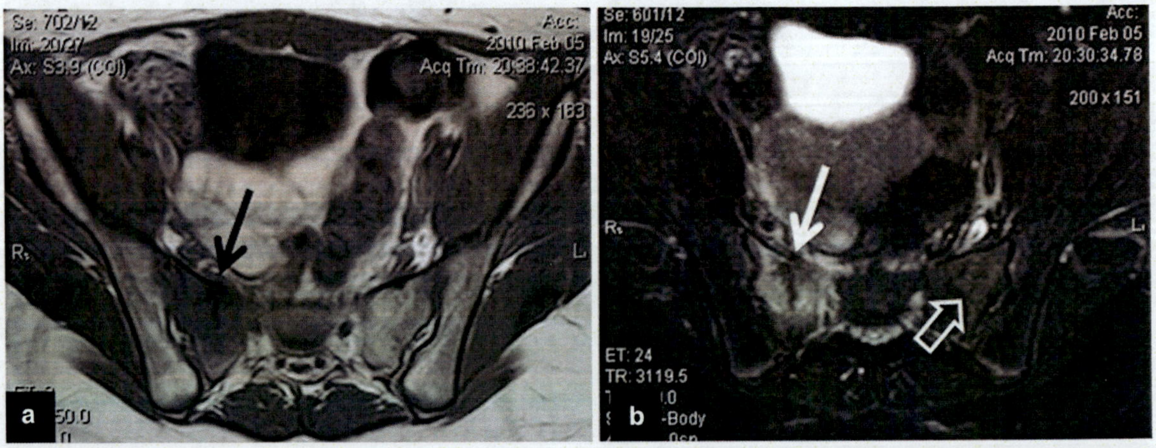

Fig. 15 Stress fracture of the right sacral wing and stress reaction of the left sacral wing, in a 16 year-old female weight lifter. The oblique axial T1-w (**a**) and fat suppressed T2-w (**b**) as well as the oblique coronal T1-w (**c**) and fat suppressed T2-w (**d**) MR images, show a low signal intensity fracture line on the right (*arrows*) with surrounding bone marrow edema. The stress reaction on the left shows only subtle marrow edema, not depicted on T1-w MR images, without any fracture line (*open arrows*)

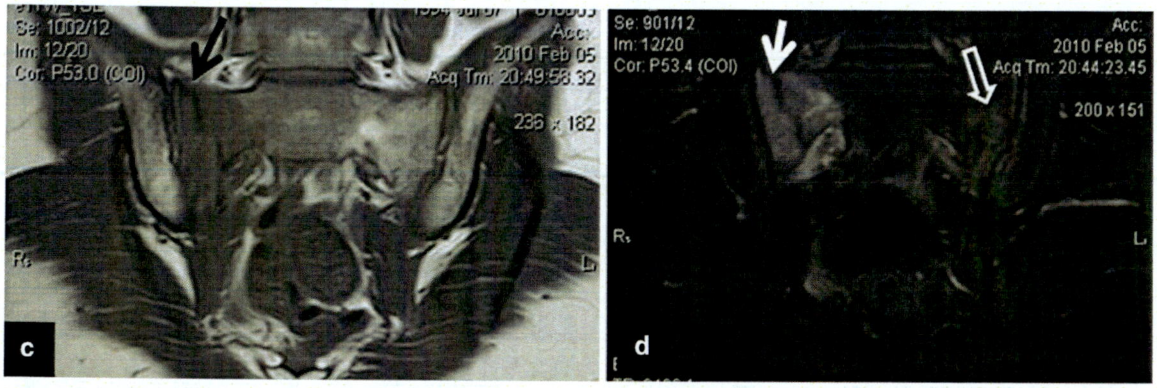

Fig. 15 (continued)

cases of delayed diagnosis or in cases that it develops on the outer aspect of the femoral neck, where tensile forces predominate and may become unstable. Surgery is the treatment of choice in the cases above.

Occasionally in children involved in sports, a bright fluid intensity T2 signal may be seen within a linear fracture line in the subchondral area. This should not be misinterpreted as a stress injury since a subchondral fracture is often the earlier finding of Legg-Calve-Perthe's osteochondrosis corresponding to osteonecrosis (Figs. 7 and 8) (Salter and Thompson 1984).

2.5 Femoroacetabular Impingement–Herniation Pit

Femoroacetabular impingement (FAI) is widely accepted to be associated with premature osteoarthritis, with symptoms presenting as early as the second decade in the athletic population. Two types of FAI have been recognized.

In the "*cam*" type FAI, there is a femoral waist deficiency with a bump projecting in the outer aspect of the head and neck junction, also called "pistol-grip" deformity (Fig. 16). A relationship to pervious SFCE has been suggested by many authors. Articular cartilage injury and labral tears tend to occur in the anterior and superolateral acetabular rim.

In the "*pincer*" type FAI, overcoverage of the femoral head and neck may be caused by acetabular retroversion or congenital global overcoverage. In normal individuals, the acetabulum has its lateral opening directed slightly anteriorly. In the abnormal case, the

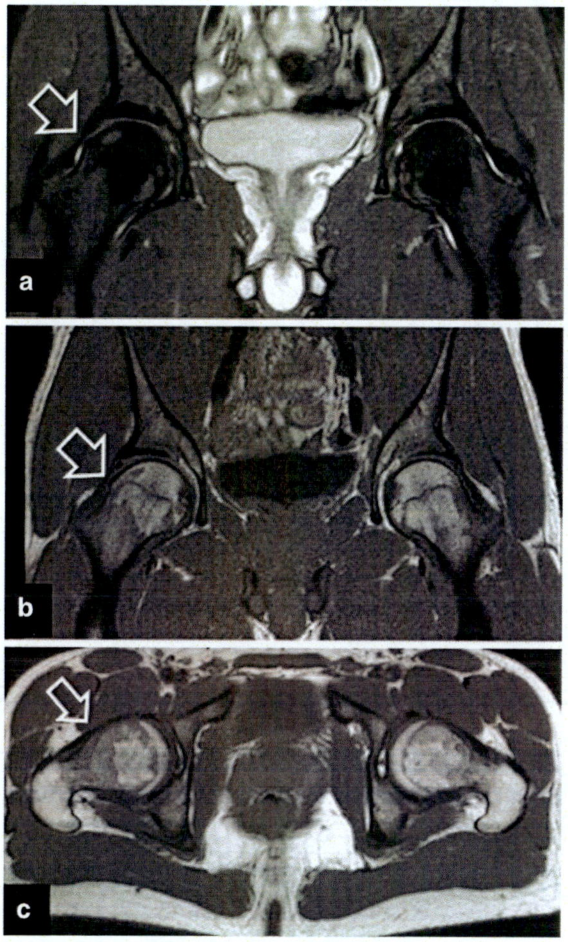

Fig. 16 CAM type femoroacetabular impingement in a 16 year-old male athlete with right hip pain in flexion. The coronal fat suppressed PD-w (**a**), coronal T1-w (**b**) and transverse T1-w (**c**) MR images, show the abnormal lateral projection of the head-neck junction (*arrows*), also called "pistol grip" or "tilt" deformity

acetabular opening is directed posteriorly. With plain AP radiographs, this is visualized as the acetabular "crossover" sign. The "crossover" sign is present when the anterior lip of the acetabulum crosses over the posterior lip on a standard frontal view of the pelvis (Fig. 17) (Jamali et al 2007). In cross sectional imaging, the anterior acetabular wall lies lateral instead of medial, to the posterior one, with respect to a perpendicular line to the horizontal plane. The ischial spines may also be prominent (Kalberer et al. 2008). MR arthrography is helpful to assess the posterior and postero-inferior acetabular articular cartilage injury seen with this type of FAI.

Synovial *herniation pits* in the femoral neck, formerly thought to be a normal variant, are highly correlated with FAI (Leunig et al. 2005). Herniation pits represent an ingrowth of fibrocartilagineous tissue through cortical erosion resulting in a subcortical cavity of the proximal femur. This lesion is located within the anterosuperior lateral quadrant of the femoral neck and is considered as an anatomical variation as it occurs in 5% of the population (Pitt et al. 1982). Plain

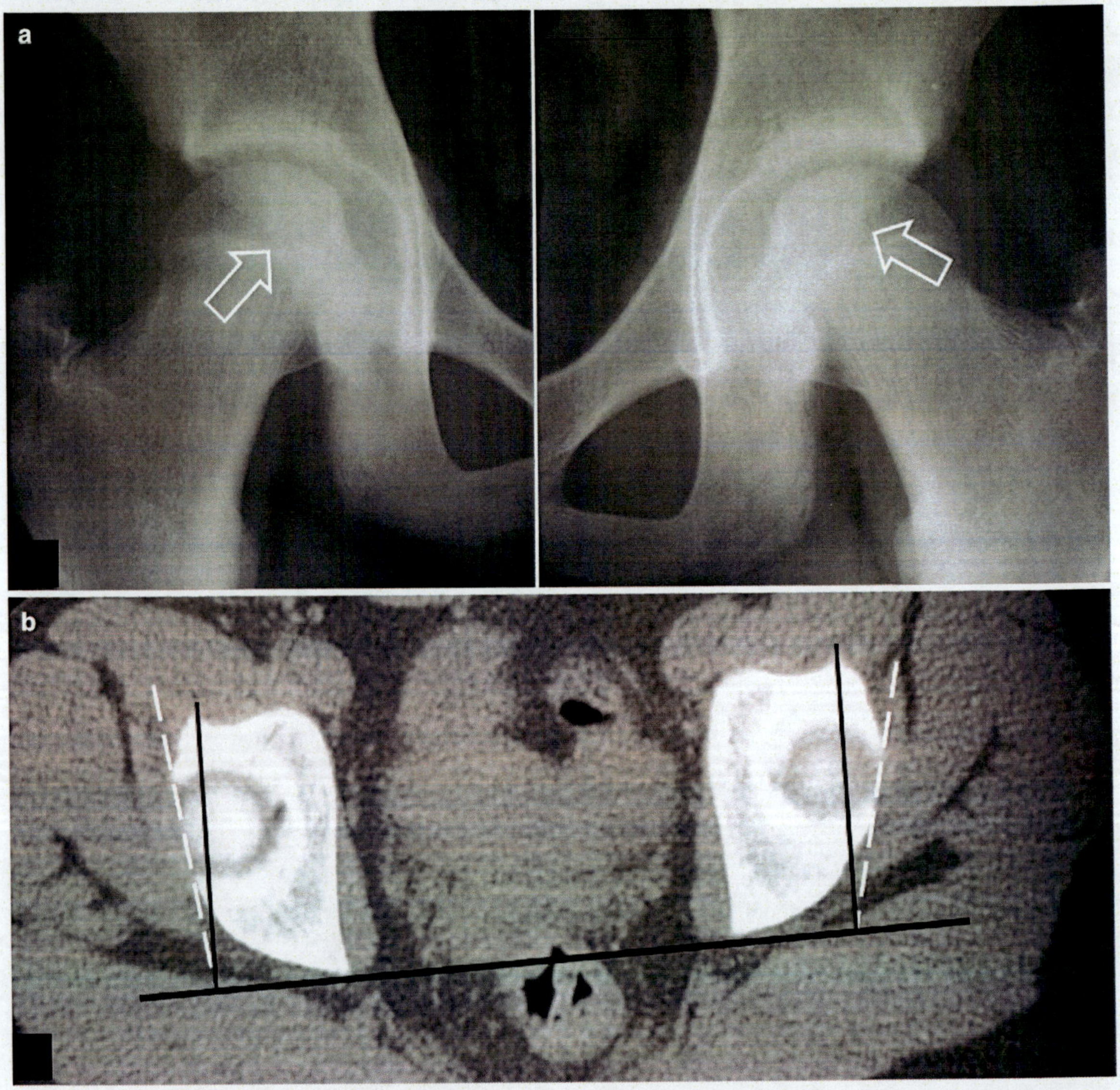

Fig. 17 Femoroacetabular impingement (pincer type) in a 14 year-old female track athlete. (**a**) The AP plain radiograph shows the crossover sign (*arrows*). (**b**) The axial CT image in the superior level of the hip joints shows that the anterior acetabular wall lies lateral to the posterior wall. This finding is diagnostic of acetabular retroversion

radiographs reveal a well-described lytic lesion with surrounding sclerosis. On CT, the lesions show sclerotic margins and the overlying cortex may be thinned or broken. On MR imaging, herniation pits exhibit signal intensity low on T1-w and high on T2-w, rarely with associated bone marrow edema. With certain MR imaging sequences, the synovial fold herniation within the lysis, may mimic the nidus of an osteoid osteoma. In subjects with intense athletic activity, herniation pit may enlarge and become symptomatic (Crabbe et al. 1992; Daenen et al. 1997). In our experience, herniation pits are extremely rare in the growing skeleton.

It has to be pointed out, that abnormal hip joint morphology in the pediatric age group may not reflect the fully formed pathologic abnormalities seen in adults. Although impingement conditions may start in the growing skeleton, degenerative changes are not usually seen before adulthood, even in highly competitive athletes. Radiologists should be able to depict subtle changes in the hip joint morphology and to suggest regular follow-up in terms of prompt depiction of FAI and prevention of degenerative changes. Joint preserving surgery is no longer possible in athletes with advanced cartilage delamination and joint degeneration who had long-lasting FAI during their athletic life.

2.6 Pathologic Fractures

Pathologic fractures may occur during normal sports activities when there is an underlying lesion. Common pathologic fractures around the hip area include avulsion of the lesser trochanter resulting from a femoral fibrous dysplasia (Fig. 18), and complete fracture with angulation of the femoral neck usually due to fibrous dysplasia or aneurysmal bone cyst (Figs. 19 and 20). Rarely, malignant lesions such

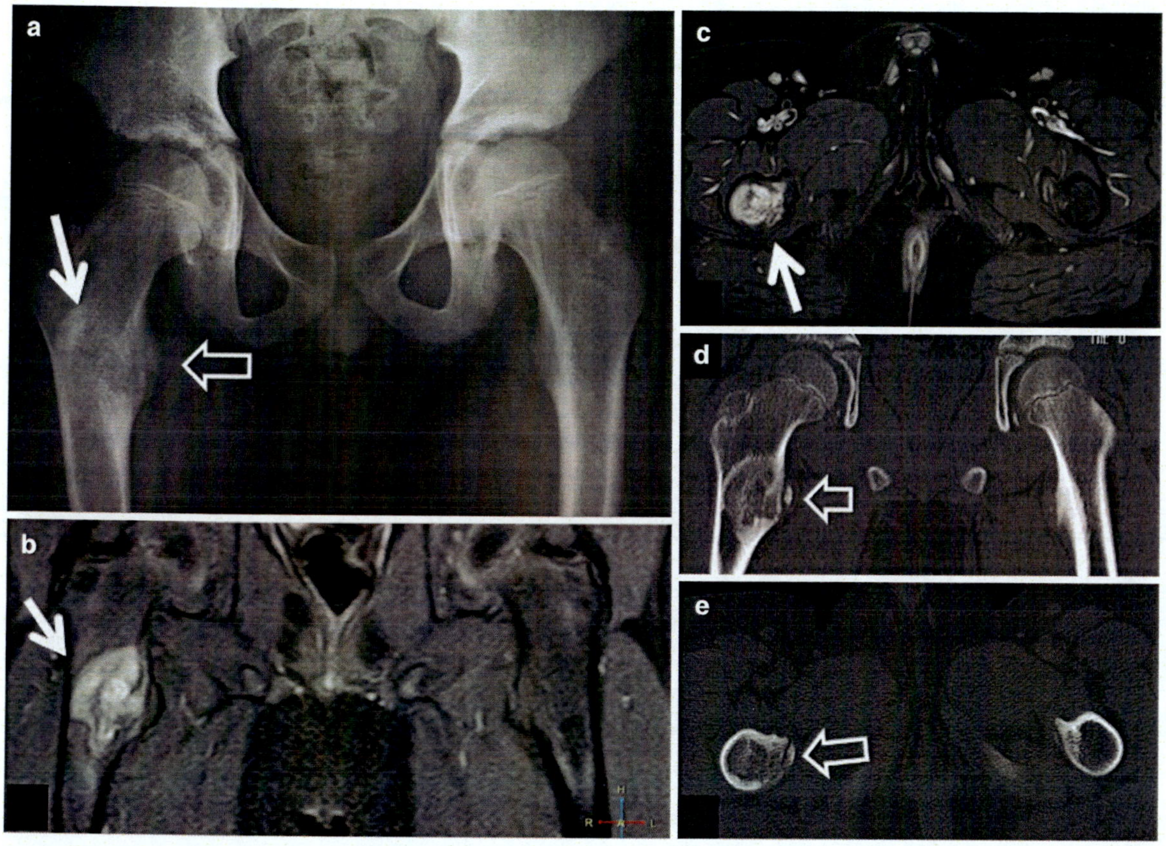

Fig. 18 Fibrous dysplasia in 11-year-old male athlete who presented with limp after a football game without any distinct injury. The plain radiograph (**a**) and the coronal (**b**) and axial (**c**) fat suppressed MR images, show the abnormality with the typical ground-glass radiographic appearance and increased bone marrow signal intensity (*arrows*). *Open arrow* in (a), shows poorly defined cortical margins of the lesser trochater suggesting avulsion. The coronal (**d**) and axial (**e**) multi-detector CT images show to better advantage the avulsion of the lesser trochanter (*open arrows*)

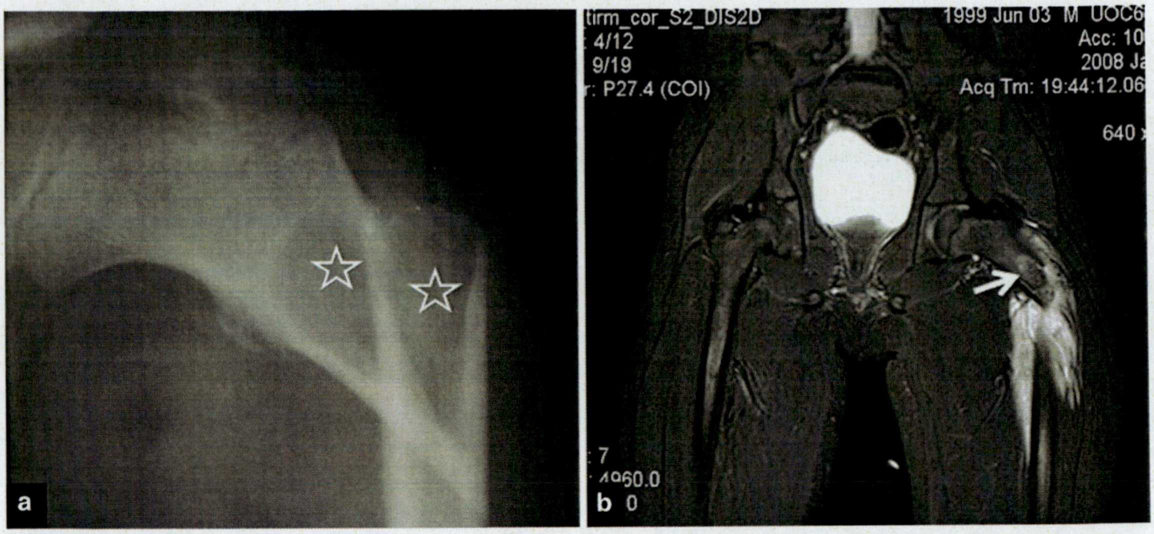

Fig. 19 A 9 year old male tennis player, with a proximal femoral fracture following a sudden deceleration. (**a**) The plain radiograph shows the fracture with various angulation, and the underlying fibrous dysplasia on both sides (*open stars*). (**b**) The coronal STIR MR image confirms the presence of the moderately high signal intensity fibrous dysplasia (*arrow*) and in addition shows soft tissue edematous changes

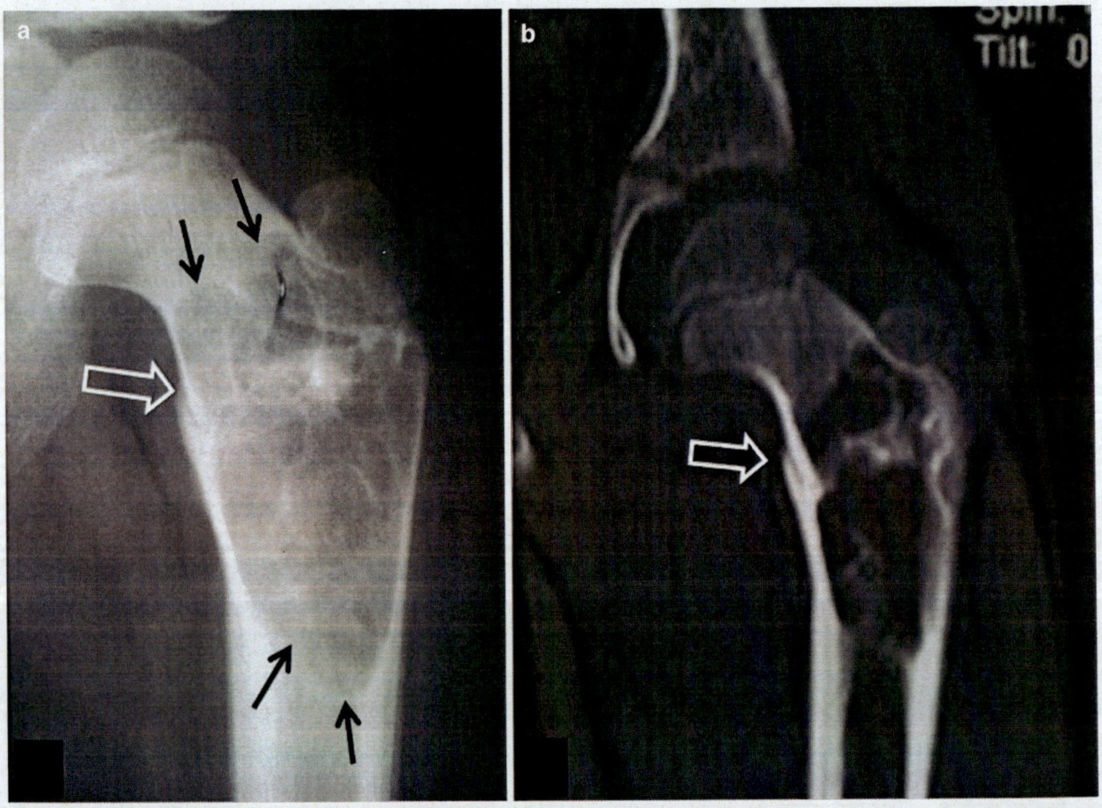

Fig. 20 Pathologic fracture because of aneurysmal bone cyst, in a 8-year-old male athlete, after a fall during mountain skiing. (**a**) The plain radiograph shows a large lytic, well defined lesion, with internal septa, in the metaphysis and proximal diaphysis of the left femoral bone (*arrows*). A fracture line is also shown (*open arrow*). (**b**) The coronal CT reconstructed image confirms the presence of the non-displaced fracture (*open arrow*)

as proximal femoral osteosarcoma and Ewing's sarcoma may be complicated with fractures during athletic activities.

3 Articular Injuries

The differential diagnosis of intraarticular hip pain in athletes includes labral degeneration and tears, intraarticular loose bodies, synovitis, chondral injuries, and early degenerative joint disease (Petersilge et al. 1996). Any MRI examination in a young athlete with hip pain should include at least one cartilage-sensitive sequence as the thick articular cartilage is demonstrated non-invasively (Fig. 21).

3.1 Chondral–Osteochondral Injuries–Loose Bodies

Focal *chondral* lesions of the hip joint result from impaction injuries and rarely from subluxation or dislocation of the hip. These lesions can be depicted only by MR arthrography because articular surfaces are closely apposed. Even with MR arthrography, only advanced lesions can be shown with confidence (Palmer 1998; Bohndorf 1999). Acute *osteochondral* injuries can be depicted by plain MR imaging because of the presence of the subchondral bone marrow edema. Early diagnosis and treatment of osteochondral lesions in elite athletes is important as degenerative joint disease can result in untreated cases. Acute osteochondral injuries do usually occur in high energy sports and thus they are rarely seen in young athletes.

Loose bodies may present clinically with chronic joint pain, locking and limited range of motion. In young athletes, loose bodies are seen in advanced cases of osteochondritis dissecans, which is supposed to result from chronic repetitive trauma. CT is diagnostic in the intra-articular presence of osseous or osteochondral loose bodies (Figs. 22 and 23). Cartilaginous loose bodies are better seen on T2-w MR images after intra-articular injection of diluted contrast, as the fragments decrease in signal intensity compared with the hyperintense signal of the contrast solution (Palmer 1998; Bencardino and Palmer 2002).

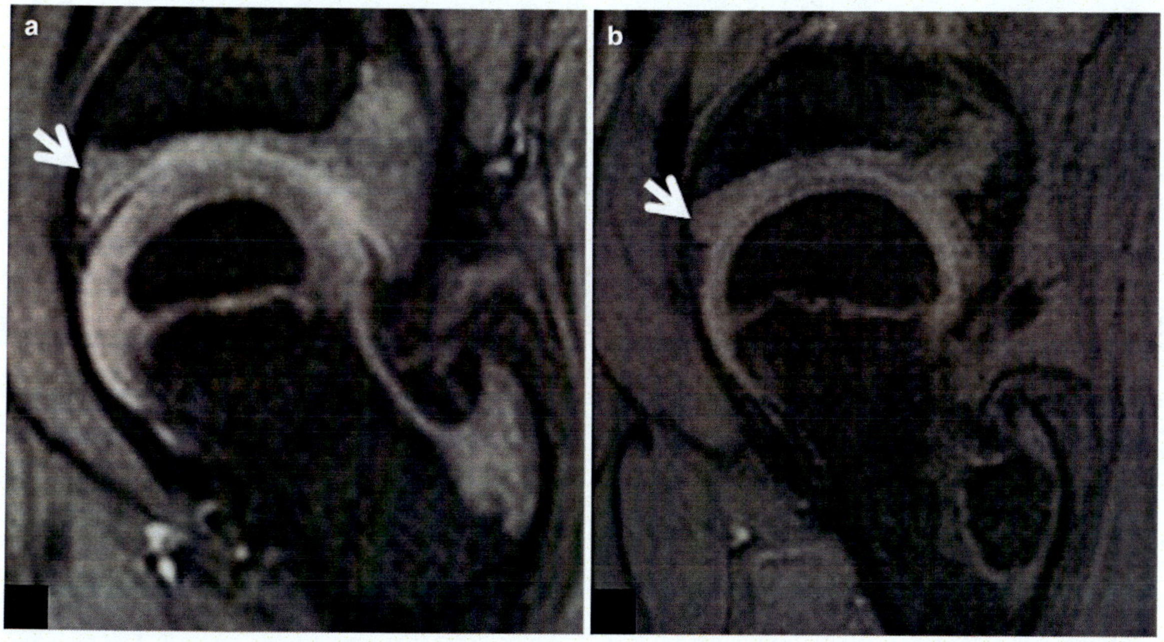

Fig. 21 (**a**) Oblique axial 3D T1-w GRE MR image shows the normal high signal intensity articular cartilage in a 3 year old boy. (**b**) Oblique axial T2* MR image in a 7 year-old boy, shows reduced cartilage thickness compared to (a). In both cases, there is normally extension of articular cartilage within the base of the labrum (*arrows*) which is not demonstrating the low signal intensity it exhibits in adults

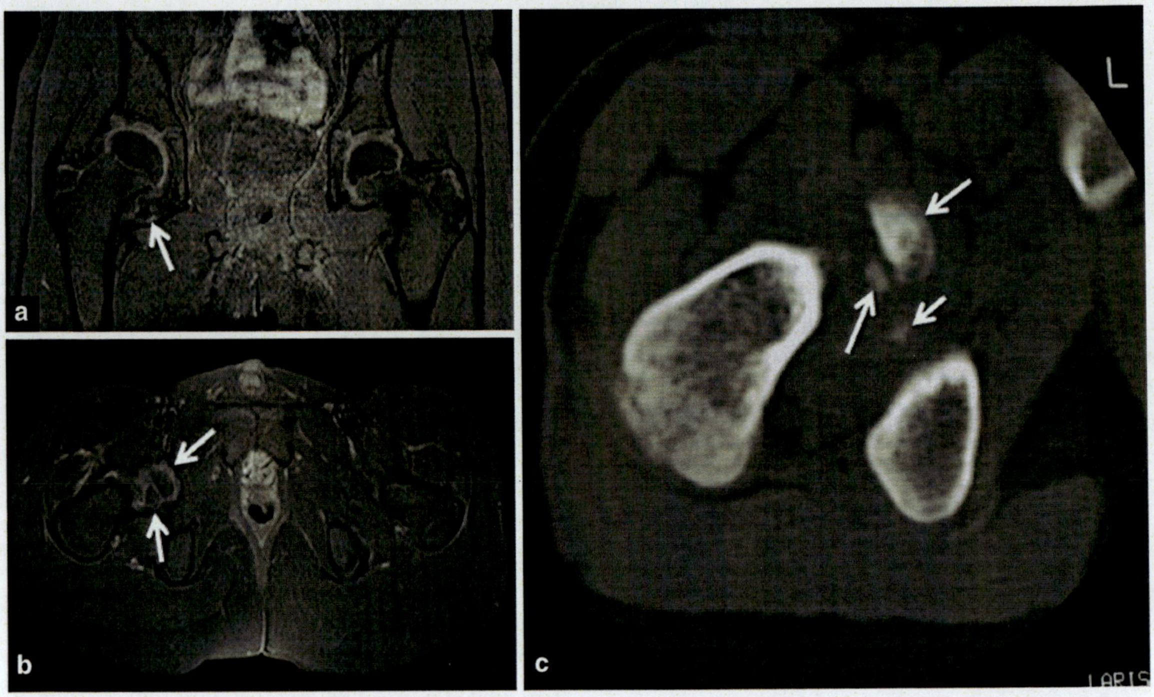

Fig. 22 Loose intra-articular bodies (*arrows*), in an 11-year-old male (mountain biking athlete) with previous hip dislocation. (**a**) Coronal and (**b**) axial fat suppressed contrast-enhanced MR images and (**c**) axial CT image

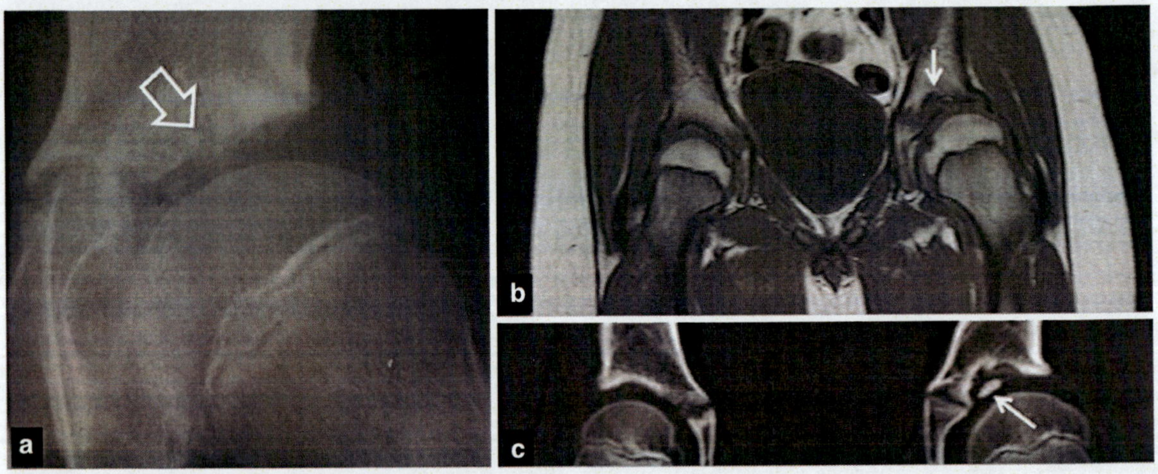

Fig. 23 Osteochondritis dissecans of the acetabulum in an 11-year-old male tennis player who reports mechanical problems of the left hip joint. (**a**) The plain radiographs shows irregularity in the acetabular roof (*arrow*). (**b**) The coronal T1-w MR image shows a defect in the acetabulum and a low signal intensity lesion (*arrow*). (**c**) The coronal CT reconstructed image shows to better advantage the grade III osteochondral lesion (*arrow*). The sclerotic appearance of the detached fragment, suggests osteonecrosis

3.2 Labral Injuries

The acetabular labrum is a fibrocartilaginous structure which enlarges the articular surface area enclosing the femoral head beyond its equator and thus increasing the stability of the joint. Labral tears can be a difficult clinical problem as the symptoms, including clicking and anterior inguinal pain, are not usually specific. Nevertheless, it is important to accurately diagnose this disorder, as early degenerative changes may occur due to wrong distribution of the loading forces resulting in chondral damage (Harris et al. 1979). In general, the presence of labral tears should raise the suspicion of an underlying osseous abnormality which acts as a predisposing cause (Wenger et al. 2004)

Anterior labral tears in athletes can result from twisting injuries with associated hyperextension and femoral external rotation (Byrd 1996). Posterior labral tears result from axial loading on the flexed hip. Sports activities requiring external rotation at the hip joint include soccer and hockey (Leunig et al. 1997).

Developments in hardware and software in MR provide with the ability to achieve high resolution images. Thus, MRI by using gradient echo or fat suppressed PD-w sequences may depict labral tears (Fig. 24). MR arthrography is the imaging method of choice for labral tear depiction because of the distension of the capsule it achieves (Fig. 25). It has been shown that MR arthrography findings closely correlate with the surgical findings (Petersilge et al. 1996; Czerny et al. 1999).

3.3 Subluxation–Dislocation

Hip dislocations in sports injuries occur rarely and are usually associated with high-energy contact sports such as American football, rugby, collision in skiing and bicycling (Pallia et al. 2002). These injuries occur as

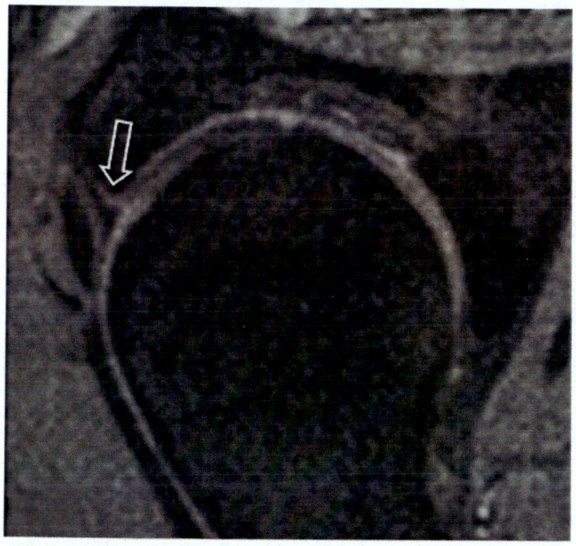

Fig. 24 The oblique axial fat suppressed PD-w MR image, shows a complete tear through the base of the anterior labrum (*arrow*) in this 15 year-old female mountain skiing athlete

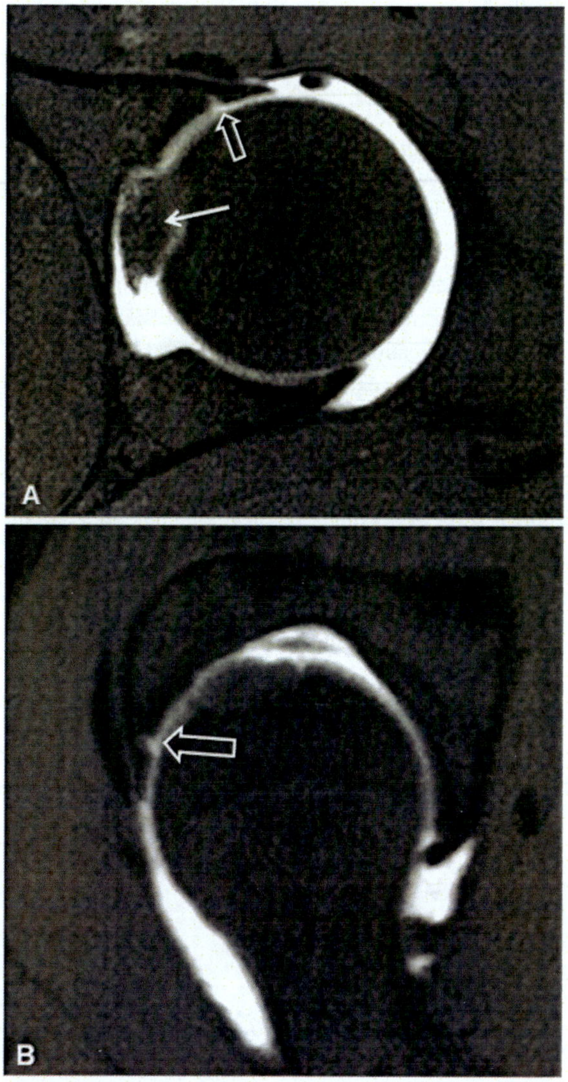

Fig. 25 Partial articular surface tear of the anterior labrum in a 14 year old football goalkeeper with a recent fall and injury on the left hip, shown with fat suppressed T1-w MR arthrogram in the axial (**a**) and oblique axial (**b**) planes (*arrows*). The ligamentous teres ligament is thickened (*thin arrow*)

the femur is forced posteriorly (Reigstad 1980). Literature reports are limited on the incidence of dislocation due to sporting injuries. In children, hip dislocation may result from minor trauma (Barrett and Goldberg 1989). The primary imaging assessment for detecting dislocation of the hip should be made with A/P radiographs of the pelvis and 45° oblique Judet views. CT, particularly with the multilevel reconstruction supplied by the multidetector technology, is able to demonstrate small intra-articular loose bodies following a dislocation, which should be removed to prevent further chondral injury and subsequent degenerative osteoarthritis (Fig. 22). In elite athletes with hip dislocation, MR imaging should be performed after successful closed reduction, to assess any associated osteochondral lesions or surrounding soft tissue injury.

The most common complication of hip dislocation is *osteonecrosis* occurring in 10–20% of patients, depending upon the patient's age, severity of injury and the delay in reduction. A recommended algorithm for early depiction of femoral head osteonecrosis following posterior dislocation of the hip is to start with an MR imaging in 4-6 weeks after trauma (Poggi et al. 1995). Patients with normal bone marrow signal intensity are at a low risk. In cases of abnormal marrow signal, another MR examination should be performed at 3 months or sooner if newer symptoms develop. The degree of cartilaginous injury following a hip dislocation cannot be appreciated currently. Thus, massive *chondrolysis* following such an injury may occur and early post-traumatic osteoarthritis may develop (Fig. 26).

Hip *subluxation* is a recently recognized sports-related injury that may be subtle in its clinical presentation and thus difficult to appreciate (Cooper et al. 1991). The mechanism of injury is either a fall onto a flexed knee with the hip adducted or a sudden stop with pivot over the weight-bearing extremity. The femoral head is forced posteriorly upon but not over the acetabular rim and therefore spontaneous reduction occurs. These injuries may be associated with bone bruise of the femoral head or the acetabulum and fracture of the posterior acetabular wall. Femoral head osteonecrosis can occur after hip subluxation (Cooper et al. 1991).

Ligamentum teres partial tear or avulsion may complicate repetitive subluxation or dislocation of the hip. The avulsed ligament may hinder complete reduction. Clinically, the athletes present with deep pain, often with mechanical symptoms. In children, radiographs may show a widened joint space but otherwise may be normal without any evidence of avulsion injury or previous dislocation. A spontaneous reduction of a dislocated hip in children is not uncommon due to softness of the articular cartilage and the ligamentous laxity. Fat suppressed MR images will show the thickening and the abnormal edema within the ligament (Fig. 27a, b). CT is better in depicting avulsion and intra-articular loose bodies (Fig. 28).

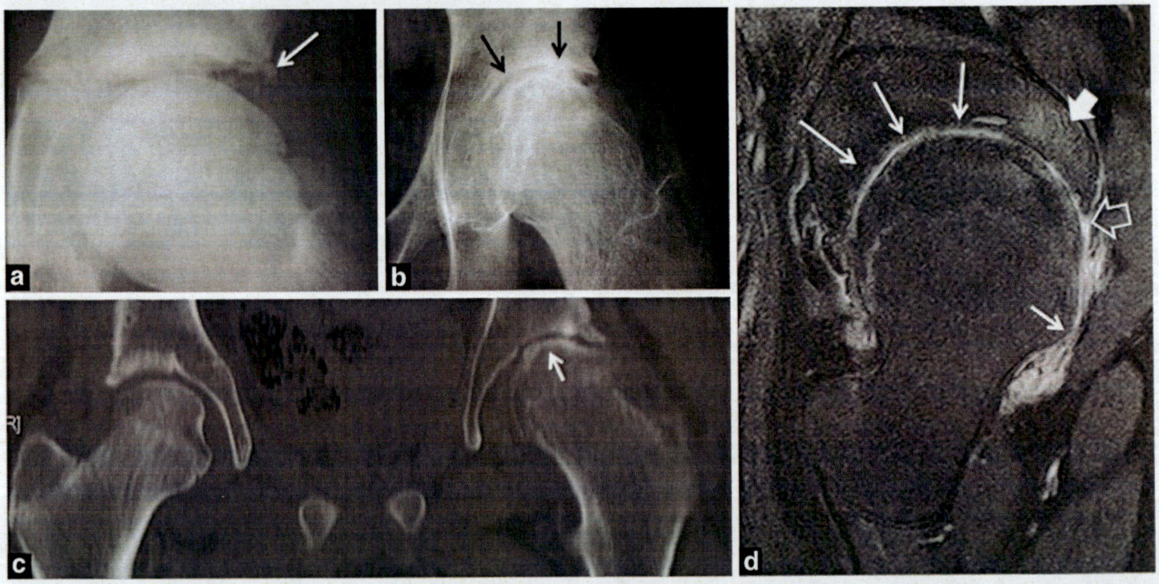

Fig. 26 Post-traumatic chondrolysis and osteoarthritis in a 15-year-old athlete who sustained a hip dislocation during mountain biking races. (**a**) The plain radiograph immediately following reduction of the dislocation, shows some cortical irregularity due to a posterior wall fracture of the acetabulum (*arrow*). The joint space is normal. (**b**) The patient complained of pain and limited function of the left hip and the 1 year follow-up radiograph shows joint space narrowing (*arrows*) and subcortical sclerosis on both sides. (**c**) The coronal CT image shows to better advantage the joint space narrowing (*arrow*). (**d**) The fat suppressed contrast enhanced oblique axial T1-w MR image confirms the joint space narrowing with global articular cartilage thinning (*long arrows*) and in addition shows bone marrow edema (*short white arrow*). The anterior labrum is degenerated (*open arrow*). The abnormal head-neck offset (*small arrow*) may have resulted from a previous slipped femoral capital epiphysis. This abnormality has probably caused the anterior labral degeneration due to "cam" type impingement

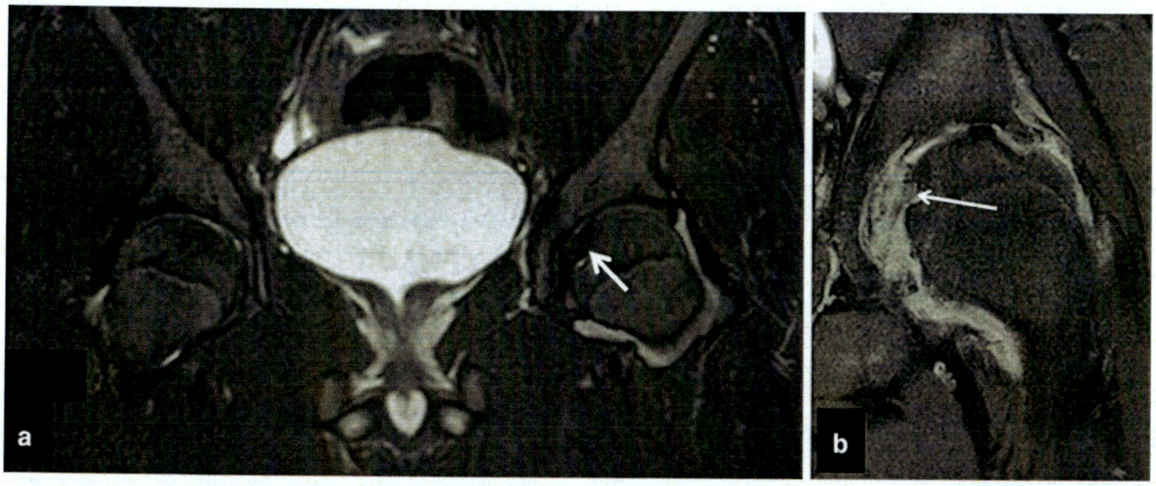

Fig. 27 Two patients with ligamentum teres injury. (**a**) Same patient as in Fig. 25. The coronal STIR image shows joint effusion and thickening and focal intrasubstance edema of the ligamentum teres (*arrow*), presumably following a subluxation of the hip joint during a reported fall injury. (**b**) Same patient as in Fig. 26. The coronal fat suppressed contrast-enhanced T1-w MR image at 1-year follow-up, shows the post-traumatic osteoarthritis and the thickened enhancing ligamentum teres (*arrow*)

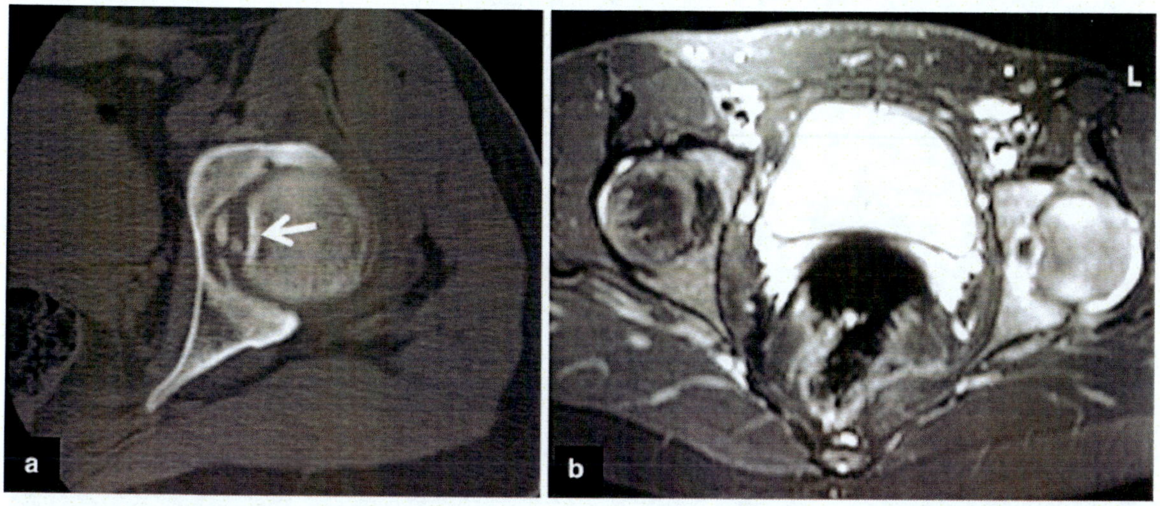

Fig. 28 Avulsion of the ligamentous teres insertion in a 16-year-old male following posterior hip dislocation during water skiing. Main complaints were related to mechanical problems with audible sounds and limitation of joint motion. (**a**) The axial CT shows the loose bony bodies in the left hip joint and the defect in the insertion site (*arrow*). (**b**) The axial fat suppressed T2-w MR image, confirms the detached ligament, nicely demonstrated within the joint effusion. In addition, extensive high signal intensity bone marrow edema is depicted which never transformed in osteonecrosis in follow-up studies

4 Soft Tissue Injuries

4.1 Muscle Strains

Muscle strains are indirect injuries following acute trauma or overuse and represent the most common injuries around the hip and groin area in the general athletic population (Palmer et al. 1999). In elite athletes and in young to middle-aged recreational athletes, strain injuries involve the musculotendinous junction whereas older subjects involved in sports activities are susceptible to tendon injuries (Speer et al. 1993). In the growing skeleton, muscle strains tend to occur in adolescents rather than in children. Strains typically occur in a single muscle within a group of synergists that cross two joints (Speer et al. 1993). The most commonly involved muscles are the hamstrings (biceps femoris, semimembranosus, semitendinosus), adductor longus, rectus abdominis, iliopsoas and rectus femoris following an eccentric contraction and stretching when the applied force exceeds the muscle strength (Garrett 1996). Strain of the quadratus femoris muscle can be clinically presented as hip pain (O'Brien and Bui-Mansfield 2007). Muscle strains have been classified into three grades as follows:

Grade I: Clinically, the pain is moderate without any functional deficit. MR imaging shows a "feathery" high signal intensity on T2-w fat-suppressed or STIR images with no discontinuity of muscle fibers (Figs. 29 and 30). T1-w images are normal (Newman and Newberg 2006).

Grade II: There is moderate disruption of muscle or musculotendinous junction with partial functional deficit. Imaging findings include high signal intensity on fat suppressed images along with partial intrasubstance tearing and often a hematoma at the musculotendinous junction, which is typical of the lesion (Palmer et al. 1999) (Figs. 31–33). T1-w images show fluid collections (hematomas) of varying signal intensity depending upon the time elapsed from injury. Gradient echo sequences might be useful to enhance the presence of blood products (Armfield et al. 2006).

Grade III: In this injury which is quite rare in the growing skeleton, there is complete disruption of the musculotendinous junction resulting in significant loss of functionality. MR imaging is able to show the torn edges of the muscle and tendon. There is almost always a hematoma present at the tear site.

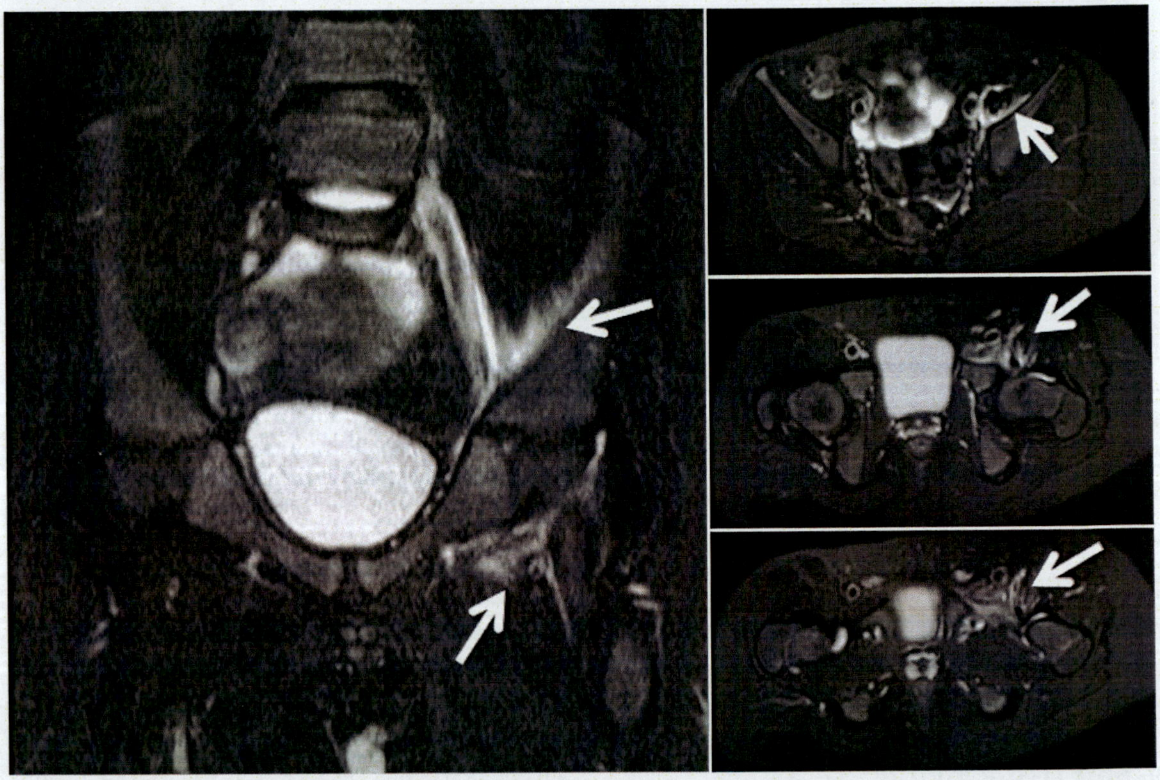

Fig. 29 Multiple muscle strain grade I, in a 14 year-old male basketball player. The coronal STIR (*left*) and axial fat suppressed T2-w (*right*) MR images show edema on the left side (*arrows*) into the muscles iliopsoas, adductors, pectineus and sartorius

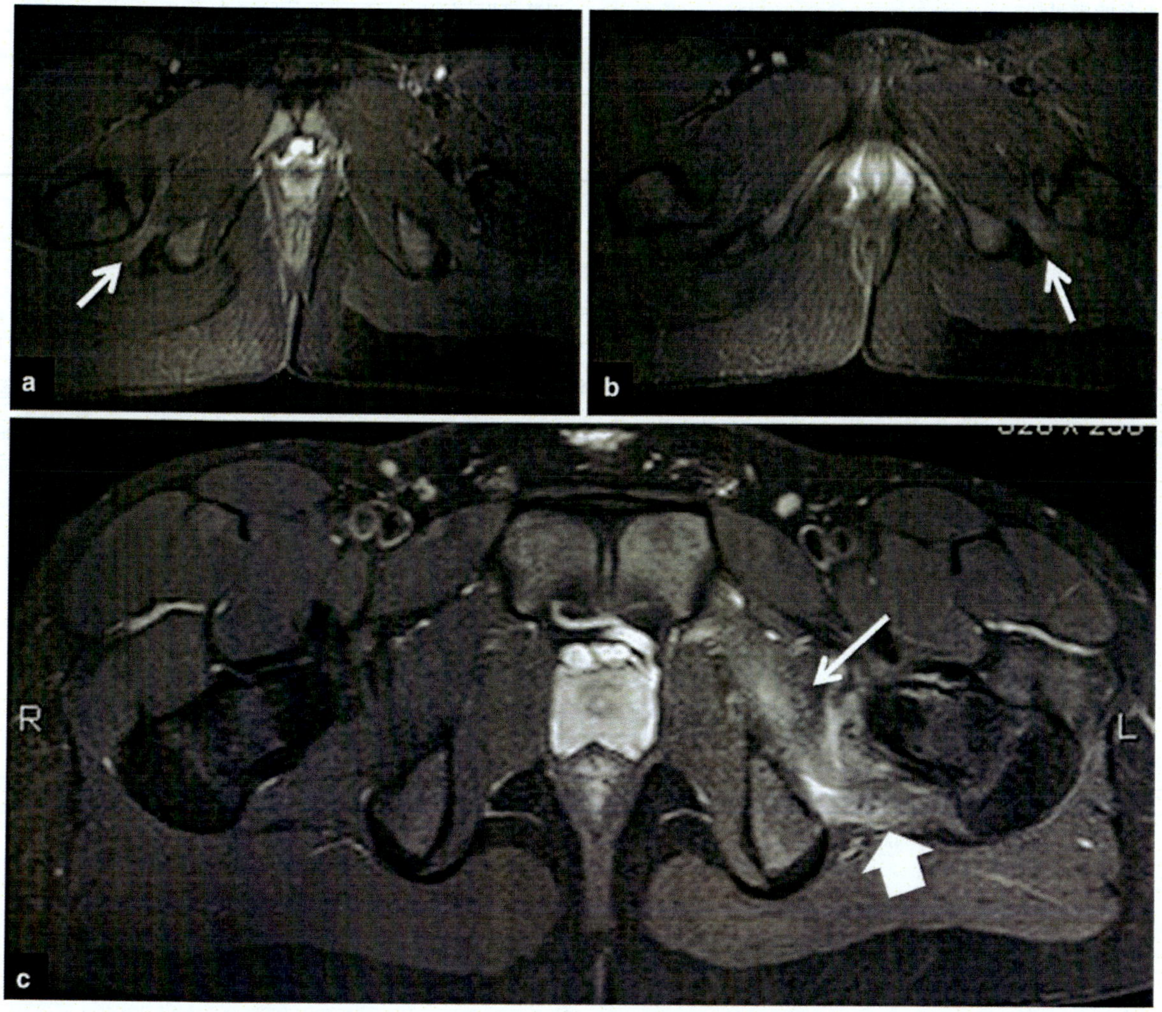

Fig. 30 Axial fat suppressed PD-w MR images. Quadratus femoris strain grade I is shown bilaterally in a 14 year-old female track athlete (arrows in **a** and **b**). (**c**) Quadraturs femoris (*thick arrow*) and external obturator (*thin arrow*) muscle strain grade I, is demonstrated in this 16-year-old elite male football player

4.2 Muscle Contusion

Muscle contusion is a direct blunt impaction injury to the muscle, usually seen in contact and collision sports such as football, hockey and skiing (Steinbach et al. 1994). Quadriceps contusions are usually the most disabling ones (Labella 2007). MR imaging applying fat-suppressed T2-w and STIR sequences show rather diffuse increased signal intensity without any significant muscular fiber discontinuity or architectural distortion (Fig. 34). Muscle contusions may be associated with hematoma formation, which can subsequently lead to development of myositis ossificans (Labella 2007).

4.3 Tendinous Injuries

Isolated tendon involvement in children and adolescents with sports injuries are rare and mainly are seen in the context of avulsion injuries at the tendon

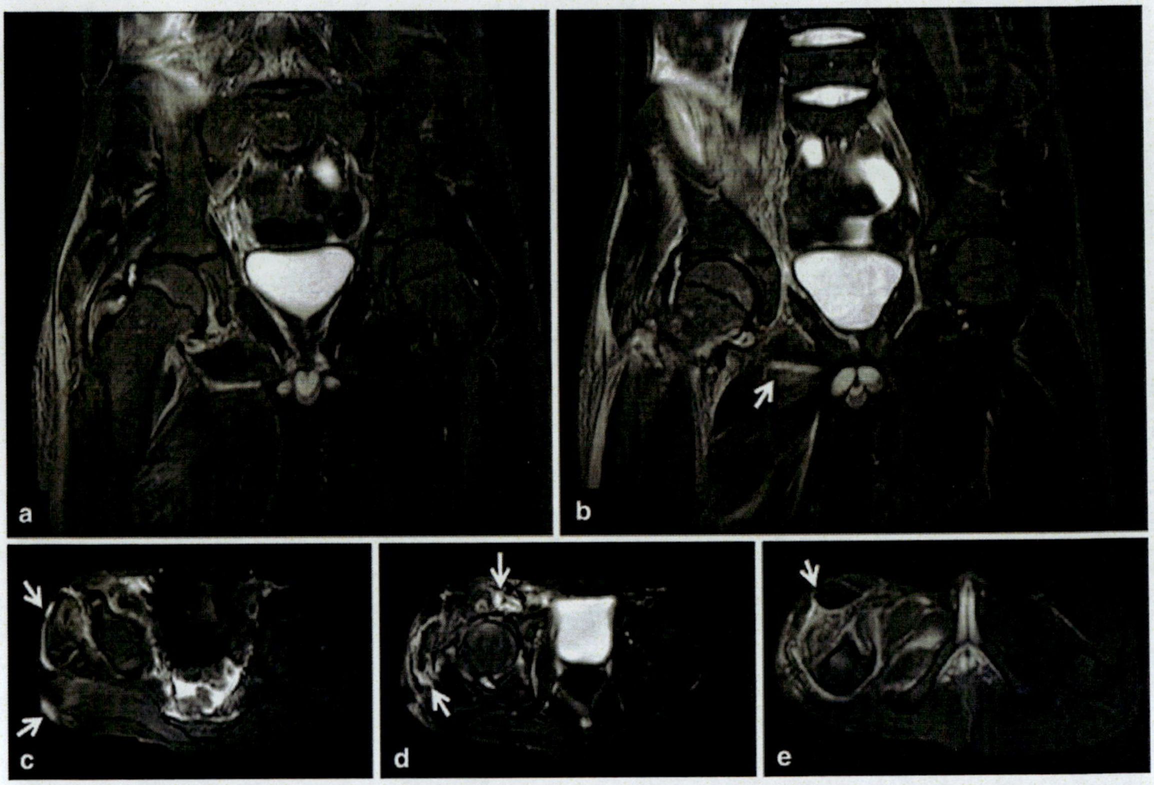

Fig. 31 Diffuse edema in the right side muscle groups in a 10-year-old male football athlete. The coronal STIR (**a**, **b**) and the axial fat suppressed T2-w (**c–e**) MR images, show diffuse edema in the anterior, lateral, posterior and adductor muscles. Small fluid collections classify the lesions as Grade II (*arrows*). Bone marrow edema in the right proximal femoral bone represents stress reaction

insertion site. Differential diagnosis problems may arise at the tendon insertion site in children, as the sports injuries may mimic infection and vice versa. A systematic approach of the clinical and biochemical data, will allow accurate interpretation of MRI findings (Fig. 35). Isolated tendon involvement in young athletes should raise the suspicion of previous steroid misuse causing quick muscle growth (Brittenden and Robinson 2005).

4.4 Bursitis

Bursitis is a disorder characterized by inflammation of a bursa. In athletes, this disorder results from excessive friction, rubbing and rarely from a direct trauma. Three main bursae can become inflamed in the region of the pelvis and hip following sports injuries: (1) trochanteric bursa, (2) ischiogluteal bursa and (3) iliopsoas bursa (Kneeland 1999). Iliopsoas bursitis is probably the most common and results from chronic rubbing of the iliopsoas tendon causing anterior hip pain (Fig. 36). The normal bursa is collapsed on MR imaging. Clinically, it may present with hip pain or symptoms from compression upon the inguinal and pelvic structures. Sports activities that have been shown to be associated with iliopsoas bursitis are competitive track and field, strength training, rowing and running uphill. Image guided, usually with US, aspiration and injection of long-lasting corticosteroids, results in relief of symptoms (Wunderbaldinger et al. 2002).

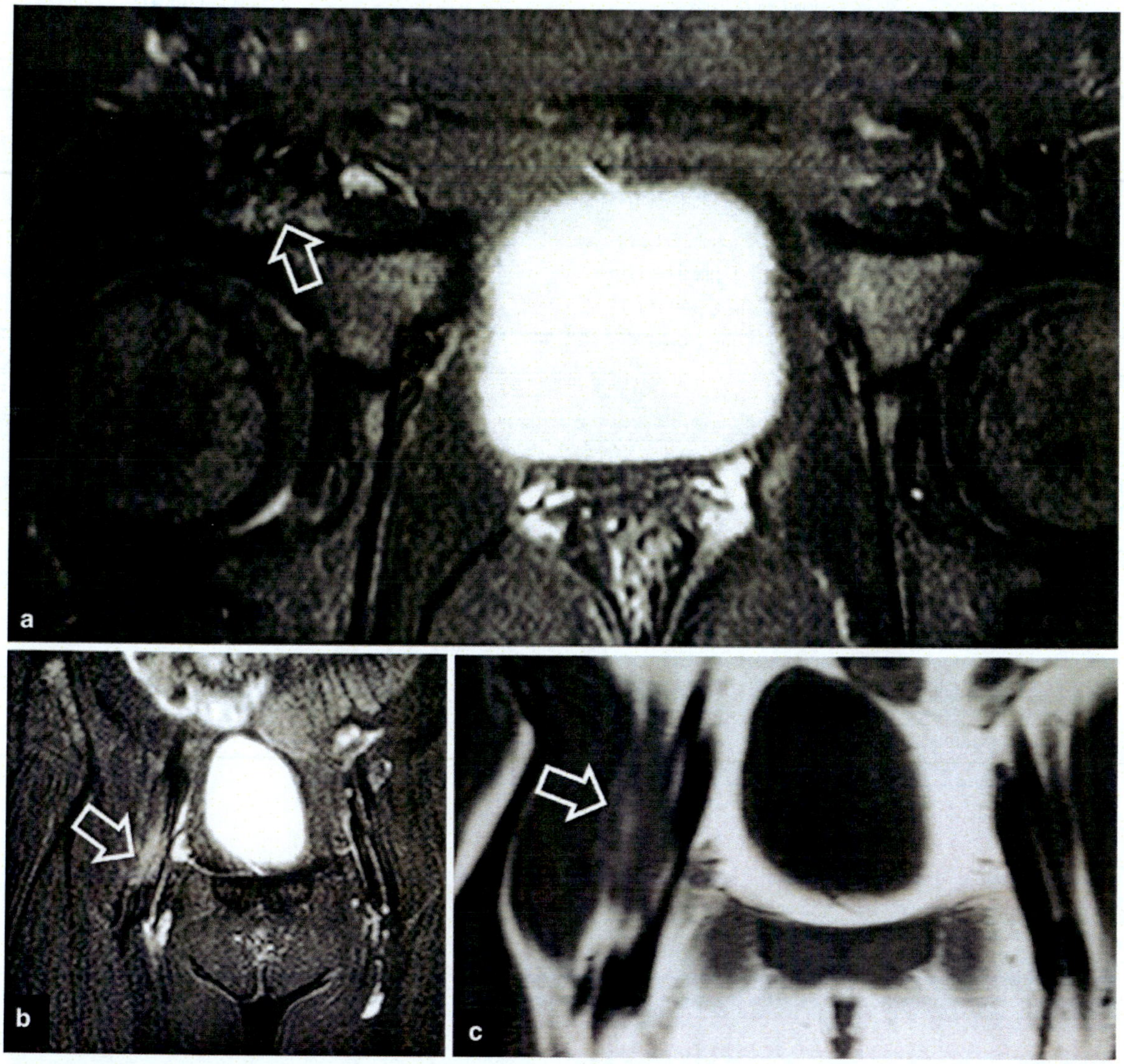

Fig. 32 Pectineus strain grade II in a 9 year-old female dancer with pain and tenderness over the anterior right hip joint. The axial (**a**) and coronal (**b**) STIR MR images, show edema within the right pectineus muscle (*arrows*). (**c**) The coronal T1-w MR image, depict hemorrhagic component within the muscle (*arrow*)

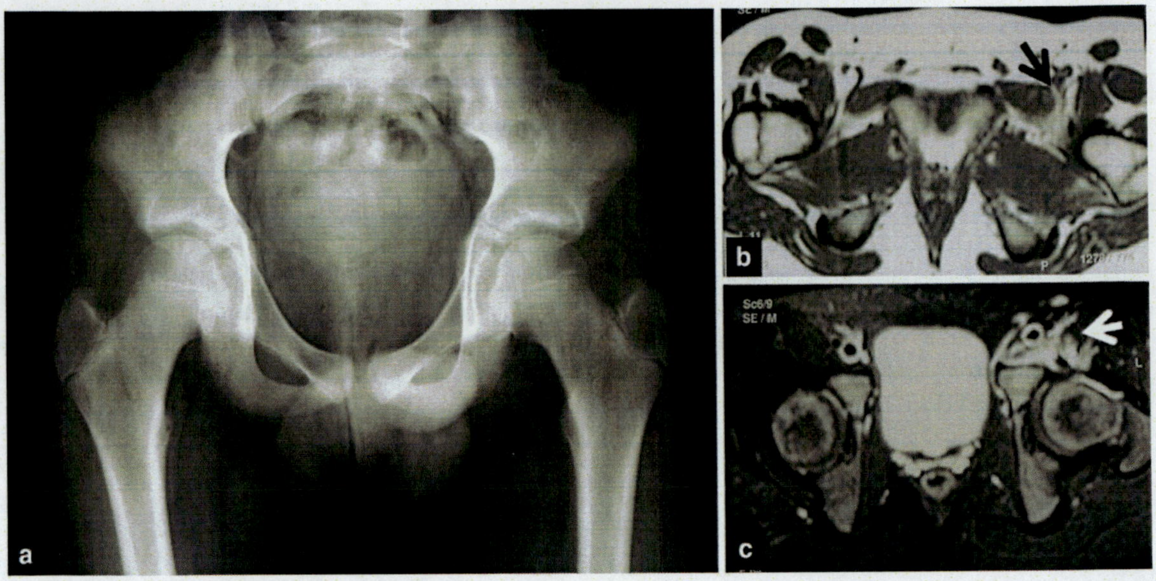

Fig. 33 A mountain climbing and football 13-year-old male athlete with muscle strain grade II. (**a**) The plain radiograph required for investigating avulsion injuries, is normal. The axial T1-w (**b**) and fat suppressed T2-w (**c**) MR images, show high signal intensity in keeping with hemorrhagic muscle strain of the left iliopsoas and pectineus muscles (*arrows*)

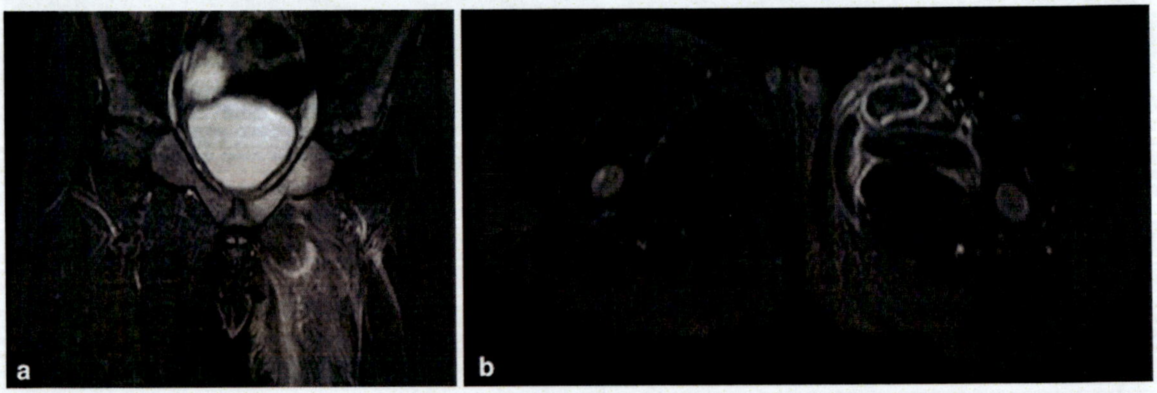

Fig. 34 Muscle contusion in a 7-year-old male while playing football in the park. The patient received a direct impaction from the knee of an older child, the day before imaging. The coronal fat suppressed T2-w (**a**) and the axial STIR (**b**) MR images, show diffuse edema in the anteromedial thigh muscles and subcutaneous tissues

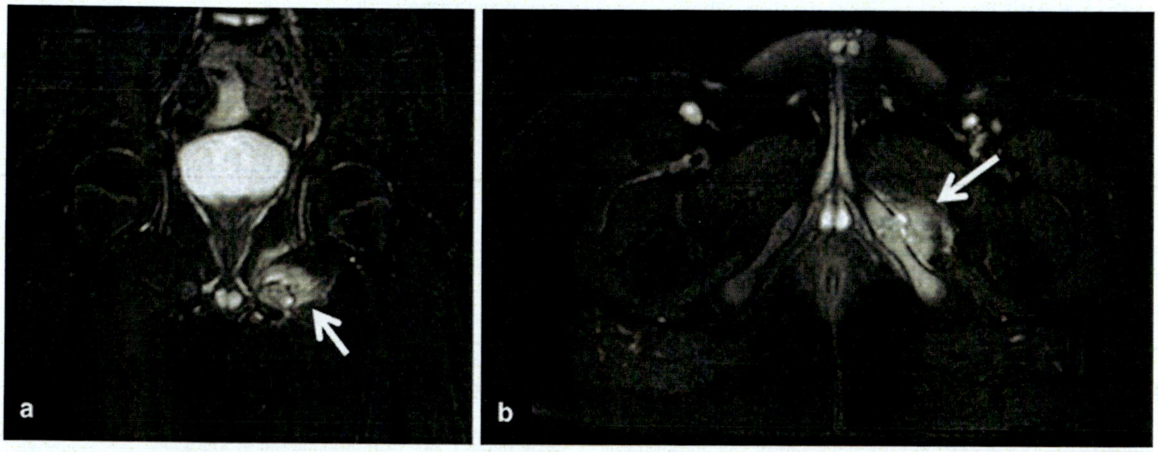

Fig. 35 Osteomyelitis of the ischiopubic ramus in a 7-year-old male patient presenting with pain and fever during the last 2 weeks. There was no history of participation in sports. The blood culture was positive for *Staphylococcus aureus*. The coronal STIR (**a**) and the axial fat suppressed T2-w (**b**) MR images, show bone marrow edema, and soft tissue edema within the external obturator muscle (*arrows*). The overall appearance could be easily mistaken for acute avulsion injury or chronic apophysitis (for comparison see Fig. 14)

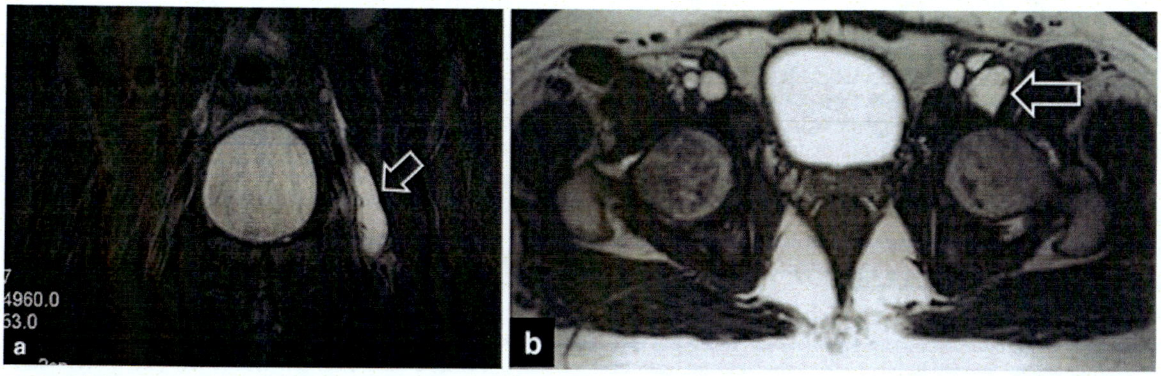

Fig. 36 Iliopsoas bursa on the left (*arrows*) depicted with coronal STIR (**a**) and axial T2* (**b**) MR images, in a 16 year-old track athlete

5 Conclusion

Sports-related hip injuries occur less commonly than in the extremities, but they can be associated with inconclusive clinical findings, long rehabilitation time and occasionally risk of permanent disability. In children and adolescents, the majority are soft tissue or apophyseal injuries that heal with conservative treatment. The available imaging modalities are effective when they are selected on the basis of a thorough history and physical examination. Plain radiographs are useful for avulsion injuries, myositis ossificans and for depicting other disorders not related to trauma. The role of ultrasonography has to be established.

CT is useful for depicting intra-articular loose bodies and chronic avulsions. MR imaging is the method of choice for identifying bone marrow disorders such as occult stress fractures and musculotendinous pathology. MR imaging of the hip following the intra-articular administration of diluted gadolinium has proven to be extremely valuable for diagnosing osteochondral lesions, labral tears and loose bodies. This is now required by the orthopedic surgeons as intra-articular lesions may be amenable to arthroscopic treatment.

References

Anderson MW, Greenspan A (1996) Stress fractures. Radiology 199:1–12

Armfield DR, Kim DHM, Towers JD, Bradley JP, Robertson DD (2006) Sports-related muscle injury in the lower extremity. Clin Sports Med 25:803–832

Barrett IR, Goldberg JA (1989) Avulsion fracture of the ligamentum teres in a child. J Bone Joint Surg 71:438–439

Bencardino JT, Palmer WE (2002) Imaging of hip disorders in athletes. Radiol Clin North Am 40:267–87, vi–vii

Bogost GA, Lizerbram EK, Crues JV III (1995) MR imaging in evaluation of suspected hip fracture: frequency of unsuspected of bone and softtissue injury. Radiology 197: 263–267

Bohndorf K (1999) Imaging of acute injuries of the articular surfaces (chondral, osteochondral and subchondral fractures). Skeletal Radiol 28:545–60

Brandser EA, El-Khoury GY, Kathol MH (1985) Adolescent hamstring avulsions that simulate tumors. Emerg Radiol 2:273–278

Brittenden J, Robinson P (2005) Imaging of pelvic injuries in athletes. Br J Radiol 78:457–468

Byrd JW (1996) Labral lesions: an elusive source of hip pain. Case reports and literature review. Arthroscopy 12:603–612

Combs JA (1994) Hip and pelvis avulsion fractures in adolescents. Phys Sports Med 22:41–49

Cooper DE, Warren RF, Barnes R (1991) Traumatic subluxation of the hip resulting in aseptic necrosis and chondrolysis in a professional football player. Am J Sports Med 19:322–324

Crabbe JP, Martel W, Matthews LS (1992) Rapid growth of femoral herniation pit. AJR Am J Roentgenol 159:1038–1040

Czerny C, Hoffman S, Urban M et al (1999) MR imaging arthrography of the adult acetabular capsular-labral complex: correlation with surgery and anatomy. AJR Am J Roentgenol 173:345–349

Daenen B, Preidler KW, Padmanabhan S et al (1997) Symptomatic herniation pits of the femoral neck: anatomic and clinical study. AJR Am J Roentgenol 168:149–153

DeLee JC, Farney WC (1992) Incidence of injury in Texas high school football. Am J Sports Med 20:575–580

Deutsch AL, Mink JH, Waxman AD (1989) Occult fractures of the proximal femur: MR imaging. Radiology 170: 113–116

Deutsch AL, Coel MN, Mink JH (1997) Imaging of stress injuries to bone: radiography, scintigraphy and MR imaging. Clin Sports Med 16:275–290

Dwek JR (2009) The hip: MR imaging of uniquely pediatric disorders. Radiol CLin N Am 47:997–1008

El-Khoury GY, Daniel WW, Kathol MH (1997) Acute and chronic avulsive injuries. Radiol Clin North Am 35:747–766

Gamble JG, Kao J (1997) Avulsion fracture of the lesser trochanter in a preadolescent athlete. J Pediatr Orthop 2:188–190

Garrett WE (1996) Muscle strain injuries. Am J Sports Med 24:S2–S8

Gomez E, DeLee JC, Farney WC (1996) Incidence of injury in Texas girls' high school basketball. Am J Sports Med 24:684–687

Harris WH, Bourne RB, Oh I (1979) The acetabular labrum: a possible aetiological factor in certain cases of osteoarthritis of the hip. J Bone Joint Surg Am 61:510–514

Hodnett PA, Shelly MJ, MacMahon PJ, Kavanagh EC, Eustace SJ (2009) MR imaging of overuse injuries of the hip. Magn Reson Imaging Clin N Am 17:667–679

Jamali AA, Mladenov K, Meyer DC et al (2007) Anteroposterior pelvic radiographs to assess acetabular retroversion: high validity of the cross-over-sign. J Orthop Res 25:758–765

Kalberer F, Sierra RJ, Madan SS et al (2008) Ischial spine projection into the pelvis: a new sign for acetabular retroversion. Clin Orthop Relat Res 466:677–683

Kneeland JB (1999) MR imaging of sports injuries of the hip. Magn Reson Imaging Clin North Am 7:105–115

Kocher MS, Tucker R (2006) Pediatric athlete hip disorders. Clin Sports Med 25:241–253, viii

LaBella CR (2007) Common acute sports-related lower extremity injuries in children and adolescents. Clin Ped Emerg Med 8:31–42

Leunig M, Werlen S, Ungersbock A, Ito K, Ganz R (1997) Evaluation of the acetabular labrum by MR imaging arthrography. J Bone Joint Surg Br 79:230–234

Leunig M, Beck M, Kalhor M et al (2005) Fibrocysticbchanges at anterosuperior femoral neck: prevalence in hips with femoroacetabular impingement. Radiology 236:237–246

Moeller JL (2003) Pelvic and hip apophyseal avulsion injuries in young athletes. Curr Sports Med Rep 2:110–115

Newman JS, Newberg AH (2006) MRI of the painful hip in athlete. Clin Sports Med 25:613–633

O'Brien SD, Bui-Mansfield LT (2007) MRI of quadrates femoris muscel tear: another cause of hip pain. AJR Am J Roentgenol 189:1185–1189

Pallia CS, Scott RE, Chao DJ (2002) Traumatic hip dislocation in athletes. Curr Sports Med Rep 1:338–345

Palmer WE, Kuong SJ, Elmadbouh HM (1999) MR imaging of myotendinous strain. AJR Am J Roentgenol 173:703–709

Palmer WE (1998) MR arthrography of the hip. Semin Musculoskelet Radiol 2:349–362

Petersilge CA, Haque MA, Petersilge WJ et al (1996) Acetabular labral tears: evaluation with MR arthrography. Radiology 200:231–235

Pitt MJ, Graham AR, Shipman JH, Birkby W (1982) Herniation pit of the femoral neck. AJR Am J Roentgenol 138:115–121

Poggi JJ, Callaghan JJ, Spritzer CE et al (1995) Changes on magnetic resonance images after traumatic hip dislocation. Clin Orthop 319:249–259

Reigstad A (1980) Traumatic dislocation of the hip. J Trauma 20:603–606

Rossi F, Dragoni S (2001) Acute avulsion fractures of the pelvis in adolescent competitive athletes: prevalence, location and sports distribution of 203 cases collected. Skeletal Radiol 30:127–131

Rupini HD, Holder LE, Espinola DA et al (1985) Three-phase radionucleotide bone imaging in sports medicine. Radiology 156:187–196

Salter RB, Thompson GH (1984) Legg-Calve-Perthes disease: the prognostic significance of the subchondral fracture and a two-group classification of the femoral head involvement. J Bone Joint Surg Am 66:479–489

Shin AY, Morin WK, Gorman JD et al (1996) The superiority of magnetic resonance imaging in differentiating the cause of pain in endurance athletes. Am J Sports Med 24:168–176

Slocum KA, Gorman JD, Puckett ML et al (1997) Resolution of abnormal MR signal intensity in patients with stress fractures of the femoral neck. AJR Am J Roentgenol 168: 1295–1299

Speer KP, Lohnes J, Garrett WE (1993) Radiographic imaging of muscle strain injury. Am J Sports Med 21:89

Spitz D, Newberg A (2002) Imaging of stress fractures in the athlete. Radiol Clin North Am 40:313–331

Steinbach LS, Fleckenstein JL, Mink JH (1994) Magnetic resonance imaging of muscle injuries. Orthopedics 17:991–999

Tehranzadeh J (1987) The spectrum of avulsion and avulsion-like injuries of the musculoskeletal system. Radiographics 7:945–974

Wenger DE, Kendell KR, Miner M et al (2004) Acetabular labral tears rarely occur in the absence of bony abnormalities. Clin Orthop Relat Res 426:145–150

Wunderbaldinger P, Bremer C, Schellenbrger E et al (2002) Imaging features of iliopsoas bursitis. Eur Radiol 12:409–415

Knee

Anastasia N. Fotiadou and Apostolos H. Karantanas

Contents

A.N. Fotiadou
Department of Radiology, Hinchingbrooke Hospital,
Huntingdon, PE29 6NT, Cambridgeshire, UK
e-mail: natfot@yahoo.gr

A.H. Karantanas (✉)
Department of Radiology, University Hospital, Stavrakia
711 10, Heraklion, Greece
e-mail: akarantanas@gmail.com

A.H. Karantanas (ed.), *Sports Injuries in Children and Adolescents*,
Med Radiol Diagn Imaging, DOI: 10.1007/174_2010_16,

Key Points

- Knee joint is commonly injured in the young athlete. The increased intensity of training and competition among young athletes is associated with increased risk for both acute and chronic injuries.
- Acute osseous injuries are usually promptly recognized with clinical examination and the diagnosis is established with plain radiographs.
- Chondral and osteochondral injuries, physeal injuries and bone bruise, are better assessed with MR imaging.
- The role of ultrasonography is evolving in the study of superficial structures, such as muscles and tendons. Of particular interest to the growing skeleton is the weaker bone compared to ligamentous or tendinous insertion and thus avulsion fractures may occur.
- Chronic injuries may demonstrate themselves clinically in a nontypical pattern. Chronic injuries include stress reactions and fractures, traction apophysitis and osteochondritis dissecans.
- Plain radiographs may be helpful but usually MR imaging is required to clarify the cause of symptoms.
- Early diagnosis and treatment of chronic injuries are critical to prevent long-term functional disability and deformity.

1 Introduction

Youth sports participation carries an inherent risk of injury, including overuse injuries which are becoming more prevalent nowadays. The knee joint is one of the most commonly injured sites in young athletes. The present chapter will focus on the imaging findings of common and uncommon knee injuries in young athletes with emphasis on variations and patterns that are unique to the growing skeleton.

2 Osseous Injuries

2.1 Bone Bruise

Trabecular bone is commonly injured as a result of trauma to the knee. MR imaging is the method of choice to assess these radiographically occult injuries. *Bone bruising* or *contusion* is demonstrated with decreased signal intensity on T1-w and increased signal intensity on T2-w or short-tau inversion recovery (STIR) images (Fig. 1) (Kapleov et al. 1993; Mandalia et al. 2005). An isolated bone bruise may account for the clinical symptoms and require only rest as its resolution will occur in few weeks depending upon the location and its original size. Bone bruises in the knee have often been used as secondary signs for detecting other associated abnormalities. A careful analysis of its pattern, will guide the investigation for associated intra-articular lesions (Sanders et al. 2000). A bone bruise extending up to the articular surface should raise the suspicion of an osteochondral injury (Fig. 2).

Pivot shift injury combined with external rotation of the tibia or internal rotation of the femur, will result in disruption of the anterior cruciate ligament (ACL). Resultant anterior subluxation of the tibia will cause impaction of the lateral femoral condyle against the posterolateral margin of the lateral tibial plateau. Bone bruising will be present in the posterior aspect of the lateral tibial plateau and the middle portion of the lateral femoral condyle (kissing contusions) (Fig. 3). Associated injuries that may occur with pivot shift injury include tear of the posterior capsule, tear of the posterior horn of the lateral or medial meniscus and injury of the medial collateral ligament (MCL) (Figs. 3 and 4).

In *dashboard* injury, bruising is found at the anterior aspect of the tibia and occasionally at the posterior surface of the patella. Associated soft-tissue injuries are disruption of the posterior cruciate ligament (PCL) and the posterior joint capsule. *Hyperextension* injury results in a kissing contusion pattern in the anterior aspect of the distal femur and proximal tibia. Resulting injuries

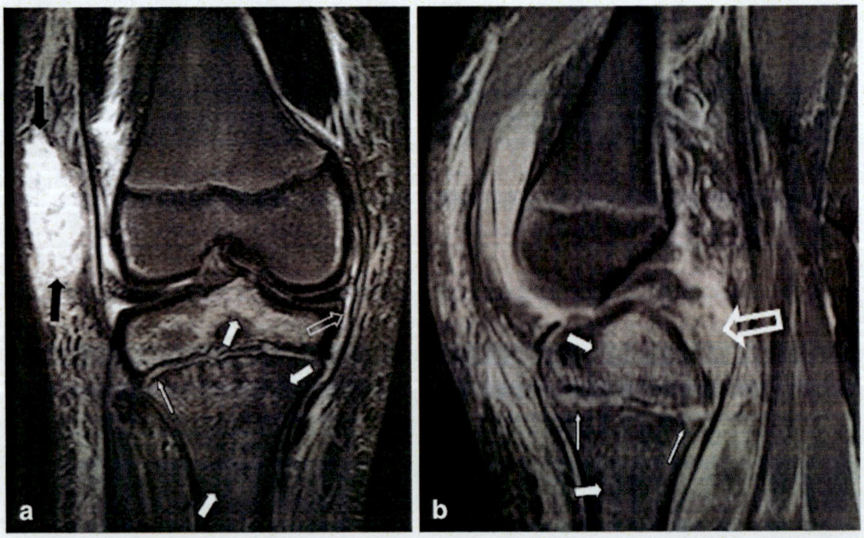

Fig. 1 Complex knee joint injury during mountain skiing, in a 10-year-old boy. The coronal STIR MR image (**a**) and the sagittal fat suppressed intermediate-w TSE MR image (**b**), show the high signal intensity in the bone marrow of the tibial epiphysis and metaphysis, in keeping with bone bruise (*arrows*). A tear of the posterior cruciate ligament (PCL) is seen at its tibial insertion (*open arrow*). The increased signal intensity and broad widening at the tibial growth plate represents an acute epiphyseal injury (*thin arrows*). Additional findings include injury of the medial collateral ligament (MCL) with meniscocapsular separation at the coronary ligament (*thin open arrow*), joint effusion and soft tissue changes with a superficial hematoma formation (*black arrows*)

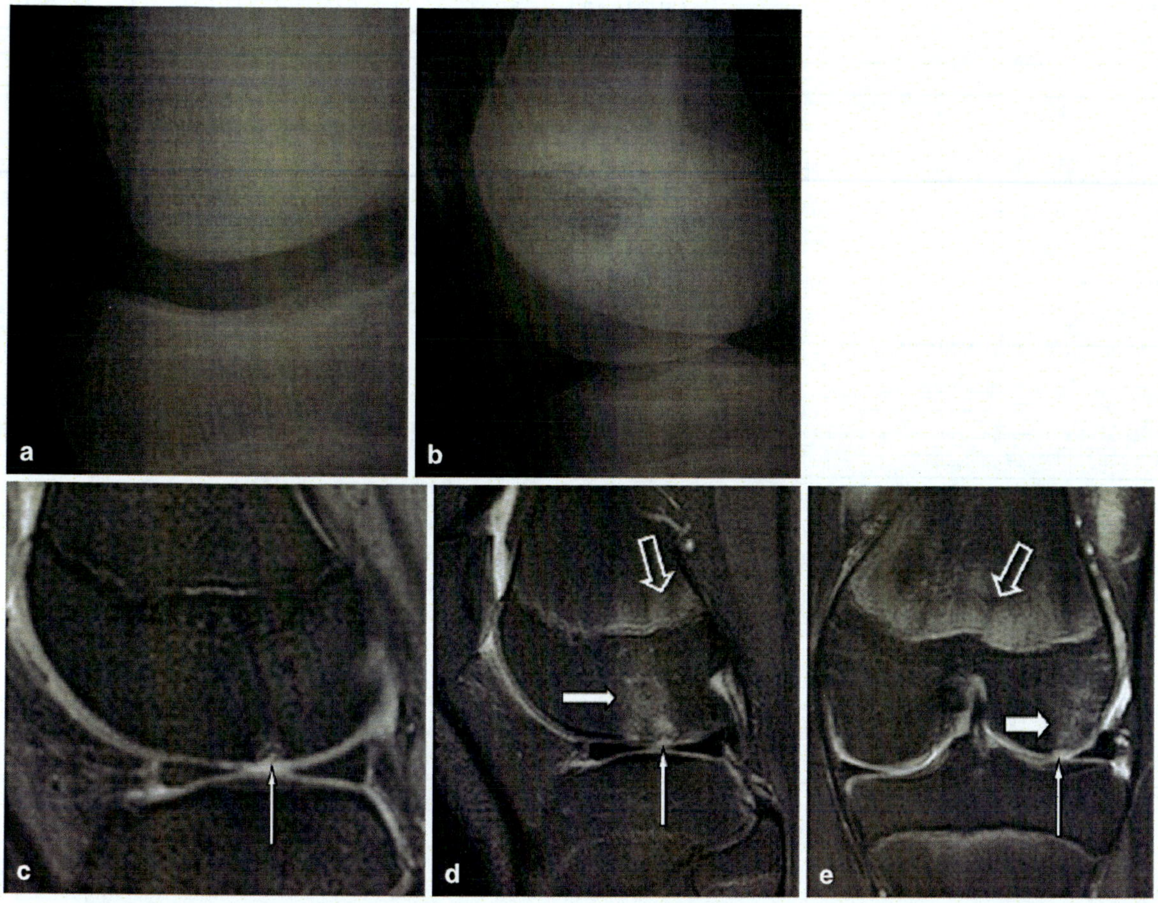

Fig. 2 A 14-year-old girl with a twisting injury during basketball. The AP (**a**) and lateral (**b**) radiographs show a normal appearance of the lateral femoral condyle. The sagittal gradient echo (**c**), and fat suppressed PD-w TSE MR images in the sagittal (**d**) and coronal (**e**) planes, reveal the focal articular cartilage disruption (*thin arrow*) and the associated bone bruise (*arrows*). The high signal intensity in the distal femoral metaphysis represents normal red marrow (*open arrows*)

may involve the ACL, PCL, or meniscus. During *clip* injury, bruising is most prominent in the lateral femoral condyle secondary to a direct blow. There may be a second smaller area of edema present in the medial femoral condyle secondary to avulsive stress to the MCL (Kaplan et al. 1999). *Patellar dislocation* is also associated with bone bruise in the lateral aspect of the lateral femoral condyle, occasionally complicated with an osteochondral injury (Fig. 5).

2.2 Fractures

Patellar fractures have an increased incidence in sporting activities in adolescents. These fractures represent less than 5% of all knee injuries and about 17% are sports-related (Ray and Hendrix 1992; Maguire and Canale 1993). Transverse fractures occur from direct trauma, whereas sleeve fractures from twisting injuries (Bruijn et al. 1993; Ray and Hendrix 1992). Longitudinal fractures are rare. Haemarthrosis with or without intra-articular fat is common. Plain radiographs are usually sufficient for diagnosis. In nondisplaced fractures or for clarifying the presence of a bipartite patella, MR imaging may be helpful (Fig. 6).

Any jumping sport resulting in a heavy twisting impaction fall may result in *tibial plateau impaction* fractures. Trampolining, is a sport commonly involved.

One of the main roles of MR imaging is to depict radiographically *occult* fractures. They are demonstrated as a line of high signal intensity on fat suppressed images and are commonly associated with subperiosteal hematoma (Fig. 7).

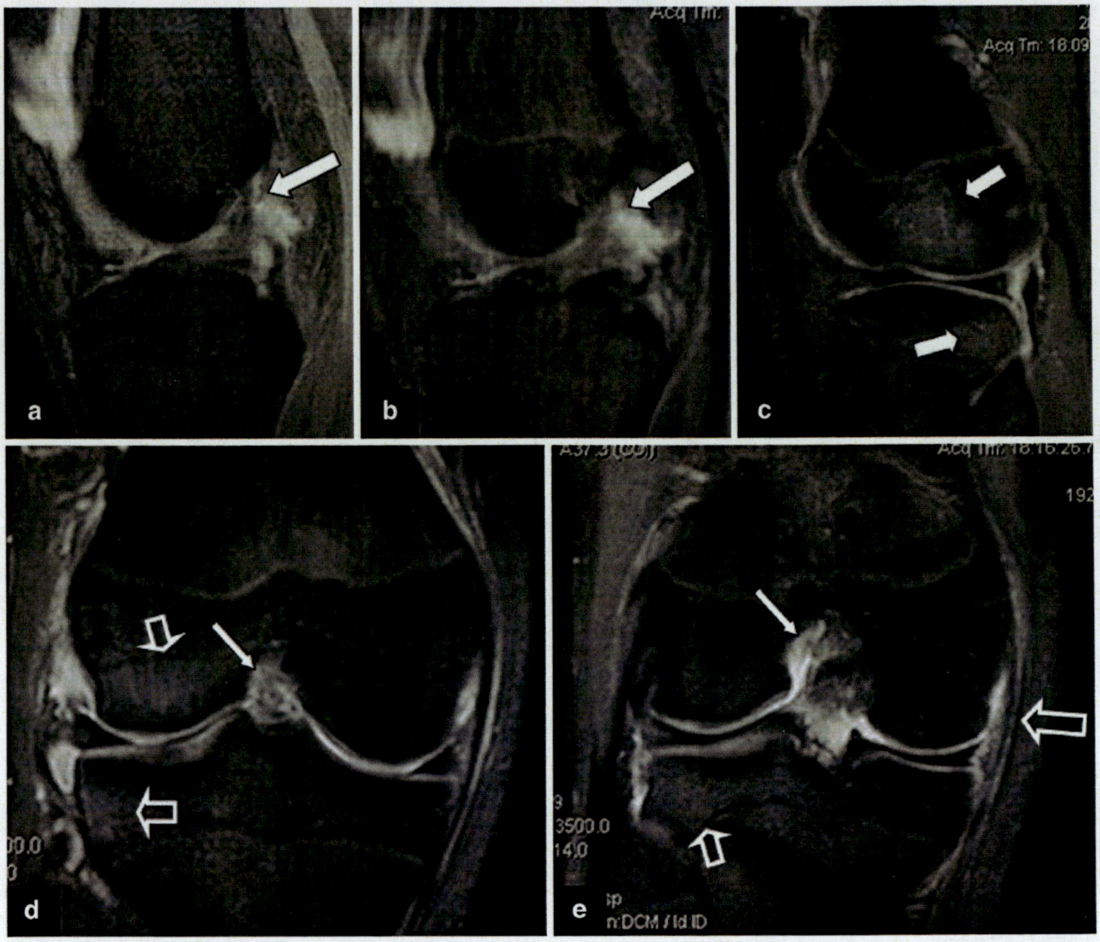

Fig. 3 A 16-year-old football player with a recent injury. The sagittal MEDIC (**a**) and fat suppressed PD-w TSE (**b, c**) MR images show the complete tear of the anterior cruciate ligament at its femoral insertion (*arrows*). The bone bruise in the posterior lateral tibial epiphysis and the lateral femoral condyle have a "kissing" pattern (*short arrows*). The coronal fat suppressed PD-w TSE (**d, e**) MR images confirm the presence of the bone bruises (*short open arrows*) and the anterior cruciate ligament tear (*thin arrow*). Sprain of the MCL is also seen (*open arrow* in **e**)

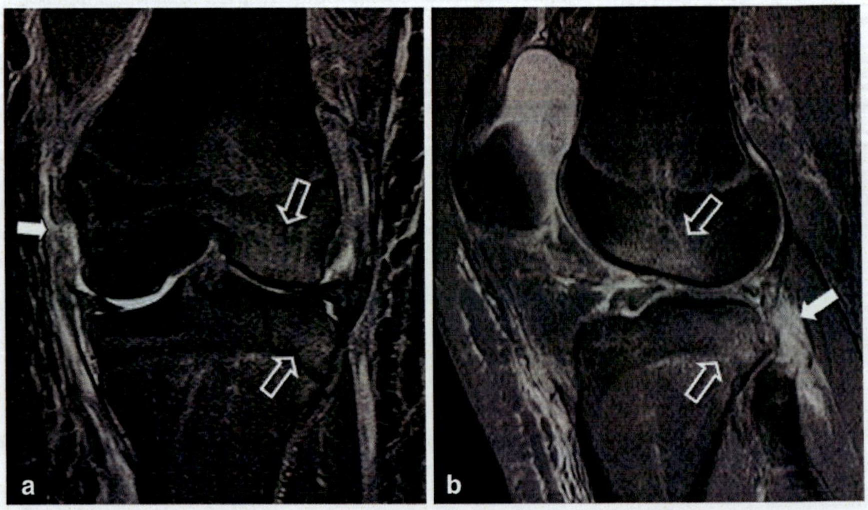

Fig. 4 A 15-year-old basketball player, with a recent pivot shift injury. (**a**) The coronal STIR MR image shows the grade III tear of the MCL (*arrow*) and the "kissing" bone bruises (*open arrows*). (**b**) The sagittal fat suppressed PD-w MR image shows the "kissing" bone bruises (*open arrows*), intra-articular effusion and a strain of the popliteus myotendinous junction (*arrow*)

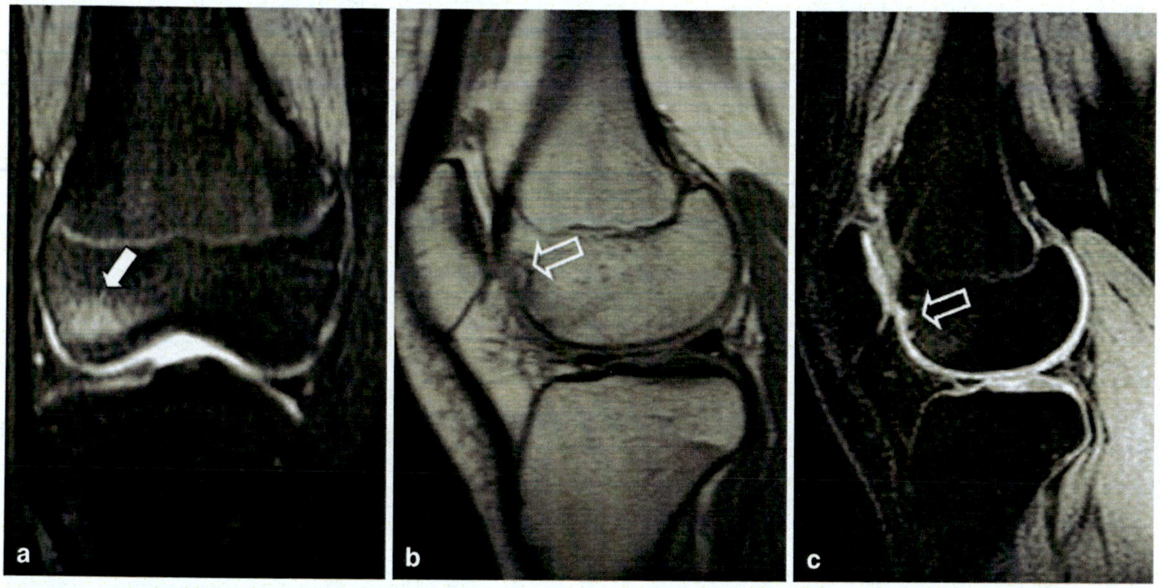

Fig. 5 A 13-year-old girl with a recent lateral patellar dislocation. (**a**) The coronal fat suppressed PD-w MR image shows the bone bruise in the anterior lateral femoral condyle (*arrow*). The sagittal PD-w TSE (**b**) and the fat suppressed 3D-T1-w gradient echo (**c**) MR images confirm the presence of the bone bruise and also reveal an impacted osteochondral injury in the lateral femoral condyle (*open arrows*)

Fig. 6 (**a**) The coronal STIR MR image shows a bipartite type II patella, simulating a longitudinal fracture in a 11-year-old boy who sustained an injury during mountain skiing (*arrow*). Cortication on both sides of the high signal intensity line favors the diagnosis of a bipartite patella. (b) The sagittal fat suppressed PD-w MR image shows bone marrow edema (*arrow*) which is often seen in painful bipartite patella

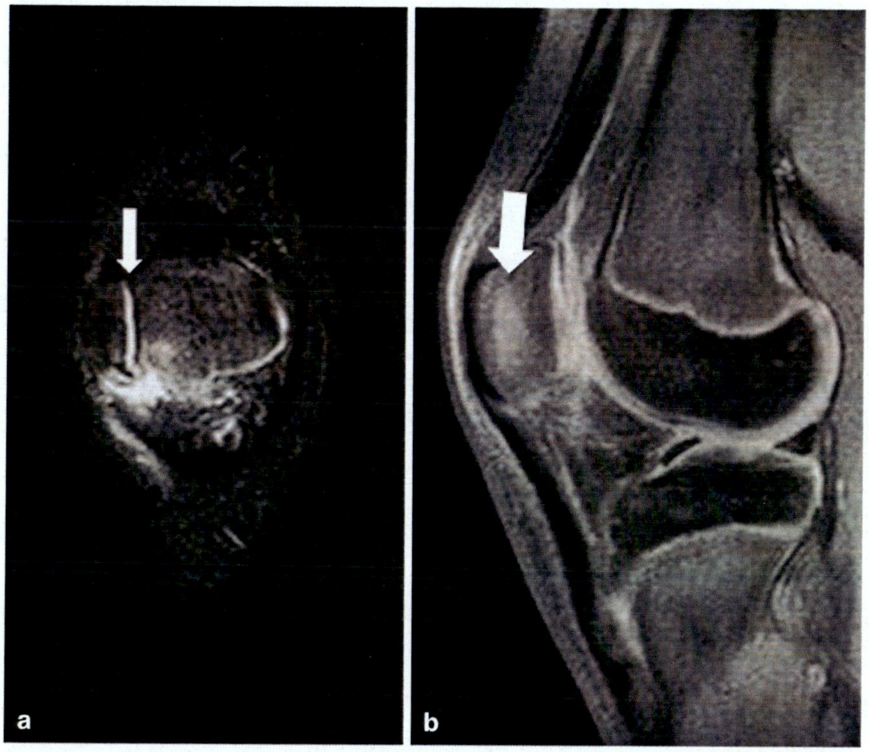

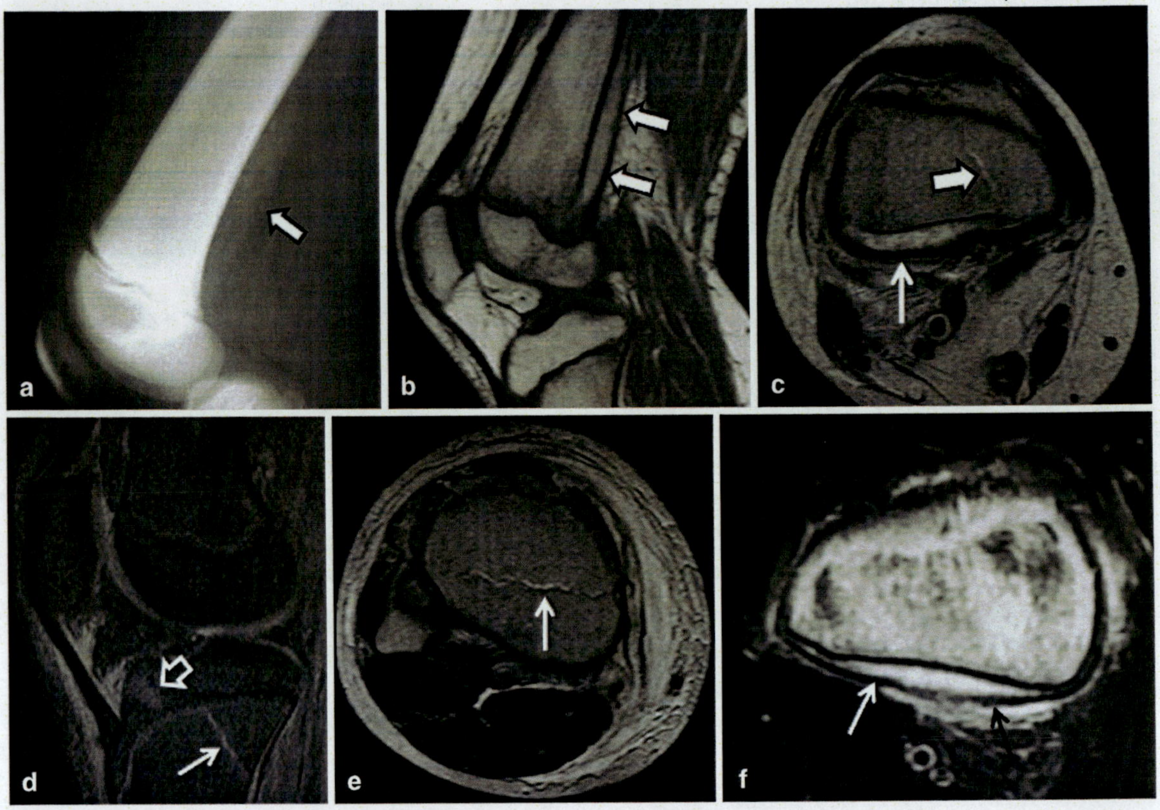

Fig. 7 Occult fractures. (**a–c**) A 9-year-old female skiing athlete after a twisting injury. The plain radiograph (**a**) shows a density posterior to the distal femoral metaphysis suggesting hematoma formation (*arrow*). The corresponding sagittal T1-w (**b**) MR image shows a high signal intensity subperiosteal hematoma (*arrows*). The axial T2-w MR image (**c**) shows the occult fracture (*arrow*) and the subperiosteal hematoma (*thin arrow*). (**d, e**) A 15-year-old male football player. The sagittal fat suppressed PD-w (**d**) image shows the fracture line (*arrow*) extending up to the growth plate. Bone bruise in seen in the anterior aspect of the epiphysis (*open arrow*). (**e**) The fracture line is seen in the transverse T2-w TSE image (*arrow*). There is also soft-tissue hematoma anteriorly and medially secondary to the direct blow. (**f**) The T2-w MR image in the transverse plane shows the bone bruise in the marrow and the subperiosteal hematoma (*arrows*) following a trauma during football in this 6-year-old male

2.3 Avulsion Injuries

Avulsion injuries include the *acute* ones which correspond to fractures of the tendon or ligament insertions and the *chronic* ones which represent incomplete avulsions due to repeated microtrauma.

2.3.1 Acute

Tibial Eminence Fractures

Before maturation, the tibial ACL insertion is weaker compared to the ligament itself and thus eminence avulsions are more common than are mid-substance tears. Children between 8 and 12 years of age are commonly affected (Iobst and Stanitski 2000). The lack of associated injuries is the most notable feature. A developmentally wider notch width may be a risk factor for sustaining a tibial eminence fracture (Kocher et al. 2004).

This injury is usually the result of forxed valgus and external rotation of the tibia or hyperflexion and internal rotation of the tibia. Clinically, these patients present with pain and limited range of motion. A large haemarthrosis and block at motion may also be present. Myers and Mc Keever's tibial eminence fracture classification is based on displacement. *Type I* fractures are displaced <3 mm. In *type II* fractures, the anterior one third to one half of the fracture is elevated with an intact posterior hinge. In *type III* fractures, the fragment is completely avulsed from the proximal tibia. A *type III+* fracture is a type III with rotation of the fragment. A *type IV* fracture is complete displacement with rotation and comminution of the fragment. Radiographs usually confirm the diagnosis. However, they often underestimate the size of the avulsed fragment, which is mostly cartilaginous in young athletes. Computed tomography (CT) and MR imaging are performed in order to assist in complicated cases. MR imaging is useful to rule out other associated injuries and assess the integrity of the ligaments (Kocher et al. 2003, 2004) (Fig. 8). Treatment varies and is based on the classification/displacement of the fracture. Types I and II are usually treated nonoperatively whereas types III and IV are treated arthroscopically with reduction and fixation with K-wires (Vaquero et al. 2005).

Posterior Tibial Fracture

Avulsion fractures of the PCL tibial insertion are rare. They result either from hyperextension or from forceful displacement when the knee is flexed. If the fragment is not significantly displaced, plain radiographs may be inconclusive. CT or MR imaging is diagnostic (Fig. 9).

Tibial Tuberosity Fractures

The tibial tuberosity physis injuries are commonly encountered in boys and result from eccentric quadriceps muscle contractures, such as those seen with jumping sports. Tibial tuberosity acute avulsion is most

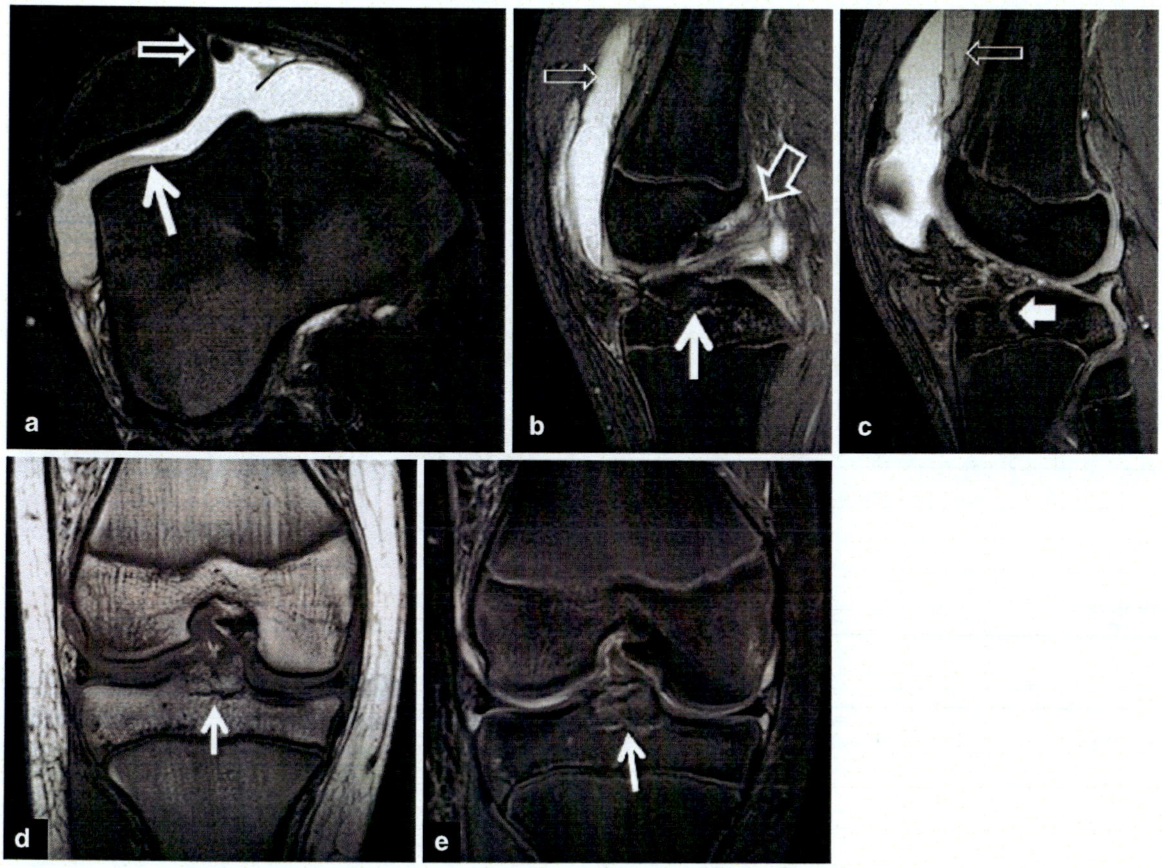

Fig. 8 MR imaging of the knee of a 14-year-old football player with a recent injury. (**a**) The transverse T2-w TSE image shows haemarthrosis (*arrow*) and a round fatty deposit (*open arrow*) suggesting the presence of an intraarticular fracture. The sagittal MEDIC images (**b**, **c**) show the nondisplaced avulsed tibial eminence (*white thin arrow*), a tear in the proximal anterior cruciate ligament (*open arrow*) and a transepiphyseal fracture (*short arrow*). The hemorrhagic effusion is also obvious (*open thin arrows*). The coronal T1-w SE (**d**) and fat suppressed PD-w TSE (**e**) images confirm the tibial eminence avulsion which is not significantly displaced (*arrows*)

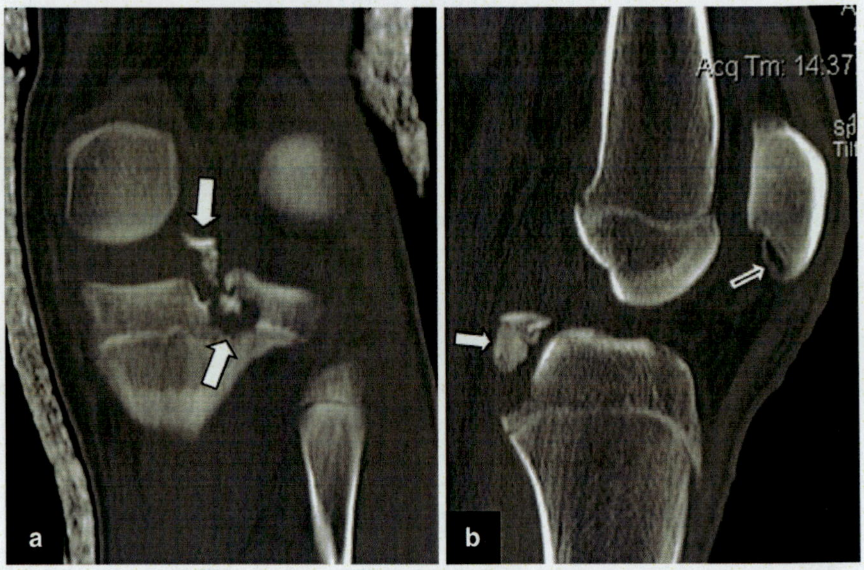

Fig. 9 A 16-year-old elite skier sustained a contact injury with a flexed knee. The coronal (**a**) and sagittal (**b**) MDCT reconstructions show the displaced avulsion fracture of the posterior tibial epiphysis, at the insertion of the PCL (*arrows*). A sleeve fracture of the inferior pole of the patella is also seen (*open arrow*)

commonly seen in athletes with preexisting Osgood–Schlatter disease. Patients present clinically with localized pain and swelling (Ogden et al. 1980). According to the Watson-Jones classification, there are three types of these injuries. In *type I*, a small fragment of the distal portion is avulsed. In *type II*, the epiphysis is lifted upwards and incompletely fractured. In *type III*, there is displacement of the proximal base of the epiphysis with the fracture line extending into the joint. Type I and II fractures tend to occur in younger athletes aged 12–14, whereas type III in older ones (15–17 years of age) (Watson-Jones 1955).

Plain radiographs are sufficient for diagnosis. Slight internal rotation of the tibia allows a better demonstration of the tubercle on the lateral view. MR imaging findings in chronic avulsive injuries may show the avulsed fragment as well as the thickening of the patellar tendon at its insertion without any associated edema in or around the tendon (Fig. 10) (Ogden et al. 1980).

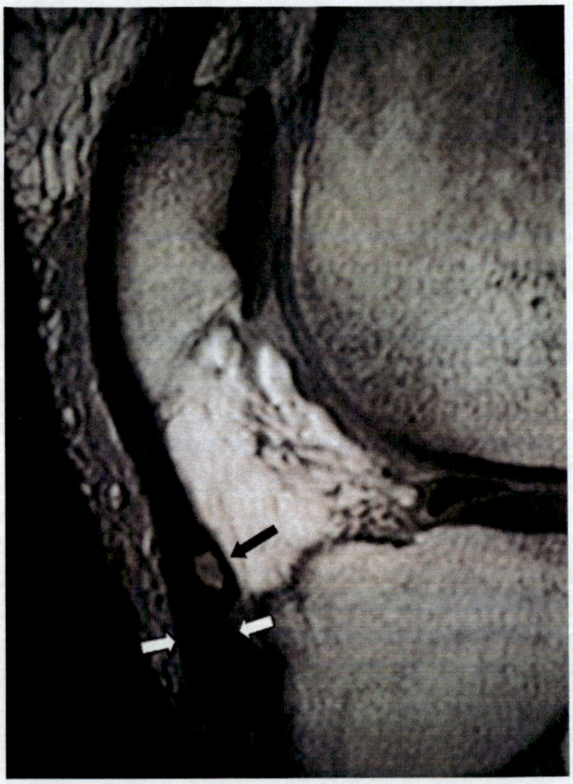

Fig. 10 A young adult elite basketball player, with a history of an acute injury at the anterior aspect of the knee during adolescence. The PD-w TSE MR image in the sagittal plane shows the chronic avulsion of the tibial tubercle (*black arrow*) associated with thickening of the distal patellar tendon insertion (*arrows*)

Patellar Sleeve Fractures

Sleeve fractures of the inferior pole of the patella occur in athletes 9–12 years and represent acute cartilaginous avulsion injuries with the periosteum being stripped downwards in continuity with the tendon (Ray and Hendrix 1992). Radiographs may show one or more bone fragments in close proximity to the lower pole of the patella but also may be negative if the fragment is not ossified. MR imaging may be required for accurate demonstration of the cartilaginous injury. CT is also helpful in depicting minimally displaced fragments (Fig. 9). Rarely, sleeve fractures may occur in the upper pole (Maripuri et al 2008).

2.3.2 Chronic

Osgood–Schlatter Disease

Osgood–Schlatter disease represents a chronic avulsion injury and is most commonly encountered in young athletes 10–15 years of age, usually boys. The exact cause of this condition is unknown. It is considered to result from repetitive microtrauma or a traction apophysitis of the tibial tuberosity in jumping sports requiring repeated flexion and forced extension of the knee (Outerbridge and Micheli 1995). The different growth rates of the bone and the soft tissue also contribute to its pathogenesis. The usual presentation is with anterior knee pain localized to the tibial tubercle and swelling. Up to 50% of patients the symptoms are bilateral. Examination reveals tenderness and swelling at the tibial tubercle. Radiographs are rarely indicated unless there is suspicion of more serious lesions, including cysts and tumors about the knee. When performed, they may reveal fragmentation and irregular ossification at the tibial tubercle (Fig. 11) (Outerbridge and Micheli 1995; Wall 1998). This finding however may represent a normal ossification center. MR imaging may be helpful by demonstrating soft-tissue swelling anterior to the tibial tubercle, thickening and edema of the distal patellar tendon, and infrapatellar bursitis (Fig. 11). The disease usually is self-limited. In a minority of patients, both the symptoms and imaging findings persist to adulthood (unresolved disease) (Fig. 12).

Sinding–Larsen–Johansson Syndrome

This syndrome is similar to Osgood–Schlatter disease involving the distal patellar pole at the insertion of the patellar tendon. It is seen in boys aged between 11 and 13 and results from repeated pull of the quadriceps extensor mechanism (kicking and jumping sports). Plain radiographs may show fragmentation of the inferior

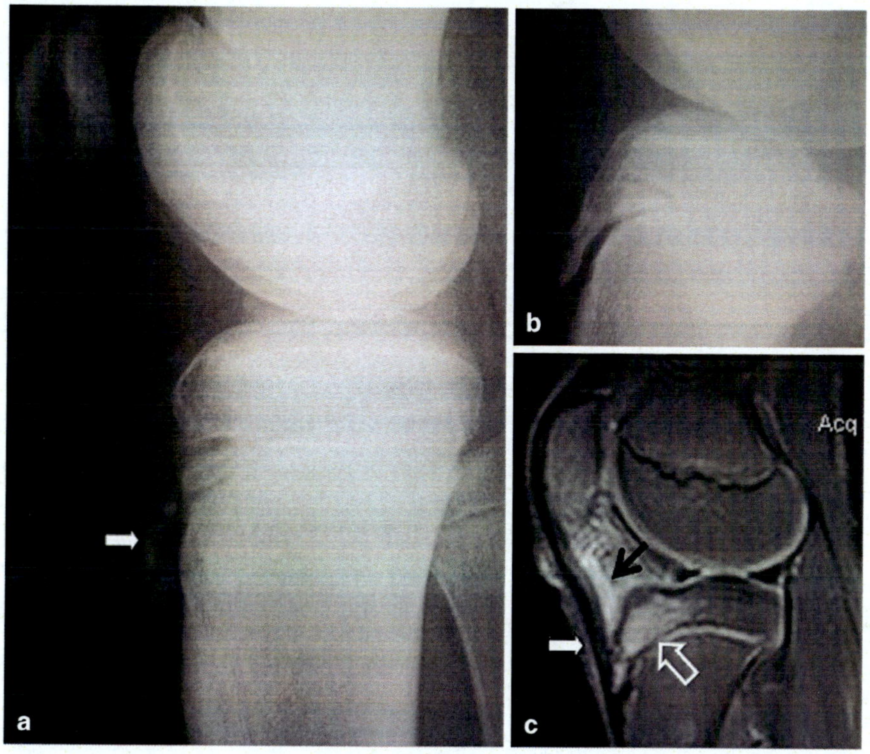

Fig. 11 Osgood–Schlatter disease in two young athletes. (**a**) The lateral plain radiograph shows the fragmentation of the tibial tubercle (*arrow*). (**b**) The plain radiograph in a 12-year-old football male athlete with anterior knee pain does not show any fragmentation. (**c**) The corresponding fat suppressed sagittal PD-w MR image shows infrapatellar bursitis (*black arrow*), increased signal intensity in the patellar tendon (*thin arrow*) and bone marrow edema into the tibial epiphysis and tubercle (*open arrow*)

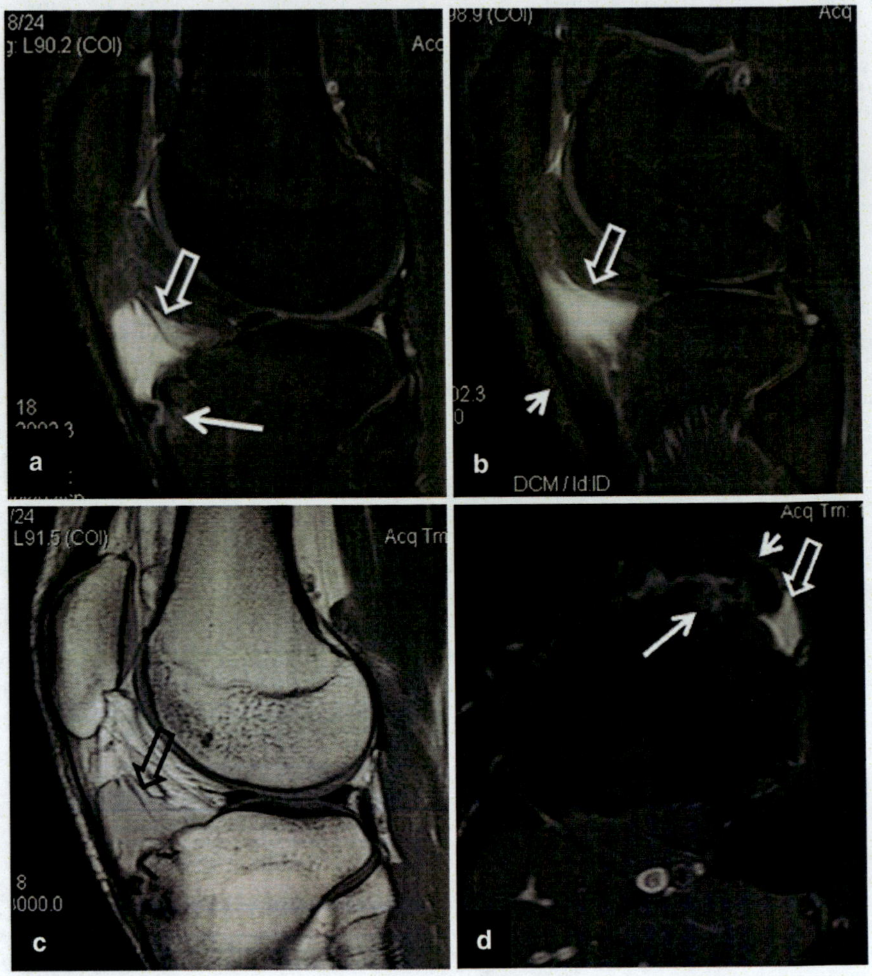

Fig. 12 A 20-year-old tennis athlete, with persistent anterior knee pain for the last 5 years, despite conservative treatment (unresolved Osgood–Schlatter disease). The sagittal fat suppressed (**a**, **b**) and plain PD-w TSE (**c**) as well as the fat suppressed axial T2-w TSE (**d**) MR images show persistent retropatellar bursitis (*open arrows*), fragmentation of the tubercle with subchondral marrow edema (*long arrows*) and thickening with focal signal hyperintensity of the distal patellar tendon (*arrowheads*)

patellar pole. MR imaging will show bone marrow and soft tissue edema (Figs. 19–21 chapter 17) (Outerbridge and Micheli 1995). A similar disorder may involve the upper pole of the patella, seen mainly in sports requiring jumping and kicking.

Jumper's Knee

Jumper's knee is a syndrome characterized by pain either at the distal or the proximal insertion of the patellar tendon. It is caused by repetitive microtrauma seen most often in adolescent boys participating in basketball, volleyball, or football. MR imaging shows thickening of the tendon with increased signal intensity on T1-w and T2-w images. Ultrasonography is also diagnostic by demonstrating not only the thickening of the tendon but also the neovascularization.

2.4 Stress Fractures and Reactions

Stress or fatigue injuries represent a spectrum of disorders, ranging from a stress reaction of bone marrow to a frank fracture. Stress injuries in children, once considered rare, are seen with increasing frequency, presumably due to increased participation in sports (Coady and Micheli 1997). Stress injuries result from repetitive compression and bending forces on a bone or from prolonged muscular action on a bone that has not been used to that stress. They are usually seen in jogging, aerobics, racquet games, long distance running and football (Courtenay and Bowers 1990).

Stress reactions are radiologically occult injuries. On MR imaging they are demonstrated as high signal intensity areas on fat suppressed images in the absence of a recognizable traumatic event (Fig. 13). Stress reactions are on MR imaging similar to bone bruises. It is

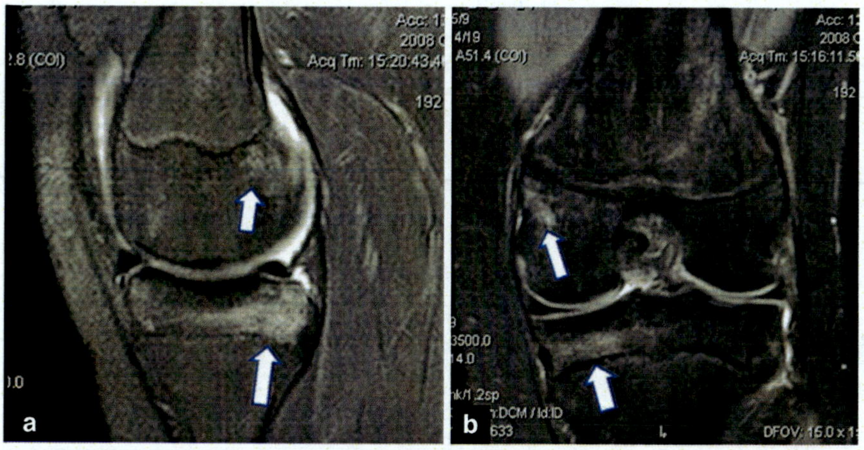

Fig. 13 Stress reaction in a 15-year-old amateur football player without any history of trauma. The sagittal (**a**) and coronal (**b**) PD-w fat suppressed MR images show the bone marrow edema in the medial-posterior tibial epiphysis and the posterior and medial femoral condyle (*arrows*). The high signal intensity area in the lateral aspect of the distal femoral metaphysis represents normal red bone marrow

the history indeed of a previous traumatic event which favors the diagnosis of a bone bruise or the absence of trauma which suggests a stress reaction. The latter, if not treated with rest, will proceed to stress fracture.

Stress fractures in young athletes occur in about equal proportions in males and females and most commonly involve the tibia. Most tibial stress fractures close to the knee joint are seen postero-medially. These fractures are on the compression side of the tibia allowing early response to rest and activity modification with an early return to sports. Clinically, stress fractures present with bone pain, particularly on exertion. Radiographic examination should be the first imaging study in the evaluation of a patient with suspected stress injury. However, the sensitivity of early radiographs is as low as 15% and delayed radiographs reveal findings only in 50% of patients. The earliest radiographic manifestation of a stress fracture is localized periosteal and endosteal thickening, with or without a sclerotic fracture line (Fig. 14) (Carty 1994). Scintigraphy with 99mTc MDP used to be the next choice of imaging. MR imaging has been demonstrated to have an equivalent sensitivity to scintigraphy and even greater specificity in diagnosing stress fractures. It also allows accurate grading of the entire spectrum of these lesions. MR imaging seems to be more accurate than scintigraphy in correlating bone changes with clinical symptoms (Fredericson et al. 1995). It is clinically important to differentiate between stress reaction and other pathology, especially when there is no clear history of trauma. STIR and fat-suppressed T2-w imaging are excellent in depicting the high signal intensity marrow edema that is associated with the stress fracture (Fig. 14). Occasionally, however, the edema pattern is difficult to differentiate from that associated with infection or an aggressive neoplasm. In these cases, long TR images and contrast-enhanced T1-w images should be applied to confirm the presence of a low signal intensity fracture line within the marrow edema (Fig. 15). This line allows the lesion to be confidently identified as a stress fracture (Anderson and Greenspan 1996). High resolution CT with long-axis reformations might be helpful to identify a linear band of lucency or sclerosis when the fracture cannot be depicted on MR images.

3 Physeal Injuries

3.1 Acute

Acute injury to the physis may result from an isolated and direct trauma or may occur after an injury to the epiphysis or metaphysis. The physes of the distal femur and proximal tibia are uncommon sites of physeal injury but are commonly associated with posttraumatic bridge formation (35 and 16%, respectively) (Ecklund and Jaramillo 2001). Proximal tibial physeal fractures are approximately three times less common than those of the distal femoral epiphysis, perhaps due to protection of the collateral ligaments insertions (Mann and Rajmaira 1990). Transphyseal and physeal fractures of the lower femur are seen more frequently in team contact sports. The risk of growth disturbance following a physeal fracture is dependent on the severity of the injury, the patient's remaining growth potential, the anatomic site involved, and the type of fracture. Significantly displaced or comminuted fractures are at greatest risk for growth

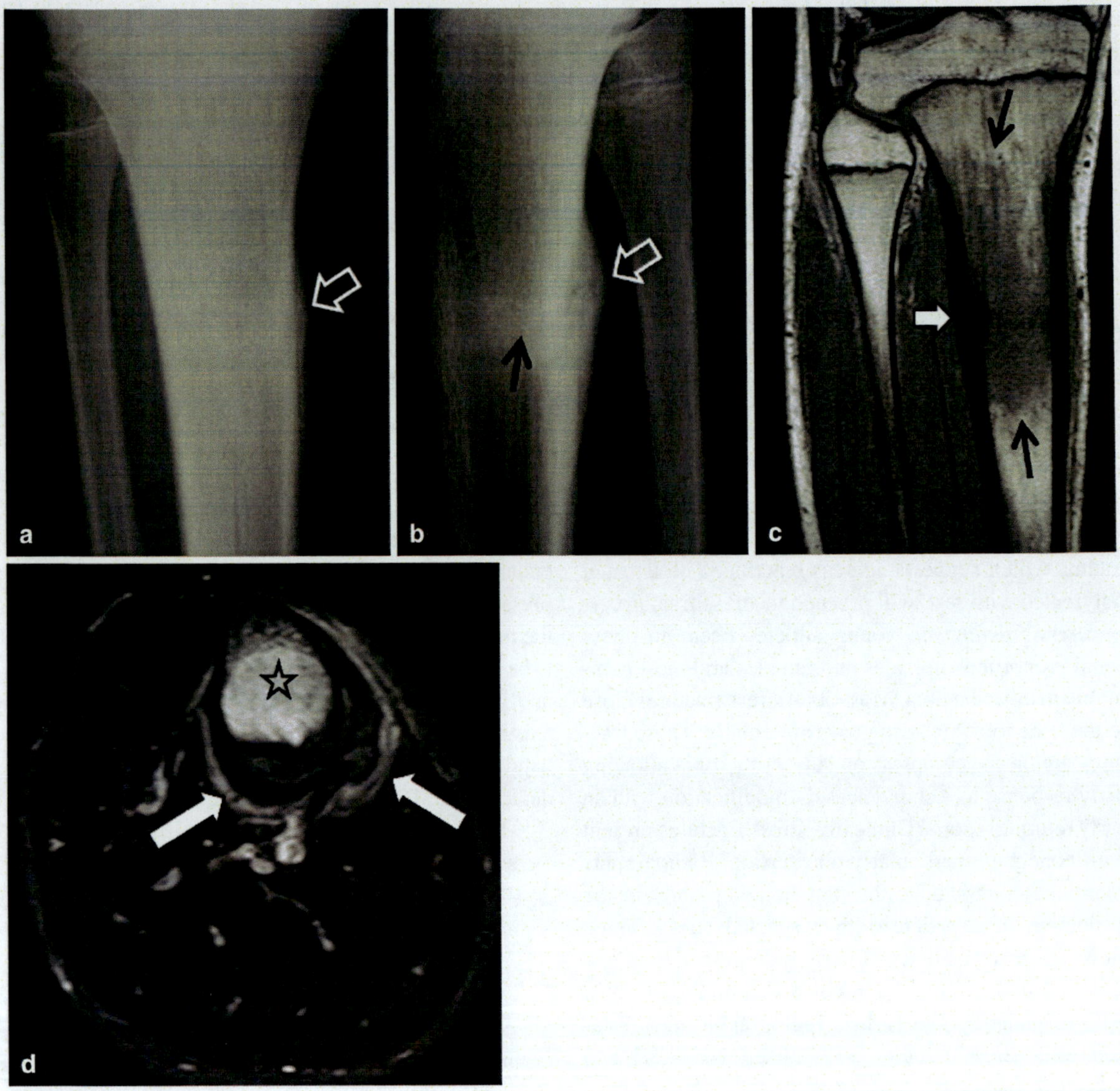

Fig. 14 A 14-year-old male track athlete presenting with a 5-week history of proximal tibial pain. The PA (**a**) and lateral (**b**) plain radiographs show a thick periosteal reaction (*open arrows*). Trabecular sclerosis suggesting the presence of a stress fracture is hardly seen (*black arrow*). (**c**) The coronal T1-w MR image shows extensive bone marrow edema (*arrows*) and periosteal reaction (*white arrow*). (**d**) The transverse fat suppressed T2-w MR image shows the edema into the bone marrow (*asterisk*) and the periosteal thickening with soft tissue edema (*white arrows*)

arrest. Younger patients have a poorer prognosis because there is more time for deformity to develop. Undulating multiplanar physes, such as those of the proximal tibia and distal femur, are particularly prone to growth arrest. Peripheral bridging may cause focal growth arrest and consequently angular deformity. Central bridging may lead to leg length discrepancy (Moran and Macnicol 2006; Al-Otaibi and Siegel 1998).

Physeal fractures are usually easier to see on the lateral view but may be missed at all on radiographs. A tunnel view is a useful additional projection if an injury is suspected and not visible on the anterior–posterior and lateral view.

MR imaging in *acute physeal injury* is not routinely performed, although it can demonstrate the cartilaginous path of the fracture, as well as possible associated findings (Fig. 1). The information concerning the pathway of the fracture is of prognostic value since a vertical physeal fracture permits bone formation across the cartilage, which results in a bridge of bone across the

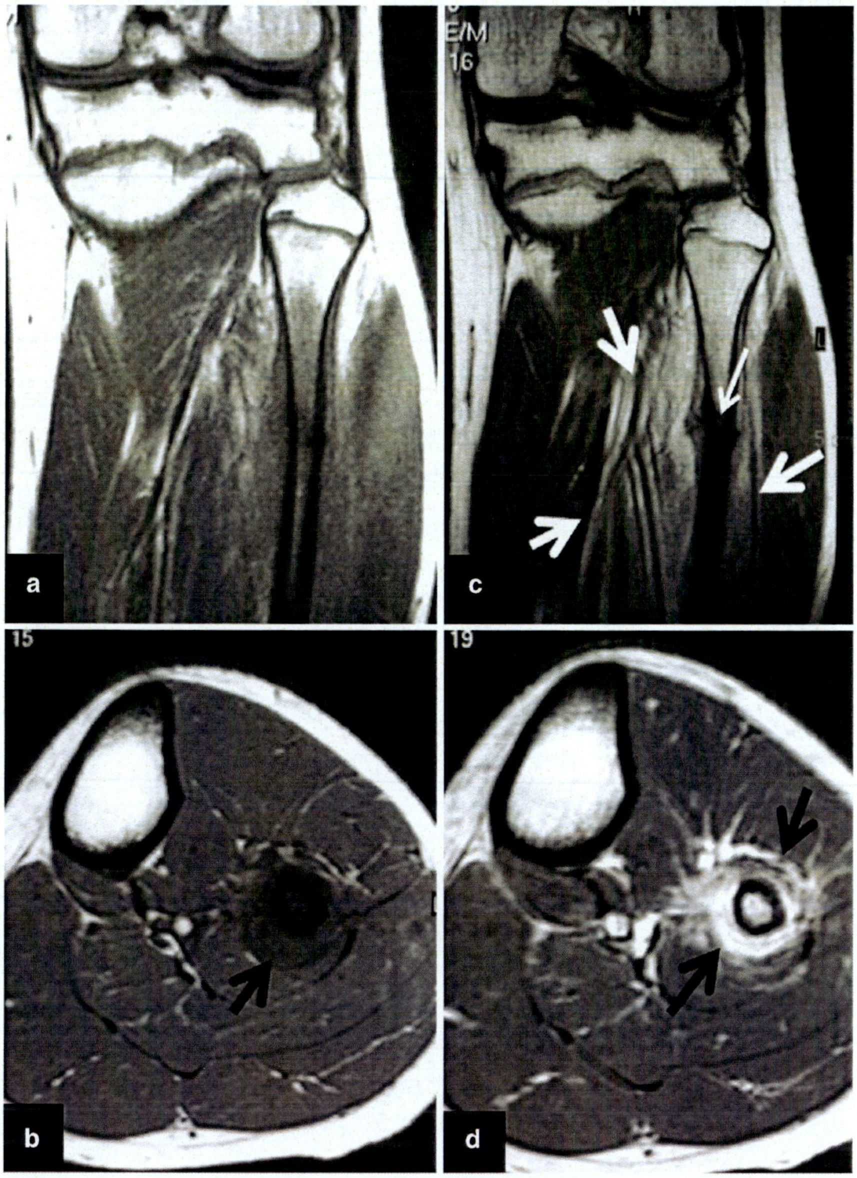

Fig. 15 A 15-year-old male footballer with stress fracture of the proximal fibula. The coronal (**a**) and axial (**b**) T1-w and contrast enhanced coronal (**c**) and axial (**d**) T1-w MR images, show a periosteal reaction in the fibula, with bone marrow edema and reactive soft tissue changes that enhance after contrast medium administration (*arrows*). The low signal intensity fracture is better seen on the coronal enhanced T1-w image (*thin arrow* in **c**)

physis (Busch 1990). The thin axial sections provided by 3D T2* MR sequences, allow an estimation of the bridge-to-physis ratio, which has been used for treatment planning. Physeal fractures can be seen on fat suppressed PD-w, STIR and T2*-w GRE images. *Bony bridges* complicating acute injuries occur most frequently near the areas of normal physeal closure (Ogden 1984). They can be depicted up to 3 m after injury with radiographs and earlier with MR imaging. The proper MR sequences for assessing the bridging, depicted as a low signal intensity area interrupting the high signal physis, are the high resolution T2* or the fat suppressed PD-w TSE (Fig. 16). Small bridges show low signal intensity on T1-w images (Fig. 16) but the larger ones may be isointense with the fatty marrow.

3.2 Chronic

Overuse or stress injuries of the physis due to repetitive trauma, has been implicated as a cause of extension of physeal signal intensity into the adjacent metaphysis, demonstrated on fat suppressed MR images. This finding though has also been described in asymptomatic children. The *widening* of the physis, focal or generalized, in the absence of a single traumatic event, has been

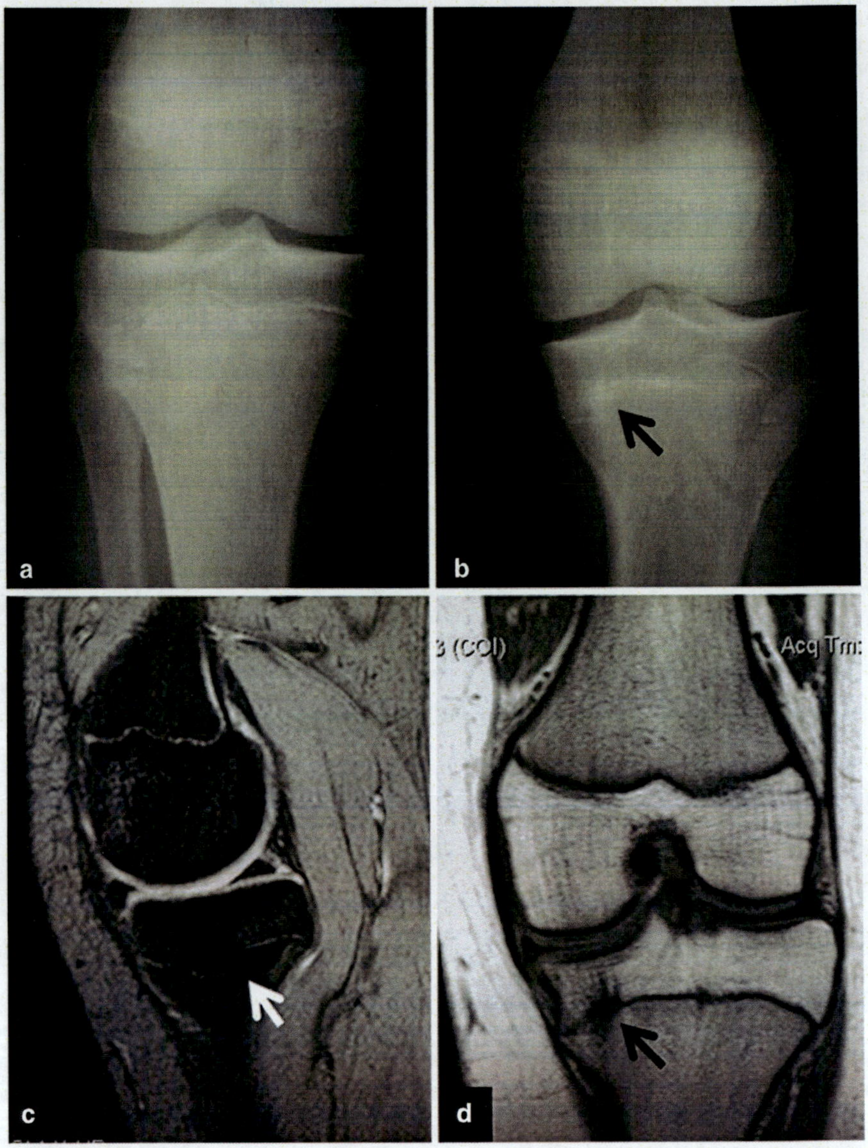

Fig. 16 Growth arrest of the tibia. An 11-year-old female skiing athlete with a previous epiphyseal injury. The plain radiographs (**a**, **b**) show the normal tibial epiphyseal plate on the right knee and the abnormal bridging with a sclerotic line on the left (*arrow*) resulting in angular deformity. The sagittal T2* (**c**) and the coronal T1-w (**d**) MR images, show on the medial side the low signal intensity bone bridge interrupting the normal growth plate (*arrows*)

attributed to stress injury of the physis (Laor et al. 2006). The role of radiologists in depicting promptly this lesion is important because excellent prognosis is expected with rest and immobilization.

4 Articular Injuries

4.1 Chondral and Osteochondral Injuries

Chondral lesions are more prevalent than meniscal or ligamentous injuries in the skeletally immature patients. They are the most common lesions, seen in up to 34%, in children examined with MR imaging for evaluation of internal derangement of the knee (Oeppen et al. 2004).

The distribution of chondral injuries depends on skeletal maturity: proportionally more femoral lesions are seen in skeletally immature patients, and more patellar lesions are seen in skeletally mature patients (Oeppen et al. 2004). Chondral injuries are significant because they may predispose a patient to premature osteoarthritis (Conaghan 2002). This tendency is especially true in patients with full-thickness cartilage injuries, which may be amenable to the newer cartilage-repair treatments, such as the autologous chondrocyte transplantation (Brittberg et al. 1994).

Articular cartilage is in general difficult to image due to its small size and location on curved surfaces. However, the newer developments on MR imaging hardware and software, allow for an adequate and easy depiction of normal and abnormal cartilage. Together with the proper knee coil, two sequences are used most commonly for this purpose: a) a fat-suppressed 3D T1-w spoiled gradient-recalled echo and b) a fat suppressed intermediate-w (TE: 40–45 ms on 1.5 T) high-resolution turbo (fast) spin-echo. The latter is very sensitive to depict associated lesions in and around the knee joint area. With the former, the articular cartilage shows high signal intensity and with the latter lower signal intensity than the adjacent joint fluid. In the presence of joint effusion, T2-TSE (FSE) images are useful as they are able to show the cartilage as a low signal intensity structure and then an abnormality is seen as a discontinuity (Fig. 17). Subchondral bone marrow edema is frequently seen with cartilaginous injuries (Figs. 2 and 18).

MR imaging findings in osteochondral injuries include cartilaginous thickening in grade I lesions, superficial ulceration or fissuring in grade II, deep ulceration or fissuring in grade III, associated bone bruise in grade IV and separated fractures in grade V. Impaction fractures may also occur (Fig. 18). Osteochondral injuries are usually associated with joint effusion, occasionally hemorrhagic (Fig. 17). Thus, the need for MR arthrography is very limited as most of the chondral

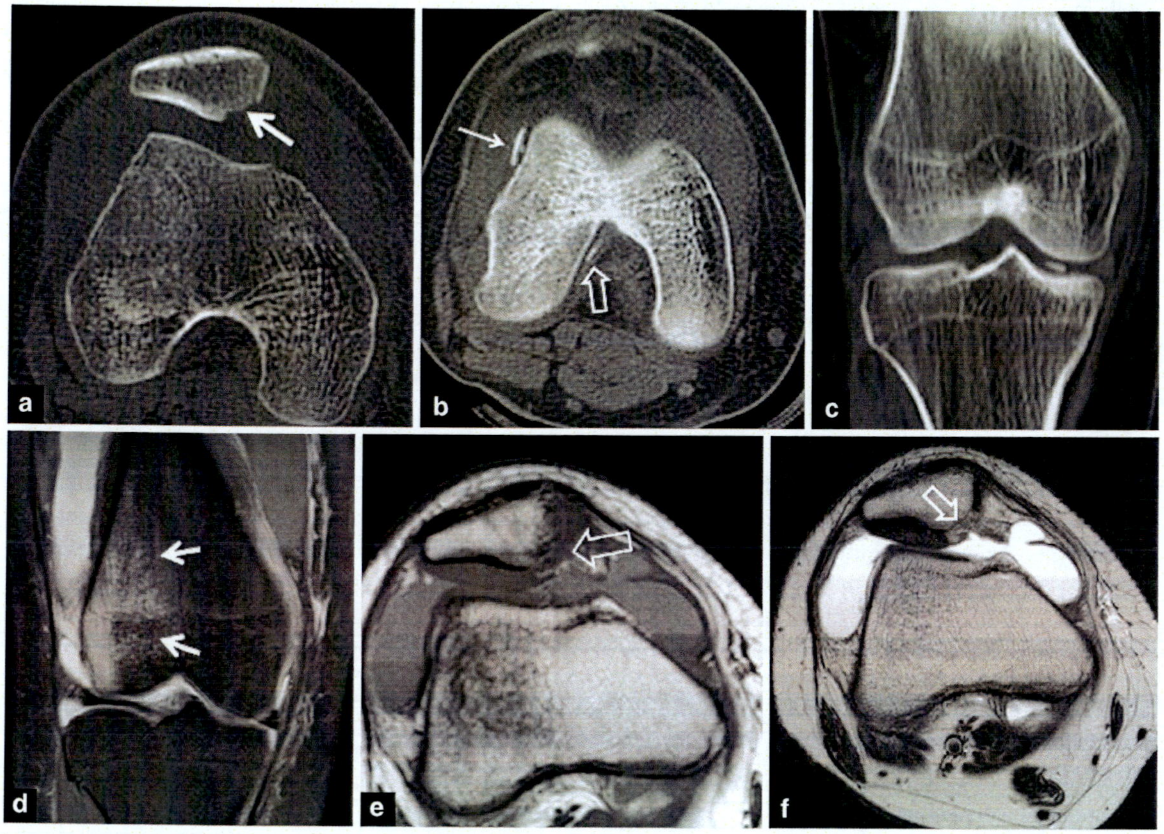

Fig. 17 A 15-year-old female basketball player, with a twisting injury 1 day before imaging. The axial CT images (**a**, **b**) show a cortical irregularity in the medial articular surface of the patella (*arrow*) and a chip bony fragment by the lateral femoral condyle (*thin arrow*). There is also joint effusion and a possible small loose body posteriorly (*open arrow*). (**c**) The coronal MPR CT image shows a loose body into the medial joint space. (**d**) The coronal fat suppressed PD-w MR image, shows the joint effusion and in addition the bone bruise in the anterior lateral femoral condyle (*arrows*). This pattern suggests previous lateral patellar dislocation. (**e**) The axial T1-w MR image shows hemorrhagic joint effusion with fluid-fluid levels, and irregularity of the patellar cartilage (*arrow*). (**f**) The axial T2-w MR image, shows to better advantage the grade IV cartilage defect in the patella (*arrow*), exposing the bone. The hemorrhagic joint effusion provides an "arthrographic" effect

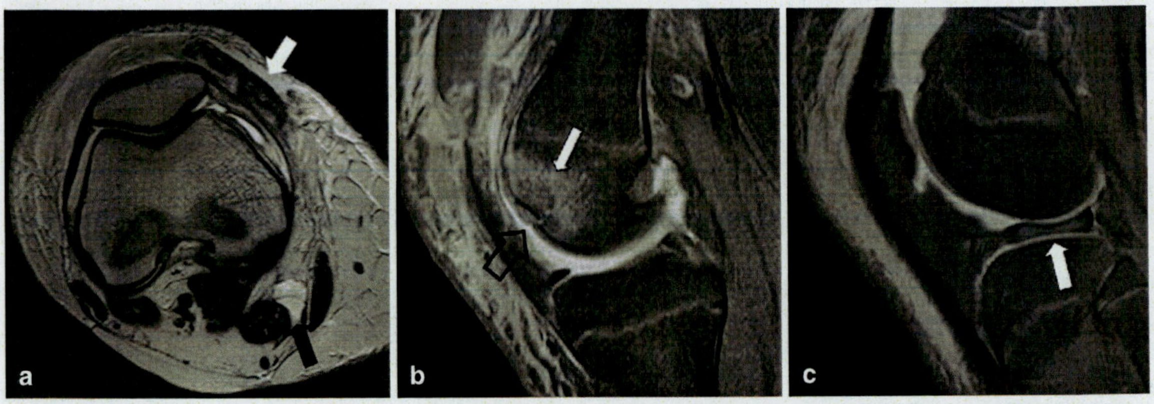

Fig. 18 Meniscal contusion. A 14-year-old skier who was injured during slalom 2 days before imaging. (**a**) The axial T2-w TSE MR image shows hematoma formation in the subcutaneous tissue on the medial aspect of the knee (*arrow*) and a ruptured baker cyst posteriorly (*black arrow*). (**b**) The sagittal fat suppressed proton density MR image shows an impacted osteochondral fracture in the medial femoral condyle (*open arrow*), the associated bone bruise (*thin arrow*) and the prepatellar hematoma. (**c**) The sagittal fat-suppressed proton density MR image shows joint effusion and extensive intra-meniscal high signal intensity in keeping with a contusion of the lateral discoid meniscus (*arrow*)

lesions will be accurately classified because the effusion is helpful for depicting loose bodies. A cartilaginous loose body will follow the signal intensity of the normal cartilage on all pulse sequences.

4.2 Meniscal Injuries

In children younger than 12 years of age, the menisci are highly vascularized. As a result, a horizontal line of increased signal intensity originating from the capsular attachment most probably represents a nutrient vessel rather than a tear (Oeppen et al. 2004). Although the incidence and age distribution of meniscal injuries is not known, they are uncommon in children under 10 years of age (Iobst and Stanitski 2000). The *meniscal contusion* is unique for this age group of athletes (Fig. 18). This lesion is characterized by a generalized increased signal intensity following an acute injury without any distinct linear component (Cothran et al. 2001). In follow up MR imaging, there is a self limited resolution of the abnormal signal intensity.

Meniscal tears are most commonly seen in running, jumping, cutting, and pivoting sports. They are generally associated with a discoid lateral meniscus. The most typical tear morphology is that of peripheral longitudinal tear, involving the posterior portion of the meniscus (Busch 1990). Meniscal detachments are more common in younger children whereas substance tears, often of the bucket-handle pattern, tend to occur in adolescents. Meniscal tears often occur in combination with other injuries such as ACL and MCL sprains or chondral injuries (Busch 1990). The presentation is similar to that in adults, with pain and mechanical symptoms. Non acute injuries may present with poorly defined generalized knee pain. McMurray's test is not in children as sensitive as it is in adults regarding clinical diagnosis (Siow et al. 2008).

Lateral notch view radiographs are obtained to rule out unsuspected fractures, osteochondral lesions, and loose bodies. Signs of discoid meniscus may also be noticed on a standing anterior–posterior radiograph. These include widening of the lateral joint space, squaring of the lateral femoral condyle, and cupping of the lateral tibial plateau (Fig. 19). There also may be hypoplasia of the lateral tibial spine (Takeda et al. 1998). Three types of discoid meniscus have been recognized: (1) *complete* when the disc occupies the entire tibial plateau; (2) *incomplete* with a concave or convex rim; and (3) *Wrisberg type* when there is no posterior attachment of the meniscus to the tibia. Discoid menisci cause clicking or joint locking and due to their morphology, they are more vulnerable to trauma with the tear usually occurring in the posterior or central zone.

MR imaging modality of choice for diagnosing a torn meniscus or a discoid meniscus. The MR appearances of meniscal injuries in children are similar to those in adults, perhaps with a lower overall accuracy, and do not require further description (Figs. 20–22).

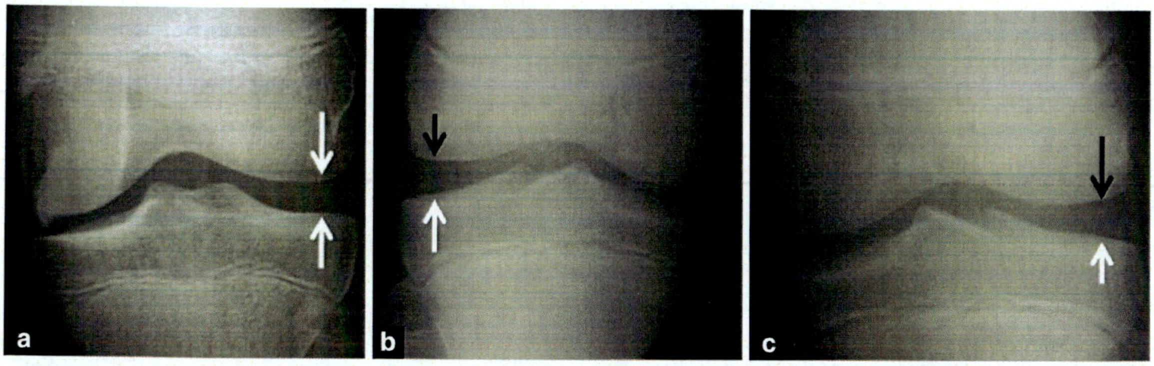

Fig. 19 Discoid meniscus in two young athletes with knee pain on exercise. The AP radiographs show widened lateral joint space (*white arrows*) in the left knee of a 14-year-old girl (**a**) and bilaterally in a 12-year-old boy (**b**, **c**). There is also squaring of the lateral femoral condyles (*black arrows*)

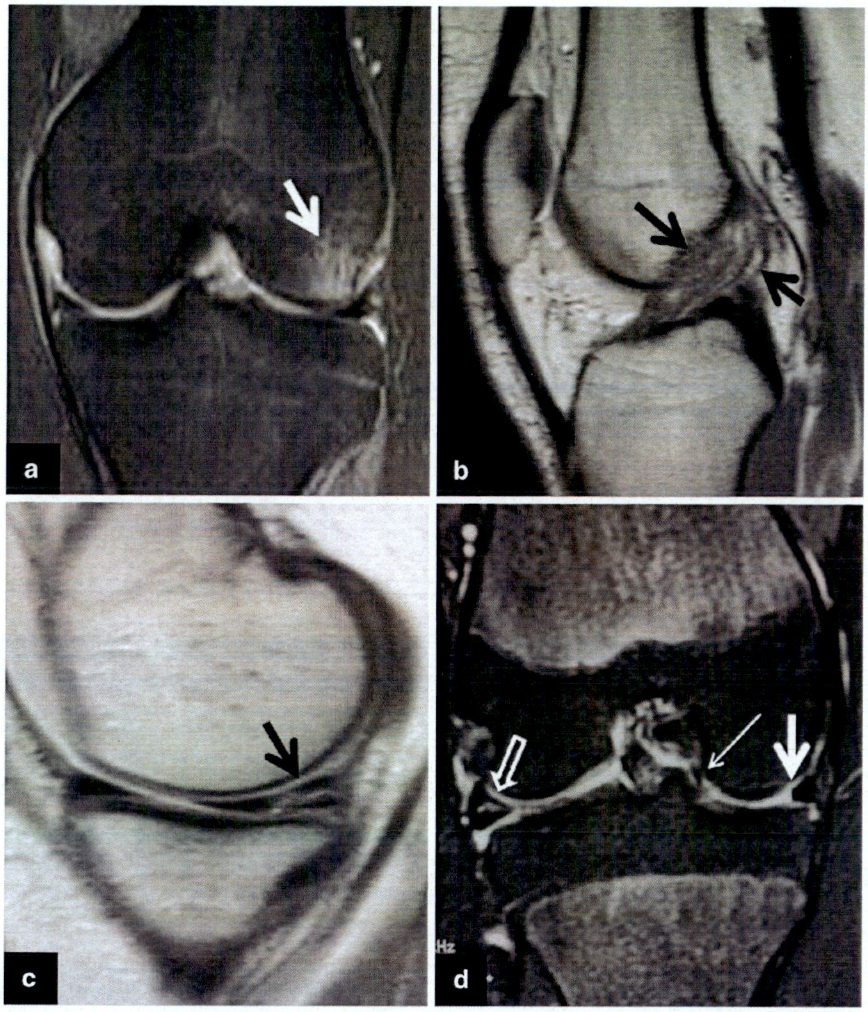

Fig. 20 A 15-year-old female skier, with recent twisting injury. (**a**) The coronal fat suppressed PD-w MR image shows bone bruise (*arrow*) in the lateral femoral condyle. The sagittal PD-w MR images (**b**, **c**) show a torn anterior cruciate ligament and a vertical and horizontal tear of the medial meniscus (*arrows*). (**d**) The coronal fat suppressed PD-w MR image in another female athlete, 11-year-old, shows an amputated medial border of the medial meniscus (*white arrow*), a loose body representing the detached meniscus (*thin arrow*) and degeneration grade II in the lateral meniscus (*open arrow*)

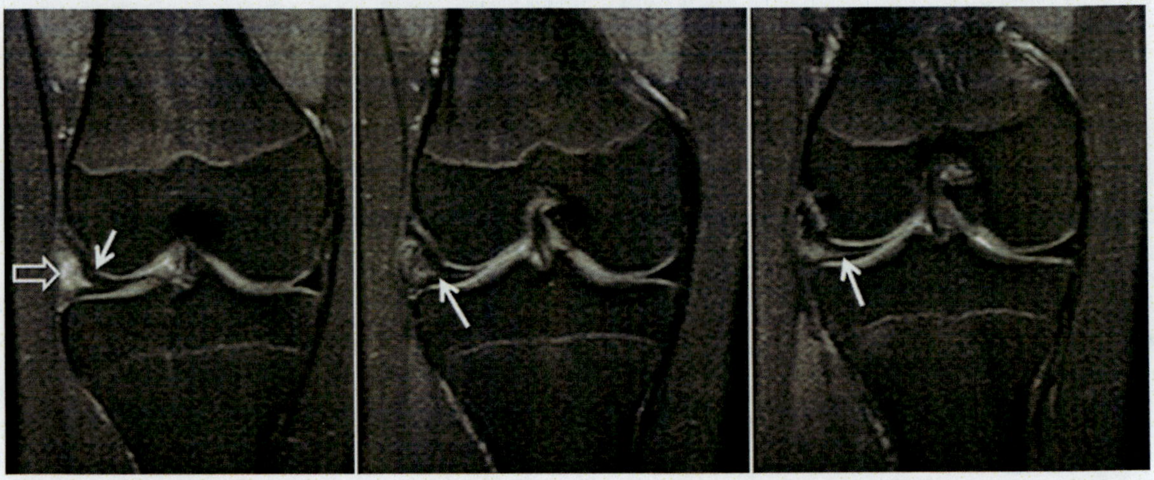

Fig. 21 A female track athlete, with pain in the lateral aspect of the knee. The coronal fat suppressed PD-w images show a torn discoid lateral meniscus (*arrows*) with cyst formation (*open arrow*)

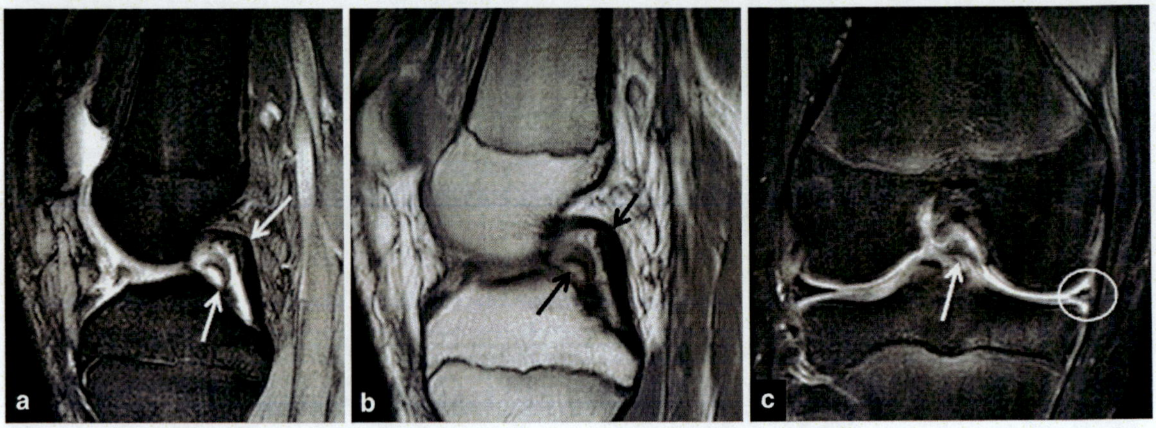

Fig. 22 A 15-year-old basketball player, with a history of recent locking in the knee joint. The sagittal MEDIC (**a**) and PD-w (**b**) MR images show the typical "double" PCL sign (*arrows*) suggesting a "bucket-handle" medial meniscus tear. (**c**) The fat suppressed coronal PD-w MR image, shows the displaced fragment (*thin arrow*) and the amputated medial meniscus (*circle*)

The postoperative meniscus after repair may show abnormal signal intensity and enhancement, for months or years following arthroscopic repair, similar to adults (Hantes et al. 2004). This is a normal postoperative finding (Fig. 23).

4.3 Chondromalacia Patella

Chondromalacia patella is a frequent cause of retropatellar pain in athletic children, particularly girls. Plain radiographs are usually normal but rarely may show an ill-defined posterior patellar border, osseous defects and sclerosis locally at the latest stages (Raissaki et al. 2007). On MR imaging there may be an increased thickness of the retropatellar cartilage along with abnormal signal intensity on cartilage-specific sequences (Fig. 24). This may be seen in association with a "saucer" shaped bony defect, on the rear surface of the patella, known as the *patellar dorsal defect* (Smith and Tao 1995). The latter is considered by many authors, to represent a developmental anomaly consisting of fibrous tissue and is typically asymptomatic. MR imaging features include a subchondral osseous defect located usually in the superolateral aspect of the deep surface of the patella, with intact overlying cartilage, unless chondromalacia coexists (Fig. 25) (Ho et al 1991).

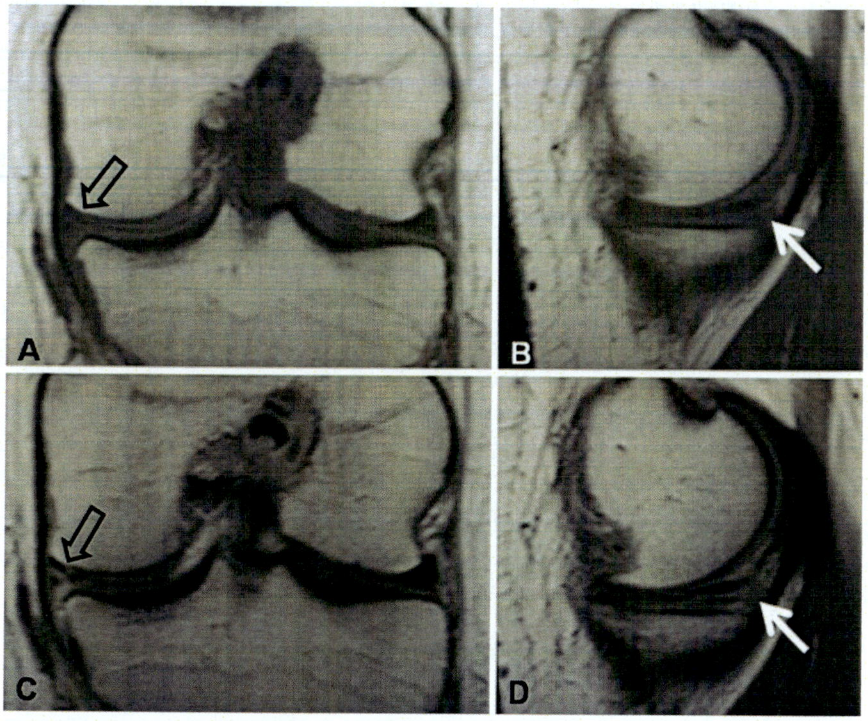

Fig. 23 Asymptomatic 16-year-old female tennis player with bucket handle tear repair and ACL reconstruction 1 year before imaging. The coronal and sagittal T1-w MR images, before (**a**, **b**) and after (**c**, **d**) contrast administration, show abnormal medial meniscus signal and abnormal enhancement (*arrows*). These are normal postoperative findings

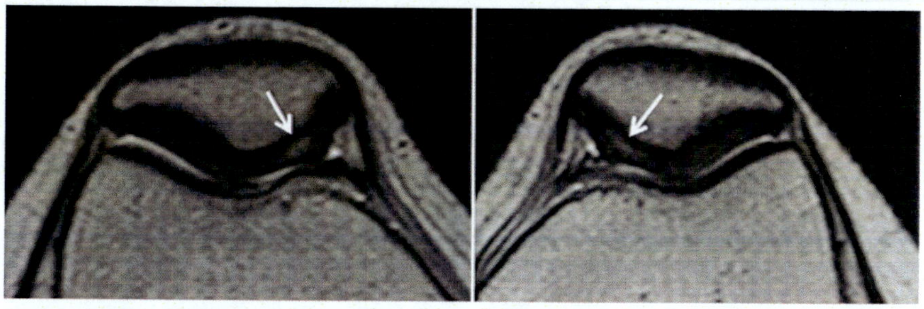

Fig. 24 Chondromalacia patella in a 15-year-old female tennis player. The axial T2-w TSE MR images show bilaterally focal thickening and high signal intensity within the medial articular cartilage of the patella (*arrows*)

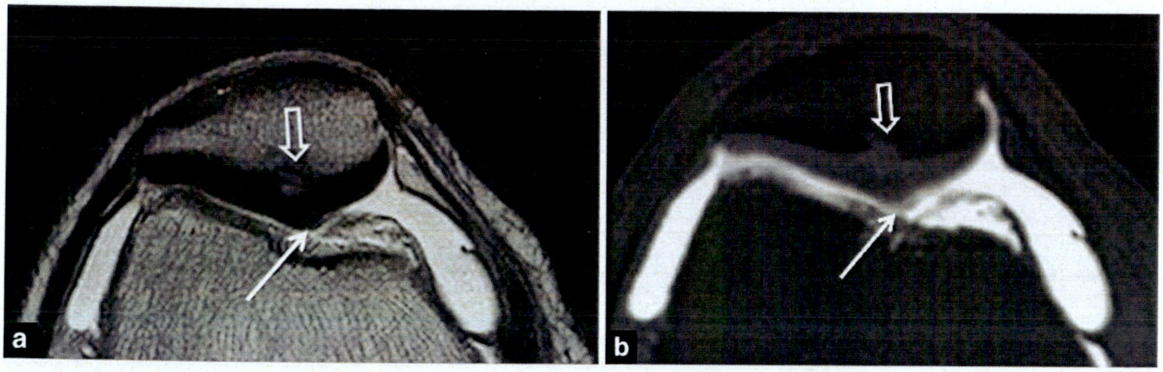

Fig. 25 Dorsal patellar defect and chondromalacia in a 16-year-old elite tennis player with mild anterior knee pain since adolescence. The axial T2-TSE (**a**) and fat suppressed T1-w following arthrogram (**b**) MR images, show the dorsal patellar defect not communicating with the joint (*open arrow*) and the focal thickening of the articular cartilage in keeping with mild chondromalacia (*thin arrow*)

4.4 Patellar Subluxation-Dislocation

Patellar subluxation or dislocation is seen in contact sports and occurs following valgus stress to the knee with internal rotation of the femur or via a direct blow. Predisposing causes include patella alta, ligamentous laxity, genu valgum, trochlear dysplasia, increased Q angle and tear of the medial patello-femoral ligament. The patient usually presents with obvious displacement of the patella, as well as with anterior knee pain and swelling. Patello-femoral hemarthrosis and tenderness along the medial patella may also be suggestive of patellar dislocation. Most dislocations occur in a lateral direction and are associated with injury to the medial retinacular tissues and the medial patello-femoral ligament. Medial, superior and intra-articular dislocation also can occur but are rare (Carr 2003).

Repeated episodes of subluxation or dislocation occur in up to 49% of patients. Persistent instability may result in unrecognized intra-articular injury, usually an osteochondral fragment from the medial facet of the patella or from the lateral femoral condyle. Anteroposterior, lateral, and Merchant view radiographs can evaluate for patella alta/baja, or osteochondral fractures of the patella or intercondylar groove or lateral femoral condyle. Avulsion injuries may be seen of the medial aspect of the patella and may be best depicted on Merchant view radiographs. Radiographs are limited in the ability to identify osteochondral injuries (Bharam et al. 2002). MR imaging can provide significant information with regard to the location and magnitude of soft-tissue and the commonly seen osteochondral injury (up to 79%), the patellar deformity and the anatomy of the trochlea (Figs. 5, 17, and 26). Small osseous avulsions which might migrate as loose bodies are better seen with CT.

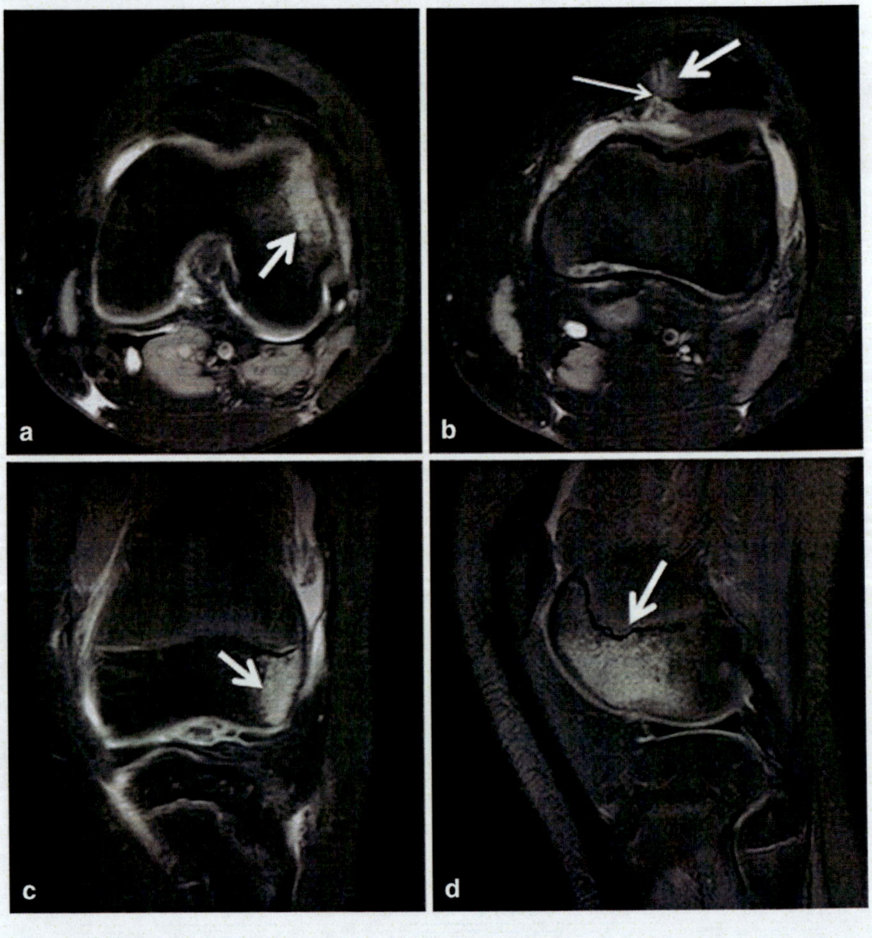

Fig. 26 A 14-year-old male volley ball athlete was injured during landing. The fat suppressed PD-w MR images in the axial (**a**, **b**), coronal (**c**) and sagittal (**d**) planes, showed bone bruise in the anterolateral femoral condyle and medial patella (*arrows*). An osteochondral injury of the medial articular surface of the patella with cartilage delamination is seen (*thin arrow*). The pattern of the bone bruise suggests a previous, temporary, lateral dislocation of the patella

4.5 Patello-Femoral Syndromes

Patello-femoral syndromes represent the most common cause of chronic knee pain in young athletes. Causes include overuse, direct trauma and poor patellar tracking (Fig. 27). These patients often have associated anatomic malalignment, consisting of genu valga, tibia vara, femoral anteversion, patella alta and increased Q-angle. Patients usually present with pain related to increased pressure on the patello-femoral joint from activities such as running hills or sprinting. Symptoms are often intermittent and commonly bilateral.

Radiographic evaluation of patello-femoral pain is not routinely necessary. When performed, radiographs should include Merchant and skyline views of the knee. Plain films can reveal the level of skeletal maturation, bony variants such as bipartite patella and developmental malalignment (Fig. 27). MR imaging may show associated meniscal and articular cartilage abnormalities and is helpful to rule out other causes of anterior knee pain such as Osgood–Schlatter disease, Sinding–Larsen–Johansson syndrome, patellar tendonitis, quadriceps tendonitis, and plica syndrome (Harvey 1982).

4.6 Osteochondritis Dissecans

Osteochondritis dissecans is thought to result from repetitive trauma to the weight-bearing areas and is usually seen in the lateral aspect of the medial femoral condyle. Radiographs may initially be normal, whereas in the later stages a subarticular lucency, with or without loose bodies, may be demonstrated. MR imaging is more sensitive than plain radiographs. Signs on fat-suppressed MR images that suggest instability include: a fragment outlined by fluid, an articular fracture passing through the subchondral bone plate and a 5-mm or larger cyst deep to the lesion (Fig. 28). The criteria above have high specificity for lesions in adults, but not in juveniles (Kijowski et al. 2008).

5 Muscular and Ligamentous Injuries

5.1 Muscular Injuries

Injuries to muscles and the myotendinous unit are encountered with increasing incidence in children. They deserve special attention because their appearances can

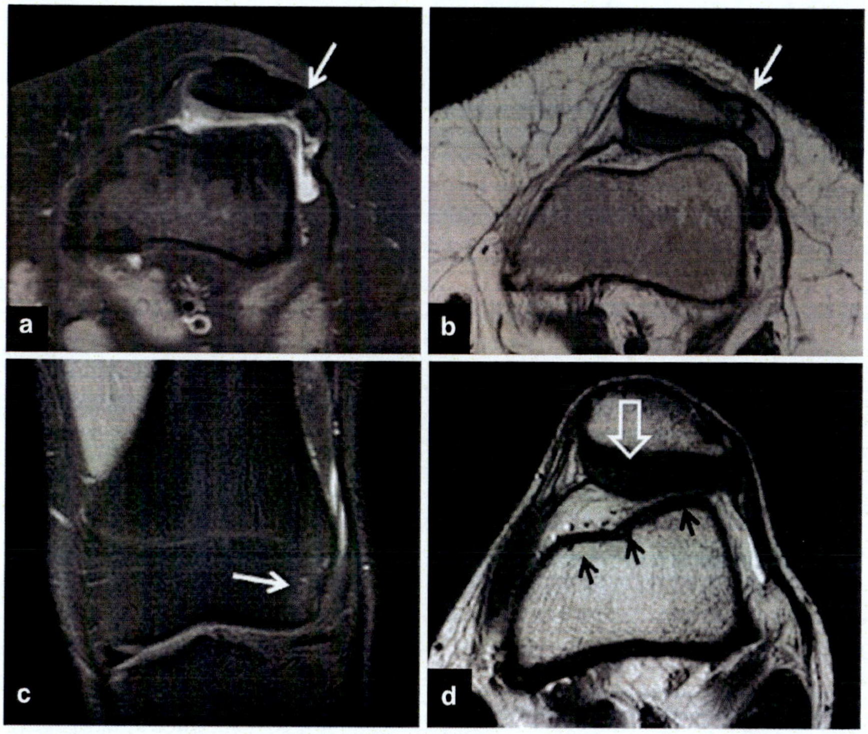

Fig. 27 The axial fat suppressed PD-w (**a**) and T1-w (**b**) MR images show the bipartite patella (*arrows*) associated with thinning of the articular cartilage and minor joint effusion. The coronal fat suppressed PD-w (**c**) and axial T2-w (**d**) MR images of a 15-year-old football player, show a bone bruise in the lateral femoral condyle (*arrow*) and a lateral subluxation of the patella which has a Wiberg III appearance (*open arrow*). The trochlea is quite steep (*small arrows*). The combination of a weak bone bruise, subluxation and a deformity of the patellofemoral joint, suggest mal-tracking and recurrent dislocations of the patella

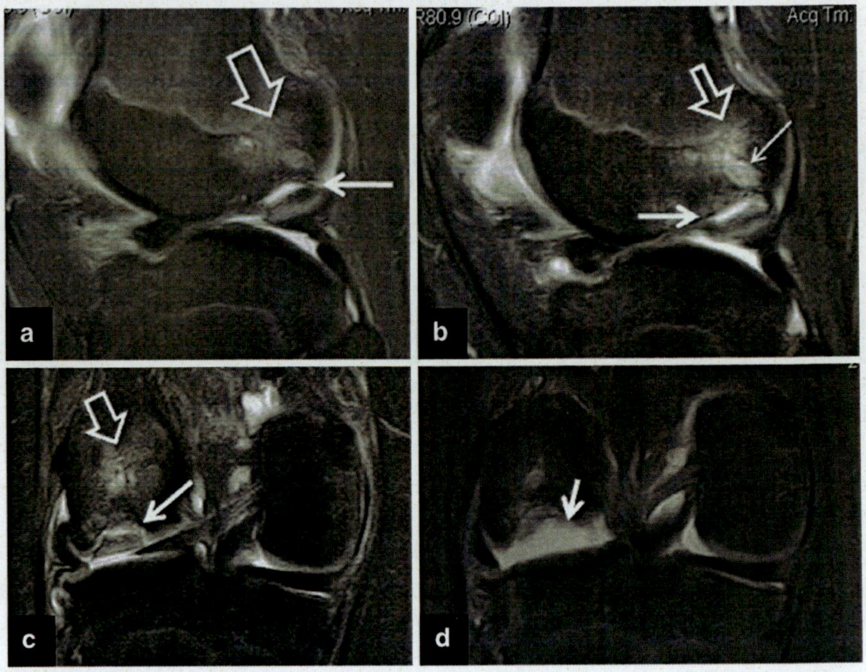

Fig. 28 Unstable osteochondritis dissecans in a 15-year-old football player. The sagittal (**a**, **b**) and coronal (**c**) fat suppressed PD-w MR images, show the osteochondral fragment surrounded by fluid (*arrows*). There is also bone marrow edema (*open arrows*) and cyst formation deep in the subchondral bone (*thin arrow*). As the bone marrow was still viable, the clinicians suggested rest and conservative treatment. The athlete did not reduce the athletic activities and 3 months later the fragment was detached (*arrow* in **d**)

be misinterpreted. The three categories of acute myotendinous injury include muscle contusion, myotendinous strain, and tendon rupture. *Contusions* typically result from direct trauma and exhibit intramuscular edema and hemorrhage at MR imaging. Ultrasonography is able to depict such lesions by demonstrating edema and hemorrhage. *Myotendinous strains* are associated with inadequate warm-up, previous injuries, overuse and irregular surface. They are classified as grade I (stretch injury), grade II (partial tear), and grade III (complete rupture). MR imaging demonstrates high signal edema on T2-w and STIR images at the myotendinous junction, as well as associated hemorrhage (Figs. 4 and 29). Third-degree lesions with myotendinous rupture and tendon retraction can have a mass-like presentation on physical examination. MR imaging demonstrates the edema, hemorrhage, and the location of the retracted tendon, thus assisting operative repair (Bencardino et al. 2000; Palmer et al. 1999).

Myositis ossificans may complicate moderate and severe muscle contusions affecting athletes in the second decade and radiologically becomes apparent 2–4 weeks after injury. This complication is rarely seen in the knee joint region.

5.2 Ligamentous Injuries

5.2.1 Anterior Cruciate Ligament Injuries

ACL injuries were traditionally considered to be rare in children and adolescents with still open physis. Currently, there is an increase in these injuries, because children are involved in high intensity athletic activities at a younger age. In children younger than 11 years, tibial spine fracture is more common and after 12 years ACL injury far exceeds it in frequency (Vaquero et al. 2005). ACL injuries are encountered more frequently in boys, but as the skeleton matures, girls are affected more often (Prince et al. 2005). The mechanism of injury is a flexion, twisting, or hyperextension injury with immediate pain and haemarthrosis. ACL sprain is commonly associated with MCL sprains and meniscal tears. The patterns of ACL injury depend on the degree of skeletal maturity. Complete ACL tears have been described to be more common in the partially and fully mature groups.

Radiographs are not routinely used for suspected ACL injuries. However, in skeletally immature patients, due to the imbalance between ligaments and epiphyseal strength, a lateral radiograph may show avulsion of the tibial eminence where the ACL attaches. Since the clinical tests are as effective as MR imaging, the latter is performed mostly for depicting associated lesions.

The primary findings for ACL tear include abnormal signal intensity, abnormal course defined as a Blumensaat angle greater then 9.5°, and discontinuity (Figs. 3, 8, 20, and 30). Bone bruise, anterior tibial displacement (>5 mm compared to femur), uncovered posterior horn of lateral meniscus, PCL buckling (angle < 105°) and an abnormal posterior cruciate line (parallel to the distal PCL, not dissecting the medullary cavity within the distal 5 cm of the femur) are among the secondary findings. Bone bruising is the most important secondary sign (Brandser et al. 1996). The sensitivity of MR imaging for the diagnosis of an ACL tear in children, has been reported to be 95% and the specificity 88%, when based on both the primary and secondary findings (Lee and Yao 1988). Prevalence of bone bruises in children with ACL injuries appears to range from 70 to 80% which is similar to that reported

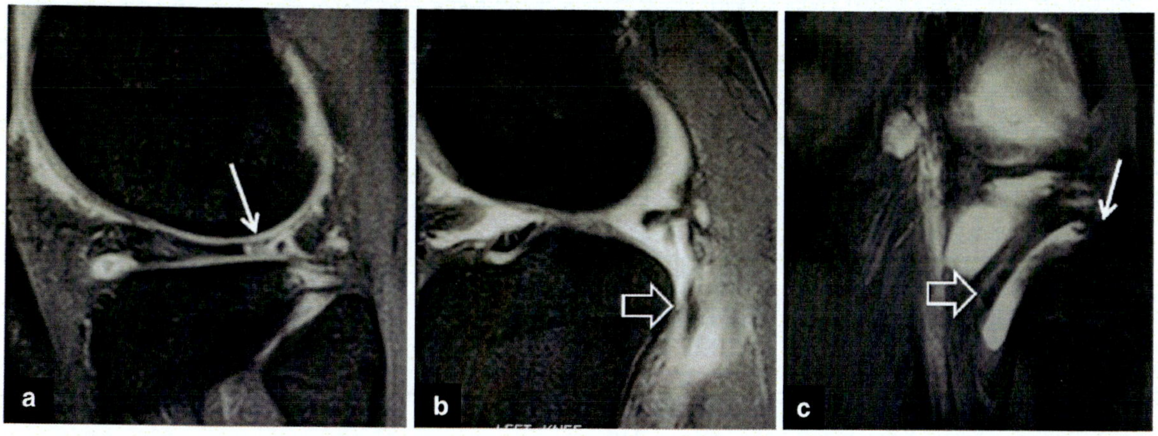

Fig. 29 A 16-year-old football player with a history of a hyperextension knee injury during football and resulting posterolateral corner injury. The sagittal MEDIC MR images, show lateral meniscal tear (*arrow* in **a**) and grade II popliteal musculotendinous strain (*open arrow* in **b**). (**c**) The coronal fat-suppressed PD-w TSE MR image demonstrates fluid surrounding the popliteal tendon which shows increased signal intensity in keeping with a grade II strain (*open arrow*). The popliteofibular ligament is intact (*thin arrow*)

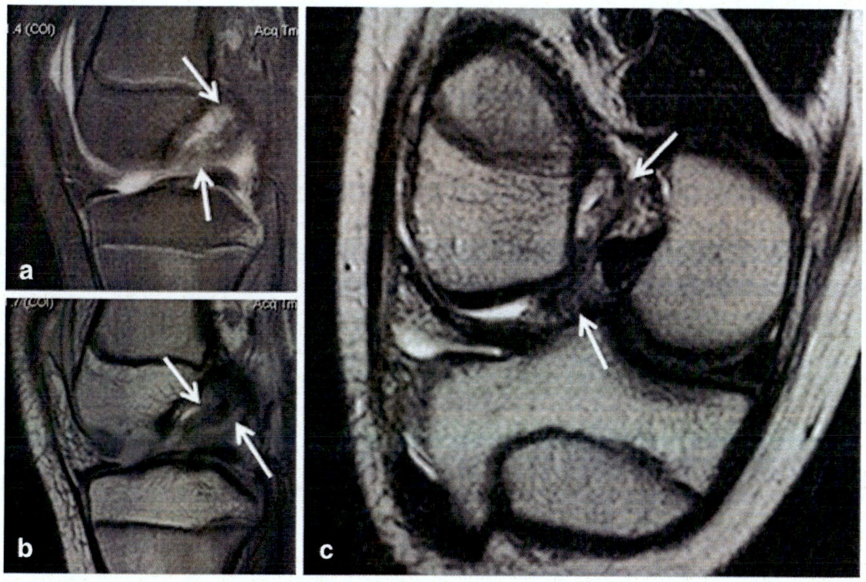

Fig. 30 A 12-year-old girl who sustained a twisting injury during a basketball game, 2 days before imaging. The sagittal fat suppressed intermediate-w (**a**) and PD-w (**b**) TSE MR images, show swollen and edematous anterior cruciate ligament which has an abnormal course, particularly at its proximal insertion (*arrows*). (**c**) The high resolution oblique axial (parallel to the presumed course of the ligament) T2-w TSE MR image, shows to better advantage the torn ligament which has a wavy appearance with attenuated fibers (*arrow*)

for adults. Regarding associated findings, it seems that medial meniscal tears are more common than lateral, as in adults, but with a lower prevalence. Other associated lesions as well as secondary signs in favor of a diagnosis of ACL tear, are probably as common as in adults (Prince et al. 2005). In general, a potential source of false-negative MR imaging for ACL tear, is the delay between the injury and imaging.

Differentiation of partial from complete tears with MR imaging might be difficult. It has been suggested that the absence of bone bruising may indicate a partial ACL tear. In one study, bone bruising of the postero-lateral tibia (94%) and lateral femoral condyle (91%) was common with complete tears, whereas only 17% of patients with partial tears had bone bruises. In addition, 80% of partial tears with bone bruises are high-grade injuries that lead to complete rupture within 6 months (Zeiss et al. 1995).

5.2.2 Posterior Cruciate Ligament Injuries

Injury of the PCL is uncommon in children. The most common mechanism of injury is posterior displacement of the tibia in a flexed knee and hyperextension. MR imaging findings of PCL injury include complete rupture, intrasubstance abnormal signal intensity, and avulsion of the insertion site (Fig. 1). Avulsion fractures are best evaluated with CT (Fig. 9). Meniscal injuries are commonly seen. Associated bone marrow edema may reflect the mechanism of injury (Sonin et al. 1995).

5.2.3 Lateral Collateral Ligament Injuries

Injuries of the lateral collateral ligament (LCL) are uncommonly diagnosed in the pediatric population. MR imaging findings of LCL injury include discontinuity, morphologic disruption, increased intrasubstance signal, and loss of demarcation between the ligament and adjacent fat. LCL injuries are usually associated with injury to the cruciate ligaments and to other postero-lateral corner structures (Figs. 4 and 29) (King et al. 1996).

5.2.4 Medial Collateral Ligament Injuries

MCL injuries occur from a valgus stress to an extended knee while the foot is planted or from a direct blow to the lateral aspect of the joint. Skiers are mostly prone to MCL injury. MR imaging is required mainly for depicting concurrent injuries of the menisci and/or ACL. The possibility of a distal femoral epiphyseal injury is the primary reason to consider radiographs as part of the evaluation of medial knee instability.

MCL injuries seen on MRI can be graded as a sprain (grade 1), a partial tear (grade 2), or a complete tear (grade 3). The MR findings of MCL injury are similar to those described for LCL (Figs. 1, 3, and 4). The location of the bone bruising in patients with MCL injury is usually located on the lateral side of the knee joint (Yao et al. 1994).

6 Various Disorders: Incidental Findings

MR imaging may depict other irrelevant pathology in athletes with locking or painful in general symptoms (Figs. 31 and 32). Pigmented villonodular synovitis may present with local or diffuse form and often symptoms are related to recurrent joint effusions. The application of T2* MR sequences enhances the diagnostic confidence as it reduces the signal from the lesions due to magnetic susceptibility effects of haemosiderin. Gaglion cysts and synovial hemangiomas may rarely occur in this age group. Finally, known or previously undiagnosed osteochondromas, may result during sports activities in repetitive injuries over the popliteal artery.

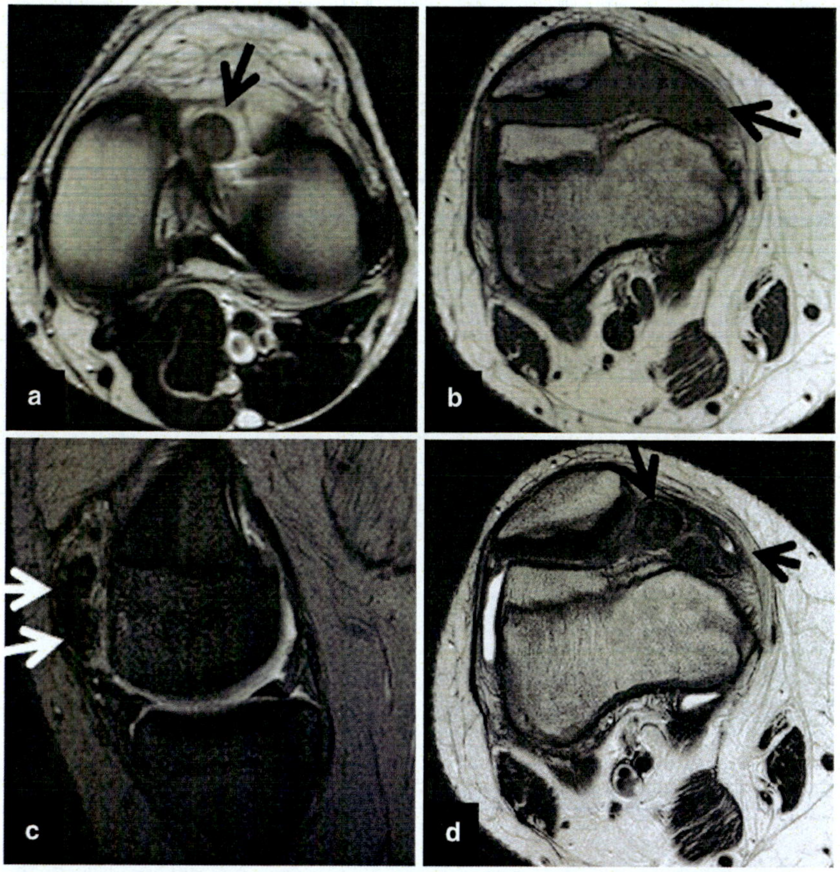

Fig. 31 Two athletes with a final histologic diagnosis of pigmented vilonodular synovitis (PVNS). (**a**) A 16-year-old football player with limited extension in the left knee, shows on the axial T2-w MR image, a round lesion of intermediate signal intensity in the anterior joint space (*arrow*), in keeping with focal PVNS. A 14-year-old male tennis player with swelling and pain of his right knee joint, mainly during playing. The axial T1-w (**b**), sagittal T2* (**c**) and axial T2-w (**d**) MR images, show a diffuse mass into the medial joint space (*arrows*), with lower signal intensity on T2 and T2* compared to T1-w MR images, in keeping with diffuse PVNS

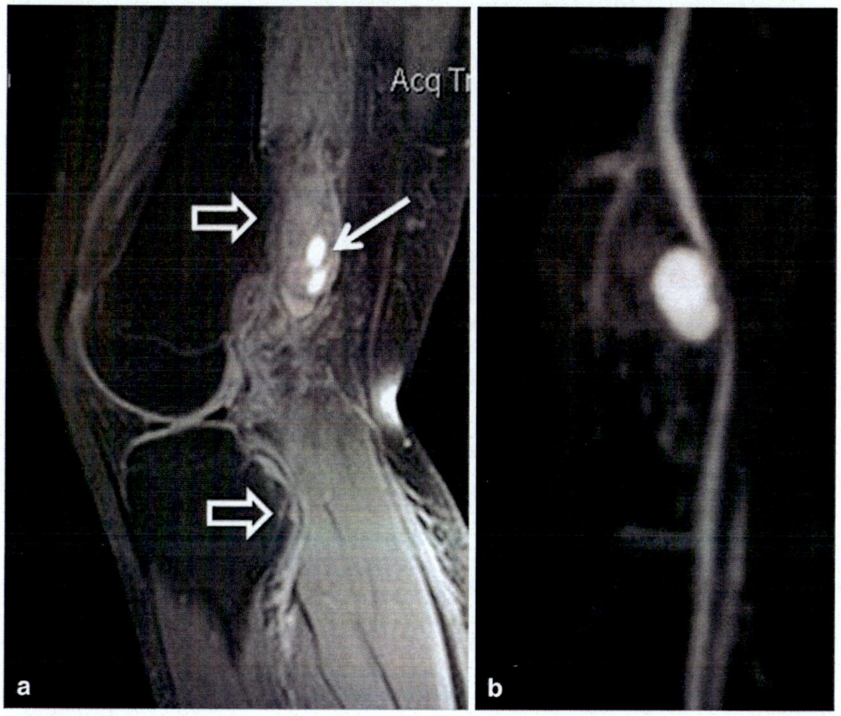

Fig. 32 A 14-year-old female track athlete, with known hereditary multiple osteochondromatosis. During exercise, the girl felt sudden pain in the popliteal fossa. (**a**) The sagittal fat suppressed T1-w MR image shows osteochondromas in the posterior distal femoral metaphysis and posterior proximal tibia (*open arrows*). A cavity with fresh blood is seen, demonstrating high signal intensity (*arrow*). (**b**) The MIP from a 3D T1-w arteriography following bolus injection of contrast medium shows an aneurysm of the popliteal artery. A rupture of the popliteal artery was confirmed at surgery

References

Anderson MW, Greenspan A (1996) Stress fractures. Radiology 199(1):1–12

Al-Otaibi L, Siegel MJ (1998) The pediatric knee. Magn Reson Imaging Clin N Am 6(3):643–660

Bencardino JT, Rosenberg ZS, Brown RR, Hassankhani A, Lustrin ES, Beltran J (2000) Traumatic musculotendinous injuries of the knee: diagnosis with MR imaging. Radiographics 20:S103–S120

Bharam S, Vrahas MS, Fu FH (2002) Knee fractures in the athlete. Orthop Clin North Am 33(3):565–574

Brandser EA, Riley MA, Berbaum KS, el-Khoury GY, Bennett DL (1996) MR imaging of anterior cruciate ligament injury: independent value of primary and secondary signs. AJR Am J Roentgenol 167(1):121–126

Brittberg M, Lindahl A, Nilsson A, Ohlsson C, Isaksson O, Peterson L (1994) Treatment of deep cartilage defects in the knee with autologous chondrocyte transplantation. N Engl J Med 331(14):889–895

Bruijn JD, Sanders RJ, Jansen BR (1993) Ossification in the patellar tendon and patella alta following sports injuries in children. Complications of sleeve fractures after conservative treatment. Arch Orthop Trauma Surg 112(3):157–158

Busch MT (1990) Meniscal injuries in children and adolescents. Clin Sports Med 9(3):661–680

Carr KE (2003) Musculoskeletal injuries in young athletes. Clin Fam Pract 5(2):385–415

Carty H (1994) Sports injuries in children-a radiological viewpoint. Arch Dis Child 70(6):457–460

Coady CM, Micheli LJ (1997) Stress fractures in the pediatric athlete. Clin Sports Med 16(2):225–238

Conaghan PG (2002) Update on osteoarthritis part 1: current concepts and the relation to exercise. Br J Sports Med 36(5):330–333

Cothran RL Jr, Major NM, Helms CA, Higgins LD (2001) MR imaging of meniscal contusion in the knee. AJR Am J Roentgenol 177(5):1189–1192

Courtenay BG, Bowers DM (1990) Stress fractures: clinical features and investigation. Med J Aust 153(3):155–156

Ecklund K, Jaramillo D (2001) Imaging of growth disturbance in children. Radiol Clin North Am 39(4):823–841

Fredericson M, Bergman AG, Hoffman KL, Dillingham MS (1995) Tibial stress reaction in runners. Correlation of clinical symptoms and scintigraphy with a new magnetic resonance imaging grading system. Am J Sports Med 23(4):472–481

Hantes ME, Zachos VC, Zibis AH et al (2004) Evaluation of meniscal repair with serial magnetic resonance imaging: a comparative study between conventional MRI and indirect MR arthrography. Eur J Radiol 50(3):231–237

Harvey JS Jr (1982) Overuse syndromes in young athletes. Pediatr Clin North Am 29(6):1369–1381

Ho VB, Kransdorf MJ, Jelinek JS, Kim CK (1991) Dorsal defect of the patella: MR features. J Comput Assist Tomogr 15(3): 474–476

Iobst CA, Stanitski CL (2000) Acute knee injuries. Clin Sports Med 19(4):621–635

Kaplan PA, Gehl RH, Dussault RG, Anderson MW, Diduch DR (1999) Bone contusions of the posterior lip of the medial tibial plateau (contrecoup injury) and associated internal derangements of the knee at MR imaging. Radiology 211(3): 747–753

Kapleov SR, Teresi LM, Bradley WG et al (1993) Bone contusions of the knee: increased lesion detection with fast spin-echo MR imaging with spectroscopic fat saturation. Radiology 189(3):901–904

Kijowski R, Blankenbaker DG, Shinki K, Fine JP, Graf BK, De Smet AA (2008) Juvenile versus adult osteochondritis dissecans of the knee: appropriate MR imaging criteria for instability. Radiology 248(2):571–578

King SJ, Carty HM, Brady O (1996) Magnetic resonance imaging of knee injuries in children. Pediatr Radiol 26(4):287–290

Kocher MS, Micheli LJ, Gerbino P, Hresko MT (2003) Tibial eminence fractures in children: prevalence of meniscal entrapment. Am J Sports Med 31(3):404–407

Kocher MS, Mandiga R, Klingele K, Bley L, Micheli LJ (2004) Anterior cruciate ligament injury versus tibial spine fracture in the skeletally immature knee: a comparison of skeletal maturation and notch width index. J Pediatr Orthop 24(2):185–188

Laor T, Wall EJ, Vu LP (2006) Physeal widening in the knee due to stress injury in child athletes. AJR Am J Roentgenol 186(5):1260–1264

Lee JK, Yao L (1988) Stress fractures: MR imaging. Radiology 169(1):217–220

Maguire JK, Canale ST (1993) Fractures of the patella in children and adolescents. J Pediatr Orthop 13(5):567–571

Mandalia V, Fogg AJ, Chari R, Murray J, Beale A, Henson JH (2005) Bone bruising of the knee. Clin Radiol 60(6):627–636

Mann DC, Rajmaira S (1990) Distribution of physeal and nonphyseal fractures in 2,560 long-bone fractures in children aged 0–16 years. J Pediatr Orthop 10(6):713–716

Maripuri SN, Mehta H, Mohanty K (2008) Sleeve fracture of the superior pole of the patella with an intra-articular dislocation. A case report. J Bone Joint Surg Am 90(2):385–389

Moran M, Macnicol M (2006) Paediatric epiphyseal fractures around the knee. Curr Orthop 20(4):256–265

Oeppen RS, Connolly SA, Bencardino JD, Jaramillo D (2004) Acute injury of the articular cartilage and subchondral bone: a common but unrecognized lesion in the immature knee. AJR Am J Roentgenol 182(1):111–117

Ogden JA, Tross RB, Murphy MJ (1980) Fractures of the tibial tuberosity in adolescents. J Bone Joint Surg Am 62(2): 205–215

Ogden JA (1984) Growth slowdown and arrest lines. J Pediatr Orthop 4(4):409–415

Outerbridge AR, Micheli LJ (1995) Overuse injuries in the young athlete. Clin Sports Med 14(3):503–516

Palmer WE, Kuong SJ, Elmadbouh HM (1999) MR imaging of myotendinous strain. AJR Am J Roentgenol 173(3):703–709

Prince JS, Laor T, Bean JA (2005) MRI of anterior cruciate ligament injuries and associated findings in the pediatric knee: changes with skeletal maturation. AJR Am J Roentgenol 185(3):756–762

Raissaki M, Apostolaki E, Karantanas AH (2007) Imaging of sports injuries in children and adolescents. Eur J Radiol 62(1):86–96

Ray JM, Hendrix J (1992) Incidence, mechanism of injury, and treatment of fractures of the patella in children. J Trauma 32(4):464–467

Sanders TG, Medynski MA, Feller JF, Lawhorn KW (2000) Bone contusion pattern of the knee at MR imaging: footprint of the mechanism of injury. Radiographics 20:S135–S151
Siow HM, Cameron DB, Ganley TJ (2008) Acute knee injuries in skeletally immature athletes. Phys Med Rehabil Clin N Am 19(2):319–345
Smith AD, Tao SS (1995) Knee injuries in young athletes. Clin Sports Med 14(3):629–650
Sonin AH, Fitzgerald SW, Hoff FL, Friedman H, Bresler ME (1995) MR imaging of the posterior cruciate ligament: normal, abnormal, and associated injury patterns. Radiographics 15(3):551–561
Takeda Y, Ikata T, Yoshida S, Takai H, Kashiwaguchi S (1998) MRI high-signal intensity in the menisci of asymptomatic children. J Bone Joint Surg Br 80(3):463–467
Vaquero J, Vidal C, Cubillo A (2005) Intra-articular traumatic disorders of the knee in children and adolescents. Clin Orthop Relat Res 432:97–106
Wall EJ (1998) Osgood-Schlätter disease: practical treatment for a self-limited condition. Phys Sport Med 26:29–34
Watson-Jones R (1955) Fractures and joint injuries, 4th edn. Lippincott Williams & Wilkins, Philadelphia
Yao L, Dungan D, Seeger LL (1994) MR imaging of tibial collateral ligament injury: comparison with clinical examination. Skeletal Radiol 23(7):521–524
Zeiss J, Paley K, Murray K, Saddemi SR (1995) Comparison of bone contusion seen by MRI in partial and complete tears of the anterior cruciate ligament. J Comput Assist Tomogr 19(5):773–776

Ankle and Foot

Khaldoun Koujok, Eoghan E. Laffan, and Mark E. Schweitzer

Contents

Abstract

- This chapter reviews the common and uncommon injuries of the ankle and foot in children and adolescents in sport.
- The ankle is the most commonly injured body part during sport, with ankle sprains being the most injury seen. They are estimated to account for 20% of all sports injuries in the USA. Prevalence is highest in basketball, ice skating and soccer. The differences between injuries in children, due to the unfused physes, and adults is discussed. Ligamentous injuries are reviewed. Normal, physiologic MR signal patterns around the ankle are mentioned. The Ottawa ankle and foot rules regarding radiography in ankle and foot injuries are explained. Other injuries that are reviewed include osteochondral lesions, in particular the talus, hindfoot fractures, physeal bar and osteochondroses (Sever, Kohler, Freiberg, Mueller-Weiss). Lastly, tarsal coalition, an abnormal, congenital union between bones of the hind and midfoot are discussed.

K. Koujok
Assistant Professor of Radiology, University of Ottawa
Pediatric Radiologist, Children's Hospital of Eastern Ontario Ottawa, Canada
e-mail: kkoujok@cheo.on.ca

E. Laffan
Consultant Paediatric Radiologist,
Children's University Hospital,
Temple Street, Dublin 1, Ireland
e-mail: eoghan.laffan@cuh.ie

M.E. Schweitzer (✉)
Chief of Diagnostic Imaging,
The Ottawa Hospital,
Chair of Radiology,
Professor of Radiology,
The University of Ottawa
e-mail: mschweitzer@toh.on.ca

1 The Ankle

The ankle is the most commonly injured body part during sport, with ankle sprains being the most common injury seen. They are estimated to account for 20% of all sport injuries in the USA (Ivins 2006). Prevalence is highest in basketball, ice skating, and soccer. The most common mechanism is usually a "rollover" or lateral ankle sprain, the ankle in a plantarflexed and inverted position.

A.H. Karantanas (ed.), *Sports Injuries in Children and Adolescents*,
Med Radiol Diagn Imaging, DOI: 10.1007/174_2010_129, © Springer-Verlag Berlin Heidelberg 2011

The most common ligaments involved are the anterior talofibular ligament (ATFL), calcaneofibular ligament (CFL), and posterior talofibular ligament (PTFL). The ATFL is the most commonly torn and often the only ligament affected, as it is the weakest one. The CFL is next and is almost always seen with an associated ATFL (20% of ATFL ruptures have CFL involvement). The PTFL is rarely involved. Most sprains never require imaging and can be treated conservatively.

In the acute setting, the Ottawa ankle and foot rules should be applied to avoid unnecessary radiography in children and adolescents (Bachmann et al. 2003). Ankle radiographs are only indicated if there is pain in the malleolar zones and if there is one of the following two criteria: the child cannot weight-bear (four steps) immediately after the injury, or if there is point tenderness over the posterior edge of either malleolus. Foot radiographs are indicated if the patient has pain in the midfoot or there is one of the following criteria: bony tenderness over the navicular or base of fifth metatarsal, or inability to weight-bear (four steps).

Due to the unfused physes, Salter–Harris type I and II injuries are disproportionately common when compared with isolated ligament injuries. These fractures can be difficult to diagnose on plain radiography, but should always be suspected in the young ankle. Consequently, lateral soft tissue swelling is also an indication for plain radiographs. Although two views are now considered sufficient in adults (lateral and mortise views), this has not yet been scientifically established in children (Brage et al. 1998; De Smet et al. 1999).

MR should be considered in chronic injuries or instability to diagnose unsuspected abnormalities (such as osteochondral defects) or to aid treatment planning. Complete tears of the ATFL and CFL are associated with instability. The ATFL is easily recognized on axial imaging as a uniform low-signal thin band running from the anterior aspect of the fibula to the talus. The PTFL is seen on the same axial images as thin or striated band extending from the posterior aspect of the talus to the inner aspect of the distal fibula. The CFL is slightly harder to visualize as it runs obliquely from the calcaneus to the tip of the fibula deep to the peroneal tendons. Partial tears are recognized by high T2 signal within the ligament, with more chronic tears associated with thickening of the ligament. Complete tears are diagnosed by absence of the ligament in its expected location.

Care should be taken not to confuse normal high T2 signal changes around the foot and ankle in children, representing hematopoietic marrow, as pathologic bone marrow edema. The pattern is usually symmetric, most commonly in the calcaneus, talus, and navicular and is almost always endosteal and likely represents normal growth (Shabshin et al. 2006). A more diffuse pattern of abnormal marrow signal is seen in even younger patients and represents hematopoietic marrow.

1.1 Osteochondral Lesions

Osteochondral lesions (OCL) in the ankle are much more commonly seen in children as compared to adults. It is generally regarded as a post-traumatic lesion. Initial radiographs may be normal but an OCL should be considered in any ankle with a history of trauma and chronic pain and decreased function. Failure to diagnose and treat OCLs can lead to a stable fragment becoming unstable, greater joint dysfunction, and possibly premature osteoarthritis (Schachter et al. 2005; Naran and Zoga 2008). Medial lesions are more common than lateral lesions and both are most commonly seen at the apex of the dome (Elias et al. 2007). In the talus medial OCLs are posterior, while lateral ones are closer to the midline. They can also be bilateral in up to 30%. Medial OCLs are more often the result of repetitive injury than ones located laterally.

OCLs can also be seen elsewhere in the ankle and foot, such as the talar head, tibial plafond, cuboid, navicular, subtalar joint, and the metatarsal heads (seen in ballerinas) (Naran and Zoga 2008). MRI is the most sensitive modality for detecting and staging OCLs. Various staging classifications are reported, but the precise stage is not as important as detecting the stability of the OCL, since treatment of unstable lesions is rather different (Anderson et al. 1989). Initial imaging shows a small focus of subchondral trabecular compression, with associated bone marrow edema (Fig. 1). Fluid-like signal between the parent bone or donor site and the fragment is a direct sign of an unstable fragment (Fig. 2) (De Smet et al. 1990). Indirect signs of instability include cystic change at the donor site, marked bone marrow edema, and interval collapse of the articular surface (De Smet et al. 1990). Direct MR arthrography helps to clarify

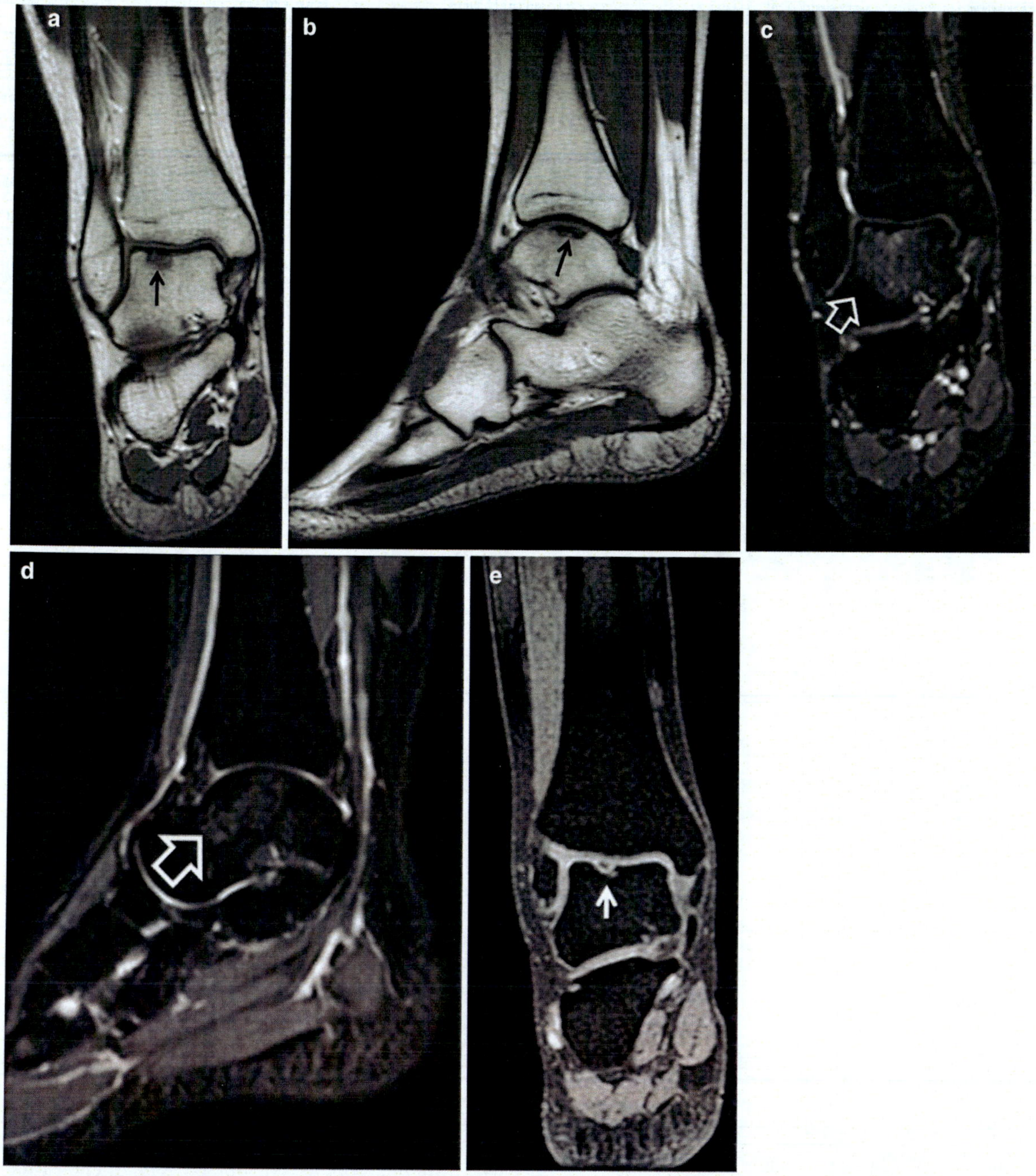

Fig. 1 (**a–e**) Coronal and sagittal T1, coronal and sagittal short tau inversion recovery (STIR) and coronal spoiled gradient echo (SPGR) imaging in a 16-year-old male with chronic ankle pain. There is a stable osteochondral defect of the lateral talar dome (*arrows*). The overlying cartilage appears intact. There is bone edema in the talus (*open arrows*), but there is no rim of high signal surrounding the lesion, cyst formation, or loose body to suggest instability

difficult cases, although is not usually needed for staging (Cerezal et al. 2008).

Stable lesions are usually immobilized with a cast for at least 1 month, whereas unstable lesions are treated surgically, with internal fixation and removal of any loose cartilage or debris. The use of allo- or autografts is becoming more common (Zengerink et al. 2010), as is the use of various cartilage transplant procedures.

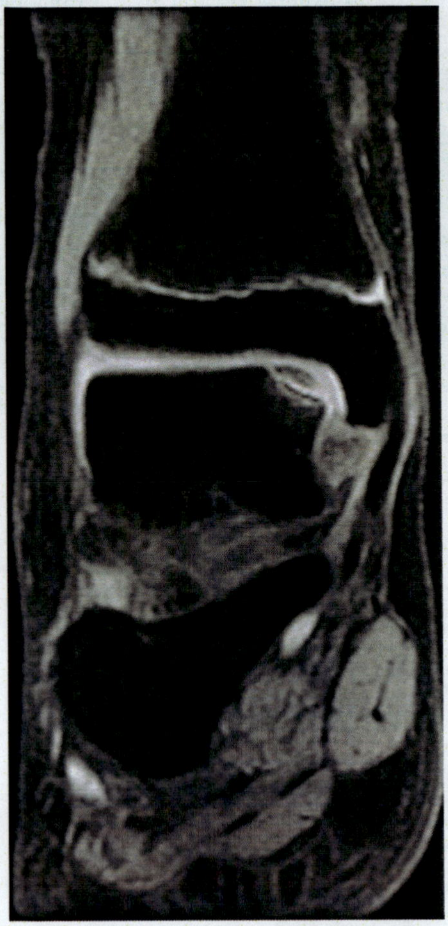

Fig. 2 Osteochondral lesion of the talus. A 12-year-old girl with a lesion of the medial aspect of the talar dome. Note the high-signal-intensity line beneath the osteochondritis dissecans, which is the most common sign of instability on MR

2 Hindfoot Fractures

Fracture of the anterior process of the calcaneus is not uncommon, and is frequently one of the occult fractures seen with ankle sprains (Figs. 3–5). It can also be seen in children with calcaneonavicular coalitions and injuries. Other occult fractures in ankle sprains are less common but occasionally involve the navicular or cuboid.

3 Physeal Bars

Fractures involving the as yet unfused physis in a child can lead to a bridging or physeal bar. This is an abnormal connection of the epiphysis and metaphysis and can be fibrous or osseous. Premature fusion results in asymmetric or halted growth of the affected limb. The lower limbs are most commonly involved, especially the distal tibia anteromedially (Ecklund and Jaramillo 2002). This region is thought to be more prone to bars due to an area known as Kump's bump, a focal wavy contour of the physis here (Ecklund and Jaramillo 2001). Bars can be suspected clinically with asymmetric leg lengths, with or without a history of trauma. They can be visible on plain radiography as focal fusion of the physis. CT and MRI can also accurately depict bars, MRI considered more advantageous due to its lack of ionizing radiation and its ability to detect both acute bars, which contain granulation tissue, and subacute and chronic bars, which consist of fibrous and osseous lesions (Loder et al. 1997). Treatment depends on the percentage of physis involved and skeletal maturity at the time of diagnosis. Resection of the bar is considered if there is less than 50% physeal involvement and/or more than 2 years left of growth.

4 Osteochondrosis

Osteochondrosis refers to any of a group of disorders involving one or more centers of ossification of the bones in children and characterized by degeneration or avascular necrosis followed by reossification (*Stedman's Medical Dictionary*, 26th edition). They have been reported since 1903. What they really refer to is an imaging appearance and a time of first discovery. The former being fragmentation and irregularity usually of an epiphysis or apophysis; the later being the first 2 decades of the twentieth century.

Approximately 40 different osteochondroses have been described. Although these disorders present with similar imaging findings there are three different pathogeneses. One is a normal variant in ossification which by definition is self-limited. This includes the majority of Kohler's diseases, Sever's disease, as well as Van Neck's disease in the pelvis. A second category includes true avascular necrosis such as Legg–Calvé–Perthes disease, Keinbocks disease, Freiberg's infraction, Preisser's syndrome, Panner's, and some patients with Kohler's. The last category is overuse conditions such as Sever's disease, Osgood–Schlatter, Sinding–Larsen–Johansson, and Scheuermann's disease, Blount disease and Panner's diseases.

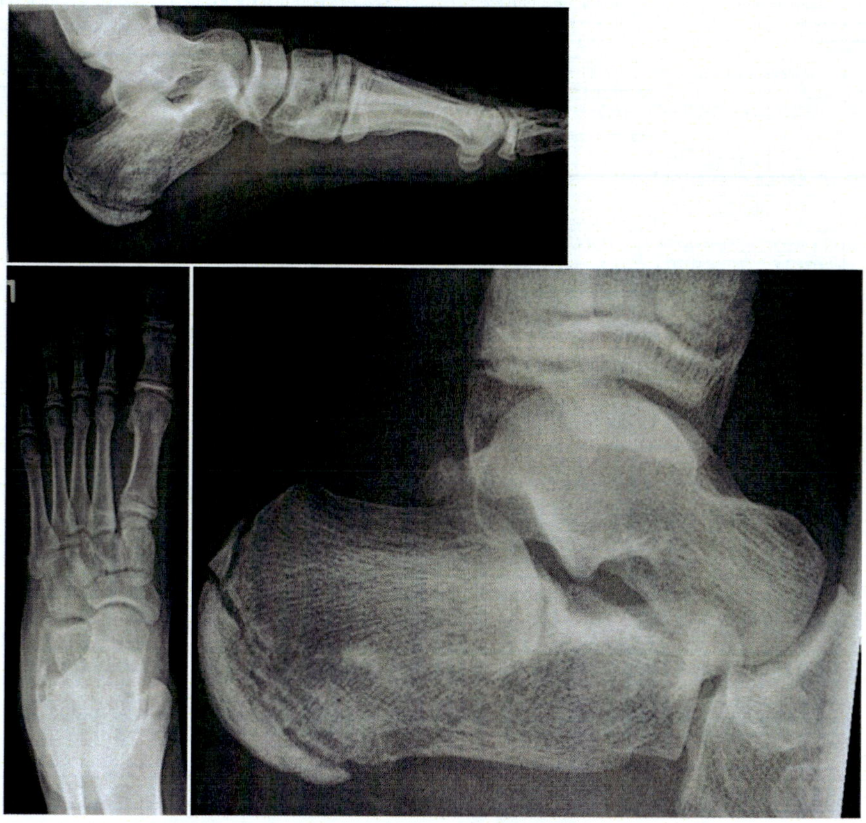

Fig. 3 Lateral and DP radiographs of the foot and lateral radiograph of the calcaneus show a fracture through the body of the calcaneus, extending to the sustentaculum tali

4.1 Sever's Disease

Also known as calcaneal apophysitis, Sever's disease or osteochondrosis of the calcaneus is the most common cause of heel pain in athletes 5–11 years (Cassas and Cassettari-Wayhs 2006). This traction apophysitis is caused by repetitive microtrauma at the bone cartilage-junction or overuse of the heel at the insertion of the Achilles tendon and plantar fascia (Adirim and Cheng 2003; Cassas and Cassettari-Wayhs 2006). It is commonly seen in athletes participating in basketball, soccer, track, and other running activities (Cassas and Cassettari-Wayhs 2006). These children have tenderness over the posterior aspect of their heel and dorsiflexion at the ankle is limited (Adirim and Cheng 2003). Sever's disease cannot be diagnosed radiographically, although marrow edema at the physis is seen by MR (Fig. 6). The condition usually resolves 2 weeks to 2 months after the initiation of conservative treatment, which may include rest, ice application, heel lifts, stretching and strengthening exercises, and, in more severe cases, nonsteroidal anti-inflammatory drugs (Madden and Mellion 1996).

Sever's disease must be differentiated clinically from asymptomatic radiographic changes. The calcaneal apophysis normally is more sclerotic than the calcaneus on the lateral view and it is commonly fragmented (Fig. 7). In non-ambulating patients, such as cerebral palsy, the density of the calcaneal apophysis is similar to the calcaneus. When a normal child breaks his lower extremity and does not bear weight, the apophysis becomes of similar density to the calcaneus and returns to be sclerotic when the child resumes his weight-bearing activities.

4.2 Köhler's Disease

This is a rare osteochondrosis of the tarsal navicular, tends to affect children from 3 to 10 years and is usually unilateral (Figs. 8 and 9). Köhler's disease is far more common in boys than in girls; however, girls

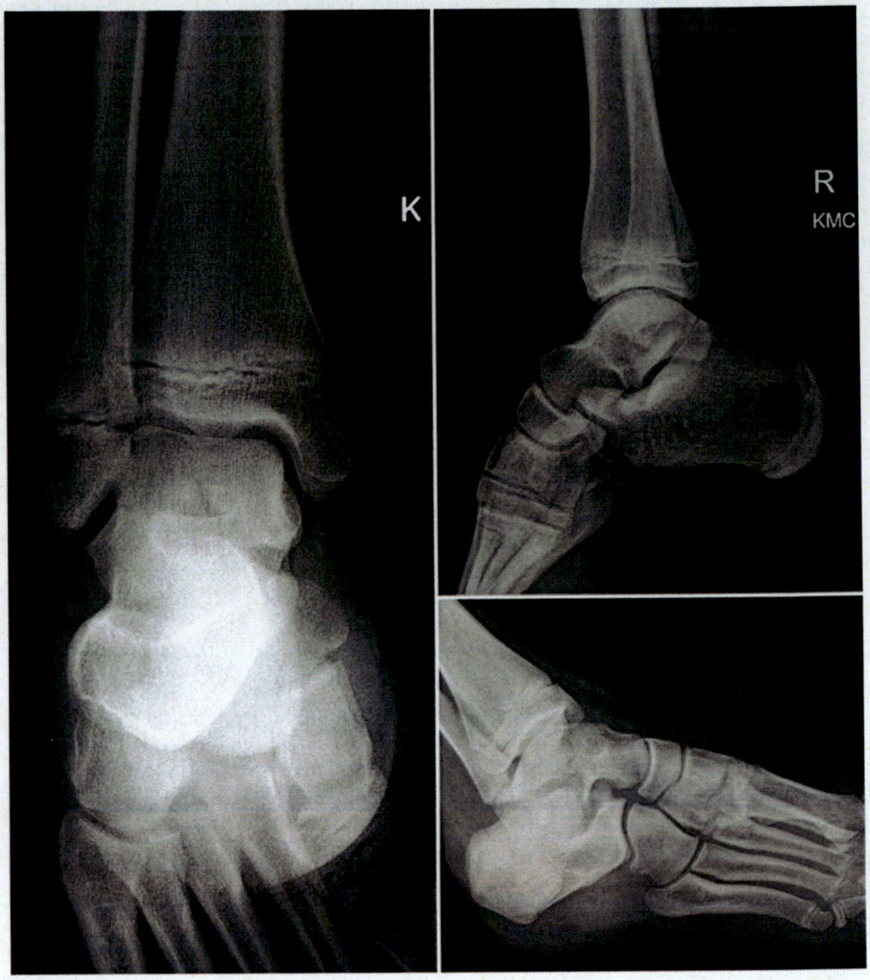

Fig. 4 Mortise, lateral, and oblique radiographs of the ankle. There is a vertical fracture through the dome of the talus. On the mortise view, the fracture looks comminuted, but undisplaced

with this condition are often younger than are boys with the disease (Cox 1958). Children present with local tenderness on the medial side of the foot in the area of the navicular. It is a benign, self-limited disease. The treatment is indicated on the basis of the symptoms and the prognosis is excellent. Disability or degenerative changes in the tarsal joints are not present at long-term follow-up as shown by Borges et al. who followed their patients on average for 31 years (24–44 years) (Borges et al. 1995).

The diagnosis may be missed because of the usual mild clinical symptoms and the difficulty in distinguishing the radiographic findings from the normal changes of bone growth. Köhler's disease must be differentiated clinically from asymptomatic radiographic changes resembling Köhler's osteochondrosis. The only imaging way to definitively differentiate true avascular necrosis from the normal variant is to have a normal radiograph that becomes abnormal on follow-up.

4.3 Freiberg Infarction

Freiberg infarction is a disorder affecting the metatarsal head (usually the second or third) and is characterized at pathologic analysis by collapse of the subchondral bone, osteonecrosis, and cartilaginous fissures. The cause of Freiberg infraction is controversial and is probably multifactorial. A traumatic insult in the form of either acute or repetitive injury and vascular compromise are the most popular theories. Freiberg infraction is much more common in women and usually manifests during adolescence. High-heeled shoes have been implicated as a causative factor (Zengerink et al. 2010).

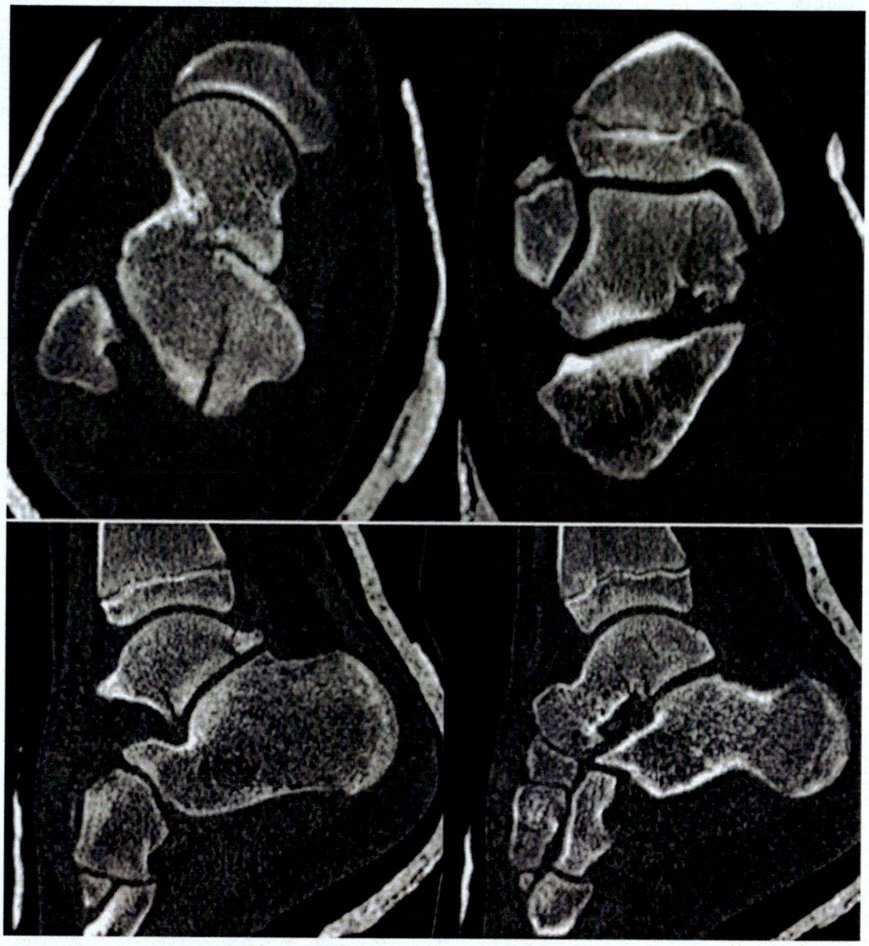

Fig. 5 Same patient as in Fig. 4. Axial, coronal, and two sagittal images confirm the comminuted fracture through the talus, extending to the ankle joint superiorly and the talocalcaneal joint inferiorly. No step defect is seen in either joint

Patients may present with pain and limited motion, although symptoms may not begin until degenerative arthrosis has developed.

Radiographically there is flattening of the metatarsal head, occasional sclerosis, and rare fragmentation (Fig. 10). It should be noted that most patients who as adolescents or adults have flattening of the metatarsal head probably never had Freiberg's as there seems to be variation in the convexity of the metatarsal heads.

Early MR imaging findings include low-signal intensity changes in the metatarsal head on T1-w images with increased signal intensity on corresponding T2-w and STIR images (De Smet et al. 1999). These changes are nonspecific and may also be seen in a stress response of the metatarsal head. There may in fact be overlap between these conditions (Elias et al. 2007). With disease progression, flattening of the metatarsal head occurs, and low-signal intensity changes, optimally crescentic develop on T2-w images as the bone becomes sclerotic.

4.4 Müeller–Weiss Disease

It is a rare condition characterized by spontaneous atraumatic osteonecrosis of the tarsal navicular bone in adults. This is the adult analogue of true Kohler's. It is often bilateral and it occurs predominantly in women (Haller et al. 1988). Müeller–Weiss disease is a debilitating condition and differs from the benign self-limiting Köhler disease occurring in children. The cause is unknown; patients may have severe and sometimes devastating pain, disability, and progressive deformity. On radiographs, odd deformation of the tarsal navicular is apparent with medial or dorsal protrusion of part or all of the navicular bone and a comma-shaped deformity due to collapse of the lateral portion of the bone. The navicular appears squeezed and occasionally fragmented between the talar head and the lateral cuneiforms.

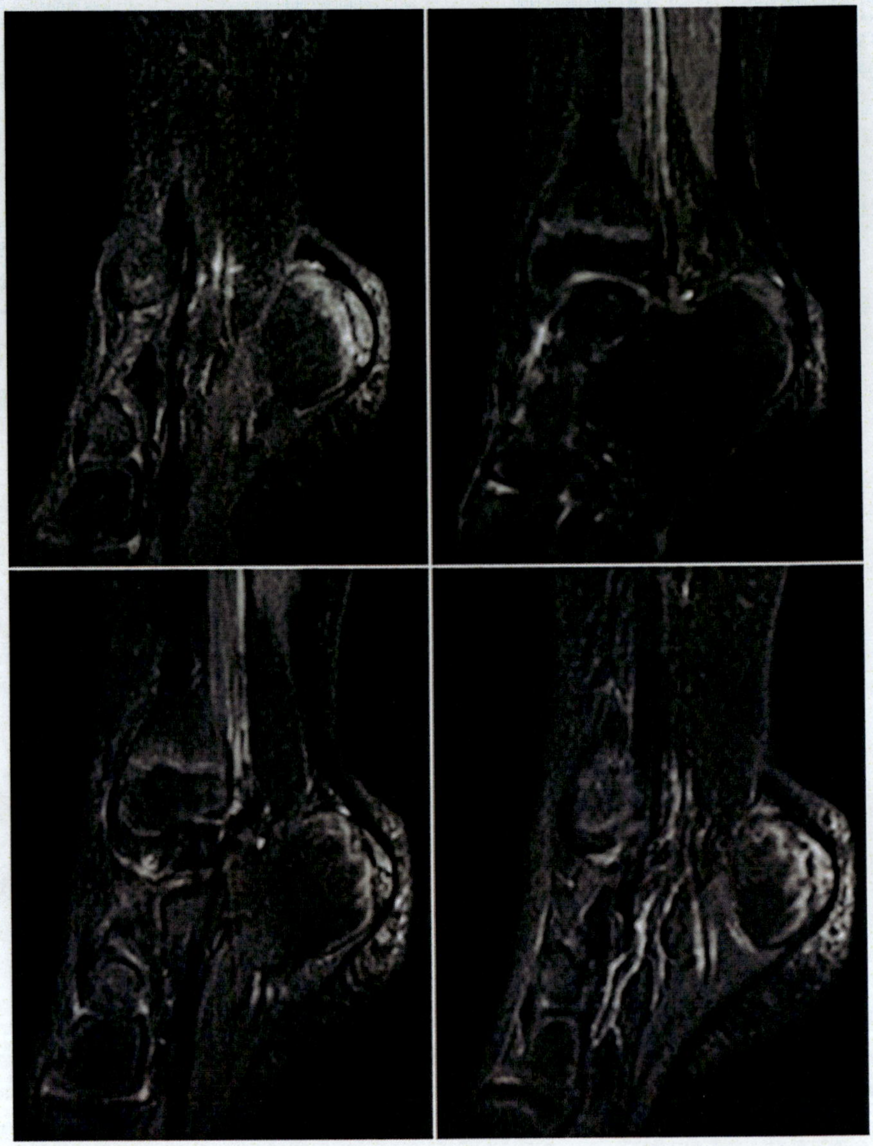

Fig. 6 A 12-year-old male with known juvenile idiopathic arthritis and longstanding heel pain. Sagittal STIR through both ankles shows increased signal in both calcaneal apophyses, the subjacent metaphyses, and in the surrounding soft tissues, consistent with calcaneal apophysitis

5 Tarsal Coalition

Tarsal coalition (TC) is an abnormal, congenital union between two or more bones of the mid- and hindfoot (Crim and Kjeldsberg 2004). It can be cartilaginous, fibrous, or bony. The most common unions (90%) occur between the calcaneus and either the talus (talocalcaneal/subtalar joints) or navicular (calcaneonavicular) bones (Newman and Newberg 2000). It is thought to affect around 1–2% of the population, although the exact prevalence is unknown and debated (Crim 2008;

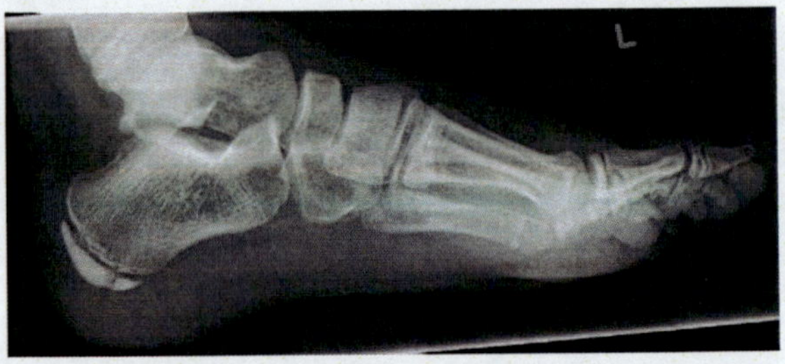

Fig. 7 Normal calcaneal apophysis. Normal appearance of the calcaneal apophysis in an 8-year-old girl. It is normally always sclerotic and often fragmented

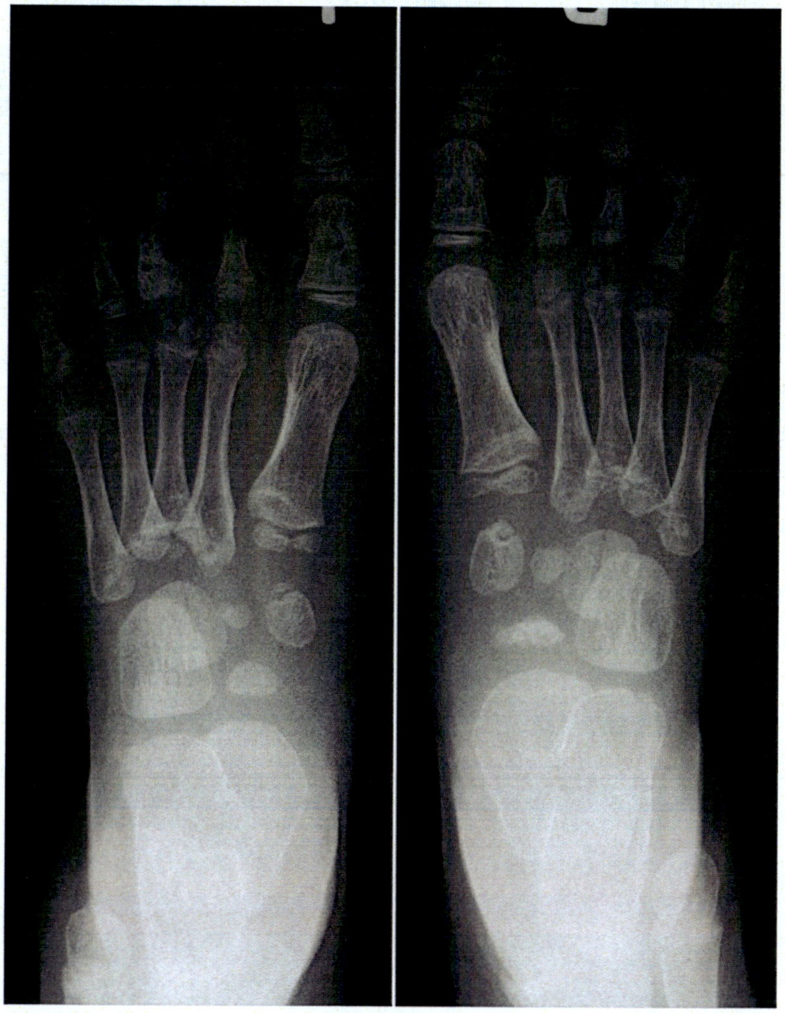

Fig. 8 Kohler's disease in a 5-year-old boy. There is sclerosis and collapse of the right navicular. The left navicular is normal

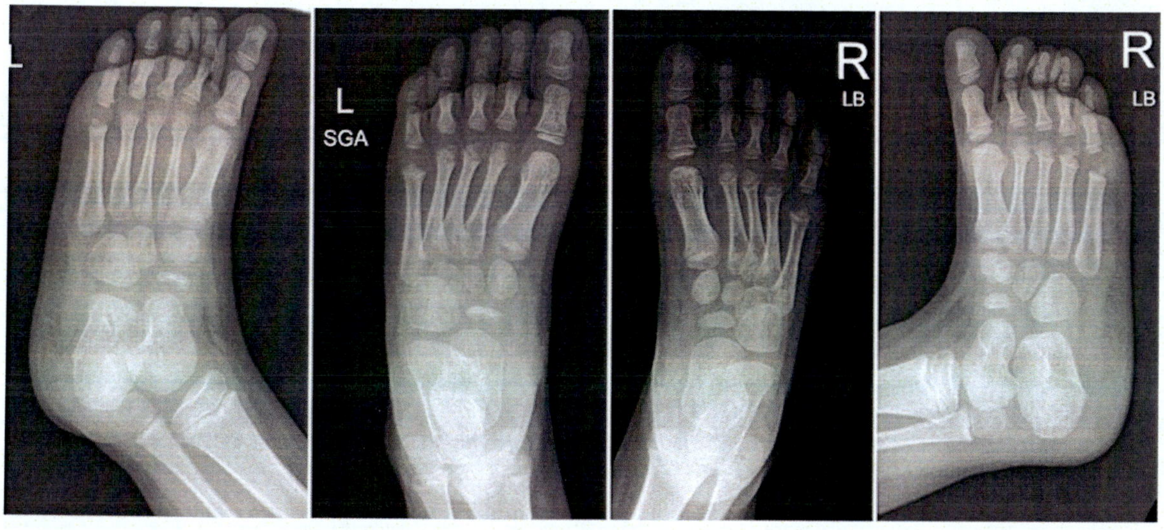

Fig. 9 5 year-old female who presented with left mid-foot pain. There is flattening and sclerosis of the navicular, consistent with Kohler's disease. The right foot was obtained for comparison

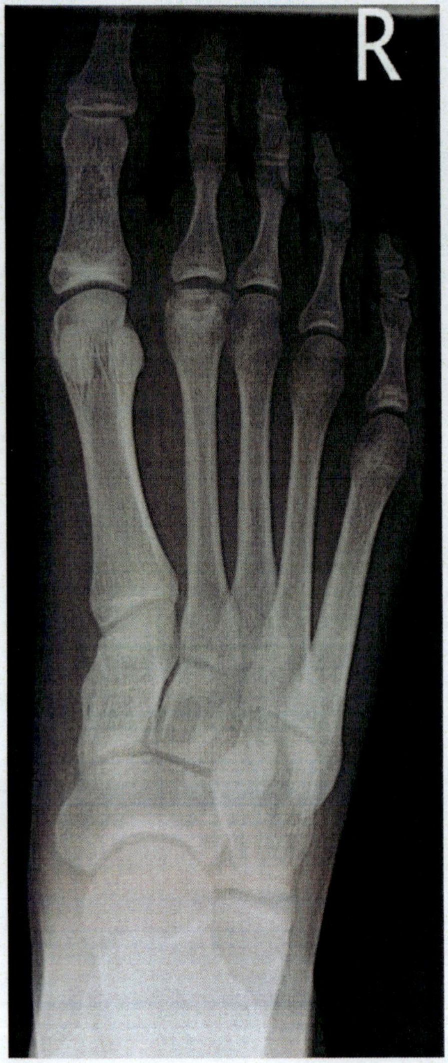

Fig. 10 Freiberg's disease. A 15-year-old girl presented with foot pain. There is fragmentation, sclerosis, and collapse of the second metatarsal head. Note a minute loose body on the medial side of the second metatarsophalangeal joint

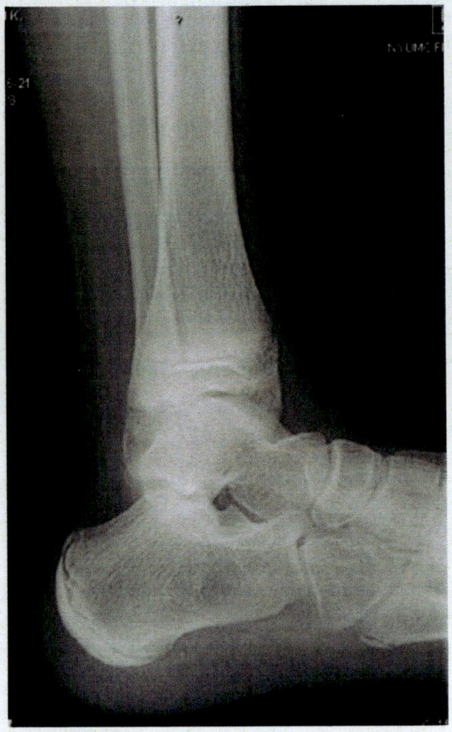

Fig. 11 Lateral view of a 14-year-old female with talocalcaneal coalition. Note the anterior beaking of the talus, the C sign and irregular sustentaculum tali

Stormont and Peterson 1983). Other locations for coalitions have been described, such as talonavicular, calcaneocuboid, and cubonavicular and navicular – first cuneiform, all much rarer (Crim 2008). Many of these unusual locations for coalitions occur as a consequence to prior injury or infection. There is also a reported association with carpal coalition, fibular hemimelia, and symphalangism (Crim 2008).

TC limits movement of the subtalar region, including eversion, inversion, and anterior gliding. Signs and symptoms include pain, flatfoot, tarsal tunnel syndrome, and peroneal tendon spasm. Symptoms usually begin in the second decade but the diagnosis is often made late, especially if patients are not highly active. The symptoms are often misinterpreted as ligament or tendon injury (Varner and Michelson 2000). Many individuals, especially those with fibrous coalitions, remain asymptomatic throughout life. For these reasons, diagnosis is often made unexpectedly by imaging.

Calcaneonavicular coalitions can be seen fairly easily on conventional radiography in adults, but can be difficult to diagnose in small children without well-developed ossification centers in the bones of the foot. The oblique view of the foot is usually the optimal view for this diagnosis. Subtalar coalitions are quite difficult to diagnose via radiography. The Harris–Beath view of the hindfoot is not routinely acquired, but can show abnormality medially, with bony overgrowth and abnormal morphology of the sustentaculum tali and adjacent talus, suggestive of talcalcaneal coalition. We have found the "C" sign described on lateral conventional radiography to be nonspecific.

Consequently, both CT and MRI have been advocated as alternate modalities. CT should be acquired in the axial plane, with sagittal and coronal images reformatted.

Although both CT and MR have reasonable accuracy, characterization as to fibrous, cartilaginous, or

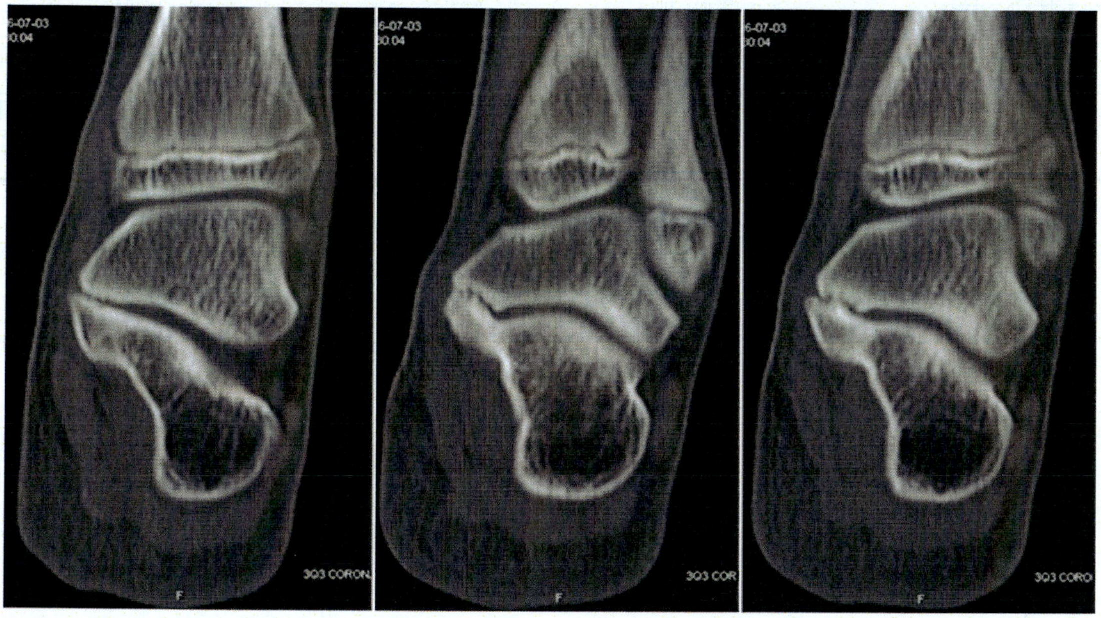

Fig. 12 Coronal CT reconstructions in the same patient as in Fig. 11. Note the non-bony coalition between the talus and sutentaculum

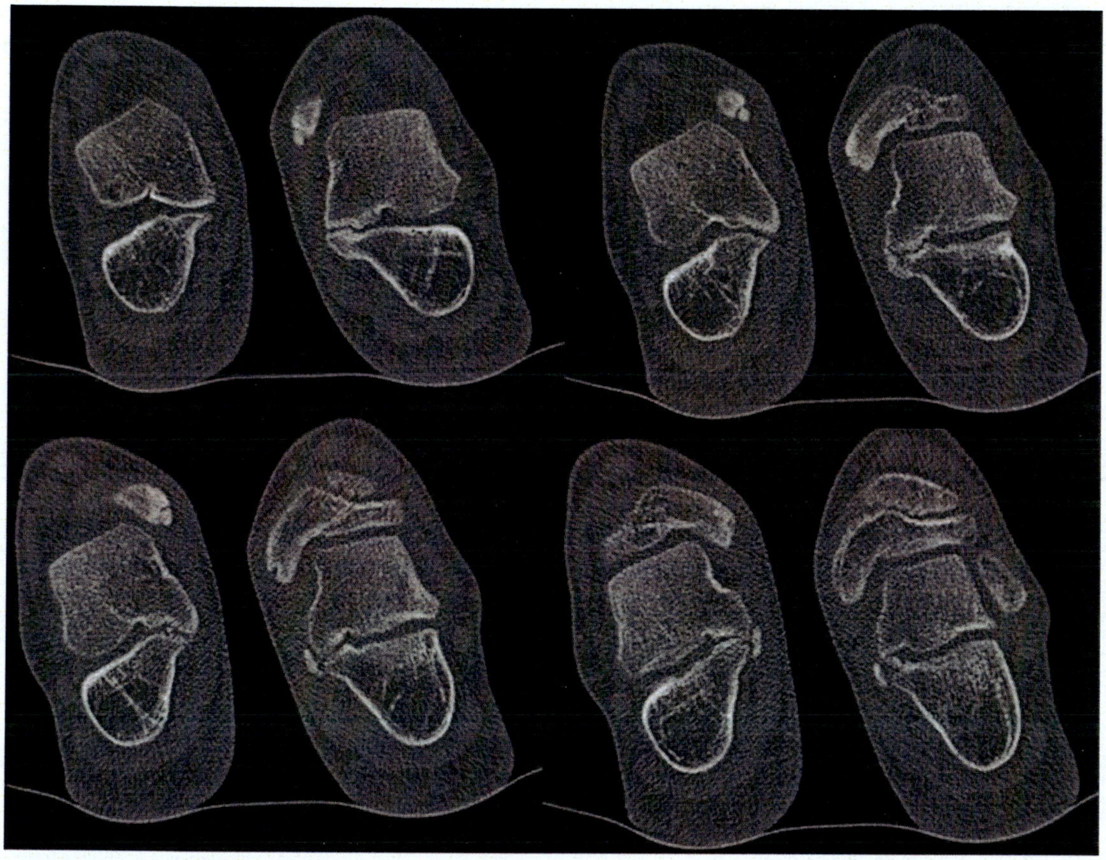

Fig. 13 A 12-year-old girl with bilateral foot pain. Coronal CT reconstructions display bilateral non-bony subtalar coalitions. Note the narrow irregular cleft between the talus and sustentaculum and the rounded inferior border of the sustentaculum, giving the C sign on lateral radiographs

osseous is best done by MR. Some authors suggest that MR is superior to CT as non-osseous unions are more common and MR is also more readily able to detect ancillary findings, such as bone marrow edema and tensosynovitis. One caveat is that without thin slice MR, when assessing for a coalition in the coronal plane there are not infrequent false-positive results. Further discussion will focus on the two most common coalitions, talocalcaneal (TCC) and calcaneonavicular (CNC).

5.1 TCC

TCC classically involves the middle subtalar joint, resulting in bony overgrowth of the sustentaculum tali and corresponding talus, irrespective of whether the union is osseous or non-osseous. Several signs have been described on lateral radiographic views. Sensitivity and specificity vary, but all should raise the suspicion of TCC. They include the talar beak, C sign, dysmorphic sustentaculum tali, blunted lateral process of talus, and absent middle facet sign (Fig. 11).

The talar beak is an abnormal bony overgrowth of the anterior superior aspect of the talonavicular joint, secondary to stress and increased movement in this joint relative to decreased motion in the subtalar joint. The C sign is a continuous, reversed C shape projected over the calcaneus, formed by continuity of a rounded inferomedial talus and abnormal sustenaculum tali (Lateur et al. 1994). The C sign is also seen in flatfoot deformities in the absence of TC (Brown et al. 2001).

A dysmorphic sustentaculum tali has a rounded, enlarged appearance, quite different when compared to the normal rectangular-shaped joint.

The blunted lateral process of the talus is also described on lateral radiographs but is considered an infrequent finding. Instead of the normal pointed inferior appearance, the lateral process develops a blunted or rounded appearance. The middle subtalar joint should be readily seen on a well-centered lateral radiograph. Its absence either implies TCC or an off-center radiograph, the latter can be determined by the absence of the posterior subtalar joint (Crim 2008).

CT and MRI are considered the most appropriate investigations in the diagnosis of TCC (Figs. 12 and 13). Both modalities can easily identify osseous coalitions.

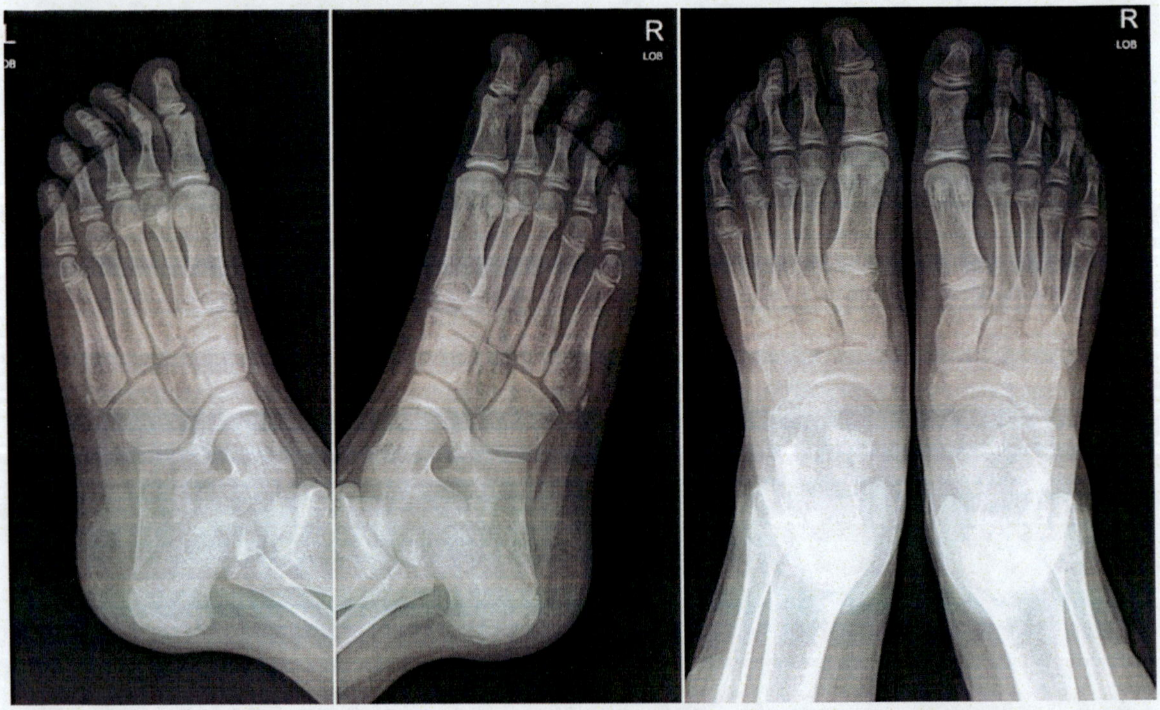

Fig. 14 Oblique and DP plain radiographs in a 10-year-old male with bilateral foot pain-bilateral osseous calcaneonavicular coalitions. Note the anteater's sign on the oblique views (elongated anterior process of the calcaneus attached to the navicular), elongated navicular and short talar neck on the DP view. A talar beak has not yet developed

Cartilaginous or fibrous TCC can be more difficult to diagnose. Unlike the normal middle subtalar facet, the abnormal TCC joint is narrow, irregular, and slopes downward. MRI has the added advantage of being able to show bone marrow edema on either side of the joint or associated synovitis.

5.2 CNC

Perhaps the most common sign associated with tarsal coalitions is the anteater sign. This sign refers to the abnormal elongation and "snout" shape of the anterior process of the calcaneus. It was originally described on oblique radiographs but can also be detected on true lateral radiographs (Fig. 14). Another sign of CNC is the elongated navicular, seen on AP radiographs of the foot. The navicular is elongated laterally beyond its normal boundary. The medial portion of the navicular is also larger than the lateral portion.

Sagittal reformatted CTs and MRI sequences are best for showing the anterior process and elongated navicular (Fig. 15). The shape, however, of both bones is more important than their proximity. There may be associated subchondral cysts and bone marrow edema, the latter seen on MR.

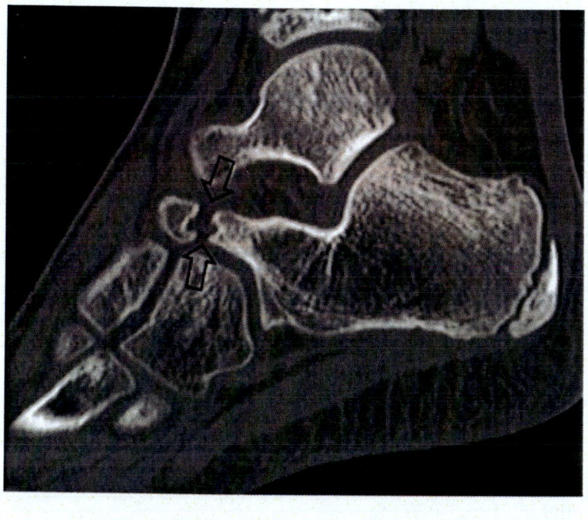

Fig. 15 Calcaneonavicular coalition. Sagittal CT reformatted image of the foot showing fibrous or cartilaginous coalition (*open arrows*). Note the vertical orientation, the proximity of the two bones, and the absence of the fat plane between them

References

Adirim TA, Cheng TL (2003) Overview of injuries in the young athlete. Sports Med 33:75–81

Anderson IF, Crichton KJ, Grattan-Smith T, Cooper RA, Brazier D (1989) Osteochondral fractures of the dome of the talus. J Bone Joint Surg Am 71:1143–1152

Bachmann LM, Kolb E, Koller MT, Steurer J, ter Riet G (2003) Accuracy of Ottawa ankle rules to exclude fractures of the ankle and mid-foot: systematic review. BMJ 326:417

Borges JL, Guille JT, Bowen JR (1995) Kohler's bone disease of the tarsal navicular. J Pediatr Orthop 15:596–598

Brage ME, Rockett M, Vraney R, Anderson R, Toledano (1998) Ankle fracture classification: a comparison of reliability of three X-ray views versus two. Foot Ankle Int 19: 555–562

Brown RR, Rosenberg ZS, Thornhill BA (2001) The C sign: more specific for flatfoot deformity than subtalar coalition. Skeletal Radiol 30:84–87

Cassas KJ, Cassettari-Wayhs A (2006) Childhood and adolescent sports-related overuse injuries. Am Fam Physician 73:1014–1022

Cerezal A, Llopis E, Canga A, Rolón A (2008) MR arthrography of the ankle: indications and technique. Radiol Clin North Am 46:973–994, v

Crim J (2008) Imaging of tarsal coalition. Radiol Clin North Am 46:17–26, vi

Crim JR, Kjeldsberg KM (2004) Radiographic diagnosis of tarsal coalition. AJR Am J Roentgenol 182:323–328

Cox MJ (1958). Kohler's disease. Postgrad Med J; 34 (397): 588–591

De Smet AA, Fisher DR, Burnstein MI, Graf BK, Lange RH (1990) Value of MR imaging in staging osteochondral lesions of the talus (osteochondritis dissecans): results in 14 patients. AJR Am J Roentgenol 154:555–558

De Smet AA, Doherty MP, Norris MA, Hollister MC, Smith DL (1999) Are oblique views needed for trauma radiography of the distal extremities? AJR Am J Roentgenol 172: 1561–1565

Ecklund K, Jaramillo D (2001) Imaging of growth disturbance in children. Radiol Clin North Am 39:823–841

Ecklund K, Jaramillo D (2002) Patterns of premature physeal arrest: MR imaging of 111 children. AJR Am J Roentgenol 178:967–972

Elias I, Zoga AC, Morrison WB, Besser MP, Schweitzer ME, Raikin SM (2007) Osteochondral lesions of the talus: localization and morphologic data from 424 patients using a novel anatomical grid scheme. Foot Ankle Int 28:154–161

Haller J, Sartoris DJ, Resnick D et al (1988) Spontaneous osteonecrosis of the tarsal navicular in adults: imaging findings. AJR Am J Roentgenol 151:355–358

Ivins D (2006) Acute ankle sprain: an update. Am Fam Physician 74:1714–1720

Lateur LM, Van Hoe LR, Van Ghillewe KV, Gryspeerdt SS, Baert AL, Dereymaeker GE (1994) Subtalar coalition: diagnosis with the C sign on lateral radiographs of the ankle. Radiology 193:847–851

Loder RT, Swinford AE, Kuhns LR (1997) The use of helical computed tomographic scan to assess bony physeal bridges. J Pediatr Orthop 17:356–359

Madden CC, Mellion MB (1996) Sever's disease and other causes of heel pain in adolescents. Am Fam Physician 54:1995–2000

Naran KN, Zoga AC (2008) Osteochondral lesions about the ankle. Radiol Clin North Am 46:995–1002, v

Newman JS, Newberg AH (2000) Congenital tarsal coalition: multimodality evaluation with emphasis on CT and MR imaging. Radiographics 20:321–332; quiz 526–527, 532

Schachter AK, Chen AL, Reddy PD, Tejwani NC (2005) Osteochondral lesions of the talus. J Am Acad Orthop Surg 13:152–158

Shabshin N, Schweitzer ME, Morrison WB, Carrino JA, Keller MS, Grissom LE (2006) High-signal T2 changes of the bone marrow of the foot and ankle in children: red marrow or traumatic changes? Pediatr Radiol 36:670–676

Stormont DM, Peterson HA (1983) The relative incidence of tarsal coalition. Clin Orthop Relat Res 181:28–36

Varner KE, Michelson JD (2000) Tarsal coalition in adults. Foot Ankle Int 21:669–672

Zengerink M, Struijs PA, Tol JL, van Dijk CN (2010) Treatment of osteochondral lesions of the talus: a systematic review. Knee Surg Sports Traumatol Arthrosc 18:238–246

Spine

Radhesh Lalam and Victor N. Cassar-Pullicino

Contents

R. Lalam (✉) and V.N. Cassar-Pullicino
Department of Radiology, Robert Jones and Agnes Hunt Orthopaedic Hospital, Oswestry, UK
e-mail: radhesh.lalam@rjah.nhs.uk

Key point

› Sports with the greatest risk of spinal injury in this age group include American football, rugby, ice hockey, wrestling, diving, skiing, cheerleading, baseball and horse riding. Disabling spinal injuries are more likely to result from cervical spine injuries than with thoracolumbar injuries. The most common mechanism for neurological injury is axial loading on a flexed neck. The spinal cord does not share the same degree of tolerance to mechanical insults as the vertebral column and SCIWORA may occur. The spine at this age has a great potential for remodelling and even severe deformities may recover over time. MRI should be performed in all cases with neurological deficit. The physis is the weakest portion of the growing skeleton and is susceptible to tensile forces. The Saltewr-Harris classification may be extrapolated to classify these physeal injuries.

1 Introduction

Injuries in sport are the third most common cause of spinal injury after motor vehicle accidents and violence. Approximately 8.7% of all new cases of spinal injury are due to sport in the USA (National spinal cord injury statistical centre. Spinal cord injury: facts and figures, 2006). The annual incidence of spinal injury in sport is 1.95 per million in Japan. The mean age at injury was 28.5 years with 88% occurring in males (Katoh et al. 1996).

A.H. Karantanas (ed.), *Sports Injuries in Children and Adolescents*,
Med Radiol Diagn Imaging, DOI: 10.1007/174_2010_130, © Springer-Verlag Berlin Heidelberg 2011

In children and adolescents sport is the second most common cause of spinal injury. Spinal injuries in children and adolescents are uncommon and account for 1–9% of total reported spinal injuries. Spinal fractures represent 1–2% of all paediatric fractures and the cervical spine is the commonest region involved accounting for 60–80% of paediatric spinal injuries (Kokoska et al. 2001). Nevertheless, children and adolescents are particularly vulnerable to sport related injuries due to the very high involvement in sports in this age group.

Sports with the greatest risk of spinal injury include American football, ice hockey, wrestling, diving, skiing, snowboarding, rugby, cheerleading and baseball (Boden and Prior 2005). Horse riding is another sport with a potential for significant spinal injury. The majority of spinal injuries in sport can be managed conservatively. Injuries leading to death, permanent disability and significant morbidity are fortunately less common. Disabling spinal injuries are more likely to result from cervical spine injuries than with thoracic or lumbar injuries. The most common mechanism of injury leading to neurological injury is an axial loading force on a slightly flexed neck.

It is well known that the growth plates and apophyses are particularly susceptible to injury in the appendicular skeleton. This is also true with the vertebral column where there are a number of ossification centres and apophyses, which are vulnerable to injury.

2 Embryology and Ossification

It is important for all clinicians dealing with spinal injuries in children to be aware of the embryology and ossification of the vertebral column for three reasons. Firstly, this avoids false positive diagnosis of spinal injuries when apparent traumatic appearances may be due to normal developmental phenomena. Secondly, knowledge of ossification helps to identify areas of the vertebral column that are particularly susceptible to injury in children. Thirdly, some normal variants may be secondary to previous trauma.

The vertebral column and the associated musculature develop from the paraxial mesenchyme which is found lateral to the notochord and neural tube in early embryonal development. The paraxial mesenchyme undergoes segmentation and then somitogenesis. The sclerotomal cells from the somite of each segment enclose the notochord and this forms the blastemal centrum of each vertebra. The neural tube that lies posteriorly is then enclosed by two neural processes arising from the posterolateral corners of this blastemal centrum forming the neural arches. The neural arches are composed of the pedicles, laminae and the spinous processes. The notochord lying between the vertebrae forms the nucleus pulposus and the surrounding mesenchyme forms the annulus fibrosis.

The occipito-cervical junction however develops from the occipital sclerotomes. The development of the upper cervical spine (up to C2) is therefore more closely related to the basiocciput, and anomalous developments therefore often affect both these regions together.

A typical vertebra ossifies from three primary centres, one in the centrum and one for each neural arch. Ossification centres appear as early as the ninth week. Generally, the arches unite between 1 and 3 years of age while the centrum unites with the arches at the neurocentral synchondrosis between 3 and 6 years of age. This union usually progresses in a craniocaudal direction.

The upper two cervical vertebrae not only develop uniquely to the rest of the spinal column but also have unique ossification compared to the rest of the vertebrae.

C1 has three primary ossification centres, one for the anterior arch and one each for the neural arches (Fig. 1a). The anterior arch is only ossified in 20% at birth and becomes ossified by 1 year of age. The neural arches fuse between 3 and 6 years and the anterior arch fuses with the neural arches by 7 years of age.

C2 has the most complex ossification process of all vertebrae (Fig. 1b). There are four ossification centres at birth: one for each neural arch, one for the body and one for the odontoid process. The neural arches fuse with each other by 2–3 years of age and with the body between 3 and 6 years of age. The body of C2 fuses with the odontoid process by 3–6 years of age. This fusion line (sub-dental synchondroses) can be seen until about 11 years of age and can be confused with a fracture. A secondary ossification centre appears at the apex of the odontoid process (os terminale) between 3 and 6 years of age, which fuses by 12 years of age. This, however, may not appear at all.

The C3–C7 vertebrae and the thoracolumbar vertebrae exhibit similar development with three primary ossification centres: one for the body and one each for

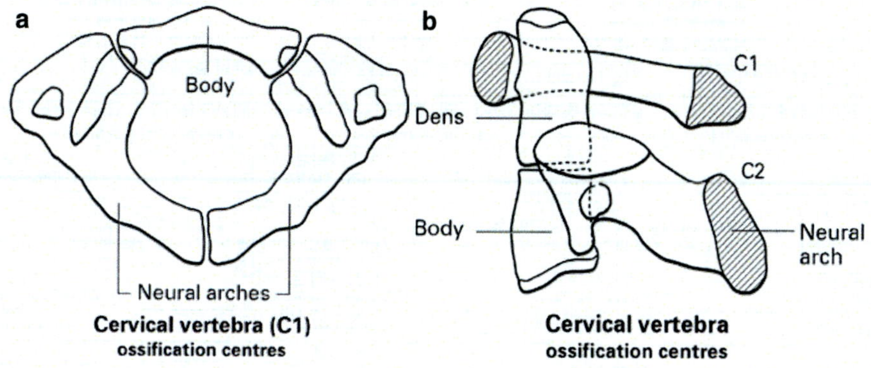

Fig. 1 (**a**) Demonstrates the ossification centres of the C1 vertebra which include one for the vertebral body and a centre on each side for each posterior neural arch. (**b**) Demonstrates the complex ossification of C2 vertebra; one centre for the body, one centre for each neural arch, one centre for the odontoid process and a centre for the apex of the dens (os terminale)

each neural arch. The neural arches fuse posteriorly by 2–3 years of age and the body fuses with the neural arches between 3 and 6 years.

When tensile forces are applied to the spine, it is usually the physis that fail first. Partial or complete physeal separations can occur before the physis fuse. Therefore before 6–8 years of age, the physis associated with the primary ossification centres may fail. After this age the physeal weakness exists at the apical odontoid physis, ring apophysis and the other secondary ossification centres. This should be remembered when assessing radiographs in children and adolescents as these physeal injuries can be subtle and easily missed.

3 Anatomy

The spinal column is composed of 32–33 vertebrae: 7 cervical, 12 thoracic, 5 lumbar, 5 sacral and 3–4 coccygeal segments.

The joints in the vertebral column include the intervertebral disc (IVD), facet joints and in the cervical spine, uncovertebral joints. The individual sacral and coccygeal vertebrae are usually fused together with almost no motion between the individual segments. The IVD is the major joint throughout the spinal column. The disc is composed of the central gelatinous nucleus pulposus and the peripheral annulus fibrosis which is arranged in a concentric 'onion skin' arrangement around the nucleus. Each vertebra typically has two facets posteriorly on each side of the midline: superior and inferior. The superior facet of each vertebra articulates with the inferior facet of the vertebra above to form the synovial facet joints. The alignment of the facet joints (coronally in the cervical spine and sagittally in the lumbar spine) varies in different parts of the spinal column to allow movements in certain directions while restricting movements in other directions. The uncovertebral joints are specific to the cervical spine and are formed on the lateral aspect of the disc by the uncinate process of one vertebra with the concavity seen in the adjacent vertebra. These synovial joints are not present at birth and are formed in childhood.

The ligaments in the spinal column from the anterior to the posterior aspect include the anterior longitudinal ligament, posterior longitudinal ligament, ligamentum flavum, interspinous and supraspinous ligaments. There are multiple other ligaments at the craniocervical junction which are important in injuries to this region (Fig. 2). The anterior and posterior atlanto-occipital membranes extend from the anterior and posterior arches of C1 to the anterior and posterior margins of the foramen magnum. The tectorial membrane is a superior extension of the posterior longitudinal ligament and attaches to the anterolateral aspects of the foramen magnum. Anterior to the tectorial membrane is the cruciate ligament which has a vertical component extending superiorly to the occiput and a horizontal component, the transverse ligament. The transverse ligament extends from the tubercle on the inner aspect of one side of the atlas to the tubercle on the other side passing posterior to the odontoid process. The transverse ligament helps to control anterior movement of the atlas with respect to the axis. The apical ligament lies between the clivus and the apex of the dens. This ligament has an accompanying artery and vein. The vertical component of cruciate and the apical ligaments are weak ligaments and do not contribute significantly to atlanto-occipital stability. The alar

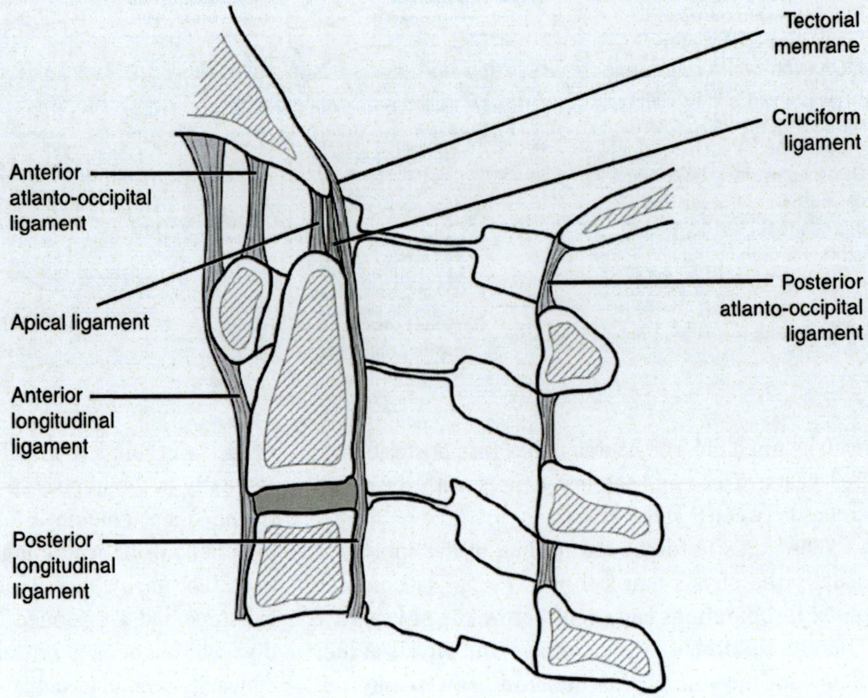

Fig. 2 Ligaments at the craniocervical junction

ligament typically extends superiorly from the lateral aspect of the upper dens to the medial inferior aspect of the occipital condyles. The alar ligament limits the atlanto-axial rotation to the contralateral side. Alar ligament tear can therefore result in a higher degree of contralateral rotation. The tectorial and alar ligaments are the main restrictors of atlanto-occipital extension. The anterior atlanto-axial ligament extends from the anterior mid portion of the dens to the inferior aspect of the anterior arch of C1.

Atlanto dens interval (ADI) is the distance between the anterior aspect of the dens and the posterior aspect of the anterior ring of the atlas. While the normal ADI in adults is normally 3 mm, in children this can be up to 5 mm. An ADI of >5 mm in flexion and >4 mm in extension is abnormal. The distance is wider in children due to the lucent cartilage in the interval combined with the hypermobility. The dens may be slightly posteriorly tilted in up to 4% of normal children and should be differentiated from acute fractures (Hernandez et al. 2004). The posterior tilting may result in a spuriously increased atlanto dens interval in the cranial aspect due to a V shaped appearance to the joint. Normal atlanto dens interval is noted at the caudal aspect of the joint in such cases.

The pre vertebral soft tissue thickness is increased in children. A pre vertebral space of less than 6 mm at C3 level is normal. Widening of the pre vertebral space can be seen in expiration and in crying. A repeat radiograph in extension and inspiration would help to exclude this. The pre vertebral space is unreliable in isolated posterior injuries to the spine.

4 Children Versus Adults

The interpretation of paediatric spine imaging can be difficult in the traumatic setting due to the complexity in development and ossification. The paediatric vertebral column has a greater degree of elasticity compared to the cord. Therefore, children can tolerate greater degree of mechanical insult to their vertebral column without sustaining an injury. However, even in the absence of vertebral injury, there may be underlying cord injury as the cord does not share the same degree of tolerance to mechanical insults and a spinal cord injury without radiographic abnormality (SCIWORA) may result. SCIWORA is more common in children than adults.

Areas of lucency seen on radiographs may be due to cartilaginous development and not due to fractures. Epiphysis, apophysis and synchondrosis occur in predictable locations, have smooth well-corticated margins and can usually be differentiated from traumatic lesions. A clear anatomical knowledge is essential to avoid errors in interpretation.

Injuries to the paediatric spine should be followed up over a long time. The paediatric spine has a great potential for remodelling and even gross deformities may recover significantly by the time the child attains maturity. However, they may also develop progressive deformity especially during adolescent growth spurt.

The pattern of injuries to the spine in children varies from that of the adult spine due to a number of factors. Whilst cervical spine injury accounts for 30–40% of all spinal injuries in adults, 60–80% of all spinal injuries in children are in the cervical region (Rekate et al. 1999).

Clinical examination can be difficult in children adding to the difficulty in assessment. Older children and adolescents are more likely to sustain spinal injuries from active sports. Younger children and infants, on the other hand, sustain spinal injuries mainly from motor vehicle accidents and not sports. In a review of 406 patients, Cirak et al. have found that motor vehicle accidents account for 71% of spinal injuries in infants (Cirak et al. 2004). Falls were the leading cause of injury in toddlers and school age children, while in the adolescent population sports related injuries were the commonest.

The upper cervical spine is more susceptible to injury in young children due to the large head size, underdeveloped neck musculature and the unique pattern of development of the upper C-spine compared to the rest of the vertebral column. Moreover, the fulcrum of movement of the c-spine is located in the upper c-spine in very young children due to the disproportionately large size of the head and the weak neck musculature. Previous studies have demonstrated that the maximum flexion in the cervical spine occurs at the C2/C3 level in infants, C3/C4 level by school age and C5/C6 level in adolescents (Athey 1991; Pang and Wilberger 1982). The cartilage endplates of the vertebrae are sites of attachment of ligaments at the margins of the vertebral bodies. Until fusion in the second decade, these are potential zones of weakness through which injuries can occur.

After 8 years of age, the bony components of the spinal column assume adult morphology and proportions, and the patterns of injury follow adult patterns. Whilst the mortality is increased with a younger age at injury, overall the prognosis is better in children compared to adults. This is due to the capacity of the paediatric spine for growth and remodelling.

5 Normal Variants

A number of normal variants are seen in the paediatric spine. These are usually due to variations in ossification and also due to hypermobility of the spine. Consequently, these are more common in the upper cervical spine due to the hypermobility and complexity of ossification in this region.

1. The normal *cervical lordosis* may be reduced or absent in children up to 16 years of age with the neck in neutral position. The posterior inter-spinous distance is a good indicator of posterior ligamentous integrity and should not be more than 1.5 times the inter-spinous distance at either the immediately superior or inferior level (Naidich et al. 1977) and has been validated by Pennecot (Pennecot et al. 1984). Additionally due to the tight ligamentous attachment between the occiput and C1, the C1–C2 inter-spinous distance can be increased on flexion, which is a normal finding.
2. *Pseudo-subluxation* at the C2–3 level was seen in 46% of children under 8 years of age in one study on lateral flexion and extension radiographs. This can also be seen in about 14% of children at the C3–4 level to a lesser degree. Pseudo-subluxation of up to 4 mm is acceptable in a child. Hypermobility of the paediatric spine, ligamentous laxity and a horizontal orientation of the articular surfaces in the upper cervical spine are thought to be responsible for this phenomenon. In some cases this can be so profound that it can be confused with a true injury. The posterior cervical line helps to differentiate this from true injury (Fig. 3) (Hernandez et al. 2004). The posterior cervical line is drawn from the anterior aspect of the spinous processes of C1 to the anterior aspect of the spinous process of C3. The anterior edge of the spinous process of C2 usually lies posterior to and within 1 mm of this line. However, it is important to note that the posterior cervical line is only useful when there is malalignment of the C2 and C3 vertebral bodies and should not be used when the alignment is normal. If the anterior aspect of the C2 spinous process is posterior and more than 2 mm away from the posterior cervical line, a Hangman

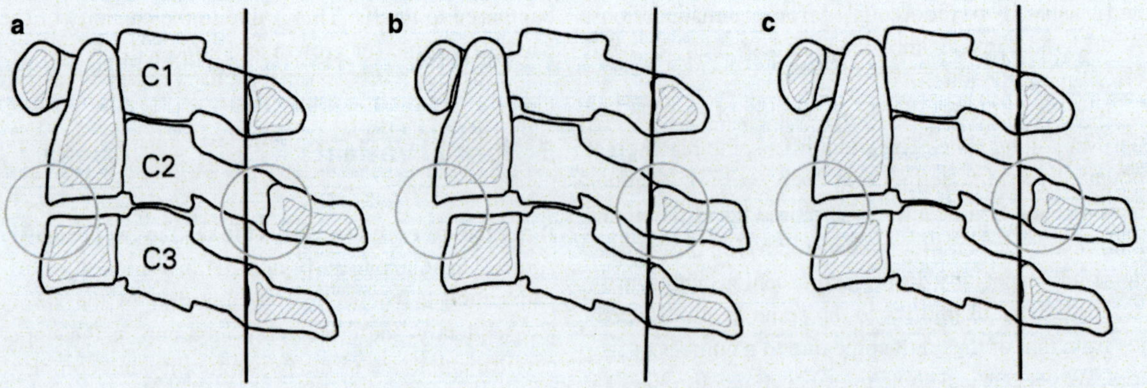

Fig. 3 Pseudo-subluxation of C2 over C3. (**a**) There is no anterior subluxation of C2 vertebral body over C3. In these cases, the posterior cervical line is not useful. (**b**) There is anterior subluxation of C2 over C3. The anterior border of the C2 spinous process lies slightly anterior to the posterior cervical line and therefore may be abnormal. (**c**) There is anterior subluxation of C2 over C3 and the anterior border of C2 spinous process lies posterior to the posterior cervical line and within 2 mm of the line. This is in keeping with pseudo-subluxation. If this distance is more than 2 mm, this is suspicious for a Hangman's fracture

fracture is present. An abnormal posterior cervical line also occurs when the anterior aspect of the C2 spinous process lies anterior to the posterior cervical line indicating an injury to the facet joints and posterior ligament complex which promote a true C2/C3 subluxation. Further imaging is however warranted in children with persistent clinical symptoms and suspicion even when pseudo-subluxation is considered.

3. *Pseudo-Jefferson fracture* or pseudo-spread of the atlas on the axis can be seen on the open mouth radiographs. The ossification of the lateral masses of C1 in young children often exceeds that of C2 . The lateral masses of the atlas therefore may overhang the axis by as much as 6 mm and is commonly seen in children less than 4 years of age and may be seen up to 7 years of age.
4. *Pseudo-wedging*: In early infancy vertebral bodies are ovoid in appearance. They become rectangular with advancing age. This is due to the fact that a radiograph demonstrates bony detail and therefore only the pattern of ossification rather than a true morphological appearance. Anterior wedging of vertebrae of up to 3 mm can be a normal variation and should not be confused with compression fractures. Some infants and children develop actual wedging of the ossification centres at C3 and rarely at C4 (Hernandez et al. 2004). This wedging can be particularly prominent at the C3 level. This is thought to be due to the hypermobility of the paediatric cervical spine, resulting in an impaction of C2 on C3 in some children.
5. *Bipartite* (anterior and posterior) ossification centres can be seen as in a coronally cleft vertebral body which can be seen up to 4 years of age due to variation in endochondral ossification.
6. The ossification centre for the anterior arch of atlas usually appears in the first year but is present in 20% at birth. In a few cases, this may be absent resulting in a failure of anterior fusion leaving a cleft. The synchondrosis at the base of the odontoid with the C2 body fuses between 3 and 6 years of age but may be delayed. The vestigial outline of this fusion can be seen up to 11 years of age as a fine sclerotic line but can be differentiated from the lucent fracture line.
7. *Congenital spondylolysis* can be seen in the paediatric spine either during investigation for neck pain or for trauma. This is most commonly seen in the cervical spine at the C6 level. This can usually be clearly diagnosed from radiographs and CT can be performed to confirm this. The appearances include a spondylolytic defect with well-corticated margins, hypoplastic posterior elements and an occult spina bifida. This can be difficult to detect on MR scan as the pedicle may not be clearly visualised, but the diagnosis should be sought when there is an absent or hypoplastic spinous process on the sagittal sequences. A spondylolytic defect at C2 can be difficult to differentiate from a hangman's fracture.
8. *Unfused ring apophyses*, ossification centres and secondary ossification centres can be confused with fractures. Understanding the normal anatomy and development should help in avoiding

misinterpretation. Normal physeal plates are smooth, regular, have sclerotic margins and occur at predictable locations unlike acute fractures which are irregular, non-sclerotic and can occur at any location. The superior and inferior ring apophysis may not ossify simultaneously and should not be mistaken for fractures. The apical odontoid epiphysis can be seen in 26% of children between 6 and 8 years of age. The posterior ring of C1 can remain cartilaginous, become fibrous or absent throughout the course of life.

6 Indications for Imaging

Indications for initial radiological evaluation in sport are similar to other patient groups. The Canadian cervical spine radiography rules do not include children and are therefore not appropriate for this patient group. A careful clinical evaluation is needed if there is a history of facial or head trauma, loss of consciousness, high speed motor vehicle accident, or birth trauma. A radiological examination should be undertaken in these circumstances and when there is an abnormality on neurological examination. The type of radiological investigation depends on the nature of injury and the clinical findings. Although the Nexus study included paediatric injuries, they had poor specificity in this age group (Hoffman et al. 2000; Hoffman et al. 1998; Viccellio et al. 2001). In the absence of clear guidelines, each case should be approached individually. The most common symptoms in cervical spine injury are pain and torticollis. Local tenderness, muscle spasm, or contracture and asymmetry are some of the clinical signs associated with spinal injury.

The presence of protective equipment like helmets and shoulder pads may cause difficulty in assessing the cervical spine in the acute setting. In one study, none of the lateral radiographs in their 20 volunteers with protective gear were adequate and even the addition of other views made the radiographs acceptable in the range of 20–35% (Davidson et al. 2001).

There is controversy regarding the number of radiographic views in cervical spine injury ranging from one to five views. Whilst the cross table radiograph picks up the majority of injuries, it has a significant false negative (21%) rate and therefore a complete radiographic series has to be performed. The three view series has a 93% sensitivity for detecting cervical spine fractures (Streitwieser et al. 1983). Undisplaced posterior ring fractures may be missed by this approach. Hyperflexion injuries can be missed on initial radiographs and may only be picked up after the initial muscle spasm settles in a few days. So a normal plain film series does not entirely exclude spinal injury and continued clinical suspicion warrants further imaging assessment.

If one level of injury is recognised in the spine, a full evaluation of the rest of the spine should be performed to exclude injuries at other levels. The number of concomitant injuries identified in patients with spinal injury varies with imaging modality used. Studies using radiographs to evaluate the rest of the spine identified 15% had concomitant injuries, while studies using MR imaging (MRI) identified 45% of patients had concomitant injuries (Henderson et al. 1991 and Qaiyum et al. 2001). The clinical relevance of these additional injuries identified on MRI is still not clear.

Flexion/extension radiographs should not be performed in the acute setting and in obtunded patients (Fig. 4). These are associated with significant false negative rates. In addition, soft tissues like the IVD are not seen on these radiographs and can displace easily during the manoeuvre and cause further catastrophic spinal injury. We suggest that these are only performed after an MRI scan. Flexion/extension radiographs however have a role after the acute period to assess stability and healing.

CT is necessary where adequate radiographs are not possible or if there is suspicion of significant/unstable injury on the initial radiographs. In diving injuries, Kligman et al. found that CT demonstrated fractures not evident on radiographs in 57% of their patients (Kligman et al. 2001). Modern CT scanning with thin sections and multiplanar reconstructions provide exquisite detail of the bony anatomy. CT underestimates the extent of soft tissue and ligamentous injuries and is not routinely indicated in evaluation of spinal injury under the age of 5 years (Hernandez et al. 2004). However, in patients with inadequate radiographs and in those with suspicion of unstable injury, a CT scan should be performed to clearly define injury pattern and facilitate management.

MRI should be performed in all athletes with suspected spinal injury and neurological deficits. MRI provides essential information of all bony and soft tissue structures in the vertebral column and their effects

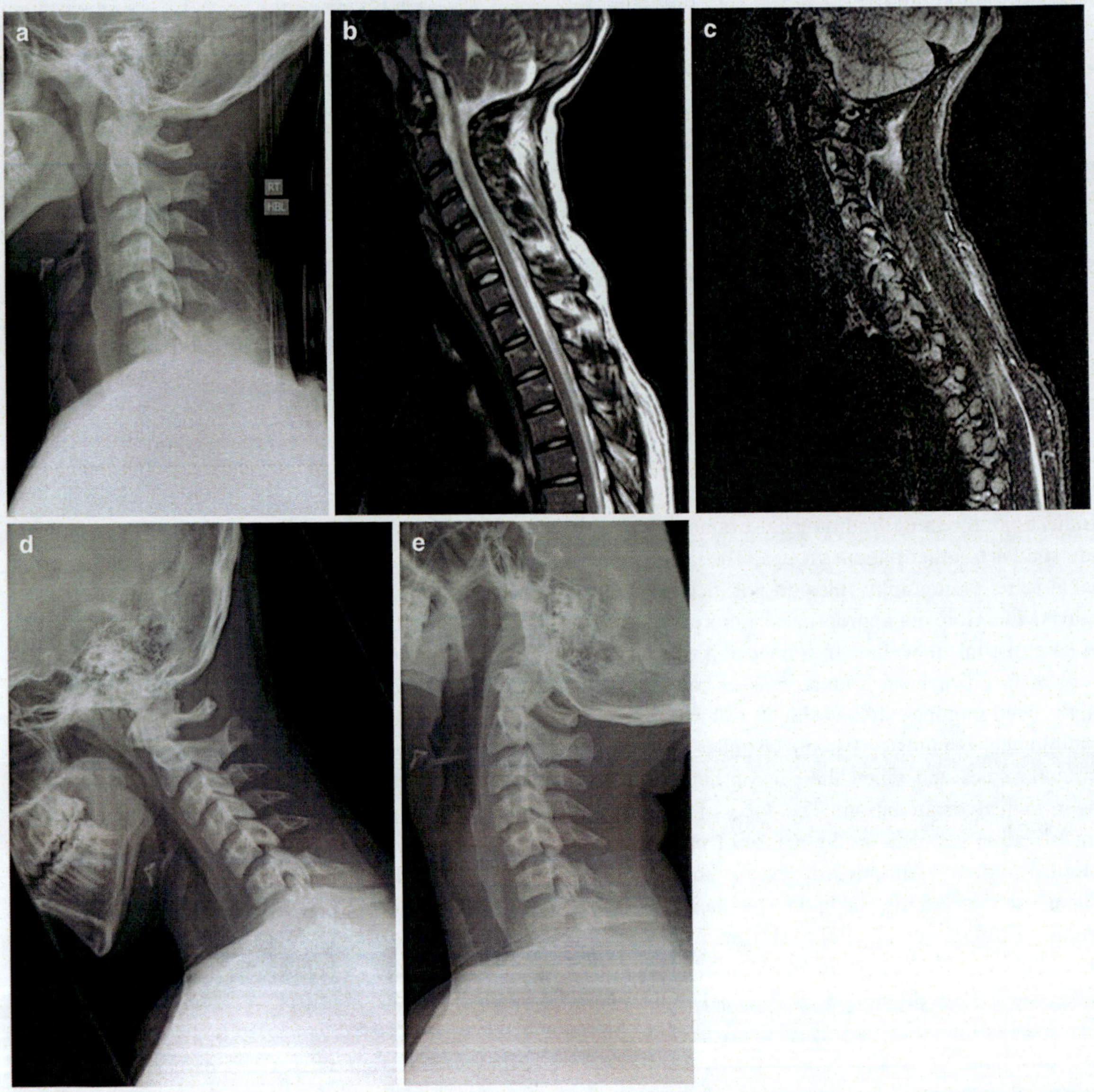

Fig. 4 Head-on rugby collision on a flexed neck in a 15-year-old boy. No neurological deficit. The lateral radiograph (**a**) shows abnormal widening of the interspinous distance at the C5/6 level. This is suggestive of posterior distracting injury despite the apparent preservation of vertebral alignment. Closer inspection does also reveal a minor compression of the anterosuperior corner of the C6 vertebra and widened facet joints. Sagittal midline T2W (**b**) image demonstrates complete rupture of the posterior ligaments including the ligamentum flavum, interspinous and the supraspinous ligaments. There is minor oedema in the anterior superior corner of the C6 vertebra. The sagittal STIR parasagittal image (**c**) shows fluid in a slightly subluxed C5/6 facet joint. This injury therefore involves the anterior and posterior columns and is a potentially unstable injury. Flexion (**d**) and extension (**e**) radiographs 2 weeks after injury demonstrate the pitfalls of this technique. Whilst on initial inspection there is satisfactory flexion/extension and the injury appears stable, closer inspection demonstrates absence of any movement at the injured level between the two radiographs making these radiographs unreliable for stability assessment

on the neurological structures including the cord and nerve roots. If a significant injury is seen at one level, it is our normal practice to evaluate the whole spinal column by means of sagittal T1-w, T2-w and STIR images. MRI distinguishes between cord contusion and compression, the distinction being useful to identify patients who may benefit from surgical decompression. The extent of injury helps to assess any potential for instability which is also necessary for patient management. The cervical cord is more susceptible to SCIWORA than any other spinal level. MRI scan is necessary in all patients with neurological signs after injury, even if radiographs and CT are normal. In addition MRI also demonstrates any significant underlying anatomical abnormalities like fusion/segmentation anomalies, Chiari malformation, developmental spinal stenosis and basilar invagination, some of which may preclude further participation in contact sport for the affected athlete.

However, it is important to realise that the appearances of the spinal column during any of these imaging examinations is that seen at the resting state of the spinal column and not the state of the spinal column at the time of impact. In other words, the maximum disruption occurs at the moment of impact following which the spinal column achieves a resting state. Studies have previously demonstrated that the maximum spinal canal compromise occurs at the time of impact and is probably 85% more than that seen at the time of imaging long after the impact.

7 Imaging Evaluation

Spinal stability is dependant on both bony and soft tissue structures. Radiographs only demonstrate bony detail. Soft tissue injury is implied by the alteration in relationships between bony structures and should be carefully sought. Any minor malalignment, angulation, displacement, abnormal bony relationships should be thoroughly interrogated requiring advanced imaging with CT or MRI.

The radiographic assessment includes assessment for alignment. Lines drawn along the anterior vertebral margins, posterior vertebral margins and the spinolaminar junctions should normally curve gently. Any sudden steps in these lines should be carefully interrogated further. Some normal variations in alignment however occur in children as discussed earlier. The prevertebral soft tissue thickness is an important indicator of spinal injuries. It should be noted that radiographs only demonstrate the ossified elements, and non-ossified normal cartilaginous elements may be misinterpreted as injuries. The interspinous distance should be uniform. An increase in the interspinous distance of more than 1.5 times the adjoining interspace is abnormal and suggests posterior ligamentous injury (Fig. 4). Radiographs of the upper thoracic spine can be difficult to obtain. This area of the thoracic spine is further obscured by the overlap of the ribs and scapula. Fortunately, injuries in this area are uncommon. However, if there is clinical suspicion, further cross-sectional imaging may be necessary. Flexion/extension radiographs are assessed for any acute change in the gentle curvature and for any displacement or widening of the joint spaces between the various vertebral levels. An acute angulation of more than 10 degrees at any level compared to the adjacent levels is abnormal.

CT with multiplanar reformatting demonstrates exquisite bone detail and has a crucial role in spinal trauma. The bony detail is far better demonstrated by CT compared to MR. Newer advances in multislice imaging allow isometric imaging. With the advances in technology, there is often a tendency to resort to CT even before plain radiographs. However, CT is not recommended for routine screening in children to avoid excessive radiation. Therefore, clinical evaluation plays an important role. Whilst routine CT of the cervical spine included at the time of imaging the head with a CT scan for blunt trauma in adults has been proven to be effective in various studies (Barba et al. 2001), the same is not true in children. Furthermore, Hernandez et al. have demonstrated in their review of 606 children that CT only showed significant findings in patients where the abnormal findings were already seen on the initial plain radiograph (Hernandez et al. 2004). They went as far as to suggest that in children under 5 years of age, CT did not contribute any further for diagnosis of new spinal injuries. Studies in obtunded trauma patients utilising MDCT alone to assess cervical spine have found that no unstable injuries were missed (Hogan et al. 2005). However, ligaments and soft tissues are not adequately seen on CT. MRI based studies demonstrate a higher incidence of ligamentous injuries than the CT based studies.

MRI is excellent at demonstrating soft tissue and cord injuries although radiography and CT may show indirect signs of significant soft tissue injury like widening of the interspinous distance, widening of the disc space or divergence of articular processes. Plain films and CT form the main stay of imaging in the acute situation. MRI is most often used as a second-line investigation mainly to exclude paediatric spinal injury in the absence of plain film and CT abnormality but with persistent clinical suspicion, and also to further evaluate injuries already detected on initial imaging, particularly for assessing soft tissues and cord. MRI is also performed to assess the cord prior to surgery and to evaluate for complications and sequelae. MRI can be difficult to perform in the very young due to their inability to stay still during the examination, and sedation may be necessary. MRI can also be difficult to perform in the multiple injured patients in the acute setting due to the difficulty in monitoring the patient while in the scanner. MRI should also be employed in cases of suspected soft tissue injury with normal radiographs before resorting to flexion/extension views in children.

8 Screening

The use of screening in sport is still controversial. Screening involves assessing for any potential background stenosis of the bony spinal canal that might make these athletes more susceptible to serious cord injury. This is commonly performed on radiographs and involves measuring the anteroposterior canal diameter (the distance between the posterior vertebral body margin and the spino-laminar junction). The Pavlov–Torg ratio is obtained by dividing the spinal canal diameter by the anteroposterior width of the vertebra and a value of less than 0.8 indicates potential stenosis. There are problems with using this method. Firstly, professional athletes have large vertebral bodies and even with normal canal dimensions may cause a spuriously low Pavlov–Torg ratio. Secondly, radiation risk and cost make screening all athletes prohibitive. Lastly, most of us use MRI for assessing stenosis and are well aware of the limitations of radiographs at assessing spinal canal dimensions. Screening is, however, acceptable in athletes with a previous history of cervical cord neuropraxia, but this group should probably be screened with an MRI scan to adequately assess the soft tissue structures as well as vertebrae.

9 Sport Specific Considerations

Detailed description of every sport is beyond the scope of this chapter. More importantly there are constantly changes in existing sport and constant invention of new sporting activities sought after by 'adrenaline junkies'. Some newer sports associated with recent reports of spinal injuries include 'sand surfing' and diving out of a plane on to a ski slope to carry on downhill skiing. Most new sports appear to have increased degree of speed and danger making the likelihood of all injuries including spinal injuries proportionately greater. It is therefore important that the imaging radiologist keeps up to date with these newer activities.

Rugby: The absence of protective gear and the massive forces involved in the scrum increase the risk of spinal injury in rugby. Ten percent of serious injuries in rugby involve the cervical spine. Each side of the scrum generates weights of up to 1.5 ton during 'engagement' and the hooker, or the central player in the front row of the scrum suffers the most injuries. The hooker may encounter up to 50% of the total scrum weight, and if engagement does not occur correctly severe spinal injury may ensue. The hooker may flex the neck during contact causing significant flexion and axial compression. Additional risks in rugby involve spear tackling and stiff-arming.

American football: This sport accounts for the highest incidence of cervical spine injuries in the USA. This is partly because of the fact that there is a high rate of uptake of this sport in America. Head injuries in American football reduced in the 1970s with introduction of helmets. However, this has resulted in tacklers hitting opponents with the crowns of their heads (also known as spearing) due to reduced fear of head injury thereby increasing the incidence of cervical spine injuries.

Ice Hockey: Approximately 9% of all hockey injuries occur in the spine (Flik et al. 2005). Injuries generally occur at the C5–C7 level. 'Checking' from behind is the most common cause of spinal injury. The player not anticipating a check is looking down and is hit from behind. This sends the checked player hurtling into the side boards with the head flexed, thus axially loading the cervical spine. Whilst impact velocities as low as 1.8 m/s are enough to cause cervical spinal injury, skating speeds can exceed 12 m/s and are enough to cause cervical spine failure.

Wrestling: Most wrestling injuries occur in the low and middle weight classes (Boden and Prior 2005). The most common wrestling manoeuvre associated with these injuries is the takedown of a standing opponent in the defensive position. Wrestlers are usually injured by one of three mechanisms: (1) The wrestler is thrown to the mat with the arms held, which prevents the wrestler from protecting himself whilst landing on his head. (2) The wrestler being landed upon by the full weight of the top wrestler midway through an attempted roll. (3) Axial compression sustained by a wrestler while attempting to 'shoot' on an opponent resulting in the head hitting the opponents head, knee or other hard surface (Boden and Jarvis 2008).

Swimming/diving and other water sports: Most swimming injuries occur when the athlete jumps during the start of the race into the shallow end of the pool. The swimmer sustains an axial compression on the head causing the spinal injury. Most diving injuries are in recreational divers and are under-reported. In one study from Greece, diving injuries were most common at C5 and C6 levels. Diving contributed to 2.6% of all cervical spine injury admissions (Korres et al. 2006). Inadequate supervision, alcohol use, shallow water and inexperienced divers are risk factors (Cooper et al. 2003).

Surfing and skim-boarding are more recently popularised water sports with ever increasing extreme manoeuvres. In skim-boarding, the athlete usually operates in shallow water, and therefore the risk is similar to diving head first in shallow water. Three recent cases of cervical spinal cord injury were reported in skim-boarding (Collier et al. 2010).

Skiing/snowboarding: Skiing/snowboarding injuries have been increasing recently and are usually dependant on poorly groomed slopes, equipment failure, poor weather, overcrowding and loss of control. The distribution of spinal injuries is even across the various spinal levels. Spinal injuries in snowboarders are approximately three times more frequent than skiing and appear to be increasing with the increase in the sport's popularity. This is either related to inexperience or jumping accidents. Jumping injuries typically occur in the thoracolumbar spine.

Gymnastics/cheerleading: Cheerleading is currently not as popular in Europe as in America. However, cheerleading accounts for more than half of all catastrophic injuries in school and college female athletes in the USA. This is because of the complex gymnastic manoeuvres, athleticism and high skill required in cheerleading. Injuries occur most commonly with pyramid formations, basket toss (involving throwing the cheerleader into the air to heights of 6–20 ft, and catching them before landing on the ground), advanced floor tumbling routines or performing a mount and landing on a hard surface.

Baseball: There is a relatively high incidence of catastrophic injury in baseball. Most of these are cranial injuries which are more common than spinal injuries. These occur more commonly due to a collision between a base runner and a fielder, typically due to a base runner diving head first into a catcher sustaining an axial compression injury.

Football (soccer): Spinal injuries are fortunately extremely rare in soccer.

Cricket: It is well known that fast bowlers in cricket are susceptible to spondylolysis.

10 Spinal Injuries

10.1 Acute Catastrophic Spinal Injuries

These include unstable fractures/dislocations, transient quadriplegia and IVD herniations. Careful clinical evaluation is essential when evaluating a child with multiple injuries as spinal injuries can be overlooked. Tenderness, ecchymosis, swelling or a palpable defect posteriorly along spinous processes should alert to the possibility of spinal injury.

Catastrophic injuries are more likely to occur after cervical spine injuries than other levels of the vertebral column. Neurological injury commonly occurs from flexion or axial compression or a combination of both. The normal lordotic curve of the cervical spine allows axial forces to be dissipated through the paraspinal muscles. However with flexion, this compensatory mechanism is inadequate and an axial load results in injury to the spinal column. The spine then fails in either flexion (flexion tear drop injury) or pure compression (burst injury) with resultant fracture, dislocation, or subluxation. Encroachment of the spinal canal by bony fragments or disc retropulsion results in neurological injury.

10.1.1 Cervical Spine

Catastrophic injuries are much more common in the cervical spine than the rest of the vertebral column. Cord and neurological injury is more common with cervical injuries (40%) than injuries in the rest of the spine (4–10%). In young children (<8 years), injuries are more common in the upper cervical spine, from the occiput to the C2/3 level. In older children and adolescents, injuries more commonly involve C5–C7 levels.

It is important to confirm that all parts of the c-spine are well demonstrated as most missed injuries are at the craniocervical region and the lowest part of the cervical spine. The open mouth view can be particularly difficult to perform in children. Pulling the arms down or a Swimmer's view can help to see the C7/T1 level. When a CT scan of the head is performed following trauma for suspected cranial injury, it is reasonable to extend this scan to include the upper cervical spine as this group of patients are more likely to have spinal injury and also less likely to yield good quality radiographs.

Cervical spinal injuries can be broadly divided by the main direction of force applied at the time of injury (*flexion, extension, axial loading, flexion rotation, lateral flexion*). The patterns of injury resulting from these forces can be understood using Denis model of three columns. The anterior two thirds of the vertebral body form the anterior column. The remaining third of the vertebral body forms the middle column and the posterior elements form the posterior column according to this model. The middle column is the key to understanding this concept.

Flexion accounts for 50–75% of all injuries. Usually, the middle column acts as a fulcrum of the vertebral column. In flexion, the anterior column is subjected to compressive force and the posterior column is subjected to distraction/tension. During flexion of the head, maximum forces act between C4 and C7, which is the common site for these injuries.

The anterior injury can be seen as a *wedge fracture* or *intervertebral disc injury*. The IVD injury may be seen as disc height loss on radiographs. The posterior distraction injury can cause widened interspinous distance, *spinous process fracture* or *bilateral facet dislocation*. The combination of anterior and posterior injuries can result in unstable injury with *anterior subluxation* (Fig. 5).

Specific types of flexion injuries include:

1. *Flexion tear drop fracture*: This is one of the most severe and unstable injuries of the cervical spine. It is frequently associated with cord injury (75%). There is comminuted fracture of the vertebral body with a characteristic triangular or quadrangular fragment at the anteroinferior corner. There is also a sagittal split in the body and frequent bilateral fractures of the posterior elements. There may be variable degrees of facet dislocation and interspinous widening from ligament injury.
2. *Odontoid fracture*: Odontoid fractures can also occur with extension. The dens displaces anteriorly with flexion and posteriorly with extension. Three types: type I, an oblique fracture limited to Dens; type II, transverse fracture through the base of the dens (most common); and type III, oblique fracture at the base of dens extending into the body of axis.
3. *Clay shoveler's fracture*: Avulsion injury of the C7 spinous process.

Extension type of injuries account for 20–30% of cervical injuries. With extension, there is compression force on the posterior elements and tensile force at the anterior column. There is prevertebral swelling, *widening of the anterior disc space* and a variable degree of injury to the posterior elements including fractures of the lamina. There can be a resultant anterior or posterior subluxation.

Specific types of extension injuries include:

1. *Hangman's fracture*: Bilateral neural arch fractures of C2 (Fig. 6), prevertebral soft tissue swelling, anterior subluxation of C2 over C3, avulsion of anterior inferior corer of C2
2. *Extension tear drop fracture*: Small avulsion fragment at the anterior inferior corner
3. *Extension type odontoid fracture*

Axial loading results from compressive force applied to all three columns of the spine. This causes compression of the whole of the vertebral body. When the degree of compression is excessive, the IVD is driven into the vertebral body which explodes into several fragments and a *burst fracture* results. Radiographic features include vertebral height loss, encroachment of the spinal canal by displaced bone fragments (usually posterosuperior corner), and disruption of the posterior vertebral body cortical outline. There is variable degree of posterior element fractures and ligament injuries, the presence of which make this fracture potentially unstable.

A specific type of axial injury is the *Jefferson's fracture*, which is a comminuted fracture of the C1 ring. There are fractures involving both the anterior arch and the posterior arch of C1. The axial load causes the lateral masses of C1 to displace laterally compared to C2 on the open-mouth view.

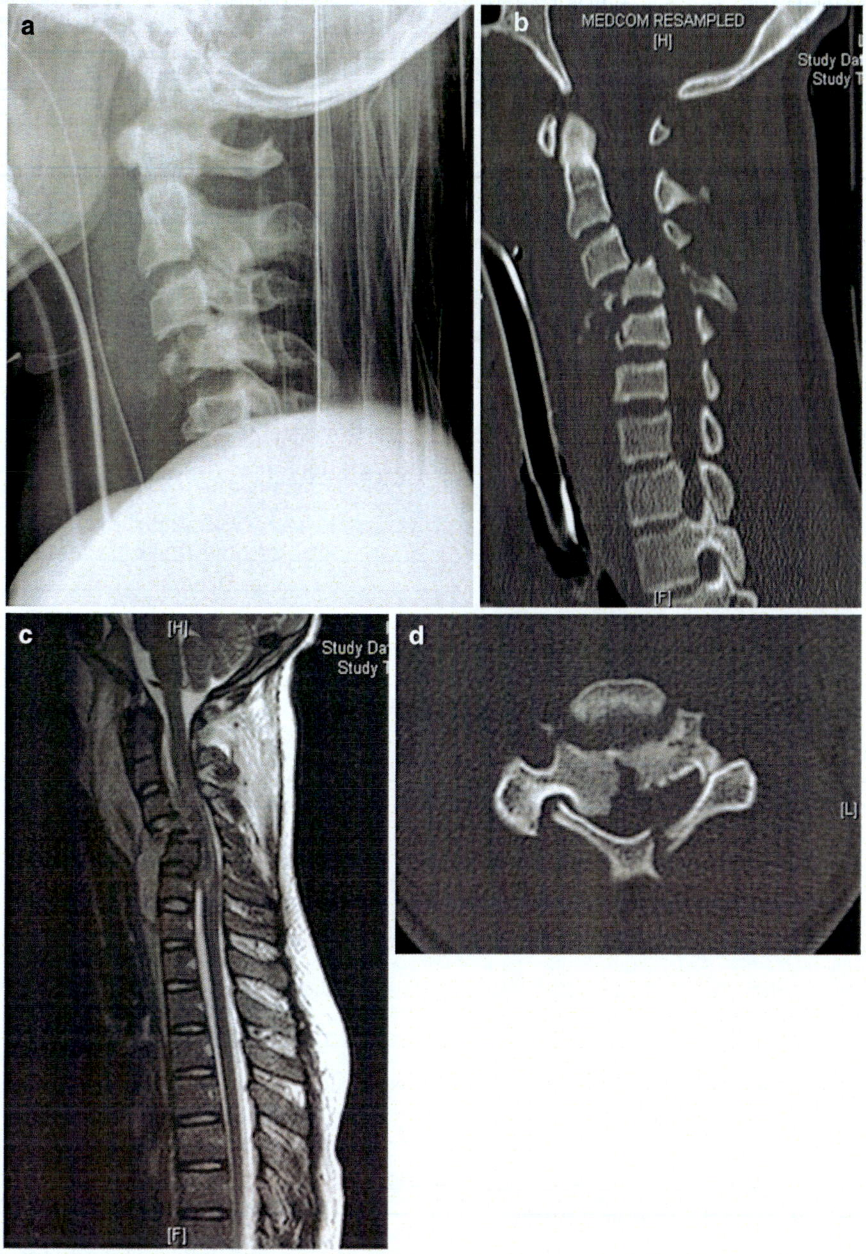

Fig. 5 A 15-year-old BMX bike rider landed on head whilst performing a back flip. Complete paralysis below C4 level (Frankel category A). The lateral radiograph (**a**) shows a C4 fracture involving the anterior part of the vertebral body, with C3/4 anterior subluxation, C5 vertebral fracture and C5/6 facet subluxation with an undisplaced fracture of the spinous process of C4. The sagittal CT reconstruction (**b**) shows the degree of canal compromise by the dislocation. The sagittal T2-w MR image (**c**) shows the extensive haematoma in the anterior soft tissues, cord compression and cord oedema. Note the low signal seen within the cord due to haemorrhage, which is a poor prognostic sign. The axial CT image (**d**) shows the characteristic sagittally oriented split in the vertebral body and the posterior element fractures

Flexion rotation: The ligaments in the spine can withstand reasonable compressive and tensile forces, but are particularly susceptible to rotational injury. A specific type of rotational injury is *unilateral facet dislocation*. There is less than 25% anterior subluxation of one vertebra over the other (>50% subluxation with bilateral facet dislocation).

Lateral flexion/shearing injuries can result in transverse process fracture, lateral vertebral compression or an uncinate process fracture.

Other specific injuries can occur due to combinations of these forces including *atlanto-axial dislocation* (hyperflexion and shearing): this is usually atraumatic and is commonly seen in rheumatoid arthritis, Down's syndrome and is due to transverse ligament rupture. Flexion/extension radiographs may be necessary to diagnose this injury. On the lateral radiograph there is increase (>2.5 mm in adults and >5 mm in children) in the distance between the anterior cortex of the dens and the posterior cortex of the

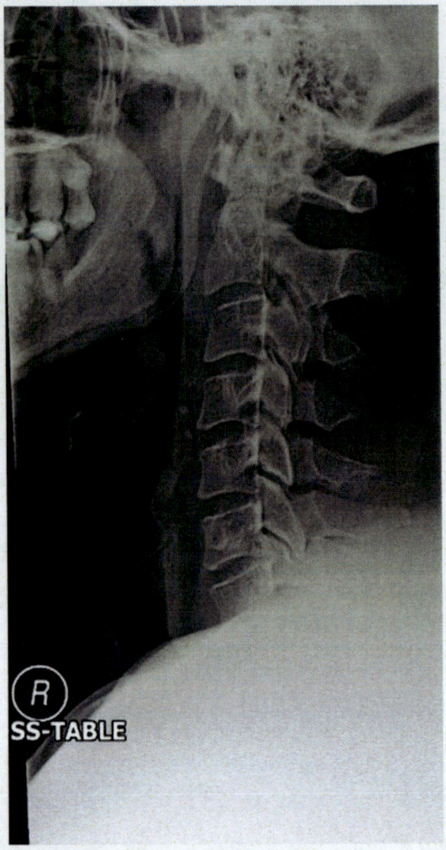

Fig. 6 Horse riding injury. Posterior arch fractures at C2 (Hangman's fracture). Note the minor anterior vertebral subluxation of C2 over C3 with disruption of the posterior spino-laminar line highlighted by posterior displacement of C2 spinous process in relation to C1 and C3 spinous processes. Also note the osteoarticular injury to the C3 articular process

anterior arch of atlas. This injury may be associated with Jefferson's fracture.

10.1.2 Thoracolumbar Injuries

Fractures of the thoracolumbar spine are less common than cervical spine and are even less commonly associated with neurological abnormalities. A number of classification systems are described, but the most frequently used system differentiates these injuries into compression, burst fractures, flexion distraction injuries and fracture/dislocations. This classification system is simple, easy to use and also has prognostic significance. Simple compression injuries are usually not associated with any neurological injury. The incidence of neurological injury increases with progression from burst fracture to flexion/distraction injuries and is almost universal with fracture/dislocations. Fortunately, flexion/distraction injuries need excessive force and are far less common than compression fractures.

Compression fractures (Fig. 7) are not strictly catastrophic injuries but are included in this section for ease of classification. With these injuries there is a loss of height of the anterior part of the vertebral body. However, the posterior vertebral body line is preserved keeping the middle column intact. No injury is seen in the posterior column in this injury.

Burst fractures are similar to burst fractures described with axial compression in the cervical spine. There is involvement of the middle column and the anterior column. There is in some cases also associated injuries in the posterior column either in the form of a sagittal fracture through the laminae and/or posterior ligamentous injury. The presence of posterior injuries makes this injury potentially unstable. Burst fractures can therefore be both stable (Fig. 8) and unstable (Fig. 9) in nature depending on the appearances of the posterior column.

The classic *Flexion distraction* injury is the *Chance* fracture. Contrary to popular belief, the fulcrum for the flexion in this type of injury is actually just anterior to the vertebral column. There is a resultant minor degree of compression anteriorly seen as a minor vertebral compression and may be associated with disc injury. The middle column is typically distracted with apparent increase in the posterior vertebral body height when compared with neighbouring vertebrae. There is always distraction injury in the posterior column seen as a combination of facet fractures, facet joint dislocation, laminar/pedicle fractures and posterior ligamentous injury. These injuries can be further classified into three types: *Type 1*, where the injuries in the three columns are bony in nature. There is therefore anterior vertebral compression with middle column distraction and the posterior column injuries are all fractures. *Type 2*, where the injuries are a combination of bone and soft tissue injuries in the three columns. *Type 3*, where the injury is completely soft tissue in nature associated with complete disruption of the IVD passing through the anterior and middle columns. There is injury to the posterior longitudinal ligament. The posterior column injury is a combination of facet dislocation/subluxation and extensive ligamentum flavum, interspinous and supraspinous ligament injuries.

The *fracture dislocations* are usually due to excessive complex mechanisms of injury with multidirectional

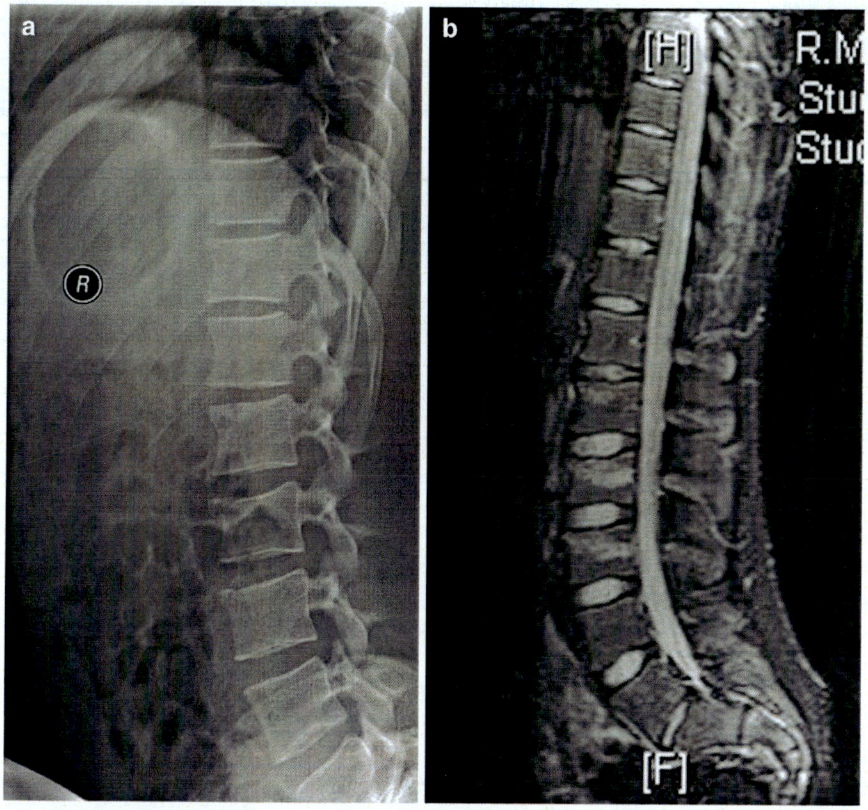

Fig. 7 Jet skiing injury in a 16-year-old. Simple lumbar wedge compression fractures. The lateral radiograph (**a**) demonstrates minor compression of the anterior superior corners of L3 and L4 vertebrae. No involvement of the middle column. A STIR (**b**) sagittal image shows minor compression of these vertebrae and also oedema in the vertebral bodies. No middle or posterior column injury. Also note the minor oedema in the anterosuperior corner of L2 vertebra in keeping a further injury here

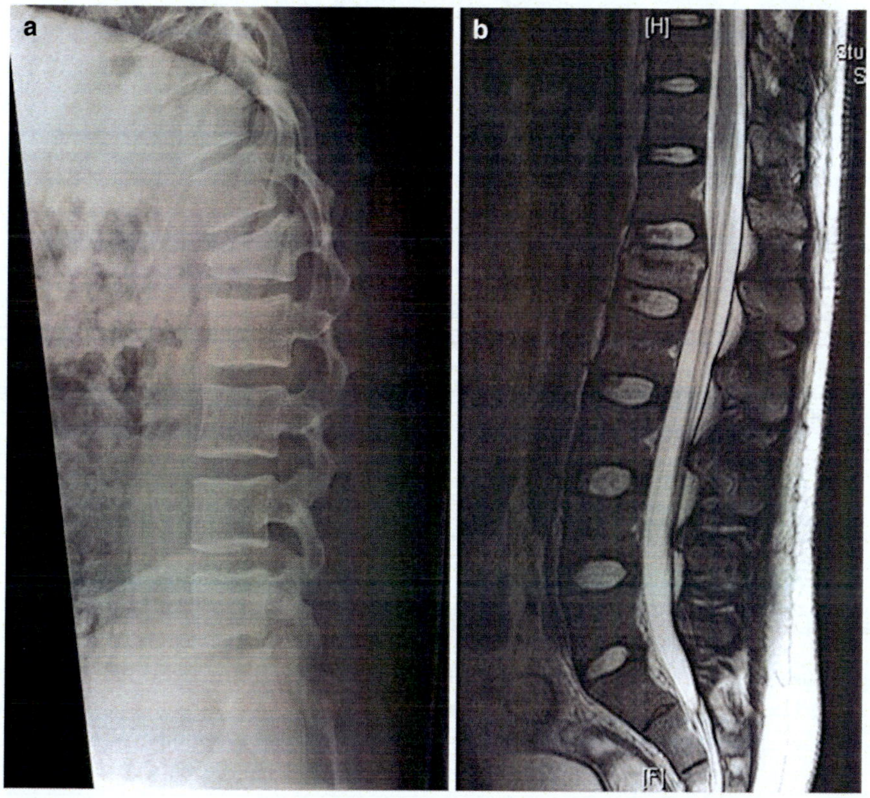

Fig. 8 Stable L1 burst fracture. Motorcross injury in a 16-year-old who came off a jump in the air and landed on his feet. The patient was neurologically intact. The lateral radiograph (**a**) shows a burst fracture of the L1 vertebra. The sagittal T2-w MR image (**b**) shows the extensive bone marrow oedema and a minor posterior retropulsion. No major canal compromise is seen. There is no evidence of any posterior ligamentous injury in keeping with a stable burst fracture. At our institution, these patients are mobilised immediately after injury with no surgery

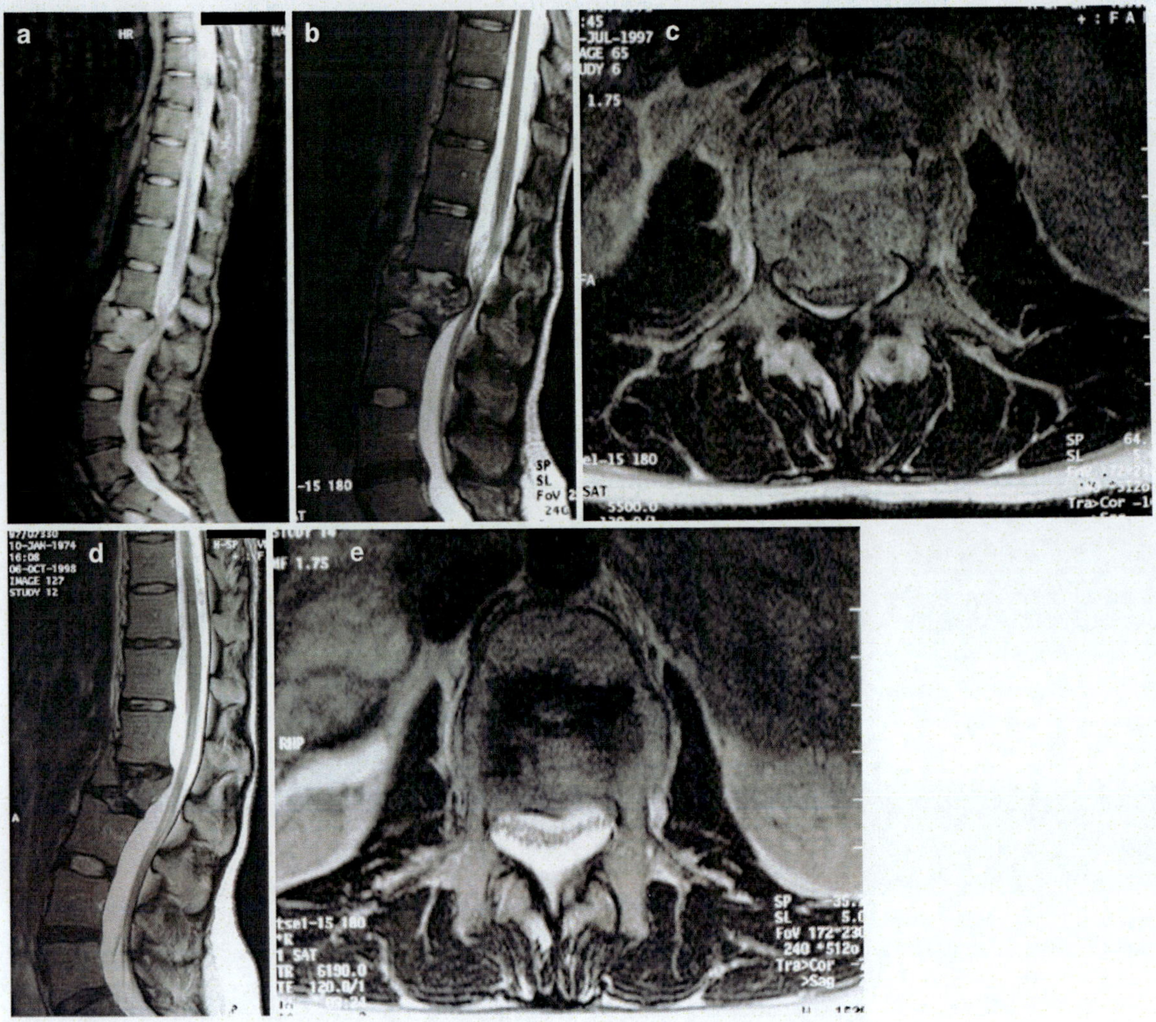

Fig. 9 Unstable burst fracture following a horse riding accident. The sagittal STIR (**a**), T2-w (**b**) and axial T2-w (**c**) MR images demonstrate a burst fracture of the L2 vertebra. Note the severe canal compromise and the sagittal fracture of the left lamina. The patient was treated conservatively. The sagittal (**d**) and axial (**e**) T2-w MR images one year later at the same level as (**b**) and (**c**) show spontaneous remodelling of the spinal canal which is now of reasonable calibre

forces resulting in severe fractures associated with malalignment. These are almost always associated with neurological injury.

10.1.3 Physeal/Apophyseal Injuries

The physis is the weakest portion of the axial skeleton to tensile forces. The ring apophysis starts to ossify at about 7–8 years of age. Before this age, injuries to the ring apophysis are difficult to ascertain. The displacement of this ossific ring apophysis is suggestive of injury to this physis. These can occur anywhere in the spine but are more common in the sub-axial portion of the cervical spine. The Salter–Harris classification used in the appendicular skeleton can be extrapolated to these injuries (Figs. 10 and 11) even though these are at the apophysis–physis junction. However, unlike Salter–Harris classification this pattern of classifying spinal apophyseal injuries does not equate to similar prognostic implications. For example, the type1 lesions in the spine appear to indicate much more severe injuries and may need surgery whilst type 3 and 4 lesions can heal conservatively. The displaced ossified apophyses are best appreciated on radiographs

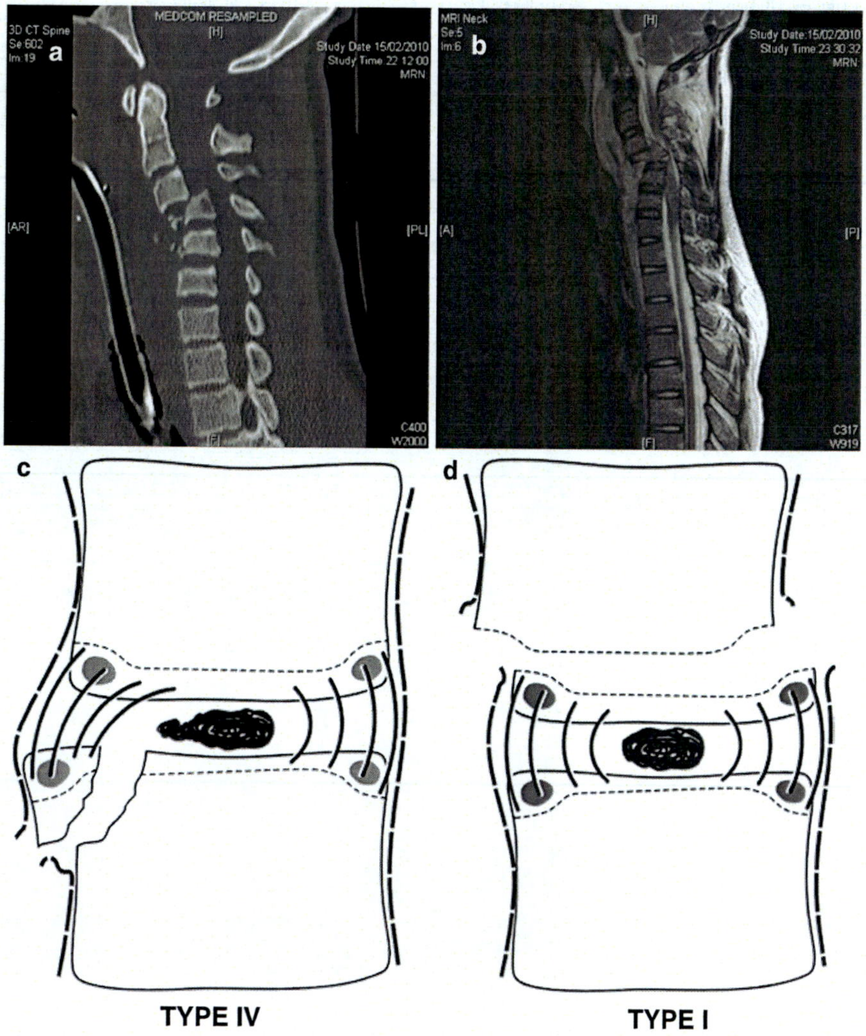

Fig. 10 Two-level physeal injury at C4 and C5 levels in a 15-year-old boy. Sagittal CT reconstruction (**a**), T2-w MR image (**b**) from the same patient as Fig. 5 show the C4 injury anteriorly passes from the anterosuperior corner of the vertebral body into the physeal junction and extends into the IVD in keeping with a type 4 injury. There is marked displacement at the fracture. The injury at the C5 level is a type 1 injury with the fracture extending through the physis without involvement of the disc or the vertebral body. Diagrammatic representation (**c**, **d**) of type 4 and type 1 physeal injuries

and CT rather than on MRI scans where the small ossific focus is difficult to identify.

Growth plate fractures can occur in the thoracolumbar spine in the adolescent population. Clinically this presents like a herniated disc if it includes the posterior disco-vertebral junction. The patient may describe a pop after lifting, fall or twisting injury. Non-operative treatment is rarely successful and surgery is frequently needed. As described in earlier sections of this chapter, the apophysis consists of a ring of ossification at the edge of the cartilaginous growth plate. Before it fuses with the vertebral body, the ring of ossification is separated from the vertebral body by a layer of hyaline cartilage which represents a relative area of weakness. Posterior apophyseal ring fractures are usually seen in the lumbo-sacral region. They commonly involve the cephalad rim of the first sacral vertebra and the L4 and L5 vertebrae less frequently. Takata et al. have classified these injuries into three categories (Takata et al. 1988):

- Type I: Simple separation of the entire margin of the apophysis
- Type II: Apophyseal injury including a portion of overlying cartilage of the annulus fibrosus
- Type III: A more localised fracture but with a larger amount of vertebral body involved. There is a round defect in the bone adjoining the fracture in this type of fracture

Epstein and associates have suggested a *fourth type* that involves a fracture of both the cephalad and caudad apophyses and involves the full length of the posterior margin of the vertebral body (Epstein et al. 1989).

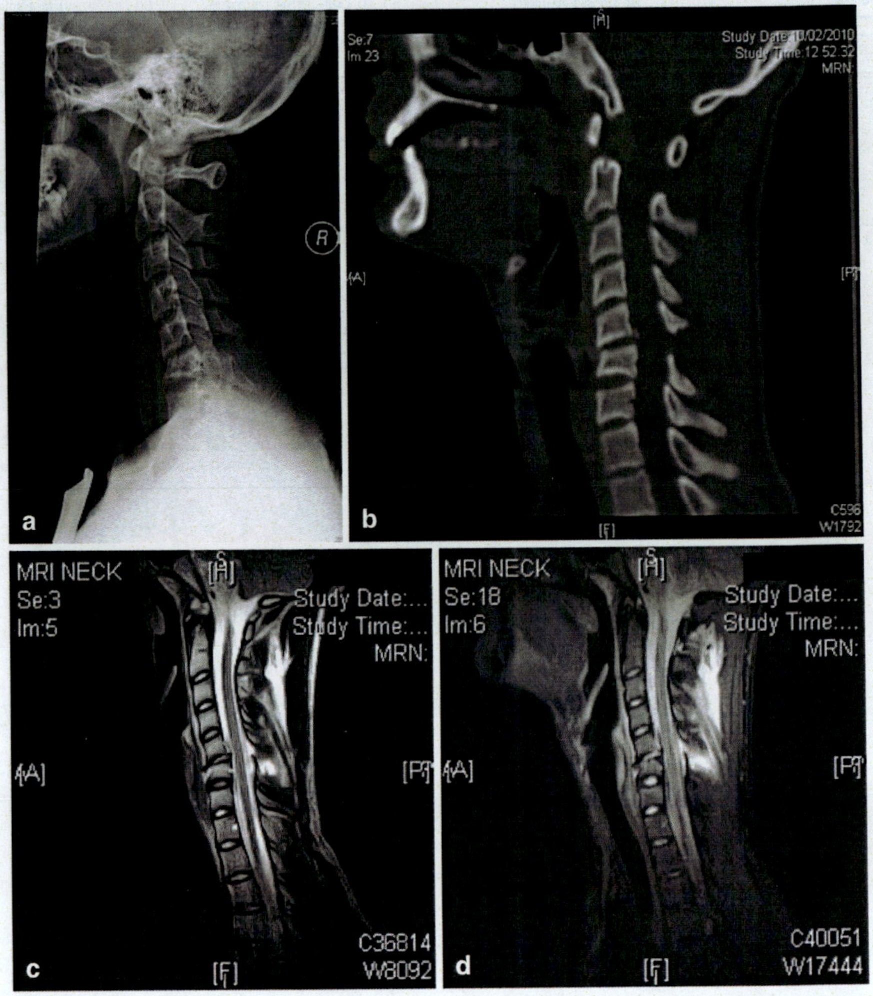

Fig. 11 Type 3 physeal injury at the C5/6 level. The displaced apophysis is difficult to appreciate on the lateral radiograph (**a**) due to bone overlap. However, the sagittal reformatted CT scan (**b**) clearly demonstrates the displaced posteroinferior C5 apophysis and the narrowed disc space. The sagittal T2-w (**c**) and STIR (**d**) MR images demonstrate the disc injury extending through the physis with displacement of the posteroinferior C5 apophysis and the posterior longitudinal ligament. The injured apophysis itself is difficult to appreciate on MRI scan and is best appreciated on CT

Type I fractures are commonly seen in children. These children present with symptoms suggestive of disc herniation. Whilst other authors have suggested that these fractures are due to trauma or strenuous activity (Handel et al. 1979), Takata et al. have not found major injuries associated with their patients. Instead they found irregularities of the end plates and suggested that fragility of the end plate is responsible for these fractures. These lesions can be difficult to see on conventional radiographs. Findings include disc space narrowing, irregularity of the posterior vertebral corner or an ossific defect displaced into the spinal canal. CT shows an arcuate fragment paralleling the posterior vertebral body outline. There is discontinuity or truncation of the normally convex posterior inferior vertebral margin on MR scans, with elevation or disruption of the posterior longitudinal ligament.

Physeal fractures can also occur through the neurocentral synchondrosis and have been described in child abuse (Vialle et al. 2006). These can be suspected on anteroposterior radiographs where there is widening of the interpedicular distance. There is anterior or posterior displacement of the vertebral body on the lateral radiographs. The fracture line may be evident and there is varying degrees of kyphosis. With anterior displacement neurological injury is unlikely and the outcome is favourable, but the risk is increased with posterior displacement of the vertebral body. MR is useful to assess cord and soft tissues but also to assess progress during healing and growth plate viability.

10.1.4 Cervical Cord Neuropraxia

Cervical cord neuropraxia (CCN) is an acute transient neurological injury associated with sensory and motor deficit in at least two extremities (Boden et al. 2006; Torg et al. 1986). CCN is classified based on neurological deficit, duration of symptoms and the pattern of injury. Clinically CCN is classified into (1) 'plegia' for episodes with complete paralysis; (2) 'paresis' for episodes with motor weakness; and (3) 'paraesthesia' for episodes that involve only sensory changes without any motor involvement. The injury is graded by the duration of symptoms: Grade 1, less than 15 min; Grade II, 15 min to 24 h; Grade III, longer than 24 h. In a study reviewing 110 patients with sports related CCN, the authors conclude that: (1) CCN is a transient neurological phenomenon and individuals with uncomplicated CCN may be permitted to return to their previous activity without an increased risk of permanent neurological injury; (2) congenital or degenerative narrowing of the sagittal diameter of the cervical canal is a causative factor; (3) the overall recurrence rate after return to play is 56%; and (4) the risk of recurrence is strongly and inversely correlated with sagittal canal diameter and it is useful in the prediction of future episodes of CCN (Torg et al. 1997). There was no correlation between classification, grading and radiologic appearances. In this study, CCN was not associated with permanent neurological injury and no permanent morbidity occurred in patients who returned to contact activities (Torg et al. 1997). There is no injury evident on the radiographs; the patient is pain free with a full range of cervical spine motion. No injury may be seen on MRI scan (Fig. 12). The injury is most common in American football players (87% of 110 patients in Torg's study). There is a prevalence of 7 per 10000 in American football players (Torg et al. 2002). Symptoms typically resolve in less than 15 min but may take up to 2 days. All mechanisms of injury including flexion, extension and axial loading can cause CCN which is thought to result from a poor technique of tackling involving the top of the head.

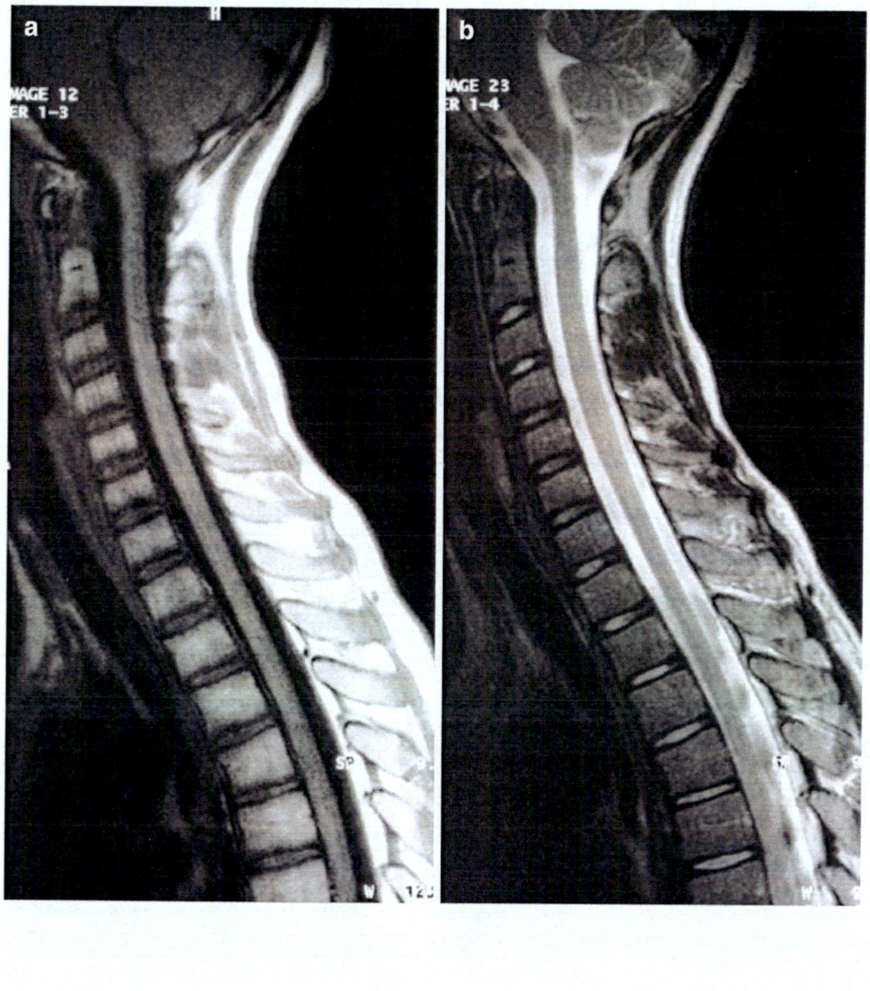

Fig. 12 Neuropraxia. A 14-year-old rugby player crashed into a tackling block during training, collapsed immediately with weakness in both right arm and left leg. The sagittal T1-w (**a**), T2-w (**b**) MR images reveal normal appearances of the cord and cervical spinal column. The patient immediately recovered full motor and sensory function although there was some residual pain

Although studies have shown no evidence of a subsequent permanent quadriplegia in athletes returning to contact sports after a CCN event, the numbers of people returning to contact sport is low. An episode of CCN is not a contraindication for return to sporting activity. However, athletes should be counselled about the significant risk of recurrent CCN (about 50%), which depends on the spinal canal dimension – the smaller the canal diameter, the greater the risk of CCN. Based on the initial assessment, those athletes with ligamentous instability, cord abnormalities on MRI, symptoms lasting longer than 36 h, and recurrent episodes, should be excluded from a return to contact sports (Torg et al. 2002).

10.1.5 SCIWORA

SCIWORA refers to spinal cord injury without radiographic abnormality. The term was first used to describe cord injury in the absence of plain radiographic abnormality (Pang and Wilberger 1982). With the evolution of imaging, two distinct definitions of SCIWORA can be identified in various publications. With the wide spread use of CT along with plain films in the initial assessment, the term is more commonly now used to describe cord injury in the absence of plain radiographic or CT evidence of injury. A majority of these patients demonstrate abnormalities on MR imaging (Fig. 13). Six percent of patients had SCIWORA by this definition in one review (Cirak et al. 2004). There is however a further group of patients where even the MR scan is normal despite definite clinical evidence of cord injury. With this definition, the incidence of SCIWORA in the same review has reduced to 1%. SCIWORA is more common in children than in adults due to the factors described earlier such as the variable elasticity of the cord and spinal column. SCIWORA makes up to 5–55% of C-spine injuries in children. It is most common before 3 years of age. The main mechanisms of this type of injury are hyperextension, flexion, distraction and cord ischaemia. There is variable neurological deficit ranging from partial cord defects to complete transection. Various incomplete cord syndromes including central cord syndrome, Brown Sequard syndrome, anterior spinal cord artery syndrome and partial cord syndrome can occur depending on the site and mechanism of insult. Recurrent SCIWORA can occur if there is inadequate immobilisation or non-compliance with advice regarding high risk activities. These children have an initial minor SCIWORA, but with a significant neurological deficit after the recurrent SCIWORA. Wide spread use of MRI and careful immobilisation has reduced the incidence of recurrent SCIWORA. Nevertheless, due to the potential for persistent instability and re-injury in patients with soft tissue injuries, these patients often need long term follow-up and assessment of instability.

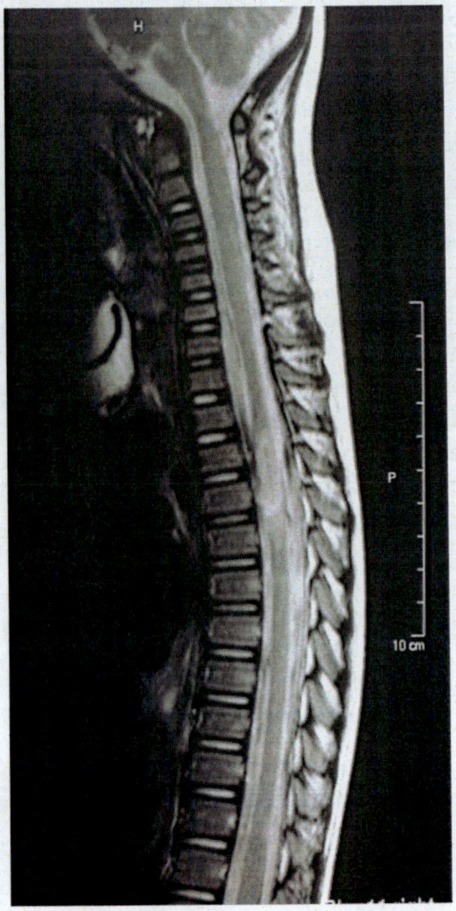

Fig. 13 A 13-year-old boy with SCIWORA. The radiographs did not show any bony abnormality. The sagittal T2-w MR image does not demonstrate any osseo-ligamentous injury of the vertebral column. Note the morphological and signal changes at the T3/4 level in keeping with intra-medullary trauma

10.2 Acute Non-catastrophic Spinal Injuries

These include strains, muscle spasms, avulsion fractures, compression fractures and some disc herniations.

10.2.1 Strains, Fractures and Disc Herniations

Strains can be caused by any low grade injury to the spine. The most common of these is the Whiplash injury – caused by a sudden extension–flexion mechanism. This is caused typically when a stationary person is shunted from the rear. These athletes present with paravertebral muscle spasm, limited range of motion and a normal neurological examination. Radiographs demonstrate a loss in the normal cervical curvature. There is however no evidence of injury to the spinal column and the alignment is normal. Treatment is conservative with muscle relaxants, physiotherapy and anti-inflammatories.

Compression fractures can occur anywhere in the vertebral column but are most common in the cervical spine from the C4 to the C7 levels and in the thoracolumbar spine from the T10 to the L2 level. Compressions of less than 25% vertebral height and with no neurological injury can be managed conservatively after simple radiographic assessment. More significant compressions may be associated with either bony or soft tissue injuries in the posterior elements of the spinal column and may need further imaging assessment including CT and/or MRI. Potentially unstable injuries may need surgical management sometimes even in the absence of neurological injury.

Avulsion fractures of the spinous process in the cervical spine, also known as Clay shoveler's fractures, usually occur in power lifters and American football players. The widely accepted mechanism is forceful flexion of the cervical spine, or forceful contraction of the trapezius and rhomboid muscles. These avulsion injuries are stable and can be treated conservatively.

Disc herniations caused by sporting activity result in pain, reduced range of motion and radicular symptoms. There may be sensory or motor neurological deficit. Radiographs usually are normal. MRI will characterise the extent of the herniation and its effect on neurological structures. Most often these athletes respond to conservative measures including a short period of rest, anti-inflammatories, physiotherapy and occasionally, epidural steroid injections. Surgery may need to be considered if these measures fail or if there is progressive neurological deficit. Often acute disc herniations are associated with a haematoma in the epidural space. It is important to identify these associated haematomas. There is a strong likelihood that these haematomas can resolve with time, and spontaneous resolution of neurological signs may occur without the need for surgery.

10.2.2 Stingers and Whiplash Injuries

A *stinger* or *burner* is classically described as a transient episode of shooting or electrical pain or paraesthesia radiating down one upper extremity after an acute event, typically one involving significant contact to the head or shoulder (Standaert and Herring 2009). There may be varying degree of associated motor weakness. Although symptoms resolve spontaneously, stingers can result in permanent neurological deficit or become recurrent, thereby limiting the athlete's ability to continue playing. This injury occurs in contact sport and is reported in up to 50–65% of collegiate American football players over the course of their career, and recurrence rates can be high (Levitz et al. 1997). Stingers are unilateral and the presence of bilateral symptoms should raise concerns for cervical cord injury rather than stingers. The neurological abnormalities are generally consistent with either C5 or C6 root pathology or an injury to the upper trunk of the brachial plexus.

There are a number of controversies with stingers, including mechanism of injury, exact location of injury, treatment, prevention and 'return to play' decisions.

Mechanism of injury controversy falls in to either the tensile or compressive categories. Tensile force is thought to occur by traction to either a nerve root or the brachial plexus and is either due to lateral flexion of the neck to the contralateral side or ipsilateral depression of the shoulder. Compressive mechanism is thought to occur on either the nerve root or brachial plexus due to either rapid extension plus ipsilateral flexion of the neck or direct compression of the brachial plexus. Levitz et al. found that the mechanism of injury in 83% of their patients was a cervical extension combined with lateral flexion to the ipsilateral side most consistent with a compressive injury to the nerve root in the spine (Levitz et al. 1997). Others have described a predominance of brachial plexus injuries in their case series (Clancy et al. 1977; Di Benedetto and Markey 1984). There is disagreement as to the exact location of injury (i.e., cervical root vs brachial plexus).

From an anatomical perspective, the cervical nerve roots appear more vulnerable than the well-protected brachial plexus, partly due to the plexiform nature of the plexus and the protective surrounding tissues (Weinstein 1998).

The indications for imaging are not well defined. Levitz et al. noted that most of these athletes (93%) demonstrated disc disease or foraminal narrowing on imaging (Levitz et al. 1997). The implications of these imaging findings are, however, not entirely clear as incidental bony and discogenic abnormalities are well documented elsewhere in the thoracolumbar spine in young athletes (Sward et al.1990). Not all athletes sustaining a stinger need imaging, but imaging should be considered for those with recurrent events, persistent symptoms and neurological deficits. A single incident that resolves rapidly with no persistent neurological deficit does not warrant imaging. In recurrent and persistent cases, radiographs including flexion/extension views may demonstrate disc space narrowing, foraminal stenosis or instability. MRI may demonstrate foraminal narrowing and root compression. Imaging of the brachial plexus may also be needed to exclude any obvious lesions including tumours or inflammatory processes. Imaging mainly plays a role in excluding significant pathology in the setting of recurrent stingers. Imaging can also aid in 'return to play' decisions. If there is a large disc herniation, the athlete may need to avoid contact sport till the symptoms completely settle. If there is significant instability, the athlete may be advised to avoid return to contact sport completely. Similarly, if an athlete has significant anatomical abnormalities in the cervical spine, there may be a need to abstain from contact sport. Although not well described in the literature with stingers, the anatomical location of the nerve injury may sometimes be evident with a combination of MRI and electrodiagnostic testing. If the injury is at the plexus level, this should spare the paraspinal muscles which should show normal appearance. The electrodiagnostic testing will demonstrate normal paraspinal conduction and a predominantly sensory conduction loss. However, if the injury is at the rootlet level, the paraspinal muscles may demonstrate acute, subacute or chronic denervation features on MRI. There may be abnormality in the paraspinal muscles on electrodiagnostic testing and correlating motor abnormalities in the distal muscles with normal sensory conduction studies.

Whiplash injuries occur typically in motor vehicle accidents during a rear-end shunt on a stationary vehicle. There is a sudden hyperextension and subsequent hyperflexion of the cervical spine associated with sudden acceleration and then deceleration of the head. This injury can also occur in sport with similar mechanisms. This injury is very common and occurs in approximately 1 million individuals in the USA, although its incidence in sports is not clear. Patients most frequently complain of headache, pain in the neck and interscapular region, paraesthesia in the arms or hands, vertigo and tiredness. Usually no abnormalities are seen on imaging. The most common abnormality described on radiographs is loss of the normal cervical curvature and kyphosis. This is thought to be a result of muscle spasm causing hypomobility and straightening of the cervical spine. The kyphosis is thought to be related to adjacent segment hypermobility. In a study involving 100 patients with whiplash injury, the authors have noted minor oedema in the anterior longitudinal ligament in only one patient (Ronnen et al. 1996). MRI is therefore not necessary in whiplash injuries.

10.3 Chronic Spinal Injuries

10.3.1 Low Back Pain and Disc Degeneration

Low back pain and disc degeneration are common problems in athletic individuals (Fig. 14). In their 5-year prospective study, Elfering et al. investigated the risk factors for the development or deterioration of lumbar disc degeneration as diagnosed by MRI (Elfering et al. 2002). Forty-one participants underwent MRI and filled out a questionnaire at baseline and at 5-year follow-up. Four classes of variables were studied: sociodemographic data (including sports), MRI identified disc abnormalities, physical job characteristics and psychosocial aspects of work. Seventeen of the 41 demonstrated deterioration of disc degeneration on MRI with only a weak correlation between disc degeneration and back pain. The extent of disc degeneration on the initial MRI, lack of sports activities and night shift work were significant independent predictors of progressive disc degeneration. In another study involving follow-up of 67 asymptomatic participants with baseline MRI scans, Borenstein et al. found that the findings on baseline MRI scan were not predictive of future development of back pain (Borenstein et al. 2001). Bartsch et al. used

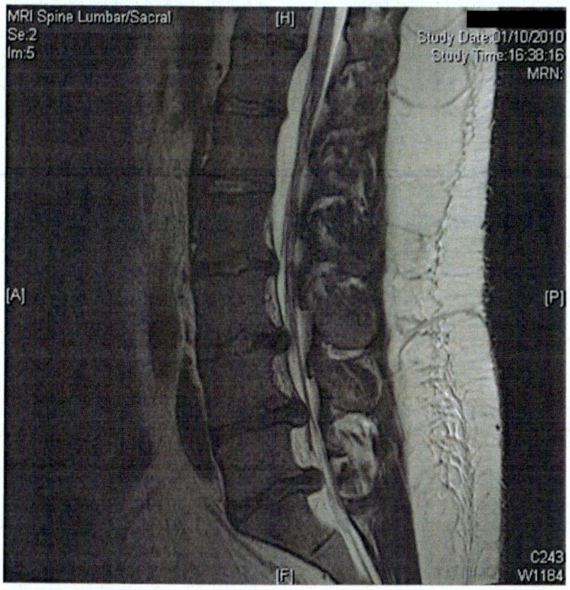

Fig. 14 Premature disc degeneration in an athlete. The sagittal T2-w MR image in a 20-year-old long-distance runner demonstrates marked disc degeneration at multiple levels with multiple disc prolapses and spinal canal narrowing

MRI to investigate cervico-thoracic disc protrusions in scuba divers and found no increase in disc protrusions in divers compared to controls (Bartsch et al. 2001) whilst other investigators found higher number of disc abnormalities in amateur divers compared to control subjects (Reul et al. 1995).

10.3.2 Stress Fractures

Stress fractures in the athletes can be either fatigue fractures or insufficiency fractures. Fatigue fractures occur when recurrent stress is applied to normal bone. Insufficiency fractures occur when there is an underlying metabolic abnormality in the fractured bone. Athletes suffering stress fractures of cancellous bone (vertebral body/sacrum) may have an underlying metabolic disorder, low oestrogen status or an eating disorder and need further assessment. Stress fractures have been reported in a number of sporting activities including running, gymnastics and track and field. Sacrum is a common site of cancellous bone stress fractures (Johnson et al. 2001). Athletes suffering cancellous bone fractures are more likely to have underlying low bone mineral density compared to those suffering cortical bone stress fractures.

10.3.3 Spondylolysis and Spondylolisthesis

Spondylolysis, defined as a fracture or defect of the pars interarticularis, has been reported in up to 47% of adolescent athletes with low back pain and is associated with sports like gymnastics, weight lifting, rowing and cricket. However, spondylolysis may be seen in both symptomatic and asymptomatic individuals. Skeletally immature individuals are at increased risk of this injury during periods of rapid skeletal growth. There is a male preponderance with a male to female ratio of up to 3:1. Racial preponderance is seen with the highest incidence in Eskimos. There is association of spondylolysis with transitional lumbar vertebra, spina bifida occulta, Scheurmann's disease, osteogenesis imperfecta and osteopetrosis. It has been proposed that this injury results from repetitive trauma and develops in stages from stress related injury to complete spondylolysis. This most commonly occurs at the L5 level (85%) with 15% occurring at the L4 level. Other levels are only affected rarely. Spondylolysis can result in varying degrees of spondylolisthesis. Whilst lateral radiographs usually demonstrate the spondylolytic defect, 45 degree oblique radiographs demonstrate the pars interarticularis without overlap from the pars on the other side. Radiographs are insensitive to early stress reaction which can be seen on MR images as high signal change in the pars on T2-w images and is best seen with fat suppression techniques. CT may show sclerosis at this stage with no cortical interruption. A classification system has been proposed for MR staging of spondylolysis (Hollenberg et al. 2002): Grade 0 (normal) with no signal abnormality of the pars interarticularis. Grade 1 denotes patients with marrow oedema but no spondylolysis. Grade 2 was assigned to patients with T2 signal abnormalities and thinning, fragmentation or irregularity of the pars. Grade 3 involved a visible unilateral or bilateral spondylolysis with abnormal T2 signal (Fig. 15). Grade 4 involved complete spondylolysis without abnormal T2 signal. In the same study, a good intra- and inter-observer reliability with this classification system was demonstrated. CT scanning with reverse gantry orientation is reliable in assessing for spondylolytic defects and sometimes stress reactions. Reversing of the gantry is not necessary with the newer multislice scanners with isometric resolution in all three imaging planes. However CT can potentially miss some patients with early stress reactions which can be seen on MR and bone scintigraphy. Scintigraphy shows increased uptake in patients with stress response and active spondylolytic defects. However, chronic inactive spondylolytic defects may not be seen on scintigraphy. Moreover, it is difficult to be specific anatomically on routine scintigraphy. Single photon emission computed tomography (SPECT) is more sensitive. It is useful to identify an early stress reaction before spondylolysis occurs as treatment is more likely to be successful at this stage. Moreover, MR demonstrates the associated disc degeneration and the effects on nerve roots. When spondylolysis is seen, serial CT scans are useful to assess healing response (Fig. 15).

Limbus vertebrae (Fig. 16) occur at the anterosuperior or anteroinferior corners of single or multiple growing vertebral bodies. This is seen as a triangular opacity at the anterosuperior or anteroinferior margin of the vertebra frequently with adjacent indentation in the vertebral body. They can simulate fractures and

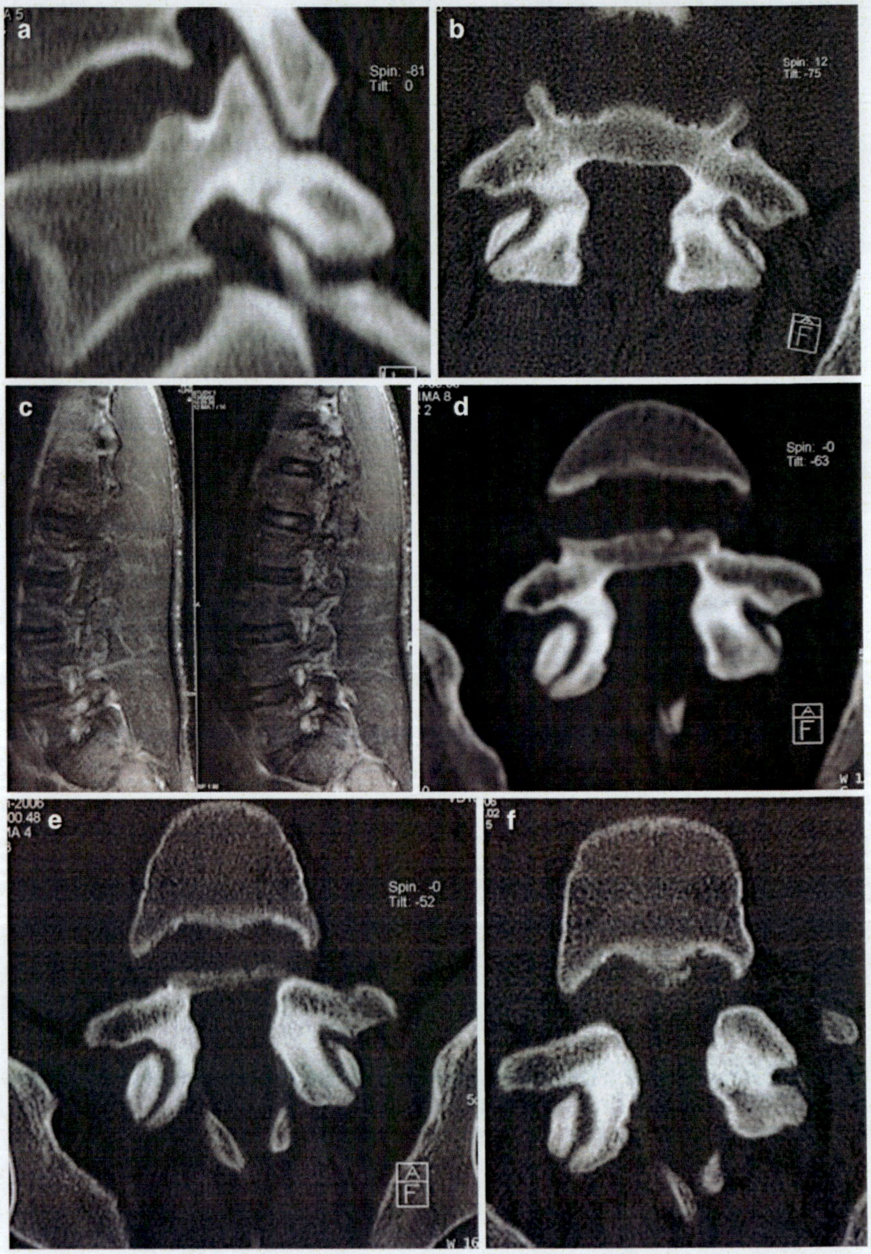

Fig. 15 Spondylolysis in a 15-year-old basket ball player. The parasagittal CT reconstruction image (**a**) and coronal oblique reconstruction image (**b**) along the L5 pars, demonstrate bilateral spondylolysis at the L5 level. The fracture ends are closely opposed and the fracture margins are 'Fuzzy', a good prognostic indicator of healing. The sagittal STIR MR image (**c**) demonstrates the oedema on either side of the pars defect. Serial CT scans at 3-monthly intervals (**d–f**) demonstrate gradual healing of the spondylolysis

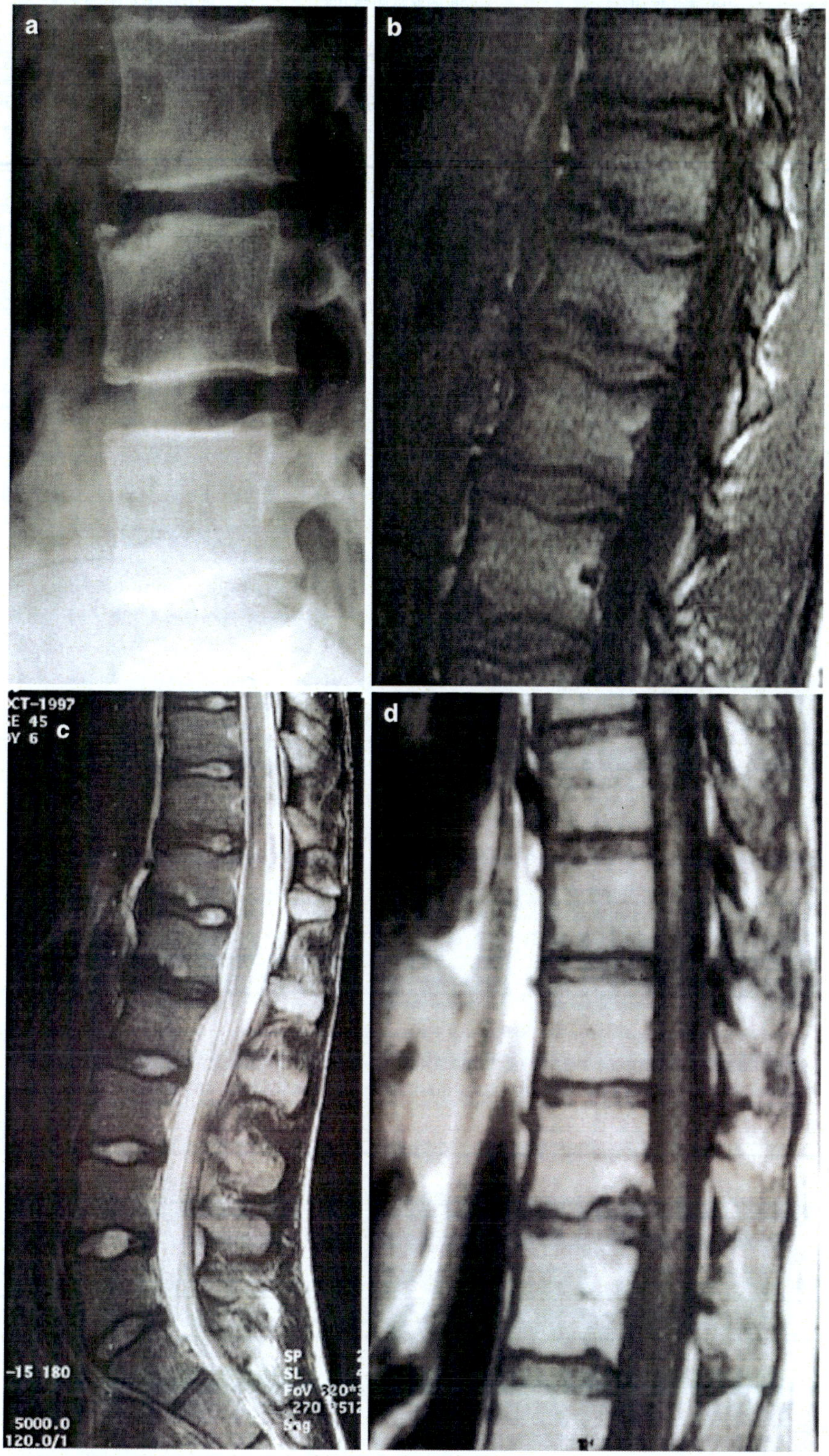

Fig. 16 Spectrum of limbus vertebrae. The lateral radiograph (**a**) shows an anterosuperior L3 limbus vertebra. The sagittal T1-w (**b**) and T2-w (**c**) images demonstrate contiguous limbus vertebrae anteroinferiorly at T12 and L1. Note degenerative changes in the adjacent discs and vertebral marrow oedema in relation to the limbus vertebrae at both levels. The sagittal T1-w (**d**) image shows limbus vertebra located posteroinferiorly at the T12 level

although often included as 'normal variants' are due to an intraosseous disc herniation usually in overuse which can be symptomatic. The bony fragment and the adjacent vertebra are well corticated with sharp margins.

11 'Return to Play' Criteria and Imaging

A number of factors play a role in the decision regarding 'return to play' (RTP) including age, experience, ability, level of participation, position played, as well as the attitudes and desires of the athlete and parents after an informed discussion about the potential risk (Torg 1997). The decision is difficult to make and athletes are commonly advised to refrain from sport as it is an easy advice to provide and to avoid potential litigation. There is also a lack of credible data regarding potential post-injury risk factors.

Torg et al. have tried to classify and advice in the decision making process on the basis of 1,200 cervical spine injuries from the national football head and neck injury registry (Torg 1997). Physicians commonly encounter three different types of lesions, divided into congenital, developmental and post-traumatic when asked to make a decision regarding RTP. Lesions are then considered to present either *no contraindication, relative contraindication or absolute contraindication.* It is however important to realise that the ultimate decision regarding RTP rests with the athlete and his/her parents.

Congenital conditions like odontoid agenesis, odontoid hypoplasia, os-odontoideum, atlanto-occipital fusion and long segment fusion in the Cervico-thoracic spine (severe Klippel–Feil anomaly) are absolute contraindications for contact sport. Spina bifida occulta on the other hand presents no contraindication. Traumatic conditions like atlanto-axial instability, atlanto-axial rotatory fixation, fractures or ligamentous injuries in the upper cervical spine and previous C1–C2 fusion constitute absolute contraindications. Healed undisplaced Jefferson's fracture, healed odontoid fractures and healed lateral mass fractures of C2 represent relative contraindications. A horizontal displacement of 3.5 mm or an angular displacement of more than 11 degrees are absolute contraindications for RTP. An acute fracture is an absolute contraindication but a stable healed fracture presents no contraindication. Unstable fractures remain absolute contraindications. All acute disc herniations and chronic 'hard disc' herniations associated with neurological findings, pain and limitation of cervical motion are contraindications.

As mentioned earlier in this chapter, athletes sustaining CCN with ligamentous instability, cord abnormalities on MRI, symptoms lasting longer than 36 h and recurrent episodes should be excluded from a return to contact sports (Torg et al. 2002). However, developmental narrowing of the spinal canal in the absence of spinal instability is neither a harbinger of nor a predisposing factor for permanent neurological injury. There is however a greater risk of recurrence of CCN with reduction in spinal canal dimensions. The presence of disc degeneration and small spinal canal however form relative contraindications for RTP.

Four criteria on MRI have been added to the 'absolute contraindication' category including the presence of Arnold–Chiari malformation, basilar invagination, spinal cord abnormality and residual cord encroachment following a healed stable sub-axial fracture.

Given the aforementioned criteria, the radiologist plays an important role in identifying these abnormalities and giving an indication as to the presence or absence of these confounding factors which affect RTP decisions.

12 Safety in Sport

Although it is difficult to estimate the exact proportion of preventable injuries, a significant proportion of all sport injuries are preventable. Prevention strategies include protective equipment, rule changes, preseason and season prevention interventions, safety measures, better coaching, societal awareness and education.

Education is the key to preventing catastrophic spinal injuries in sport. Research to identify the exact causes and mechanisms of individual spinal injuries plays a role in preventing future injuries. For example, the identification of spear tackling as a primary culprit in causing spinal injury has helped significantly in reducing the injury in American football. Education also takes the form of posters in locker rooms, slide presentations and videos. Education of coaches is also necessary in teaching safe techniques to players.

Rugby: Avoidance of physical mismatch of hookers. Avoiding untrained players from participating, banning spear tackling and stiff-arming, and sequential engagement – where the front row engage prior to the second and third rows so that the back row players do not force unprepared front row players into their opponents. The effectiveness of protective head gear in preventing spinal injury is not clear.

American football: Spear tackling injuries typically occur in defensive back players as they tackle an offensive player. 'Intentional spearing' was however banned in 1976 and the incidence of cervical injuries dropped by nearly 80% within a decade (Torg et al. 2002). Despite initial decline in incidence, the rates of quadriplegia did not show further decline in the 1990s and 2000s. It was difficult to prove 'intent' and the penalty was rarely called. The NCAA revised the spearing rule in 2005 and removed the word 'intentional' to make it easier for referees to call spearing penalties. Players are taught proper tackling and blocking techniques with the 'head up' and not with the crown of the head. Newer, lighter helmets may also help reduce cervical injuries by making it easier to keep the neck extended especially in younger players.

Ice hockey: A survey of Canadian hockey injuries demonstrated 241 spinal fractures and dislocations from 1966 to 1993 (Tator et al. 1998). The incidence worldwide was increasing in the 1980s possibly due to the increased size and speed of players and more emphasis on 'checking'. Better protective head gear may also have a role similar to football. The international ice hockey federation ruled in 1994 that 'checking from behind' is an offence and this reduced the incidence of spinal injury in international competitions.

Wrestling: Reducing wrestling injuries rests clearly with referees, coaches and athletes themselves. Referees particularly have to be aware of the vulnerability of wrestlers in certain positions and manoeuvres. Wrestlers who are off-balance have their arms held or have a potential for the opponent to land on top of them whilst the neck is flexed and the head is near the mat are particularly at risk. Referees should strictly enforce penalties for slams, which are throws involving the use of excessive force. Coaches should emphasise on safe wrestling techniques such as head-up position during any take down manoeuvre and proper rolling. Wrestlers themselves can help reduce the risk of injury by practicing safe techniques during take down, rolling and offensive tactics.

Swimming/diving: In America, there are specific rules to protect swimmers from diving injury at the shallow end of the pool. At high school level, swimmers must start the race in the water if the water depth is less than 3.5 ft. If the depth of water is between 3.5 and 4 ft, the swimmer can start the race in the water or from the deck. If the water depth is 4 ft or more, the swimmer may start the race from a raised platform of up to 30 in. from the water surface. At college level, the water depth should be at least 4 ft. Diving injuries appear to be most common in amateurs and recreational divers rather than professional divers mainly due to ignorance, reckless behaviour and intoxication. Whilst recreational diving accounts for a large proportion of all spinal injuries, competitive diving is relatively safe and catastrophic injuries are only rarely reported. Preventative strategies include not diving head first into shallow waters, adequate supervision of inexperienced swimmers and divers, avoiding alcohol and other judgement affecting substances during swimming and diving.

Skiing/snowboarding: Skiing injuries appear to occur more frequently later on in the day possibly due to skier fatigue. Safe skiing and snowboarding need to be enforced by ski patrols. Overcrowding should be avoided on the slopes. Separation of skiers from snowboarders may also help. In addition, the serious consequences of high risk jumping practices necessitate appropriate education.

Cheerleading: Currently pyramids are limited to no more than two levels in high school sport and 2.5 body lengths in college. Cheerleaders on top of the pyramids should be supported by a cheerleader at the base during dismount as they come into weight bearing contact with the performing surface. Spotters are mandatory for all persons extended above shoulder level. Any suspended persons are also not allowed to invert or rotate during dismount. Basket toss manoeuvres are also required to adhere to certain safety measures including limitation on the number of throwers, tossing from the ground level and having one of the throwers behind the flyer during the toss. The flyers are also trained to keep their head in line with the rest of the body. Stunts should be restricted in wet conditions. Coaches need to be instructed to spend as much time on safety as on accomplishment of stunts.

Baseball: Rules in baseball state that the fielder has the right of way at the base plate and the runner should avoid the fielder. It may be necessary to enforce feet-first sliding rather than head-first sliding. In little-league baseball, head-first sliding is currently not allowed.

13 Conclusion

Although the risk of catastrophic spinal injuries is very low in organised sporting activities, the physical, mental and financial cost associated with a spinal injury in these mostly young people is tremendous. The lifetime cost for the care of a quadriplegic individual can easily surpass 2 million dollars and the annual aggregate cost of care for sport related spinal cord injuries in the USA in 1995 was around $700 million (DeVivo 1997). It is therefore imperative that adequate time is spent on safety in sport even from a very early age and even in amateur sporting activities. Continued research is necessary in all sports, as we now know from experience that some changes brought in one area of a sport can affect the sportsman's chance of sustaining an injury elsewhere (e.g. increased incidence of spinal injury with better helmets in American football). This will then enable us to act swiftly to educate and, if necessary, legislate to reduce these injuries.

References

Athey AM (1991) A 3-year-old with spinal cord injury without radiographic abnormality (SCIWORA). J Emerg Nurs 17:380–384, discussion 385

Barba CA, Taggert J, Morgan AS et al (2001) A new cervical spine clearance protocol using computed tomography. J Trauma 5:652–656, discussion 656–657

Bartsch T, Cordes P, Keil et al (2001) Cervico-thoracic disc protrusions in controlled compressed-air diving: clinical and MRI findings. J Neurol 248:514–516

Boden BP, Jarvis CG (2008) Spinal injuries in sports. Neurol Clin 26:63–78, viii

Boden BP, Prior C (2005) Catastrophic spine injuries in sports. Curr Sports Med Rep 4:45–49

Boden BP, Tacchetti RL, Cantu RC, Knowles SB, Mueller FO (2006) Catastrophic cervical spine injuries in high school and college football players. Am J Sports Med 34: 1223–1232

Borenstein DG, O' Mara JW et al (2001) The value of magnetic resonance imaging of the lumbar spine to predict low-back pain in asymptomatic subjects: a seven-year follow-up study. J Bone Joint Surg Am 83-A:1306–1311

Cirak B, Ziegfeld S, Knight VM et al (2004) Spinal injuries in children. J Pediatr Surg 39:607–612

Clancy WG Jr, Brand RL, Bergfield JA (1977) Upper trunk brachial plexus injuries in contact sports. Am J Sports Med 5:209–216

Collier TR, Jones ML, Murray HH (2010) Skimboarding: a new cause of water sport spinal cord injury. Spinal Cord 48:349–351

Cooper MT, McGee KM, Anderson DG (2003) Epidemiology of athletic head and neck injuries. Clin Sports Med 22: 427–443, vii

Davidson RM, Burton JH, Snowise M, Owens WB (2001) Football protective gear and cervical spine imaging. Ann Emerg Med 38:26–30

DeVivo MJ (1997) Causes and costs of spinal cord injury in the United States. Spinal Cord 35:809–813

Di Benedetto M, Markey K (1984) Electrodiagnostic localization of traumatic upper trunk brachial plexopathy. Arch Phys Med Rehabil 65:15–17

Elfering A, Semmer N, Birkhofer D et al (2002) Risk factors for lumbar disc degeneration: a 5-year prospective MRI study in asymptomatic individuals. Spine (Phila Pa 1976) 27: 125–134

Epstein NE, Epstein JA, Mauri T (1989) Treatment of fractures of the vertebral limbus and spinal stenosis in five adolescents and five adults. Neurosurgery 24:595–604

Flik K, Lyman S, Marx RG (2005) American collegiate men's ice hockey: an analysis of injuries. Am J Sports Med 33: 183–187

Handel SF, Twiford TW Jr, Reigel DH, Kaufman HH (1979) Posterior lumbar apophyseal fractures. Radiology 130:629–633

Henderson RL, Reid DC, Saboe LA (1991) Multiple noncontiguous spine fractures. Spine 16:128–131

Hernandez JA, Chupik C, Swischuk LE (2004) Cervical spine trauma in children under 5 years: productivity of CT. Emerg Radiol 10:176–178

Hoffman JR, Mower WR, Wolfson AB, Todd KH, Zucker MI (2000) Validity of a set of clinical criteria to rule out injury to the cervical spine in patients with blunt trauma. National Emergency X-Radiography Utilization Study Group. N Engl J Med 343:94–99

Hoffman JR, Wolfson AB, Todd K, Mower WR (1998) Selective cervical spine radiography in blunt trauma: methodology of the National Emergency X-Radiography Utilization Study (NEXUS). Ann Emerg Med 32:461–469

Hogan GJ, Mirvis SE, Shanmuganathan K, Scalea TM (2005) Exclusion of unstable cervical spine injury in obtunded patients with blunt trauma: is MR imaging needed when multi-detector row CT findings are normal? Radiology 237: 106–113

Hollenberg GM, Beattie PF, Meyers SP, Weinberg EP, Adams MJ (2002) Stress reactions of the lumbar pars interarticularis: the development of a new MRI classification system. Spine 27:181–186

Johnson AW, Weiss CB Jr, Stento K, Wheeler DL (2001) Stress fratcures of the sacrum. An atypical cause of low back pain in the female athlete. Am J Sports Med 29:498–508

Katoh S, Shingu H, Ikata T, Iwatsubo E (1996) Sports-related spinal cord injury in Japan (from the nationwide spinal cord injury registry between 1990 and 1992). Spinal Cord 34: 416–421

Kligman M, Vasili C, Roffman M (2001) The role of computed tomography in cervical spinal injury due to diving. Arch Orthop Trauma Surg 121:139–141

Kokoska ER, Keller MS, Rallo MC, Weber TR (2001) Characteristics of pediatric cervical spine injuries. J Pediatr Surg 36:100–105
Korres DS, Benetos IS, Themistocleous GS et al (2006) Diving injuries of the cervical spine in amateur divers. Spine J 6:44–49
Levitz CL, Reilly PJ, Torg JS (1997) The pathomechanics of chronic, recurrent cervical nerve root neurapraxia. The chronic burner syndrome. Am J Sports Med 25:73–76
Naidich JB, Naidich TP, Garfein C, Liebeskind AL, Hyman RA (1977) The widened interspinous distance: a useful sign of anterior cervical dislocation in the supine frontal projection. Radiology 123:113–116
National spinal cord injury statistical center. Spinal cord injury: facts and figures. (2006). Retrieved 2007.
Pang D, Wilberger JE Jr (1982) Spinal cord injury without radiographic abnormalities in children. J Neurosurg 57:114–129
Pennecot GF, Gouraud D, Hardy JR, Pouliquen JC (1984) Roentgenographical study of the stability of the cervical spine in children. J Pediatr Orthop 4:346–352
Qaiyum M, Tyrrell PN, McCall IW, Cassar-Pullicino VN (2001) MRI detection of unsuspected vertebral injury in acute spinal trauma: incidence and significance. Skeletal Radiol 30: 299–304
Rekate HL, Theodore N, Sonntag VK, Dickman CA (1999) Pediatric spine and spinal cord trauma. State of the art for the third millennium. Childs Nerv Syst 15:743–750
Reul J, Weis J, Jung A, Willmes K, Thron A (1995) Central nervous system lesions and cervical disc herniations in amateur divers. Lancet 345:1403–1405
Ronnen HR, de Korte PJ, Brink PR et al (1996) Acute whiplash injury: is there a role for MR imaging? – a prospective study of 100 patients. Radiology 201:93–96
Standaert CJ, Herring SA (2009) Expert opinion and controversies in musculoskeletal and sports medicine: stingers. Arch Phys Med Rehabil 90:402–406
Streitwieser DR, Knopp R, Wales LR, Williams JL, Tonnemacher K (1983) Accuracy of standard radiographic views in detecting cervical spine fractures. Ann Emerg Med 12:538–542
Sward L, Hellstrom M, Jacobsson B, Peterson L (1990) Back pain and radiologic changes in the thoraco-lumbar spine of athletes. Spine (Phila Pa 1976) 15:124–129
Takata K, Inoue S, Takahashi K, Ohtsuka Y (1988) Fracture of the posterior margin of a lumbar vertebral body. J Bone Joint Surg Am 70:589–594
Tator CH, Carson JD, Edmonds VE (1998) Spinal injuries in ice hockey. Clin Sports Med 17:183–194
Torg JS, Corcoran TA, Thibault LE, Pavlov H, Sennett BJ, Naranja RJ, Priano S (1997) Cervial cord neuropraxia: classification, pathomechanics, morbidity, and management guidelines. J Neurosurg 87:843–850
Torg JS, Guille JT, Jaffe S (2002) Injuries to the cervical spine in American football players. J Bone Joint Surg Am 84-A: 112–122
Torg JS, Pavlov H, Genuario SE, Sennett B et al (1986) Neurapraxia of the cervical spinal cord with transient quadriplegia. J Bone Joint Surg Am 68:1354–1370
Vialle R, Mary P, Schmider L, le Pointe HD, Damsin JP, Filipe G (2006) Spinal fracture through the neurocentral synchondrosis in battered children: a report of three cases. Spine 31:E345–E349
Viccellio P, Simon H, Pressman BD, Shah MN, Mower WR, Hoffman JR (2001) A prospective multicenter study of cervical spine injury in children. Pediatrics 108:E20
Weinstein SM (1998) Assessment and rehabilitation of the athlete with a "stinger". A model for the management of noncatastrophic athletic cervical spine injury. Clin Sports Med 17:127–135

Soccer Injuries

Eva Llopis, Mario Padrón, and Rosa de la Puente

Contents

Abstract

› Soccer young player's injuries differ from those in adults players. Adolescents and indoor players have marked increased risk. Is a predominant contact sport and therefore macrotrauma lesions are more frequent than overuse injuries, the latter being related to intense training programs. Macrotrauma lesions are fractures, sprains, contusions and joint rotation injuries. The lower limb is most frequently involved and only goalkeepers have tendency for developing upper limb injuries. The high frequency of avulsion fractures is due to the growing skeleton peculiarities where the epiphyseal plate is weaker than ligament and tendons. Muscles lesions might be strains (hamstrings, quadriceps, adductor or gastrocnemius) or direct contusions. Anterior cruciate ligament rupture or avulsion is the most common serious injury, more common in females.

1 Introduction

Soccer is the most popular sport in the world, in both recreational and competitive level, with approximately 200,000 professional and 240 million amateur players. Although new training strategies have reduced the incidence of football injuries, it is a contact sport and therefore the number of injuries is still high. Biomechanics of soccer includes many different sports abilities, as speed for sprint track with changing

E. Llopis (✉)
Radiology Department, Hospital de la Ribera, Alzira, Valencia, Spain
e-mail: evallopis@gmail.com

M. Padrón
Clínica Cemtro, Madrid, Spain

R. de la Puente
Radiology Department, Hospital Universitario Marqués de Valdecilla-IFIMAV, Santander, Spain

A.H. Karantanas (ed.), *Sports Injuries in Children and Adolescents*,
Med Radiol Diagn Imaging, DOI: 10.1007/174_2010_134, © Springer-Verlag Berlin Heidelberg 2011

direction, jumping, tackling, and kicking, making a wide spectrum of injuries mechanisms. The prevalence of injuries depends on the position on the soccer field. The lower limb including all joints and calf muscles is mostly involved. On the other hand, goalkeepers have an increased number of upper limb injuries. Fatalities are associated almost exclusively with traumatic contact with goalpost, and specific recommendations from equipment manufactures are made to ensure that soccer goalposts are adequately secured during play. There is an increased participation of female players in soccer with a significant augment in the incidence of noncontact internal derangements of the knee joint (Maffulli and Baxter-Jones 1995; American Academy of Pediatrics 2000 and 2010; Yard et al. 2008).

Children are skeletally immature and susceptible to a range of injuries, which differ from those in adult players. Studies have shown that the incidence of injuries increases with the year at school and age, with a reported incidence from 7 to 65.8 injuries/1,000 h game. A previous injury is a major risk factor for future injury (Maffulli and Baxter-Jones 1995; American Academy of Pediatrics 2000 and 2010).

We are going to review common soccer injuries involving the youth population, and how biomechanics change the pattern of injury.

2 Biomechanics of Soccer

New training strategies based on stretching, appropriate cool down, use of protective equipment, as well as proper and prompt medial attention have decreased the number of injuries.

Soccer includes many different motions such as running or tacking, but from them the most specific one is kicking named as the soccer kick. The soccer-style kick lasts no longer than 5 s, depending on the length of the approach. The intensity of the kick depends on how far the kicker needs the ball to travel or how fast it has to go. Kicking is a complex motor task which we learn as children. The kicking skill develops rapidly between the ages of 4 and 6, and by the age of 9 the pattern is mature without any further development.

The most common biomechanical difference between the elite and novice footballer is that elite footballers use a refined and consistent movement pattern where novices use a variable and inconsistent one. A successful kick is usually defined in the literature either in terms of the velocity of the ball (which needs greater swing limb/foot speed), or the accuracy of direction of kick, which relies on the position of the "plant" (non-kicking) foot and hip position at impact.

Children between 2 and 3 years of age generally toddle straight into the ball to try and kick it. As they get older, they learn a paced run-up and adjust their approach to the ball from front-on to a more diagonal angle. The diagonal approach produces greater swing-limb velocity for greater ball speed. Elite athletes tend to take longer strides than novices as they approach the ball.

Numerous studies have investigated the relationship between ground reaction force on the plant foot and ball speed, for both novice and elite footballers. These show that skilled players kick faster and produce greater ground reaction forces in all directions than the unskilled.

During kicking, there is a direct relationship between the direction that the plant foot faces and the direction in which the ball travels. The optimal foot plant position for accurate direction is perpendicular to a line drawn through the center of the ball for a straight kick.

The next phase within the biomechanics of the kick is the swinging or cocking of the kicking limb in preparation for the downward motion toward the ball. During this phase, the kicker's eyes are focused on the ball; the opposite arm to the kicking leg is raised and pointed in the kicking direction to counterbalance the rotating body. As the plant foot strikes the ground adjacent to the ball, the kicking leg is extending and the knee is flexing. The purpose here is to store elastic energy as the swinging limb passively stretches to allow a greater transfer of force to the ball during the downward phase of the kick.

Before the end of the swing phase when the hip is nearly fully extended and the knee flexed, the leg is slowed eccentrically by the hip flexors and knee extensors. This is the phase of the kick where there is maximal eccentric activity in the knee extensors.

The powerful hip flexors initiate this next phase of the kick, hip flexion, and knee extension. The thigh is swung forward and downward with a concomitant forward rotation of the lower leg/foot. As the forward thigh movement slows, the leg/foot begins to accelerate because of the combined effect of the transfer of momentum and release of stored elastic energy in the knee extensors. The knee extensors then powerfully contract to swing the leg and foot forward toward the ball. As the knee of the kicking leg passes over the ball, it is forcefully extended while the foot is forcefully plantar flexed. This exposes the inside top part of the foot (medial dorsum), which is propelled at the ball. Foot speed is governed by a combination of hip rotational torque, hip flexor strength, and quadriceps strength. At the end of the swing phase, just prior to ball/foot contact, the hamstrings are maximally active to slow the leg eccentrically. This phenomenon is known as the "soccer paradox," where the knee flexors are maximally active during knee extension and the knee extensors are maximally active during knee flexion. According to various studies, the foot is in contact with the ball for 6–16 ms, depending on how well inflated the ball is. At the point of impact, 15% of the kinetic energy of the swinging limb is transferred to the ball. The rest is dissipated by the eccentric activity of the hamstring muscle group to slow the limb down. Because of the large forces involved, this stage in the kicking action is the most likely to produce injury to the hamstrings. At the instant of impact on the kicking leg, the hip and knee are slightly flexed and the foot is moving upward and forward. The follow-through of the kick serves two purposes: to keep the foot in contact with the ball for longer; and to guard against injury. The body protects itself from injury by gradually dissipating the kinetic and elastic forces generated by the swinging, kicking limb after contact. Any sudden deceleration of the limb would increase the risk of hamstring strain (Lees and Nolan 1998).

3 Physiology and Epidemiology

Adolescents are injured more often than younger children; this may be to increased risk tasking, player aggression, or determination. Those who play at indoor pitches have markedly increased risk of injury. The nature of the indoor game differs from that of the outdoor one. The size of the pitch is smaller and it is surrounded by solid walls. The playing surface is artificial and may be turf-like or smooth. There is no offside rule and referees are encouraged to play the advantage, therefore physical contact is more common (American Academy of Pediatrics 2000 and 2010).

Equipment is also important. Heavier balls are larger and with higher inflation pressures, increasing thus the risk of "goalkeeper's wrist" injuries which is a similar lesion as when falling on an outstretched hand. Head injuries secondary to impact are also increased in players. Therefore the ball size has been limited when used by younger players (Adams and Schiff 2006).

Strikers have higher rate of lower leg fractures because of higher impact injuries. The rate of injuries in female players was almost twice than in males, decreasing tremendously when training regimen improves.

There are some peculiarities of the growing skeleton and soft tissues of young soccer players that change their spectrum of injuries. Bone and muscles have higher healing ability. Bone increases its stiffness and decreases resistance to impact, and thus is suitable to bowing if overloaded. Epiphyseal growth plate is weaker than ligaments and tendons, having an increased tendency for acute avulsion fractures or overuse apophysitis. Traction epiphysis or growth plate disturbance may result from pressure on the epiphysis (Rossi and Dragoni 2001; Caine et al. 2006).

Injuries can be divided into acute associated with macrotrauma and chronic secondary to repetitive microtrauma. The most common soccer-related injuries are soft tissue contusion and bruising. Soccer is classified as a high-to-moderate intensity contact collision sport, with most injuries overall occurring from either player to player or player to ground/ball or goalpost contact rather than overuse. As a contact sport, there is an increased risk for acute trauma, fractures, sprains, and joint rotation injuries. Overuse injuries such as stress fractures, osteochondritis dissecans, apophysitis, or tendinopathies are increased with intense training programs.

4 Avulsion Fractures

Avulsion fractures occur commonly in the immature skeleton due to a sudden, forceful, or unbalanced contraction of the attached musculotendinous unit.

Pelvis avulsion fractures are particularly frequent on young soccer players. The anterior inferior iliac spine tends to fail during football when the kicking foot is suddenly blocked, as happens in a tackle. More often when the foot hits the ground, the anterior inferior iliac spine is pulled off by the reflected head of the rectus femoris. In similar circumstances the psoas muscle can avulse the lesser trochanter, but is much more infrequent. The whole apophyseal plate of the ischium can be separated through the powerful pull of the hamstrings (Figs. 1–3). Rarely, the anterior superior iliac spine can

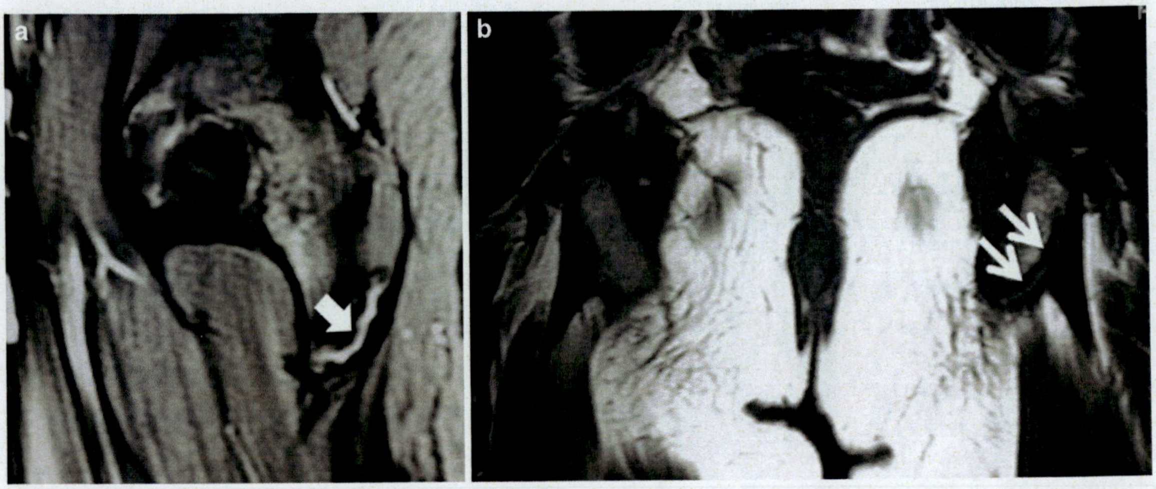

Fig. 1 Acute hamstring avulsion at its ischial insertion. The sagittal T2-w FFE (**a**) and the coronal T1-w (**b**) MR images show the abnormal signal and the minor displacement on the left side (*arrows*)

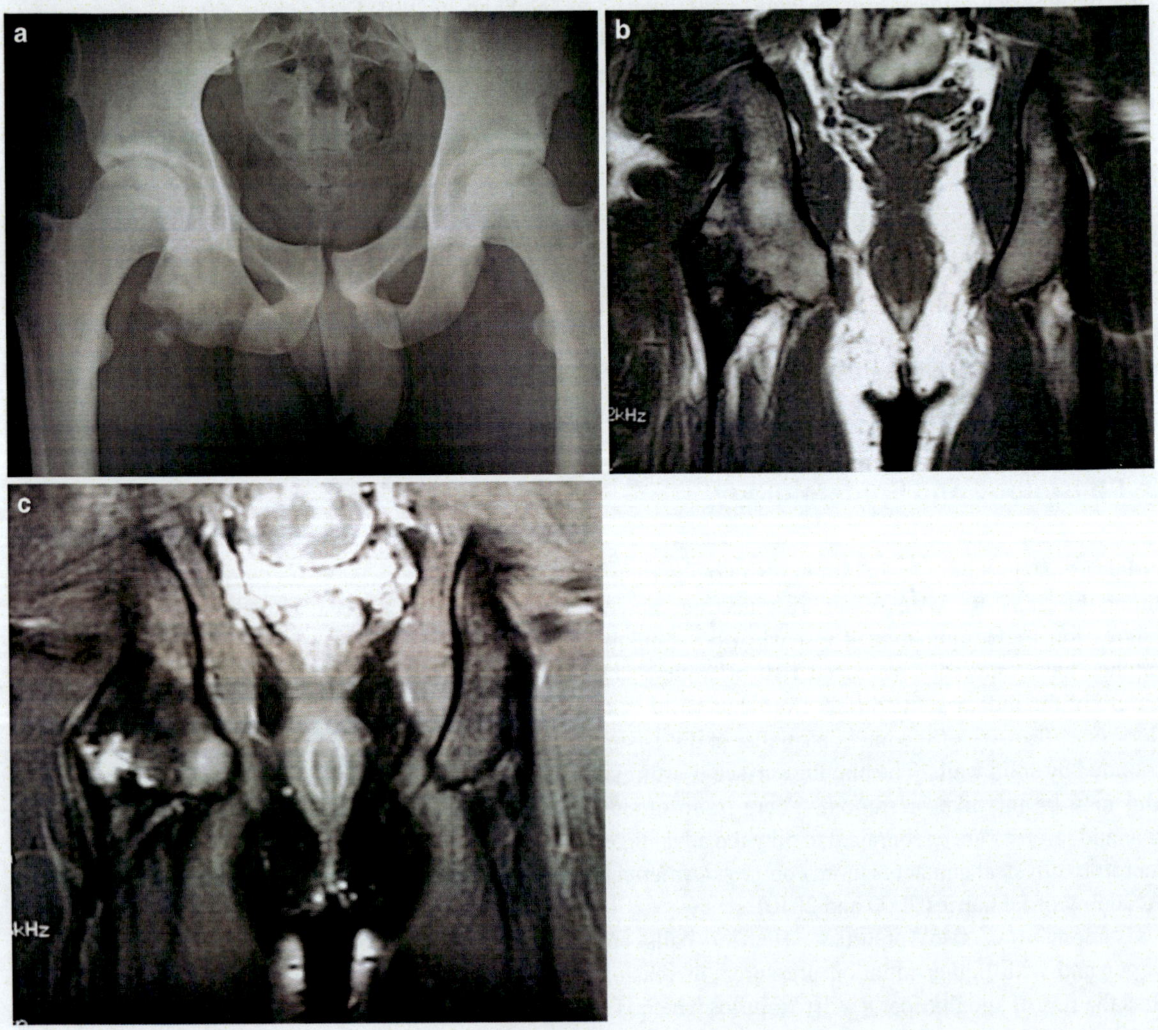

Fig. 2 Chronic avulsion of the hamstrings with pseudotumoral appearance on plain radiographs (**a**). The coronal T1-w (**b**) and fat-suppressed T2-w (**c**) MR images show the abnormal appearance of the hamstring avulsion on the right insertion site. Abnormally high signal is seen on **c**

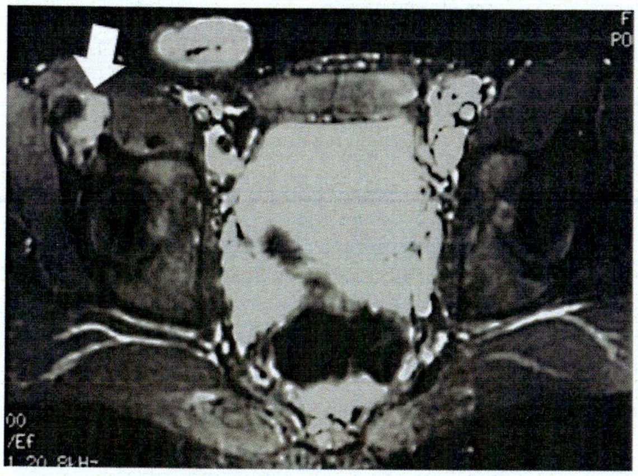

Fig. 3 Rectus femoris avulsion at its insertion on the anterior inferior iliac spine, demonstrated on axial fat suppressed T2-w MR image (*arrow*)

be avulsed by the action of the tensor of the fascia lata in a bad landing after a jump. Avulsions of the sartorius from the anterior superior iliac crest might occur after a forced extension of the hip. Some patients can sustain multiple avulsion fractures (Rossi and Dragoni 2001; Caine et al. 2006).

A similar imbalance between ligaments and epiphyseal strength has been reported to produce the classical ACL lesion in children and young athletes. In these cases, the ligament itself remains intact, but a large piece of the proximal tibia is avulsed. In 62 young patients with ACL disruptions, avulsions of the tibia were found in 80% of athletes aged less than 12 years (Fig. 4) (Fehnel and Johnson 2000).

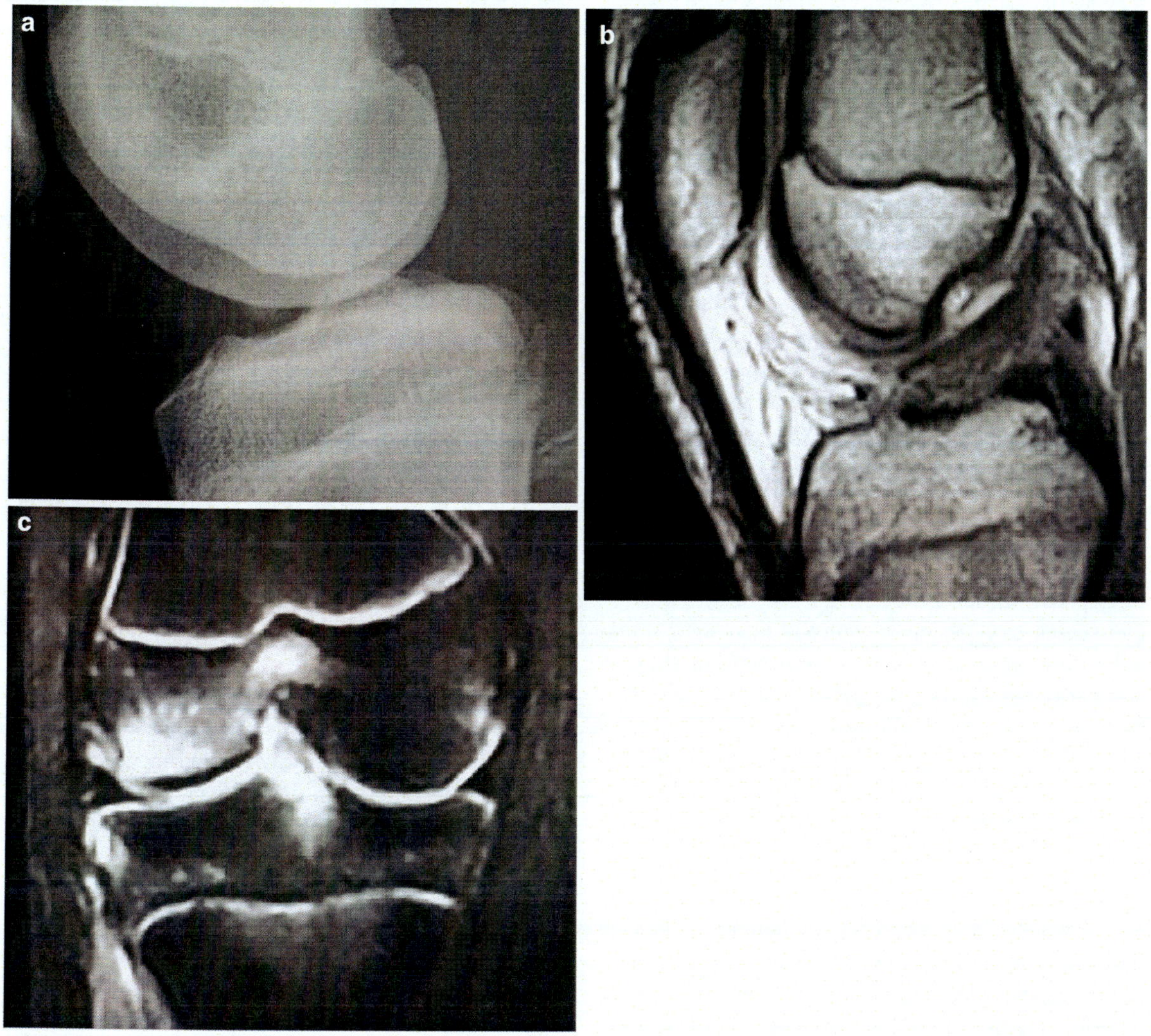

Fig. 4 A 12-year-old soccer player with ACL avulsion (**a**). The plain radiograph shows displacement of the anterior tibial spine (**b**). The sagittal PD-w MR image demonstrates the bone avulsion with a normal ACL (**c**). On coronal fat-saturated T2-w MR image, bone marrow edema of the femoral condyle in addition to the avulsion site was shown

5 Stress Fractures

Stress fractures are less frequent during childhood than in the young adult. This is due to the fact that bone regeneration is by far higher than in adults and therefore even with repetitive stresses the balance between remodeling and resorption is maintained. Soccer requires sudden stops and changes of directions during bursts of high-speed running, and might develop stress reactions and fractures on the lower extremity especially in the tibia. Changing of sports training habits in the last 6 months is seen as one of the most important risk factors.

Plain radiographs are usually normal and MR imaging is the technique of choice for an early diagnosis. Visualization of bone marrow edema and periosteal edema on fluid-sensitive sequences together with a fracture line on T1-w sequences allow an early diagnosis and treatment before a transcortical fracture develops (Niemeyer et al. 2006).

Spondylolysis is a stress fracture of the vertebral body occurring mostly at the pars interarticularis. It is rare in nonathletes, but is a common cause of back pain in adolescent athletes. Soccer players are considered to be at risk of low back pain secondary to microtrauma that results in spondylolysis or spondylolistesis. This injury appears to have both hereditary and acquired risk factors, and appears to be related to excess loading and repetitive extension of the spine. Pain is exacerbating by lumbosacral twisting and hyperextension. Patients have low back pain that worsens with extension of the lumbar spine. Symptoms initially occur in sports, but may progress to daily activity and rest. It may occur at one or multiple vertebral bodies, and it is most commonly seen at levels L4 and L5. Young athletes in an early phase of the fracture have a potential to heal. In these cases, early diagnosis with MR imaging is essential before nonunion fracture has developed (Figs. 5 and 6) (Kerssemakers et al. 2009).

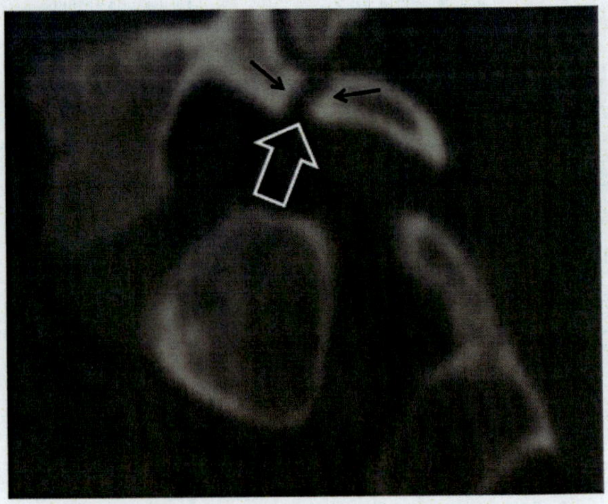

Fig. 5 Multi-detector CT (MDCT) with multiplanar reconstruction on the sagittal plane shows spondylolysis on the pars articularis of L5 (*open arrow*). The presence of cortical sclerosis (*thin arrows*) suggests a developed nonunion fracture

6 Muscle Injuries

Muscle *strains* arise from indirect trauma due to excessive stretching during rapid acceleration or deceleration that occurs particularly in soccer events. Acute muscle strain injuries are highly associated with improper warm-up before playing. In children, this type of injury tends to lead to an apophyseal avulsion fracture, due to a weaker link at the physeal plate. In young adults, biomechanical failure tends to occur at the myotendinous junction.

Adolescents are particularly prone to injuries because of the imbalance in strength and flexibility and changes in biomechanical properties of bones during the peak growth. In youth soccer players, the frequency of muscle injuries, especially contusions, are higher than in the adult population (El-Khoury et al. 1996; Raissaki et al. 2007; Paterson 2009).

The muscles most frequently involved in muscle strains are those that transverse two joints, those having a high proportion of fast twitch fibers and those undergoing eccentric contractions. The quadriceps (rectus femoris), hamstrings (semitendinous and semimembranous) (Figs. 7 and 8), adductors, and medial head of the gastronecmius are the muscles most commonly injured in soccer.

Muscle *contusions* occur secondary to direct trauma commonly by a blunt object. They are usually located in the muscle belly. MR Imaging can identify associated lesions, such as ligament tears and bone marrow injury at the myotendinous insertions (Fig. 7). However, it has difficulty in separating muscle edema, hematoma, and structural disruption, and as a result tends to overestimate the severity of injury (Barron et al. 2008). Hematomas are common in myotendinous injuries. MR imaging findings may vary depending on the time elapsed since the injury.

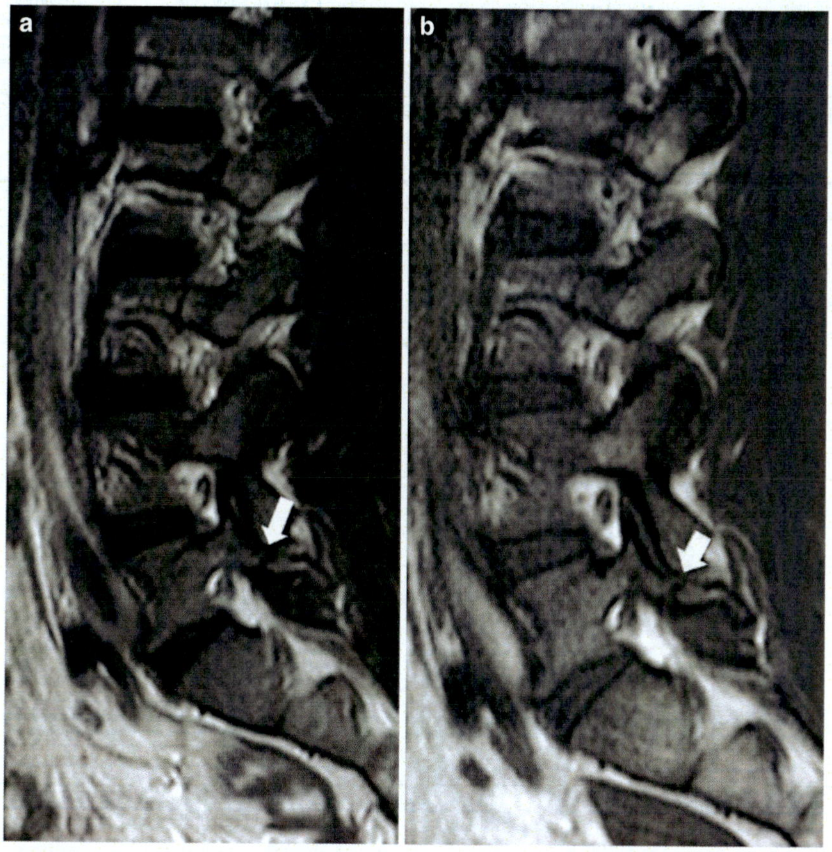

Fig. 6 The sagittal T2-w (**a**) and T1-w (**b**) MR images demonstrate stress fractures in the pars articularis of L5 vertebral body (*arrows*)

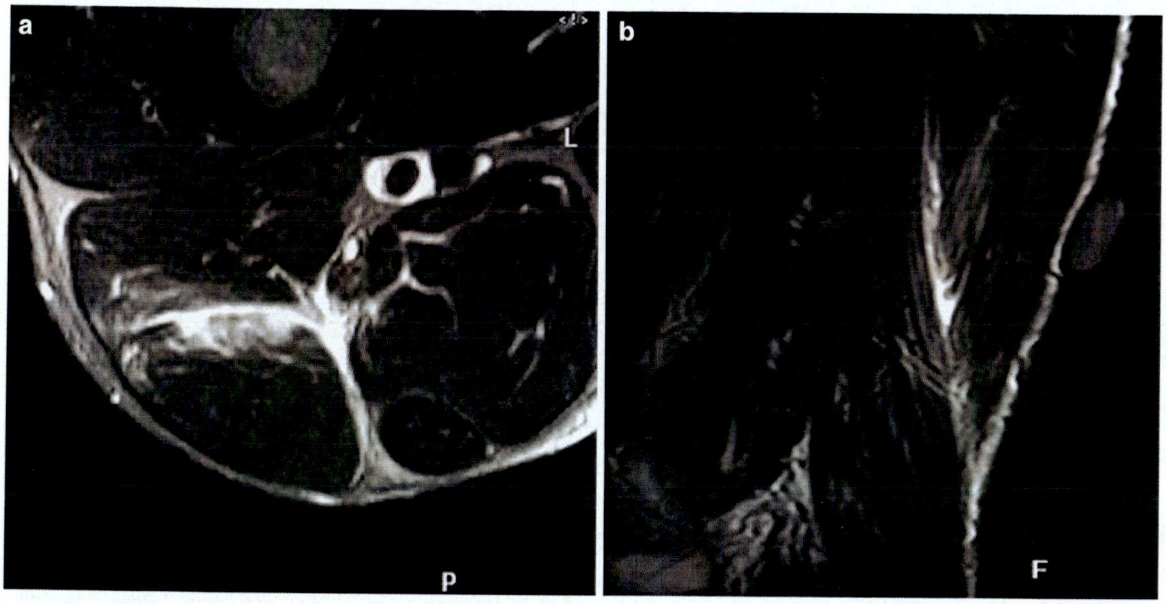

Fig. 7 The axial (**a**) and sagittal (**b**) T2-w MR images show the high signal intensity myofascial tear of the biceps tendon

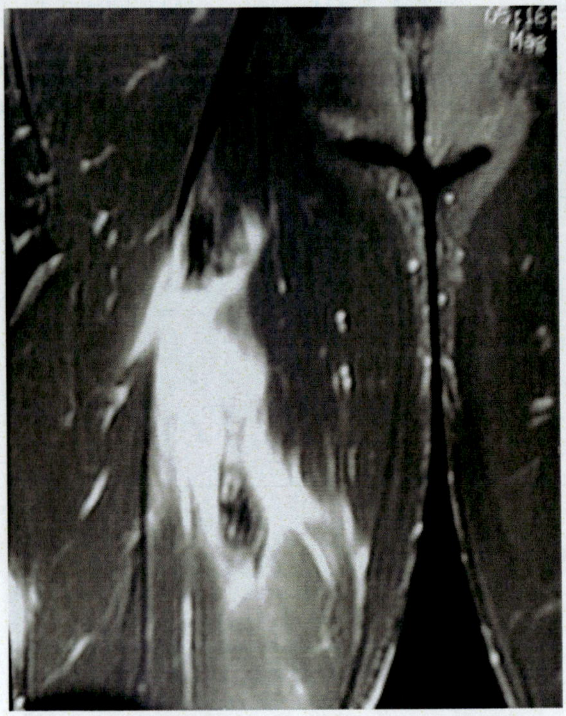

Fig. 8 The fat-suppressed coronal T2-w MR image shows a complete tear of the semitendinous myotendinous unit with hematoma

Ultrasonography (US) has some advantages, including excellent spatial resolution. Dynamic evaluation helps differentiate full from partial thickness tendon and myotendinous injuries, with active contraction giving an excellent assessment of the degree of disruption (El-Khoury et al. 1996; Raissaki et al. 2007; Barron et al. 2008; Paterson 2009).

7 Ankle

The ankle is one of the most commonly injured areas in soccer players, with a reported incidence of 17% of all injuries. The ankle is exposed to stresses during sprinting, sudden changes of direction, and with the kicking mechanism. The complex movements performed during all the phases condition repeated trauma to the anterior tibiotalar joint secondary to the repetitive dorsiflexion. Additionally, forced plantar flexion with changing directions results in overloading of the posterior structures. Posterior impingement and flexor hallucis longus pathology may progressively lead to the "footballer's ankle."

During the tacking phase, when the player is running with the ball, there is an increased load over the lateral and medial compartments of the ankle. The anteromedial tibiotalar and first metatarsal joints are the touching points where ball strikes the ankle, increasing the occurrence of injuries upon those points.

Inversion injuries affecting the lateral capsular and ligamentous structures are a frequent event in soccer. Even with a complete tear of the ligament, muscle recruitment and scar tissue can compensate for loss of ligamentous function. Differential diagnosis for acute lateral ligamentous sprain includes sinus tarsi, peroneal tendon, or retinaculum injuries. In the subacute sprain of the lateral ligaments, impingement should be included in the differential diagnosis.

Medial ligament and syndesmosis injuries, although not uncommon, are still infrequent compared to lateral injuries. Typically they respond to rehabilitation, although syndesmosis injuries do take longer to return to athletic activity.

The majority of acute ligamentous, capsular, and tendon injuries do not usually require sophisticated imaging investigation, because clinical diagnosis and functional rehabilitation provide an effective and early return to athletic activity. Imaging is reserved for acute injuries that are difficult to define or grade clinically, and players who develop chronic injuries and instability (Fig. 9).

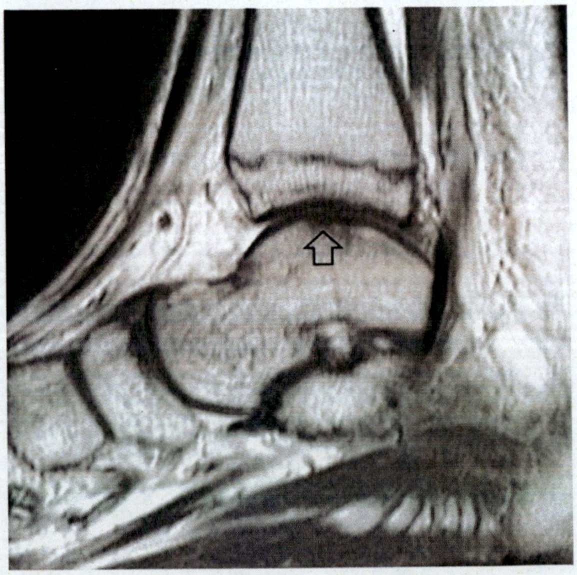

Fig. 9 The sagittal PD-w MR image shows a small osteochondral lesion in the talar dome (*arrow*), which is secondary to chronic anterolateral ankle sprains

8 Knee

The knee undergoes stresses from sprinting, jumping, cutting in, and direct impact and is frequently injured in soccer (17% of all injuries). After landing, there is a considerable translational force across the knee joint. This is increased in sports where the athlete wants to push off immediately in another direction, requiring a forceful thigh muscular contraction resulting in further rotation of the femur and ligament stress. Muscular recruitment can significantly modify the degree of knee flexion and stress directed across the joint, with the hamstrings acting to decrease tibial anterior translation. Fatigue of these muscles can precipitate a serious injury on landing when the force is transmitted through the knee ligaments alone. Knee injuries, especially anterior cruciate ligament (ACL) tears, are seen more frequently in females.

ACL tear is the most common serious injury in children who play soccer, and might end a career of the player despite expert management and surgical repair (Figs. 10 and 11). This type of injury generally occurs during deceleration, while landing or turning, and when there is a rotational force on the lower leg with the knee held semiflexed. The mechanism of injury is a flexion, twisting, or hyperextension. Player position is irrelevant to the incidence of this type of injury. ACL tears are most commonly seen in those with a history of previous injury of the knee joint, and when a talented younger player is promoted to a more senior team.

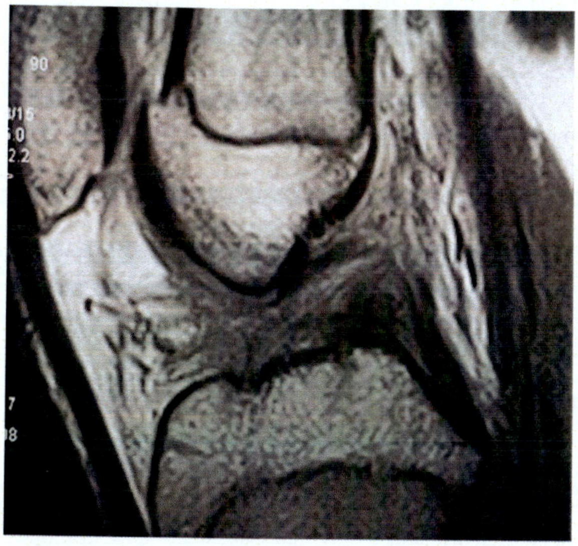

Fig. 10 The sagittal PD-w MR image demonstrates the classic appearance of an acute ACL tear

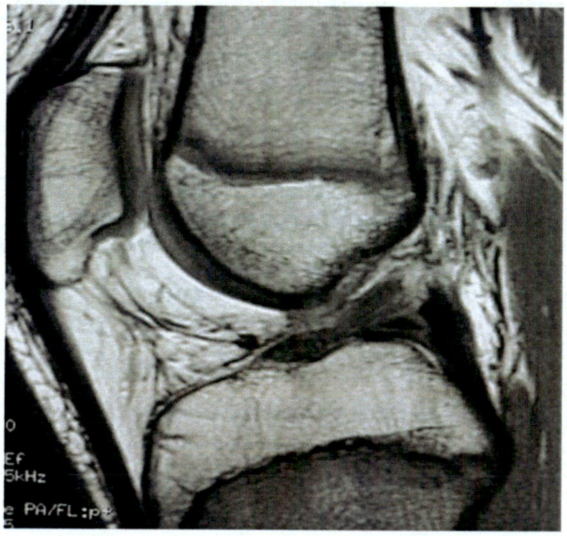

Fig. 11 The sagittal PD-w MR image demonstrates a subacute tear of the ACL

ACL tears are often associated with medial collateral ligament (MCL) tears. In one study, 90% of young athletes over the age of 12 years with ACL disruptions were found to have intrasubstance tears (Kellenberger and Von Laer 1990). MR Imaging has a good ability to predict ACL disruption, with a specificity of 95% and a sensitivity of 88% (Lee et al. 1999).Conservative treatment of ACL rupture leads to severe instability and poor knee function, and carries the risk of sustaining secondary injuries such as meniscal tears (Shea et al. 2003). However, operative reconstruction of the ACL in skeletally immature patients has the potential to cause growth arrest or result in leg length discrepancy due to physeal damage (Kocher et al. 2005). MCL injuries are treated nonoperatively as in adults.

The risk of ACL tears is increased in females due to the inherent laxity of the muscles and ligaments as well as malalignment of the knee. This can be partly compensated with additional muscle recruitment, the hamstring, thus preventing anterior tibial translation. Studies have shown that some female players have radiographically detectable osteoarthritis as early as 10–12 years after trauma.

Patellar dislocation is a relatively frequent injury in young soccer players. Predisposing factors are abnormal morphology of the patella, patella alta, or a laxed retinaculum. The common mechanism is a medial twist of the femur with the foot planted on the ground. The patella wobbles out of the patellofemoral groove to the lateral side of the knee and might be associated with soft tissue injuries. Treatment is conservative and surgery should be considered in cases of ruptured vastus medialis muscle, osteochondral lesion, or recurrent dislocations. MR imaging shows a classic bone marrow edema spectrum, with contusion on the lateral femoral condyle and medial facet of the patella, with or without loose bodies (Fig. 12).

Patellofemoral problems are also more common in females probably due to an increased valgus alignment of the knee, which causes a greater laterally directed force pulling the patella out of the groove laterally. This may contribute to patellar maltracking and instability.

Traction repetitive injuries are relatively frequent in young athletes although not specifically related with soccer. Apophysitis may occur at both distal and proximal attachments of the patellar tendon. Osgood–Schlatter disease is an apophysitis at the tibial tubercule insertion of the distal patellar tendon, while Sinding–Larsen–Johansson disease occurs at its proximal insertion. Osgood–Schlatter is related to overuse of the knee secondary to the contraction of the quadriceps muscle and the extensor mechanism during jumping, running, or cutting. It is more likely to happen during a growth spurt, and is usually bilateral. Chronic avulsion of the tendon leads to development of ossicles from the injured apophysis (Fig. 13).

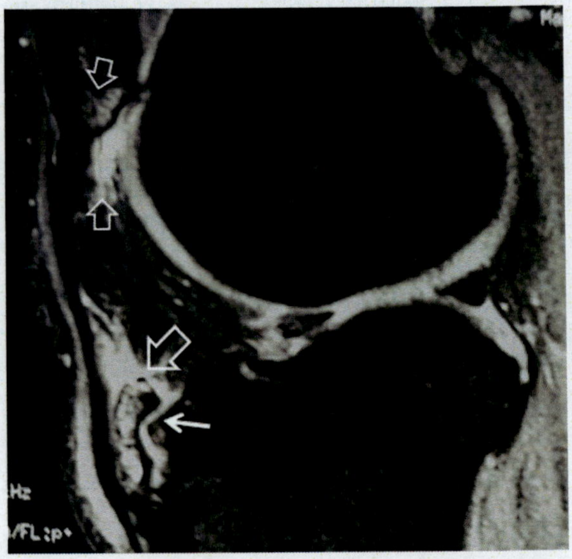

Fig. 13 The sagittal fat-suppressed T2-w MR image shows ossicles separated from the tibial tubercle (*thin arrow*), with bone marrow and soft tissue edema (*open arrow*) in keeping with Osgood–Schlatter disease. Similar findings, to a lesser extent, are seen in the proximal insertion of the tendon (*small open arrows*), suggesting Sinding–Larsen–Johansson disease

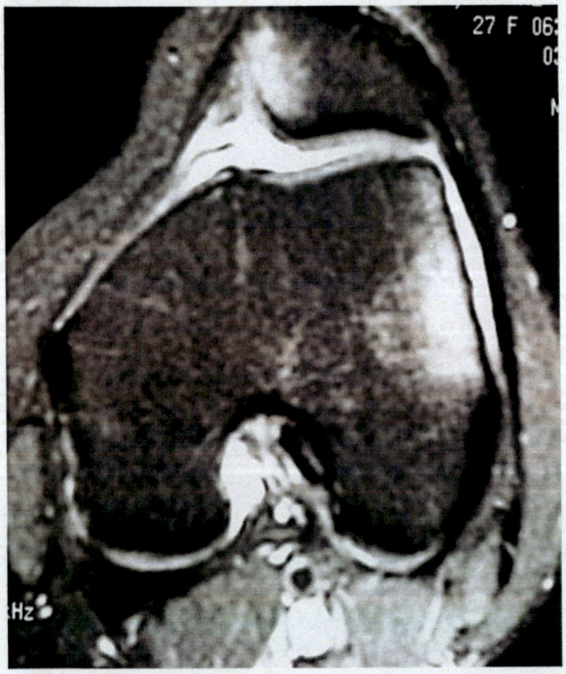

Fig. 12 The axial fat-suppressed T2-w MR image shows the classic bone marrow edema pattern of an acute patellar dislocation, located in the medial aspect of the patella and the lateral femoral condyle

Patellar tendinosis or "jumper knee" results from repetitive overloading of the extensor mechanism of the knee. Patients present with anterior knee pain.

9 Hip

Kicking, running, and jumping during soccer increase reactive forces through the anterior pelvis, in particular at the symphysis pubis, inguinofemoral aponeuroses, and parasymphyseal muscles (abdominal and adductor muscle groups). These predispose young players to develop acute and overuse injuries around the pelvis.

Muscle and myotendinous injuries are the most common injuries. Avulsion apophyseal fractures are particularly frequent around the pelvis as previously mentioned, anterior superior iliac spine, anterior inferior iliac spine ischial tuberosity, or lesser trochanter. Muscle tears occur while the muscle is being eccentrically contracted.

Hip pointer is a specific bruise in the iliac crest usually in the anterior superior iliac spine in the insertion of sartorius secondary to a direct impact.

Early development of osteoarthrosis in soccer players that have practice in their youth is a matter of concern. However, the relationship between practicing sports and femoroacetabular impingement is still under debate. Abnormal femoro-neck junction with a bump might lead to labral and cartilage lesions with hip flexion and extension movement increasing the risk of early osteoarthrosis development.

Groin pain represents a diagnostic dilemma that might result from a variety of causes with overlapping of its clinical symptoms (Fehnel and Johnson 2000; Rossi and Dragoni 2001; Morelli and Weaver 2005 ;Caine et al. 2006). This topic is discussed in detail in the relative chapters in this book.

10 Upper Limb

Upper extremity injuries represent around 2–7.7% of soccer injuries, the hand and wrist being the more frequent location in younger players. Injuries occur in roughly equal proportions from falling onto the hand, contact with other players, and ball striking the hand. Right hand is injured three times more than the left, and fractures are more common than joint injuries. "Greenstick" fractures are the most common fractures under 15 years of age (Barton 1997).

Fall on the outstretched hand or saving the ball are the usual mechanisms for distal forearm fractures, and less frequently for scaphoid fractures. Fractures of the distal radius in young goalkeepers have been related with ball size, especially if an adult is throwing a normal-sized ball to a young keeper (Boyd et al. 2001).

Scaphoid fractures are rare under 12 years of age. Its diagnosis might be challenging because athletes may show only mild symptoms and radiographs can be normal. Treatment is controversial and surgery with Herbert screw fixation is a safe option when casting is not acceptable, allowing an early return to sports (Fig. 14) (Muramatsu et al. 2002).

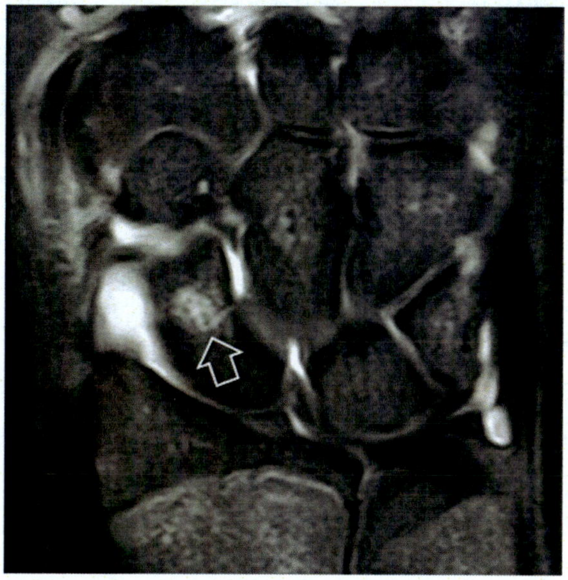

Fig. 14 The coronal fat-suppressed T2-w MR image reveals an incomplete fracture of the scaphoid with bone marrow edema (*arrow*) and joint effusion

Finger injuries, including sprains and fractures, are more prevalent on goalkeepers than in any other players of the team. Parrying and punching the ball increase the risk of injuries. Foot techniques to control the ball contribute to avoid finger injuries.

"Gamekeeper's thumb," metacarpophalangeal joint ulnar collateral ligament injury, is one of the more common injuries of a goalkeeper. It usually occurs after a fall on the ground or when the ball hits the thumb from straight ahead. The role of imaging is to rule out a complete rupture of the ligament or interposition of the abductor pollicis longus tendon, which may inhibit the healing of the ligament.

Goalkeepers in late adolescence are also subject to an uncommon but serious injury: "the goalkeeper fear of nets." This type of lesion occurs when the goalkeeper jumps to suspend the net on the hooks attached to the goalpost, and sustain ring avulsion injuries when their rings are caught on the hooks.

11 Other Injuries

Brain injury is the primary cause of fatal sport-related injuries, and in soccer players are almost always related with a traumatic contact with the goalposts. Older players (ages 15–24) experience head injuries resulting from contact with other players. It is important that young children are taught to head the ball correctly to prevent injuries, including contusions. Balls that are too large and those that are kicked with force are more likely to cause head injuries in children. Moreover, younger children have relatively weak neck muscles and large heads, with thinner skull vaults and many authors think that heading the soccer ball is better avoided in children younger than 12–14 years of age (Pickett et al. 2005).

12 Conclusions

The number of children participating in soccer at training and competition level has increased significantly, and as an inevitable consequence an increase in soccer-related injuries is occurring. Knowledge of the spectrum of injuries that might be present, depending on the age, training level, and position in the team, allows an adequate diagnosis, early treatment, and proper management.

References

Adams A, Schiff MA (2006) Childhood soccer injuries treated in US emergency department. Acad Emerg Med 13: 571–574

American Academy of Pediatrics. Committee on Sports Medicine and Fitness (2000) Injuries in youth soccer: a subject review. Pediatrics 105:659–661

American Academy of Pediatrics. Committee on Sports Medicine and Fitness (2010) Clinical report: injuries in youth soccer. Pediatrics 125:410–414

Barron D, Farrant J, O'Connor P (2008). Lower extremity injuries in children (including sports injuries). Imaging of the musculoskeletal system, vol. 1. Saunders Elsevier, Philadelphia 916–956

Barton N (1997) Sports injuries of the hand and wrist. Br J Sports Med 31:191–196

Boyd KT, Brownson P, Hunter JB (2001) Distal radial fractures in young goalkeepers: a case for an appropriately sized soccer ball. Br J Sports Med 35:409–411

Caine D, DiFiori J, Maffulli N (2006) Physeal injuries in children's and youth sports: reasons for concern? Br J Sports Med 40:749–760

El-Khoury GY, Brandser EA, Kathol MH, Tearse DS, Callaghan JJ (1996) Imaging of muscle injuries. Skeletal Radiol 25:3–11

Fehnel DJ, Johnson R (2000) Anterior cruciate injuries in the skeletally immature athlete: a review of treatment outcomes. Sports Med 29:51–63

Kellenberger R, Von Laer I (1990) Nonosseous lesions of the anterior cruciate ligament in childhood and adolescence. Prog Pediatr Surg 25:123–131

Kerssemakers SP, Fotiadou AN, de Jonge MC, Karantanas AH, Maas M (2009) Sport injuries in the paediatric and adolescent patient: a growing problem. Pediatr Radiol 39:471–484

Kocher MS, Garg S, Micheli LJ (2005) Physeal sparing reconstruction of the anterior cruciate ligament in skeletally immature prepubescent children and adolescents. J Bone Joint Surg Am 87:2371–2379

Lee K, Siegel MJ, Lau DM, Hildebolt CF, Matava MJ (1999) Anterior cruciate ligament tears: MR imaging based diagnosis in a pediatric population. Radiology 213:697–704

Lees A, Nolan L (1998) The biomechanics of soccer: a review. J Sports Sci 16:211–234

Maffulli N, Baxter-Jones AD (1995) Common skeletal injuries in young athletes. Sports Med 19:137–149

Morelli V, Weaver V (2005) Groin injuries and groin pain in athletes: part 1. Prim Care 32:163–183

Muramatsu K, Doi K, Kuwata N, Kawakami F, Ihara K, Kawai S (2002) Scaphoid fracture in the young athlete – therapeutic outcome of internal fixation using the Herbert screw. Arch Orthop Trauma Surg 122:510–513

Niemeyer P, Weinberg A, Schmitt H, Kreuz PC, Ewerbeck V, Kasten P (2006) Stress fractures in adolescent competitive athletes with open physis. Knee Surg Sports Traumatol Arthrosc 14:771–777

Paterson A (2009) Soccer injuries in children. Pediatr Radiol 39:1286–1298

Pickett W, Streight S, Simpson K, Brison RJ (2005) Head injuries in youth soccer players presenting to the emergency department. Br J Sports Med 39:226–231

Raissaki M, Apostolaki E, Karantanas AH (2007) Imaging of sports injuries in children and adolescents. Eur J Radiol 62:86–96

Rossi F, Dragoni S (2001) Acute avulsion fractures of the pelvis in adolescent competitive athletes: prevalence, location and sports distribution of 203 cases collected. Skeletal Radiol 30:127–131

Shea KG, Apel PJ, Pfeiffer RP (2003) Anterior cruciate ligament injury in pediatric and adolescent patients: a review of basic science and clinical research. Sports Med 33:455–471

Yard EE, Schroeder MJ, Fields SK, Collins CL, Comstock RD (2008) The epidemiology of United States high school soccer injuries, 2005–2007. Am J Sports Med 36:1930–1937

Common Injuries in Mountain Skiing

Carlo Faletti, Josef Kramer,
Giuseppe Massazza, and Riccardo Faletti

Contents

C. Faletti (✉), G. Massazza and R. Faletti
Trauma Center and Orthopedic Hospital, Via Zuretti 29,
10126, Torino, Italy
e-mail: carlo.faletti@cto.to.it

J. Kramer
Röntgeninstitut am Schillerpark, Rainerstrasse 6-8,
4020, Linz, Austria

Key Points

- The most common injuries that occur during the course of winter sports are mainly due to downhill skiing and snowboarding.
- In recent years it has been observed an increase in the number of accidents due also to a greater number of practitioners, especially snowboarders.
- Although head and spine injuries are often fatal, they are less common; in fact, most accidents in children and adolescents who practice winter sports involve the lower limbs.
- The role of the radiologist is essential in recognition of the lesion but also in the treatment planning using all imaging methods at his disposal by conventional radiography, ultrasound and magnetic resonance imaging especially, never forgetting the importance of clinical history and clinical examination.

1 Introduction

Downhill skiing is considered an enjoyable activity for both children and adolescents. As in almost any other sport, this is not without risk of injury. Nowadays, injury rates range from 3.9 to 9.1 per 1,000 skier days with a well documented increase in the number of traumas and fatalities associated with this sport (Meyers et al. 2007). Snowboarding is one of the fastest-growing winter sports and is thought to be associated with relatively high injury rates. According to the National Sporting Goods Association, participation in snowboarding increased by 55%, from the year 1995 to 2000 (Chan

A.H. Karantanas (ed.), *Sports Injuries in Children and Adolescents*,
Med Radiol Diagn Imaging, DOI: 10.1007/174_2010_8, © Springer-Verlag Berlin Heidelberg 2011

and Yoshida 2003). As cross-country skiing exercises most of the joints, muscles and tendons in the body, it provides the skier with an all-round workout. This, in combination with a low injury incidence, makes it an ideal recreational and competitive sport. The new skating techniques developed during the last decade have led to greater velocity. However, because cross-country skiing is practised wherever there is snow, it is difficult to establish accurate injury rates in comparison to alpine skiing, which is performed on specific terrain, in dedicated ski areas (Renstrom and Johnson 1989).

2 Epidemiology

Head and neck injuries are considered the primary cause of fatal injuries and represent 11 to 20% of total injuries among children and adolescents (Dohin and Kohler 2008). Cranial trauma is responsible for up to 54% of total hospital injuries and 67% of all fatalities, whereas thoraco-abdominal and spine injuries represent the cause of 4–10% of fatalities (Shorter et al. 1999; Skokan et al. 2003). Furthermore, upper extremity trauma is increasing with clavicular and humeral fractures accounting for most of these injuries (22–79%). However, the most common and potentially serious injuries in children and adolescents are those to the lower extremity, with knee sprains and anterior cruciate ligament (ACL) tears accounting for up to 47.7% of total injuries. Knee sprains and grade III ligamentous trauma, associated with lower leg fractures, account for 39–77% of ski injuries in this age range. Approximately 15% of downhill skiing injuries among children and adolescents are due to musculoskeletal immaturity. Other causative factors include: excessive fatigue, age, level of experience and inappropriate and/or inadequately/improperly adjusted equipment. Collisions and falls represent a significant proportion (up to 76%) of trauma and are commonly associated to excessive speed, adverse slope conditions, overconfidence leading to carelessness and gender. The type and severity of injuries are typically functions of biomechanical efficiency, skiing velocity, or slope conditions. However, a multiplicative array of intrinsic and extrinsic factors may be involved simultaneously. Despite extensive efforts to provide a comprehensive picture of the aetiology of injury, limitations have hampered reporting. These limitations include age and injury awareness, data collection challenges, poor uniformity in the definition and/or delineation of age classification as well as limited knowledge as to the predisposing factors that lead to injury. Since skill level is the primary impetus in minimising ski injuries, professional instruction focused on strategies such as collision avoidance and helmet use, fall training to minimise lower extremity trauma, adapting ski techniques and avoiding risky behaviour are, therefore, indispensible elements. Skiing equipment should be outfitted to match the young skier's height, weight, level of experience, boot size and slope conditions (Koehle et al. 2002; Lawrence et al. 2008; McCrory 2002). Moreover, particular attention should be paid to slope management (i.e. overcrowding, trail and obstacle marker upkeep) as well as to the minimising of any possibility to reach excessive speeds wherever children are present. Whether enhancing know-how, education and technology will lead to a reduction in predisposition to injury in this population remains to be seen. As with all high-risk sports, the answer may lie in increased wisdom and responsibility of both the skier and the parent to ensure an adequate level of ability, self-control and, maybe simply the use of common sense, as they venture out onto the slopes (Meyers et al. 2007).

Studies estimate the cross-country ski injury rate in Sweden to be around 0.2–0.5 per thousand skier days. A prospective study of cross-country ski injuries conducted in Vermont revealed an injury rate of 0.72 per thousand skier days. Around 75% of the injuries sustained by members of the Swedish national cross-country ski team from 1983 to 1984 were overuse injuries, while 25% were due to trauma. The most common overuse injuries included the medial-tibial stress syndrome, problems with the Achilles tendon and low back pain. The most common traumatic injuries were ankle ligament sprains and fractures, muscle ruptures and knee ligament sprains. Shoulder dislocation, acromioclavicular separation and rotator-cuff tears are not infrequent in cross-country skiing. Injuries to the ulnar collateral ligament (UCL) of the metacarpal phalangeal joint of the thumb (Stener's lesion) is the most common ski injury involving the upper extremity. Cross-country skiers, in the age range from 16 to 21, complain more frequently of mild low back pain than do similarly aged non-skiers. This may be due to the repetitive hyperextension motions cross-country skiers make during the kick phase and the recurring spinal flexion and extension during the double poling phase. Repeated slipping on hard and icy tracks often produces partial tears, or micro-trauma in the musculotendinous units of the groin (Renstrom and Johnson 1989).

3 Common Injuries with Skiing or Snowboarding

3.1 Head

Children experience more head and cervical injuries than do adults (Meyers et al. 2007; Ackery et al. 2007; Fukuda et al. 2001). The incidence of craniofacial and cervical trauma in children was reported to be twofold that observed in other age groups, with up to a quarter of traumatic injury resulting in contusion, subdural haematomas, unconsciousness, or even tetraplegia (Hunter 1999; Schmitt and Gerner 2001). Despite a higher risk of sustaining a head injury among younger skiers and boarders, older patients turn out to have more severe injuries and worse outcomes (Levy and Smith 2000). Although head injuries represent only a small fraction of the overall sum of injuries to skiers and snowboarders, it is the primary cause of fatalities (Diamond et al. 2001; Levy et al. 2002; Xiang and Stallones 2003). Facial fractures are typically associated with high speed and subsequent high impact trauma, in contrast to dental injuries, which are observed at lower velocities, as are mishaps with equipment and lifts (Gassner et al. 1999; Tuli et al. 2002). An even greater predominance of young male participants with head injuries can be observed among snowboarders compared to skiers (Abu-Laban 1991; Bladin and McCrory 1995; Prall et al. 1995; Davidson and Laliotis 1996; Sutherland et al. 1996). Although some types of injuries to skiers and snowboarders show a downward trend with the advances in technology, the incidence of head injury seems to be on the increase. The main problems are most likely associated to the current equipment, which makes skiers and snowboarders feel that they can progress from beginner slopes to intermediate slopes in just a few days.

3.2 Spine and Spinal Cord

Although a general increasing trend in the incidence of spinal and spinal-cord injuries in children and adolescent skiers has been observed over the years (Deibert et al. 1998; Levy et al. 2002), the 15–25 year age group seems to be the range mostly affected. Nowadays, spinal injuries in skiers and boarders are a major problem, especially in the young male snowboarding population and have taken an upward trend along with the increase in risk-taking behaviour (Seino et al. 2001; Koo and Fish 1999). Most spinal injuries in skiers are a consequence of jumping and fall, whilst collisions are a less common cause of spinal trauma. It has been reported that more than two thirds of spinal traumas in snowboarders are the result of jumps (Tarazi et al. 1999). However, chronic low back pain due to repetitive micro-injuries may be observed, especially in the lumbar spine. In the presence of persisting pain, even if the X-ray is negative, an MRI may show an area of bone marrow oedema of the pedicle representing stress response with or without associated spondylolysis (Fig. 1). However, advising skiers or boarders to stop jumping is not a realistic way to prevent this type of injury. Depending upon the trauma mechanism, trabecular microfractures or overt vertebral body fractures may occur (Fig. 2). Anterior and posterior endplate (limbus vertebrae) and central Schmorl's nodes have been documented in the thoraco-lumbar spine of young elite skiers. These findings are thought to be a consequence of high velocity with concomitant overload and overuse during forward postural strain at an early age (Rachbauer et al. 2001). A particular lesion in young people is that of osteochondrosis. In this case the pain is more focused and intense and an early diagnosis can be obtained by MRI if there is evidence of disc degeneration and endplate erosion associated with bone marrow oedema, better depicted with STIR (Fig. 3).

3.3 Shoulder Girdle

Although a decline in minor ski injuries has been observed over the last few decades, an increase in the proportion of upper extremity trauma has been reported in children and represent up to one third of the total number of ski injuries, excluding that of the thumb (Ueland and Kopjar 1998; Schmitt and Gerner 2001; Pecina 2002). The shoulder (rotator cuff lesions, dislocations and subluxation), the acromioclaviclar joint (separations) and the clavicle (fracture) are involved in most injuries and are mostly the consequence of a jump followed by a severe fall (Fig. 4) (Kocher and Feagin 1996). However, shoulder injuries may also

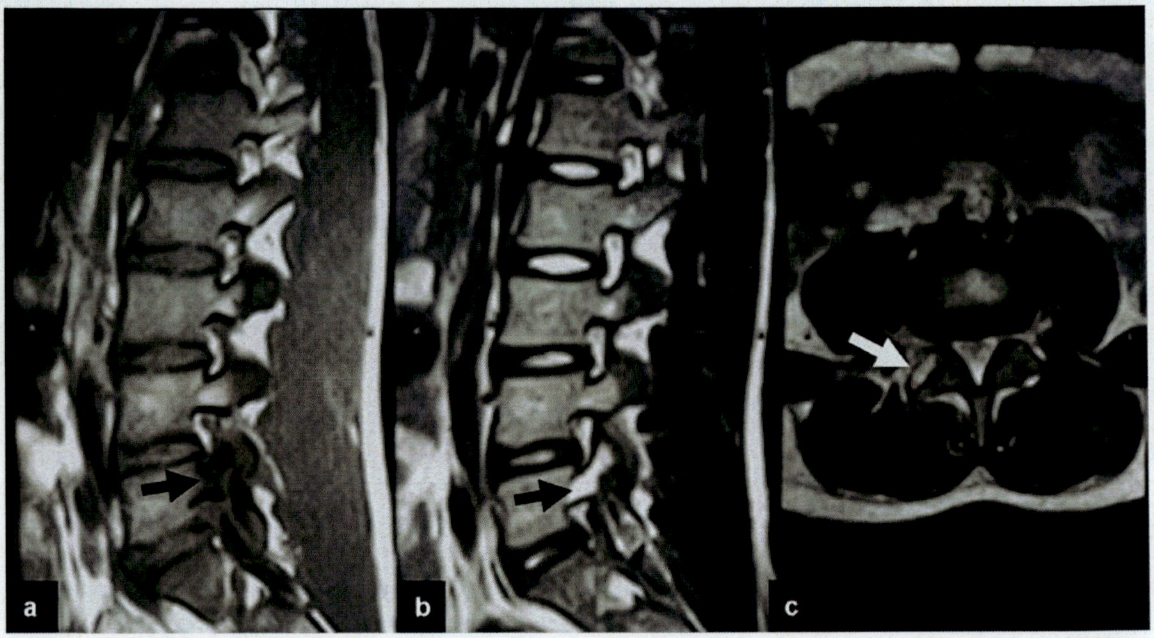

Fig. 1 A young boy skier, with right side lumbar pain. The sagittal T1-w (**a**) and T2(w) (**b**) as well as the axial T2-w (**c**) MR images, show a localized area of low signal intensity on T1-w and high on T2-w, in the right L5 pedicle (*arrows*) representing bone marrow oedema secondary to ipsilateral pars inter-articularis stress injury

result from collisions and excessive external rotation forces due to improper pole planting (Kocher et al. 1998). Prevention of shoulder injuries should be directed to general strategies that reduce falls, such as training as to the use of proper techniques and encouraging skiing with the skier in control.

3.4 Elbow, Wrist and Hand

Injury to the elbow is almost exclusively observed in snowboarders and is generally very rare. However, apophyseal separation of the distal humerus and collateral ligament injuries can be observed after falls in children and adolescents (Fig. 5). Although distal radius fractures are very common and easily diagnosed, compression injuries of the distal growth plate of the radius may be overlooked on radiographs. Therefore, MR imaging should be performed without hesitation should there be a suspicion of a growth plate injury (Fig. 6). Thumb impairment is a commonly found injury in young skiers but uncommon in snowboarders. Almost up to ten percent of trauma cases in children are confined to the thumb (Hunter 1999; Kozin 2006). The UCL sprain, or tear of the first metacarpo-phalangeal joint, the so-called skier's thumb, is caused by a fall on the outstretched hand with the pole in the palm, inducing a radial deviation stress on the UCL (Fig. 7) (Davies et al. 2002). Although the diagnosis of this injury is usually clinical, ultrasound or MR imaging may contribute to the diagnosis in equivocal cases.

3.5 Injuries to the Knee Joint

Ligamentous lesions of the knee joint are the most common ski injuries in children (up to 20%) involving the medial collateral ligament (MCL) and the anterior cruciate ligament (ACL) (Warme et al. 1995; Deibert et al. 1998). Ligamentous injuries in the knee are almost always associated with more or less severe bone contusions which show a bone marrow oedema pattern at MR imaging (Figs. 8–10). There are several trauma mechanisms resulting in ligamentous injuries of the knee. When the skier falls forward whilst catching the inside edge of one of the skis, valgus-external rotational stress leads to primarily MCL injury. On the other hand, the ACL (Ettlinger et al. 1995) may also be

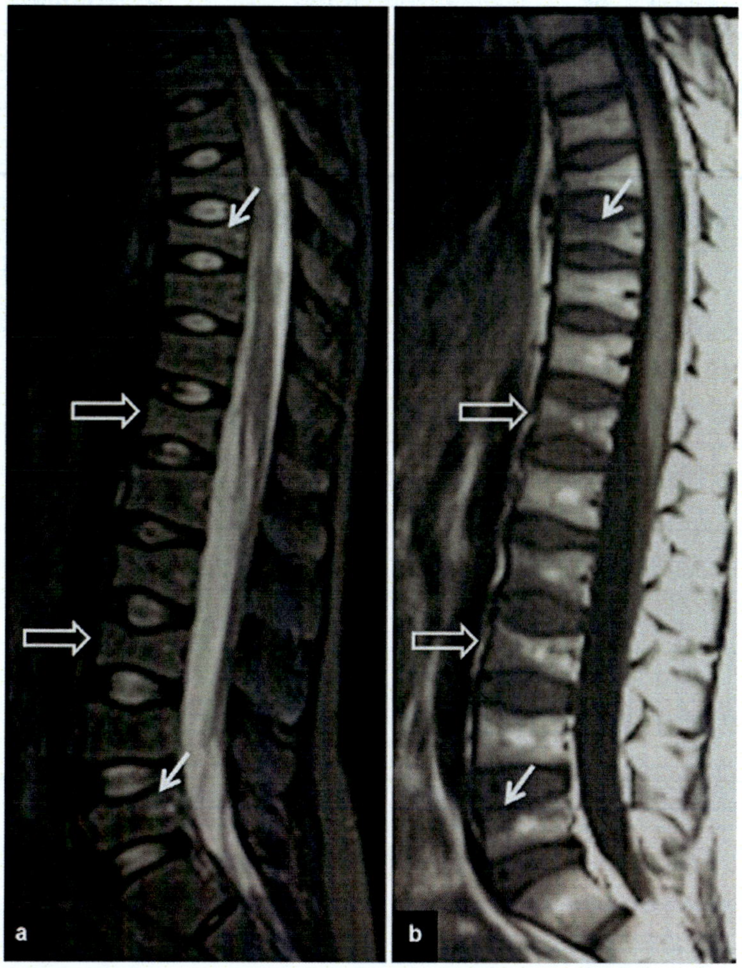

Fig. 2 A young girl skier with back pain without any history of major trauma. She had been performing high jumps over the last few years. The sagittal STIR (**a**) and T1-w (**b**) MR images showed reduced height and biconcavity in several thoracic and lumbar vertebral bodies in keeping with fractures (*open arrows*). Bone marrow oedema suggests recent overuse injuries (*thin arrows*)

involved and, in this case the loaded ski rotates outwards and forces the leg to abduct and rotate externally. Another mechanism which should be taken into consideration is when the skier lands from a jump with the knee extended and the rear of the ski comes into contact with the snow first and, therefore, acts as a lever on the boot-binding complex, which forces the tibia to be drawn forward onto the femur. Moreover, it is not uncommon, especially in beginners, for the skier to fall backwards between the skis. In this case the inside edge of the downhill ski may dig into the snow behind the skier and make the ski lever outwards, causing an internal rotation force on the hyper-flexed knee. The prevention of injuries to the knee whilst skiing is complex and involves more equipment-related adjustment and maintenance of bindings than do other areas of the body. Indeed, it is dangerous, especially for children, to make use of outdated "hand-me-down" equipment that is not tailored to their requirements. Direct trauma with anterior pain is frequently due to the direct contact of the knee with the ice. In this case, MR imaging will show the oedematous contusion of both the patellar and tibial apophysis (Fig. 11).

3.6 Lower Leg Fractures and Ankle Injuries

Fractures of the tibia, or fibula, or complete fractures of the lower leg are not uncommon in young skiers and are primarily a consequence of continual research and development in articulated boot design (Fig. 12) (Bruening and Richards 2005). In contrast to ankle

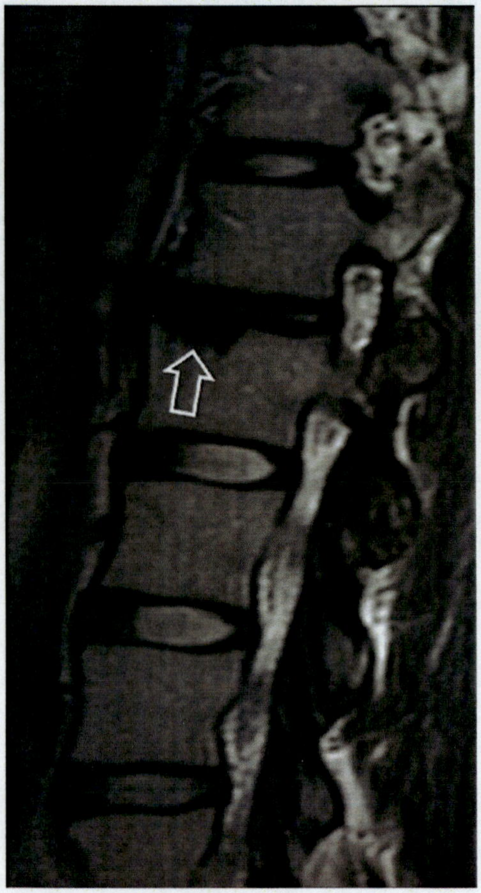

Fig. 3 A young snowboarder with lumbar pain. The sagittal T2-w MR image shows an osteochondral lesion of the superior endplate (*arrow*) and degeneration of the contiguous disc which exhibits dehydration and reduced height

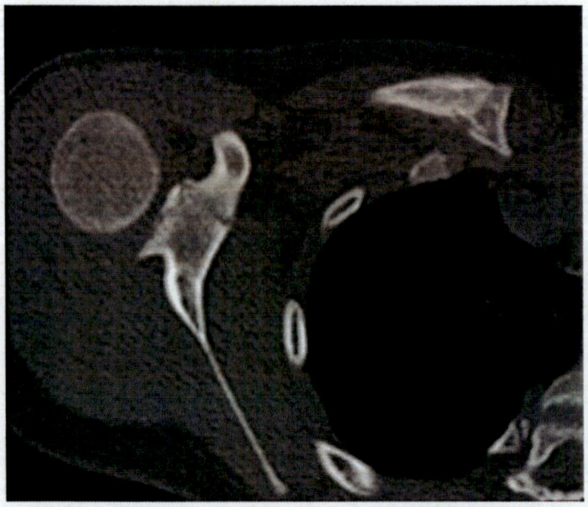

Fig. 4 A young boy after a fall whilst snowboarding. The axial CT image of the right shoulder joint shows a glenoid fracture

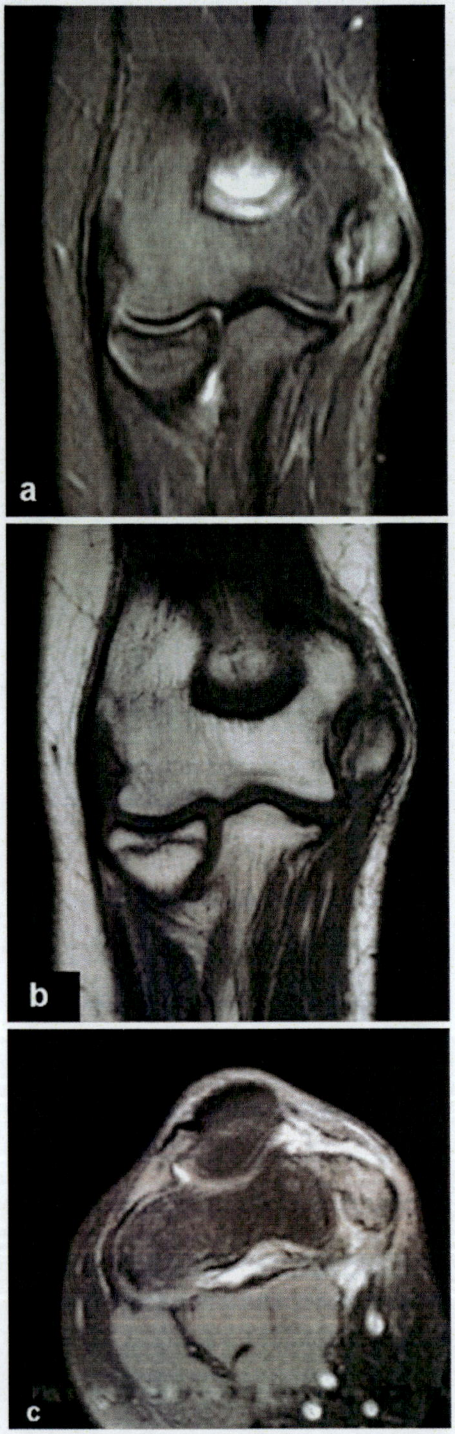

Fig. 5 A snowboarder sustained a fall and complains of elbow pain: (**a**) coronal STIR, (**b**) coronal T1-w, (**c**) axial fat suppressed PD-w MR images. There is oedema within and surrounding the ulnar humeral apophysis in keeping with minimal apophyseal avulsion

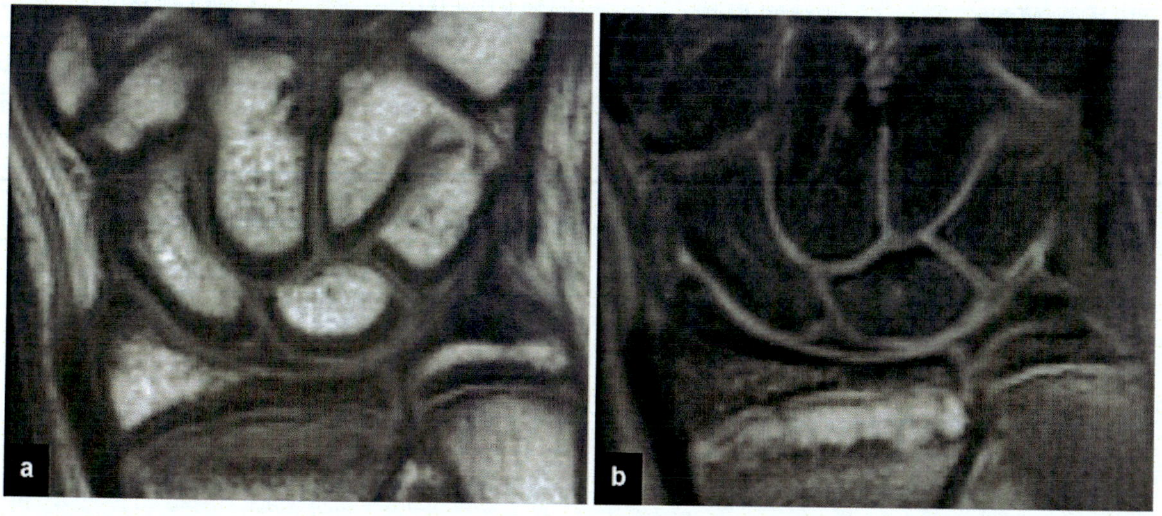

Fig. 6 A girl who fell on her hand while waiting for the lift 14 days before imaging. She reported pain in her wrist. The plain radiograph 1 day after the injury was unremarkable. The coronal T1-w (**a**) and STIR (**b**) MR images show a bone bruise proximal to the growth plate, representing trabecular microfractures

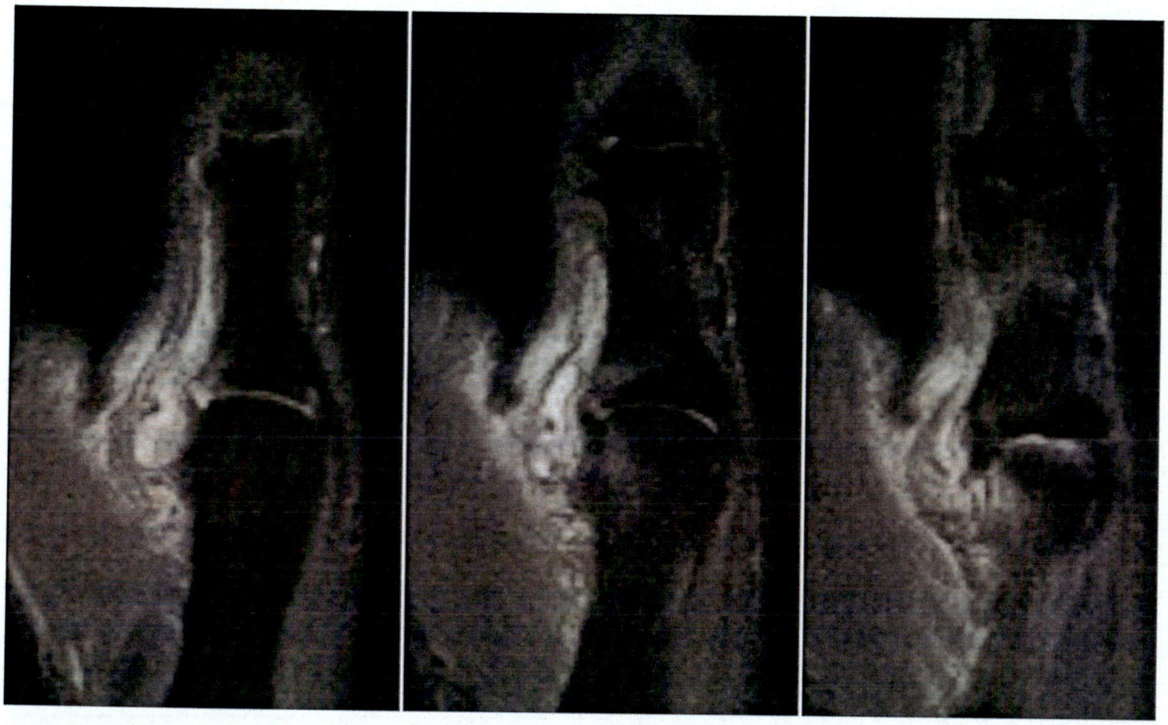

Fig. 7 The coronal STIR images of the thumb show a tear of the ulnar collateral ligament which has a weavy contour and is surrounded by soft tissue oedema

injuries in skiers, ankle joint injuries are now rare in snowboarders as snowboard boots are relatively more flexible than ski boots. Therefore, imaging should be tailored towards depicting fractures of the distal tibia, fibula, or talus (Pino and Colville 1989; Young and Niedfeldt 1999; Kirkpatrick et al. 1998).

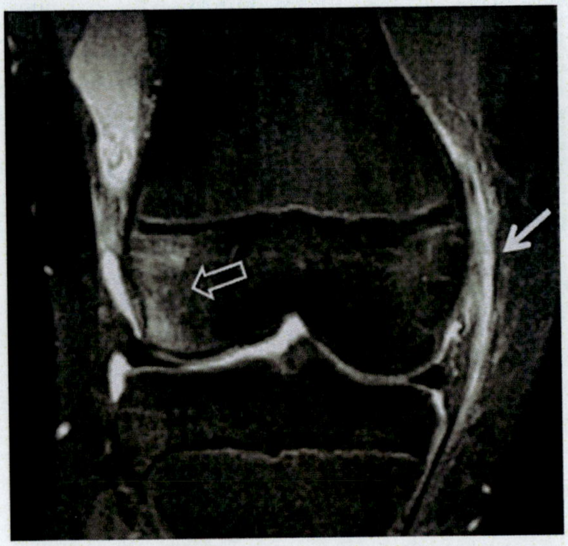

Fig. 8 A young skier after a moderate fall. The coronal fat suppressed PD-w MR image shows oedema at the medial collateral ligament suggesting grade II partial tear (*arrow*). There is also bone bruise in the lateral femoral condyle (*open arrow*) and joint effusion

4 Conclusions

To prevent skiing and/or boarding injuries the rules and regulations laid down by *International Ski Federation*, have to be followed. The use of properly adjusted equipment, specific exercise aimed at obtaining and improving the overall condition of the body and avoiding self-overestimation are prerequisites for this sport being creative and enjoyable. In cases of injuries though, radiologists play an important role both for depicting the lesion but also participating in treatment planning by means of unfolding the whole spectrum and clinical significance of the findings. History, clinical examination findings and pattern of injury, are important data which should be provided to radiologists before imaging.

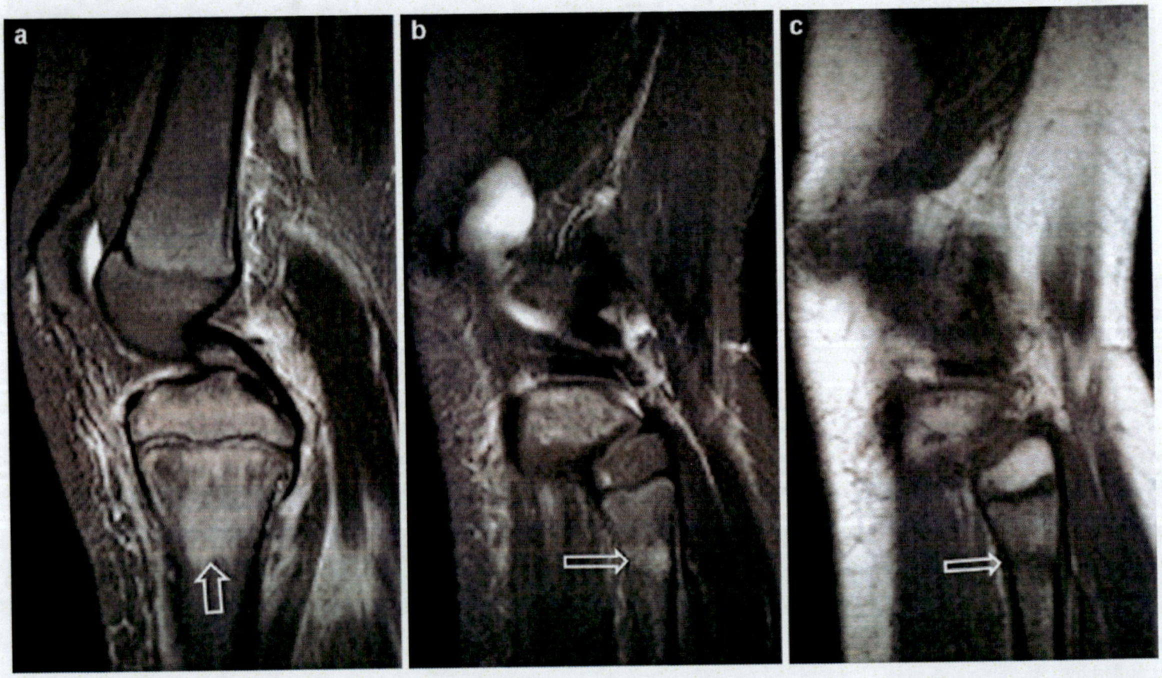

Fig. 9 A young boy after a skiing injury: sagittal STIR and T1-w MR images. Bone marrow oedema (contusion) is seen in the tibial epiphysis and metaphysis (*arrow*) (**a**). An occult to plain radiographs fracture is seen at the proximal fibula (*thin arrows*) (**b, c**)

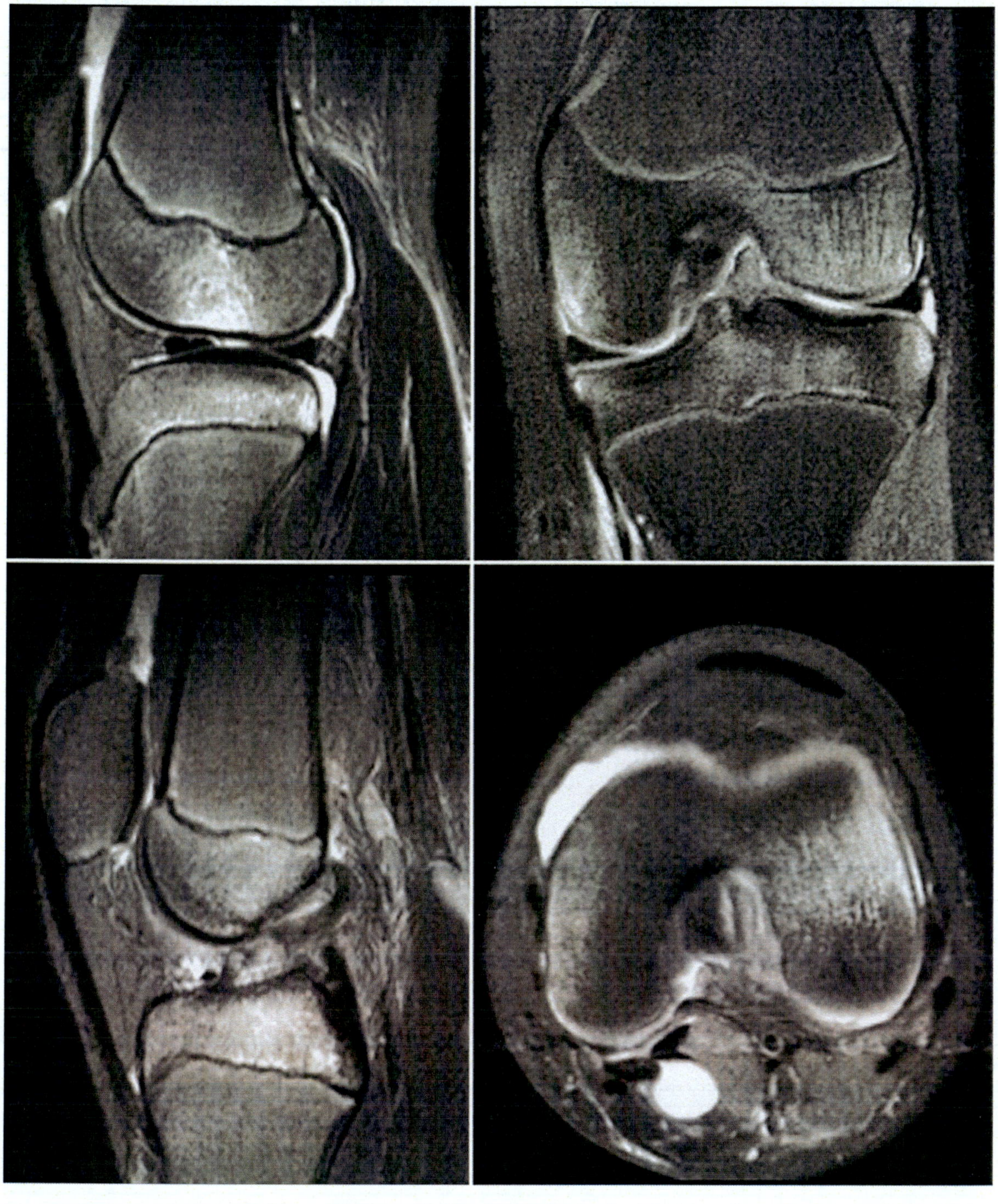

Fig. 10 The fat suppressed sagittal PD-w and coronal and axial STIR MR images, show bone bruise in the femoral condyles and proximal tibial epiphysis. There is also complete rupture of the anterior cruciate ligament and joint effusion with a Baker cyst formation

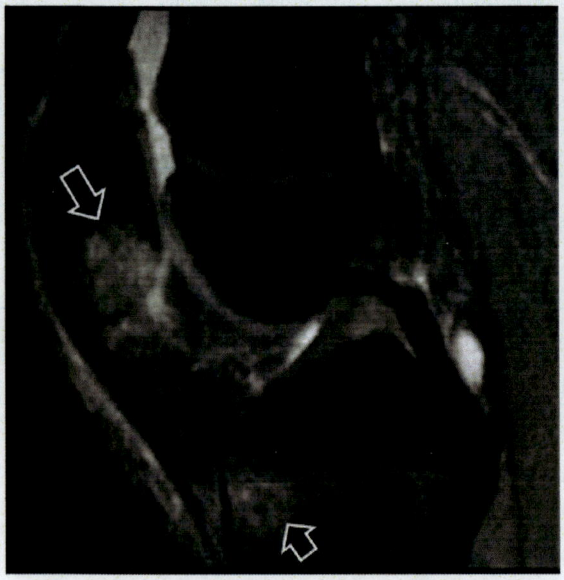

Fig. 11 A young skier with anterior pain after direct trauma on an icy slope. The sagittal STIR MR image shows bone bruising in both the patellar and tibial apophysis (*arrows*)

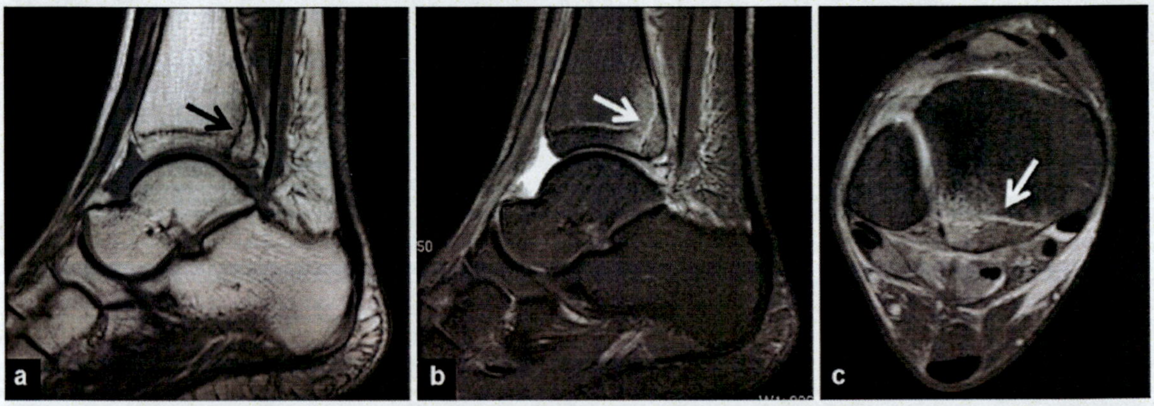

Fig. 12 A young snowboarder after jumping and falling. The sagittal T1-w (**a**), sagittal STIR (**b**) and axial STIR (**c**) MR images, show an occult fracture at the posterior malleolus of the tibia (*arrows*)

References

Abu-Laban R (1991) Snowboarding injuries: an analysis and comparison with alpine skiing injuries. Can Med Assoc J 145(9):1097–1103

Ackery A, Hagel BE, Provvidenza C, Tator CH (2007) An international review of head and spinal cord injuries in alpine skiing and snowboarding. Inj Prev 13(6):368–375

Bladin C, McCrory P (1995) Snowboarding injuries: an overview. Sports Med 19(5):358–364

Bruening D, Richards JG (2005) Optimal ankle axis position for articulated boots. Sports Biomech 4(2):215–225

Chan GM, Yoshida D (2003) Fracture of the lateral process of the talus associated with snowboarding. Ann Emerg Med 41(6):854–858

Davidson T, Laliotis A (1996) Snowboarding injuries: a four-year study with comparison with alpine ski injuries. West J Med 164(3):231–237

Davies MB, Wright JE, Edwards MS (2002) True skier's thumb in childhood. Injury 33(2):186–187

Deibert MC, Aronsson DD, Johnson RJ, Ettlinger CF, Shealy JE (1998) Skiing injuries in children, adolescents, and adults. J Bone Joint Surg Am 80(1):25–32

Diamond PT, Gale SD, Denkhaus HK (2001) Head injuries in skiers: an analysis of injury severity and outcome. Brain Inj 15(5):429–434

Dohin B, Kohler R (2008) Skiing and snowboarding trauma in children: epidemiology, physiopathology, prevention and main injuries. Arch Pediatr 15(11):1717–1723

Ettlinger CF, Johnson RJ, Shealy JE (1995) A method to help reduce the risk of serious knee sprains incurred in alpine skiing. Am J Sports Med 23(5):531–537

Fukuda O, Takaba M, Saito T, Endo S (2001) Head injuries in snowboarders compared with head injuries in skiers. A prospective analysis of 1076 patients from 1994 to 1999 in Niigata, Japan. Am J Sports Med 29(4):437–440

Gassner R, Ulmer H, Tuli T, Emshoff R (1999) Incidence of oral and maxillofacial skiing injuries due to different injury mechanisms. J Oral Maxillofac Surg 57(9):1068–1073

Hunter RE (1999) Skiing injuries. Am J Sports Med 27(3): 381–389

Kirkpatrick DP, Hunter RE, Janes PC, Mastrangelo J, Nicholas RA (1998) The snowboarder's foot and ankle. Am J Sports Med 26(2):271–277

Kocher MS, Feagin JA Jr (1996) Shoulder injuries during alpine skiing. Am J Sports Med 24(5):665–669

Kocher MS, Dupre MM, Feagin JA Jr (1998) Shoulder injuries from alpine skiing and snowboarding: aetiology, treatment and prevention. Sports Med 25(3):201–211

Koehle MS, Lloyd-Smith R, Taunton JE (2002) Alpine ski injuries and their prevention. Sports Med 32(12):785–793

Koo DW, Fish WW (1999) Spinal cord injury and snowboarding: the British Columbia experience. J Spinal Cord Med 22(4):246–251

Kozin SH (2006) Fractures and dislocations along the pediatric thumb ray. Hand Clin 22(1):19–29

Lawrence L, Shaha S, Lillis K (2008) Observational study of helmet use among children skiing and snowboarding. Pediatr Emerg Care 24(4):219–221

Levy AS, Smith RH (2000) Neurologic injuries in skiers and snowboarders. Semin Neurol 20(2):233–245

Levy AS, Hawkes AP, Hemminger LM, Knight S (2002) An analysis of head injuries among skiers and snowboarders. J Trauma 53(4):695–704

McCrory P (2002) The role of helmets in skiing and snowboarding. Br J Sports Med 36(5):314

Meyers MC, Laurent CM, Higgins RW, Skelly WA (2007) Downhill ski injuries in children and adolescents. Sports Med 37(6):485–499

Pecina M (2002) Injuries in downhill (alpine) skiing. Croatian Med J 43(3):257–260

Pino EC, Colville MR (1989) Snowboard injuries. Am J Sports Med 17(6):778–781

Prall J, Winston K, Brennan R (1995) Severe snowboarding injuries. Injury 26(8):539–542

Rachbauer F, Sterzinger W, Eibl G (2001) Radiographic abnormalities in the thoracolumbar spine of young elite skiers. Am J Sports Med 29(4):446–449

Renstrom P, Johnson RJ (1989) Cross-country skiing injuries and biomechanics. Sports Med 8(6):346–370

Schmitt H, Gerner HJ (2001) Paralysis from sport and diving accidents. Clin J Sports Med 11(1):17–22

Seino H, Kawaguchi S, Sekine M, Murakami T, Yamashita T (2001) Traumatic paraplegia in snowboarders. Spine 26(11): 1294–1297

Shorter NA, Mooney DP, Harmon BJ (1999) Snowboarding injuries in children and adolescents. Am J Emerg Med 17(3):261–263

Skokan EG, Junkins EP Jr, Kadish H (2003) Serious winter sport injuries in children and adolescents requiring hospitalization. Am J Emerg Med 21(2):95–99

Sutherland A, Holmes J, Myers S (1996) Differing injury patterns in snowboarding and alpine skiing. Injury 27(6):423–425

Tarazi F, Dvorak MF, Wing PC (1999) Spinal injuries in skiers and snowboarders. Am J Sports Med 27(2):177–180

Tuli T, Hachl O, Hohlrieder M, Grubwieser G, Gassner R (2002) Dentofacial trauma in sport accidents. Gen Dent 50(3): 274–279

Ueland O, Kopjar B (1998) Occurrence and trends in ski injuries in Norway. Br J Sports Med 32(4):299–303

Warme WJ, Feagin JA Jr, King P, Lambert KL, Cunningham RR (1995) Ski injury statistics, 1982 to 1993, Jackson Hole Ski Resort. Am J Sports Med 23(5):597–600

Xiang H, Stallones L (2003) Deaths associated with snow skiing in Colorado 1980-1981 to 2000-2001 ski seasons. Injury 34(12):892–896

Young CC, Niedfeldt MW (1999) Snowboarding injuries. Am Fam Physician 59(1):131–136

Common Injuries in Water Sports

Apostolos H. Karantanas

Contents

Key Points

- Water sports injuries are common in adolescents and uncommon in children
- The location and severity of injury depends upon the specific participation and the level of competition
- Plain radiographs, ultrasonography and MR imaging, have distinct indications
- CT is the method of first choice for imaging all serious injuries in the head and axial skeleton, followed by MRI whenever neurological deficit exists

1 Introduction

Water sports represent a wide spectrum of activities. Some of them are the same throughout the industrialized countries, and include swimming, water polo, diving, rowing, and sailing. Others are related to local particular weather conditions, and are practiced in certain periods of the year. These include wind and kite surf, jet and water ski, banana boat, snorkeling, parasailing, and various games in water parks. There is general consensus regarding the view that water spots are the most efficient way of training the whole body

A.H. Karantanas
Department of Radiology, University Hospital,
Stavrakia GR 711 10 Heraklion, Greece
e-mail: akarantanas@gmail.com

A.H. Karantanas (ed.), *Sports Injuries in Children and Adolescents*,
Med Radiol Diagn Imaging, DOI: 10.1007/174_2010_63, © Springer-Verlag Berlin Heidelberg 2011

with minimal risk of injuries (e.g., injuries among swimmers occur much rarer than among track and field athletes or football players). However, limited fitness, improper training, poor technique, and alcohol consumption, hopefully rare in the young ages, contribute to injuries related to water sports.

The present chapter illustrates common injuries occurring in children and adolescents who participate in water sports. A practical approach divides these sports as follows: in the water, under the water, and on the water. The cases discussed here were collected from referrals to a tertiary center-University Hospital, from 2004–2009 in the island of Crete.

2 Sports in the Water

2.1 Swimming

Swimming is commonly practiced at a competitive level during childhood and adolescence. Shoulder pain is a common symptom among swimmers occurring in up to 80% (Richardson et al. 1980; Colville and Markman 1999). Shoulder pain is more commonly associated with freestyle, backstroke, and butterfly with a reported incidence of 9.4% in boys and 11% in girls aged 13 and 14 years; this increased up to 21% and 25.5%, respectively, at ages 15 and 16 (McMaster and Troup 1993). The incidence of shoulder pain is related to the level of competition and the years spent in practicing the sport. Swimmer's shoulder is a multifactorial disorder resulting from a hypermobile glenohumeral joint, which allows increased motion of the humeral head. The multidirectional micro-instability leads to impingement against the undersurface of the acromion, the coracoacromial ligament, and occasionally, the coracoid process. This type of internal impingement is common in sports that require abduction and extreme external rotation (Jobe et al. 2000). MR imaging may show degeneration or tear of the posterosuperior labrum, tears of the inferior infraspinatus tendon, and subcortical cyst formation in the humeral head in advanced cases of internal impingement. In young athletes, rotator cuff tendinopathy and subcoracoid or subacromial-subdeltoid bursitis are common findings (Fig. 1). In a published case series, it was suggested that young swimmers are exposed to stresses at the proximal humeral head, which can lead to humeral head epiphysiolysis (Fig. 2) (Johnson and Houchin 2006). The differential diagnosis of shoulder

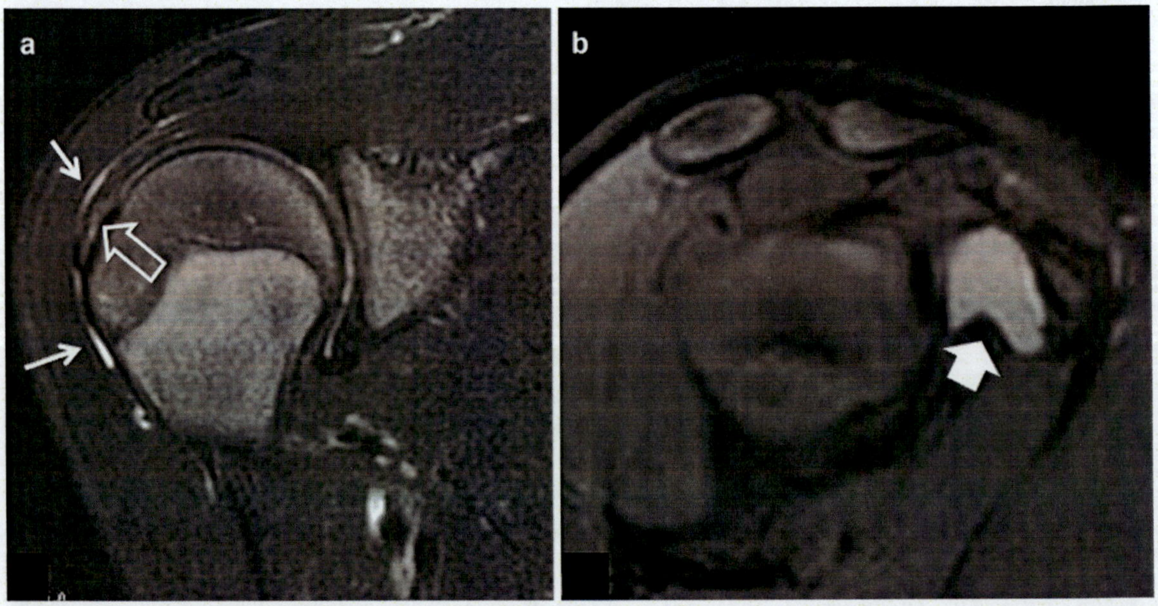

Fig. 1 An 11-year-old male elite swimmer with persisting shoulder pain despite rest. The fat-suppressed PD-w in the oblique coronal (**a**) and oblique sagittal (**b**) planes show subacromial-subdeltoid bursa (*white arrows*), supraspinatus tendinopathy (*open arrow*), and subacromial bursa (*short arrow*)

pain among swimmers should also include thoracic outlet syndrome (Richardson 1999).

Medial and/or anterior knee pain is commonly seen in swimmers, especially breast-strokers. The incidence of this symptom may be as high as 73% (Kenal and Knapp 1996). Bone marrow edema in keeping with stress reaction is a common finding (Fig. 3).

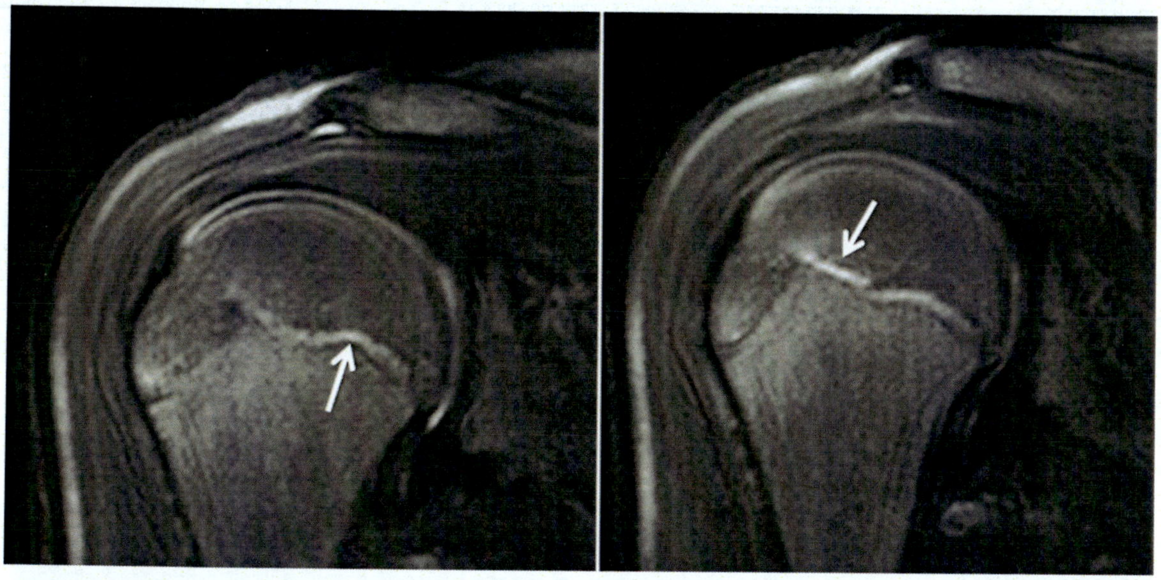

Fig. 2 The fat-suppressed oblique coronal PD-w MR images in contiguous slices show minor epiphysiolysis in a 12-year-old male elite butterfly swimmer with shoulder pain (*arrows*)

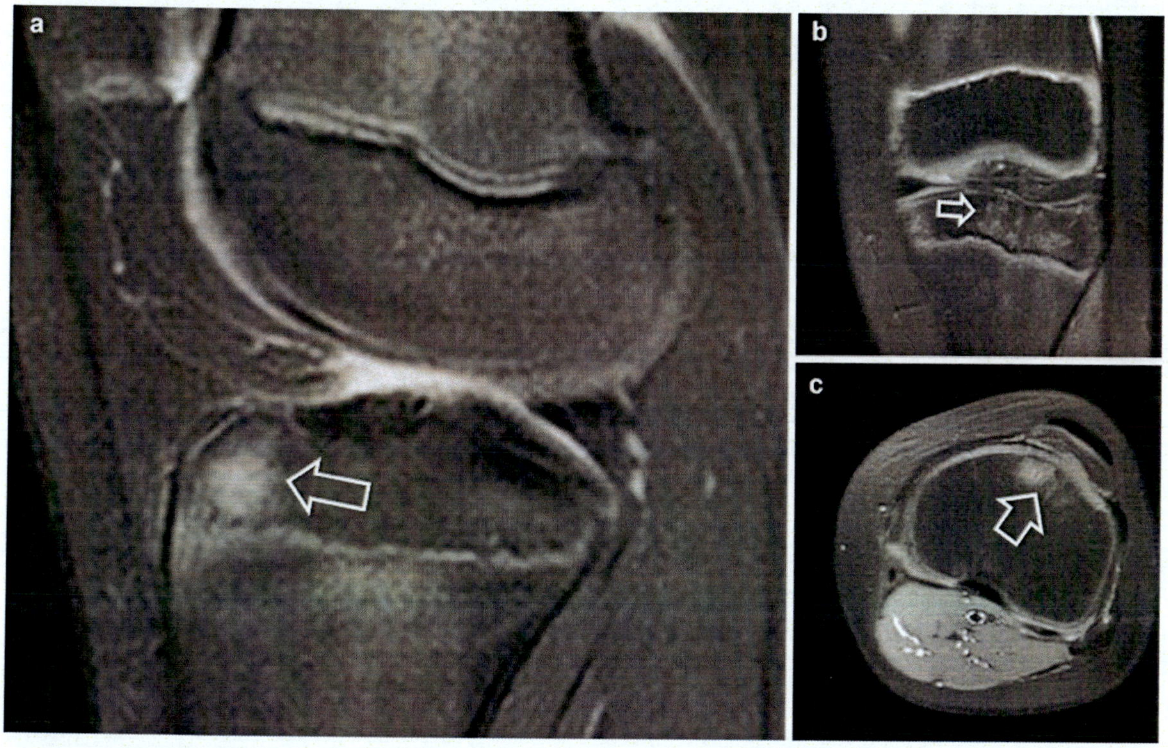

Fig. 3 A 14-year-old elite breaststroke swimmer with persistent anterior knee pain. The fat-suppressed PD-w MR images in sagittal (**a**), coronal (**b**), and axial (**c**) planes show a focal high signal intensity area corresponding to bone marrow edema-like stress reaction lesion (*arrows*)

The use of swim fins during training induces stress in the ankle and foot. Stress reaction in the bone marrow and injuries of the extensor retinaculum and tendons are common findings (Figs. 4 and 5).

In the end of winter season and during the peak of competition, stress reactions and frank spondylolysis are common among adolescent elite swimmers. Some cases of early disc degeneration and Schmorl's nodes may be observed in elite swimmers; on MRI, this finding is indistinguishable from early Scheuermann's disease (Fig. 6) (Swischuk et al. 1998).

2.1.1 Monofin Swimming

A monofin is typically used in fins-swimming and free diving. It consists of a single surface attached to foot-pockets for both the free-diver's feet. The diver's muscle power and swimming style, and the type of activity the monofin is used for, determine the choice of size, stiffness, and materials used. Technical monofin swimming at a competitive level induces significant stress in the lower spine. Disc herniations and Schmorl's nodes may occur as a result of stress fracture of the epiphyseal plate (Fig. 7).

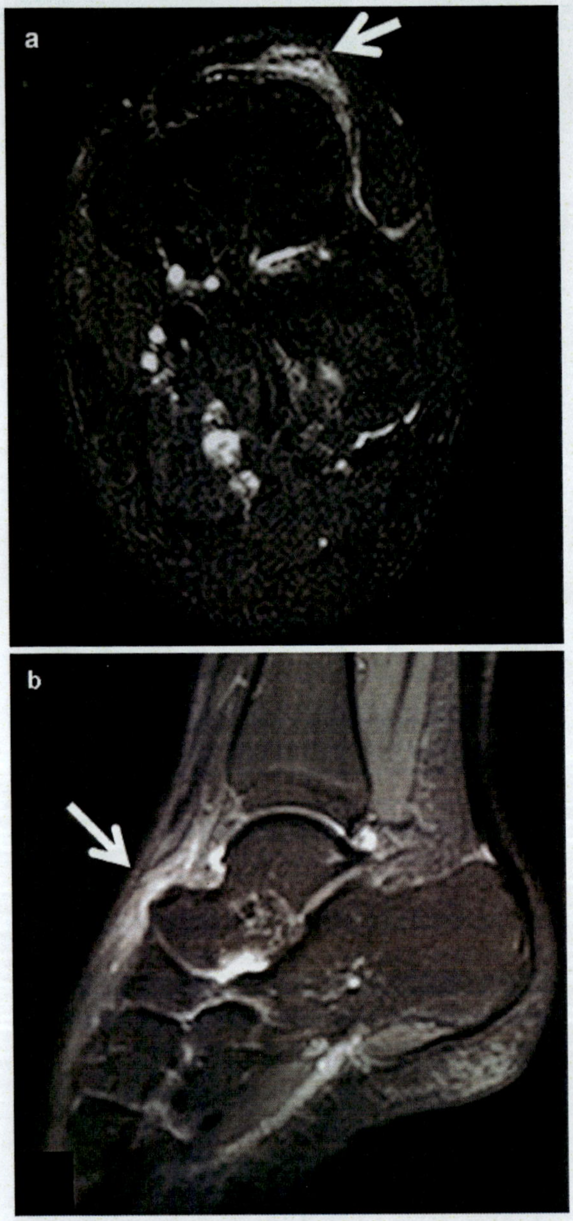

Fig. 4 A 14-year-old elite female swimmer reporting pain in the dorsal midfoot, exacerbated with use of swim fins. The oblique coronal fat-suppressed T2-w (**a**) and sagittal STIR (**b**) MR images show edematous injury of the extensor retinaculum (*arrows*)

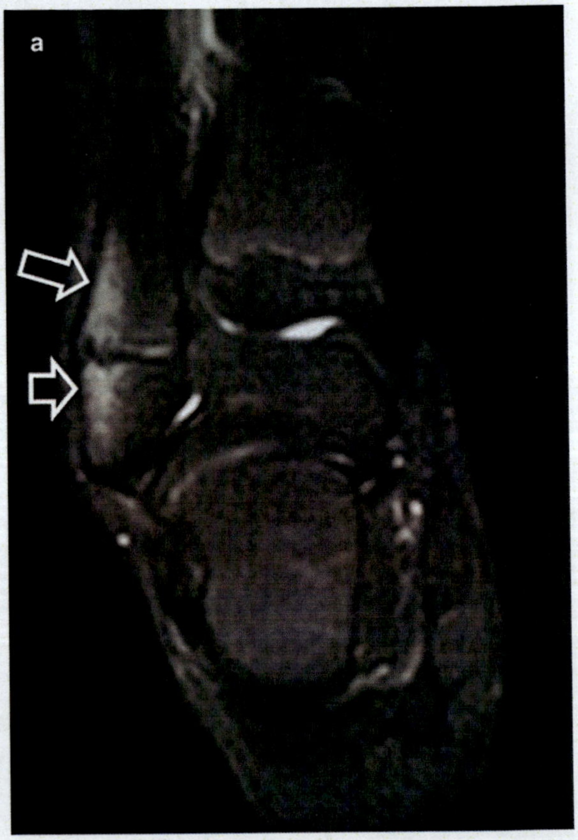

Fig. 5 A 11-year-old elite female swimmer reporting pain in the lateral ankle area, exacerbated with use of swim fins. The coronal fat-suppressed T2-w (**a**) and para-sagittal STIR (**b**) MR images show edematous changes within the bone marrow of the lateral malleolus, in keeping with stress reaction (*arrows*)

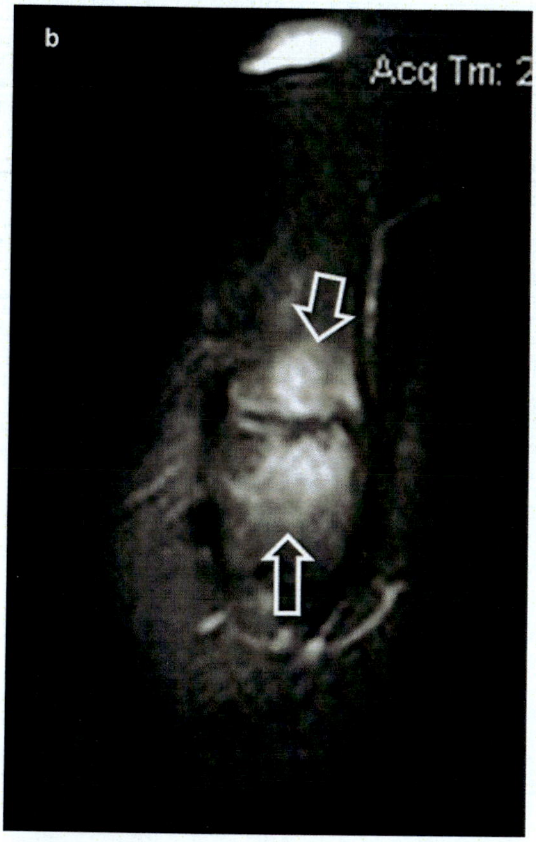

Fig. 5 (continued)

2.2 Water Polo

Water polo (WP) is a contact sport and requires continuous swimming in rapid sprints up and down with abrupt changes of direction. In between ages of 15 and 17, both male and female athletes may achieve a high level of competition. Injuries include those resulting from overuse, like in swimming, and traumatic ones, like in wrestling.

Minor injuries occur frequently in WP among adolescent athletes. Most of these injuries do not require medical aid and include skin cuts and bruising, often in the supraorbital face, due to close contact with other players and high ball velocity. *Severe injuries* may occasionally happen, mostly located in the face and head, and include fractures of the nasal bone and blowout of the orbits (Franić et al. 2007).

Low back pain is a common symptom in WP players and is the result of intense rotational movements during throwing and passing the ball. *Stress reaction* and *spondylolysis* are included in the differential diagnosis of athletes with persistent symptoms (Fig. 8). Acute nerve root compression in the lumbar region is usually the result of an acute disc prolapse. MR imaging should be applied in cases not responding to conservative treatment.

WP is associated with a high incidence of *shoulder pain* (36–38%), mainly due to intense repeated overhead activity (Webster et al. 2009). Contact with opponent players or the ball may result in dislocations and subluxations of the glenohumeral and the acromioclavicular joints. SLAP lesions result from repetitive biceps tension from overhead activity but are not usually seen in young athletes. Repetitive labral microinjuries might be demonstrated with intra-labral cyst formation (Fig. 9). Shoulder instability and labral lesions, when clinically suspected, should be studied with MR arthrography. Rotator cuff tendinopathy, partial and full thickness tears in the context of internal impingement are not common in adolescent athletes.

Elbow pain is a common complaint among WP athletes. The differential diagnosis includes ulnar collateral ligament (UCL) injuries, valgus extension overload syndrome with olecranon osteophytes/posteromedial impingement, and osteochondritis dissecans (OD) of the capitellum (Cain et al. 2003). Both MRI and US can be diagnostic in cases of UCL injuries. For the rest, MRI is the method of choice. CT is able to depict OD as well as intra-articular loose bodies. In our series, OD was the most common injury among adolescent water polo players (Fig. 10).

Stenosing tenosynovitis (*de Quervain's syndrome*) of the first dorsal compartment is the most common tendinitis of the wrist in athletes using upper extremities. *Extensor carpi ulnaris tendinopathy* is second to de Quervain's in frequency but it may affect tendons in all dorsal compartments. Commonly encountered acute injuries to the hand and fingers of WP players include lacerations, dislocations of the interphalangeal and metacarpalphalangeal joints, and fractures of the phalanges and metacarpal bones (Hutchinson and Tansey 2003; Rettig 2003). Avulsion fracture of more than 40% of the articular surface of the middle phalanx may need surgical treatment. Rupture of the collateral ligaments of the proximal interphalangeal joints may also be seen (Colville and Markman 1999).

Adductor muscle strains, demonstrated with *groin pain*, are a common injury in sports that involve sudden changes of direction like in WP. It has been documented that legwork accounts for 40% to 55% of the game,

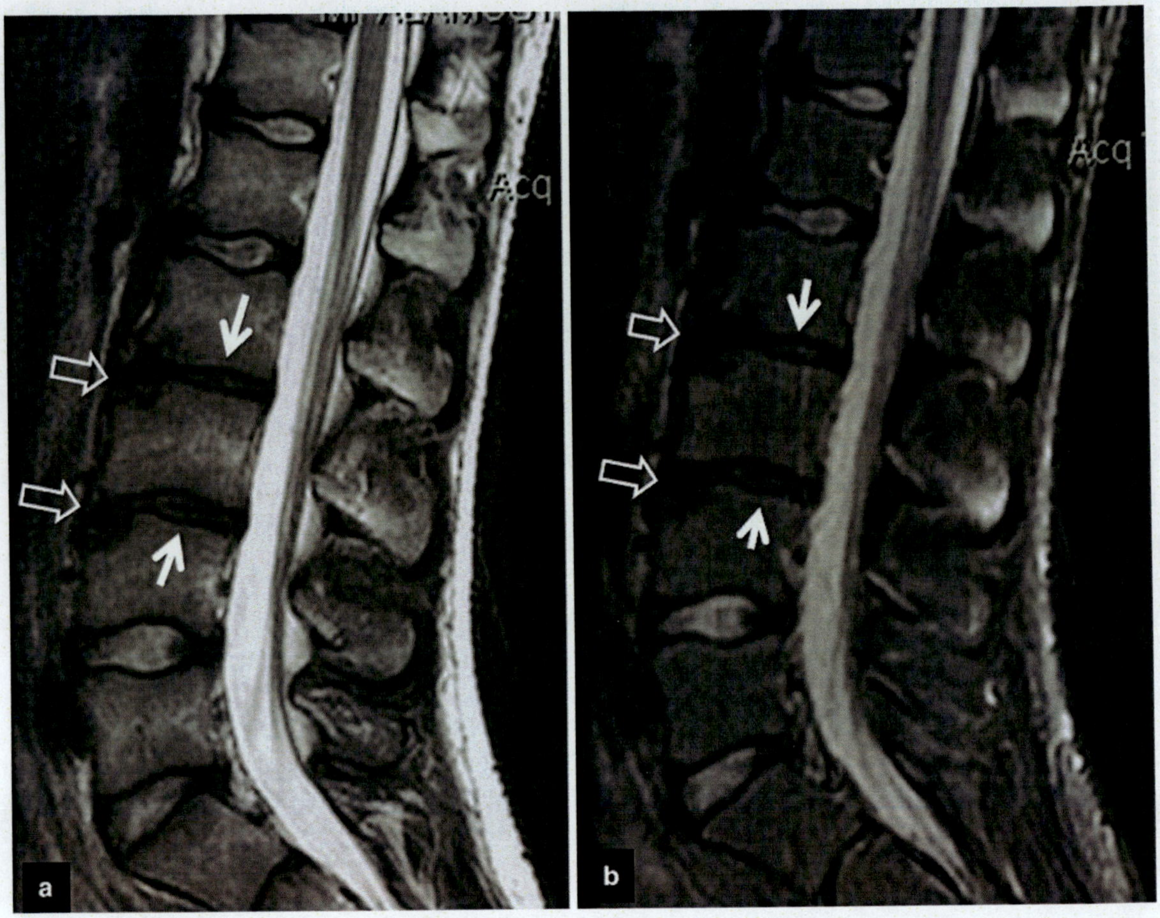

Fig. 6 A 13-year-old elite breaststroke swimmer with persistent back pain. The sagittal T2-w (**a**) and STIR (**b**) MR images show early degeneration of the discs L2-L3 and L3-L4 (*arrows*) along with anterior herniation through the upper ipsilateral epiphyseal plate (*open arrows*).The lack of presence of multiple small extrusions within the epiphyseal plates favors overuse and anterior Schmorl' node formation rather than early Scheuermann's disease

depending on the position played and game tactics. Water polo players seldom perform the breaststroke "whip kick," but instead, the right leg rotates counterclockwise while the left rotates clockwise in the "eggbeater" kick unique to water polo. The rotation of the knee, with compression on the medial aspect of the joint, causes degenerative changes. Pain along or over the origin or insertion of the medial collateral ligament is typically an overuse syndrome from the chronic stress and overuse of the eggbeater kick, but mostly it is seen in adults.

2.3 Synchronized Swimming

Synchronized swimming is a hybrid of swimming, gymnastics, and ballet. This complex activity induces high demands on the athlete often resulting in injuries unique to this sport. Most athletes enter the sport as young girls at recreational level. By the age of 13–15 years, the talented ones are chosen to train at a competitive level. Boosts and throws induce an increased risk of traumatic injuries including hematomas, contusions, sprains, acute tears of muscles and tendons, disc herniations, and fractures. Serious head injuries with post-concussive syndrome also have been reported (Mountjoy 1999). The "rocket split" move is responsible for acute groin, hamstring, and quadriceps strains. The three most common musculoskeletal overuse injuries encountered among elite and recreational synchronized swimmers are shoulder instability, lumbar pain, and patellofemoral syndrome (Weiberg 1986). Overuse may also result in tenosynovitis. Excessive pronation has been related to

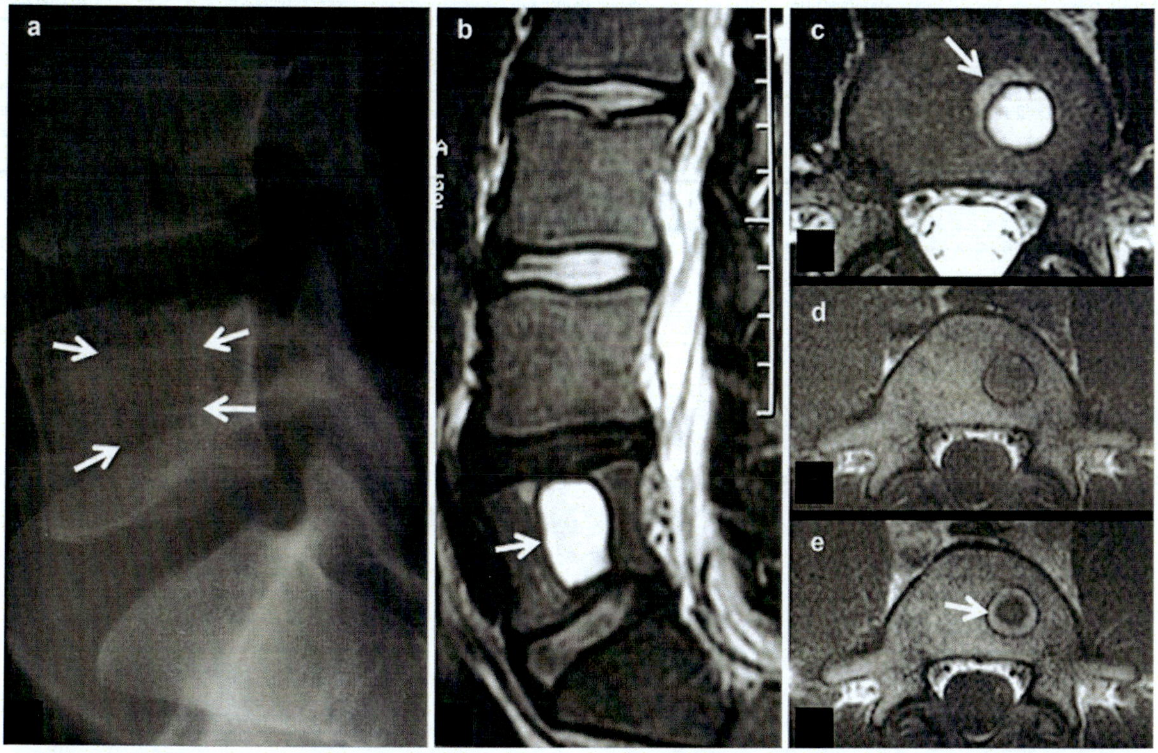

Fig. 7 A 16-year-old male elite swimmer with sudden pain during monofin swimming due to a giant Schmorl's node. (**a**) The lateral radiograph shows a well-defined large lytic lesion in the L5 vertebral body with sclerotic border (*arrows*). The sagittal (**b**) and axial (**c**) T2-w MR images show the cystic nature of the lesion, the degeneration of the L4-L5 disc, the low signal intensity border (*arrow* in b), and the reactive bone marrow edema (*arrow* in c). (**d**) The axial T1-w MR image shows the sclerotic border of the lesion. (**e**) The contrast-enhanced T1-w MR image shows enhancement medial to the sclerotic border (*arrow*), suggesting an acute lesion

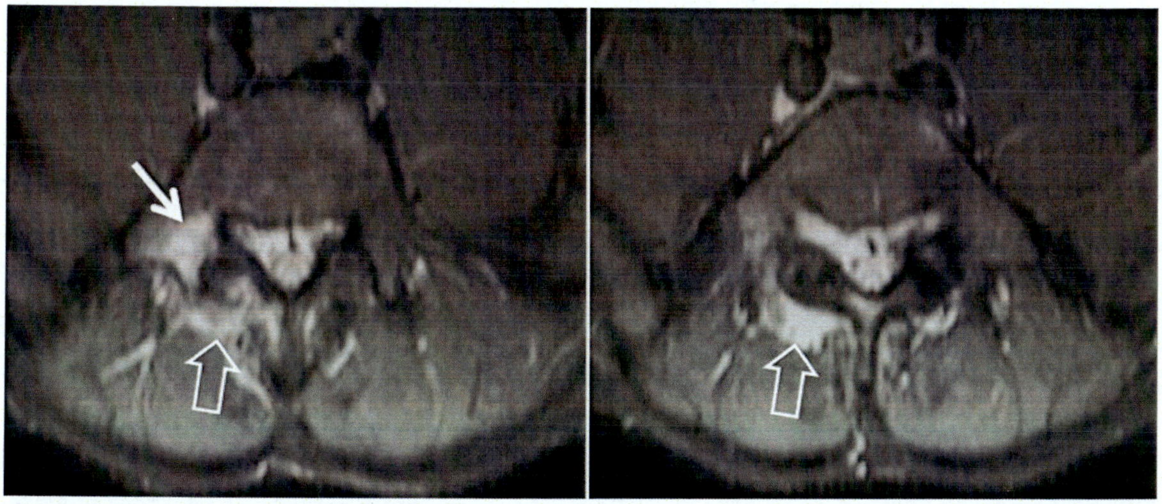

Fig. 8 A 15-year-old male water polo athlete with low back pain during the last 5 weeks. He reported 3.5 h exercise for 5 times a week. The axial STIR MR images show bone marrow edema (*arrow*) and soft-tissue (*open arrows*) edema, in keeping with unilateral stress reaction

an otherwise rare entity, tenosynovitis of the extensor longus tendon (Fig. 11).

Shoulder instability results from repetitive micro-trauma and hypermobility of the joint. No imaging findings have been described in this respect. Internal impingement may be the only clinical demonstration. As the problem is mainly muscular, there is good response to conservative treatment.

Great flexibility in the lumbar and the rest of the spine is required in this sport. *Lumbar pain* might result from facet inflammation, poor pelvic posture, and overuse together with poor muscular control. The rate of spondylolysis is not as common as in other sports. Imaging will not show any findings in these athletes with lumbar pain. Only one case of stress reaction was recorded in our database, located in the spinous processes of the lower cervical spine (Fig. 12).

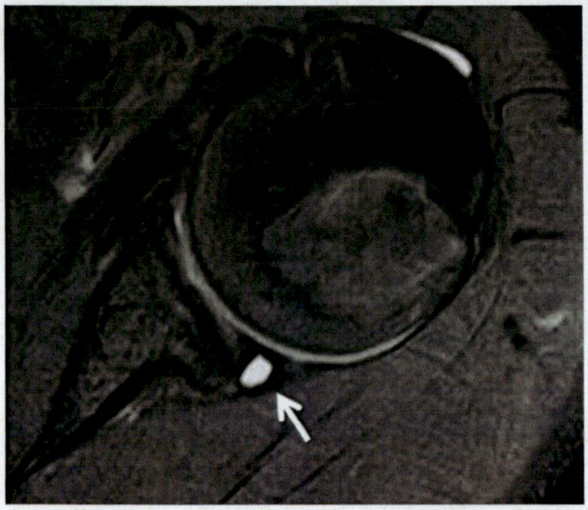

Fig. 9 A 15-year-old male water polo athlete with persistent shoulder pain particularly during throwing the ball, despite conservative treatment. The axial fat-suppressed PD-w MR image shows a labral cyst posteriorly (*arrow*)

The *patellofemoral syndrome* is mainly seen in the recreational rather than the elite athlete. Chronic strain to the medial collateral ligament may coexist. The excessive "eggbeater" motion which enables the athlete to raise the arms and body above the water is perhaps the main pathogenetic mechanism. This motion if combined with malalignment of the patella or vastus medialis oblique muscle weakness, may result in a painful syndrome.

2.4 Snorkeling

Snorkeling is the practice of swimming at the surface of the sea being equipped with a mask and a short tube called a snorkel. The routine use of swim fins allows the athlete to observe underwater for extended periods of time with relatively little effort. This kind of recreational activity is very popular among children and adolescents in the Mediterranean Sea and tropical resorts. *Delayed onset muscle soreness* has been only observed in young athletes, particularly at the beginning of holidays, and the diagnosis is clinical.

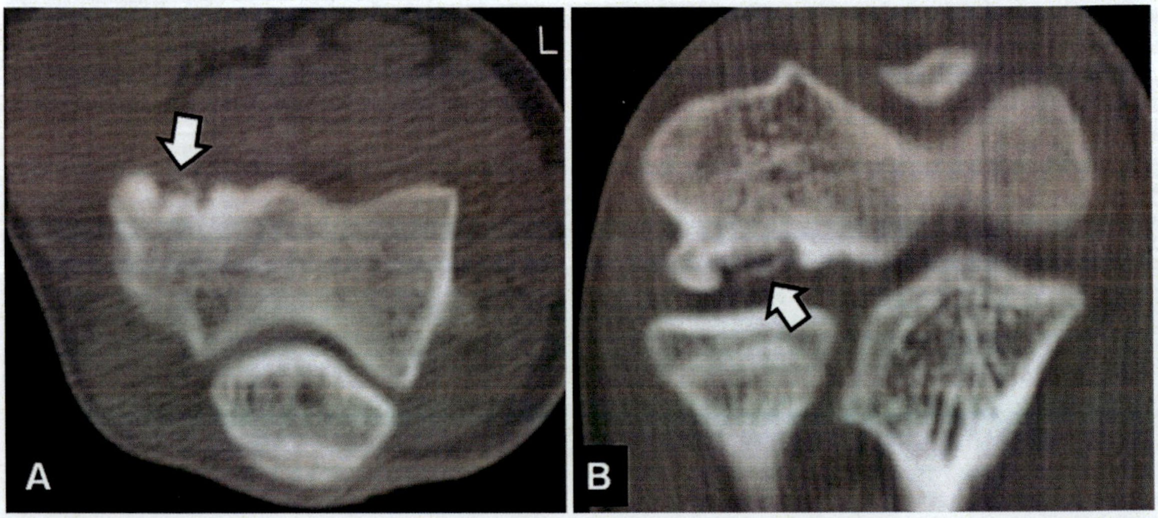

Fig. 10 Osteochondritis dissecans of the capitellum in a 15-year-old water polo male athlete. The axial (**a**) and the coronal reconstruction (**b**) CT images show the complete detachment of the osteochondral lesion without displacement (*arrows*)

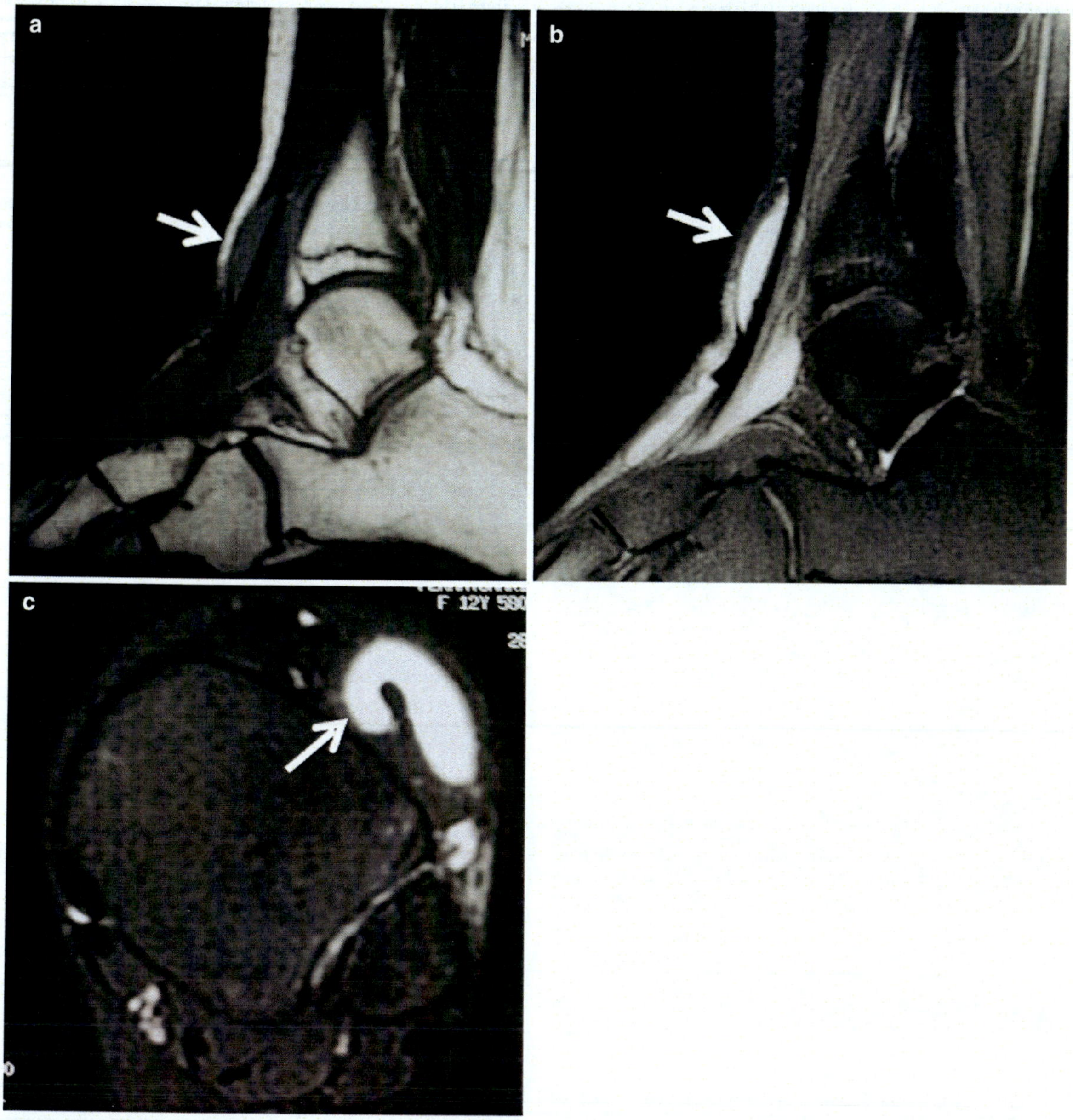

Fig. 11 Tenosynovitis of the extensor digitorum longus tendon in an elite 12-year-old female synchronized swimming athlete. The sagittal T1-w (**a**), sagittal fat-suppressed PD-w (**b**), and axial fat-suppressed T2-w (**c**) MR images show effusion (*arrows*) surrounding the tendon due to overuse

2.5 Diving

Diving is the sport of plunging into water, usually headfirst, performed with gymnastic and acrobatic stunts. There are four forms of diving: competitive, recreational, underwater (scuba), and bungee jumping related. Recreational activities are the ones mostly associated with severe injuries.

All kinds of sport account for 9–10% of all spinal cord injuries (Ouzky 2002); diving is the source of 60–80% of them (DeVivo 1997; Aito et al. 2005; Barss et al. 2008). Adolescent amateurs usually do not master the proper technique of diving. Misjudgment of the water depth, reckless behavior, and/or alcohol consumption are well-recognized risk factors (Korres et al. 2006). Male youths are mainly

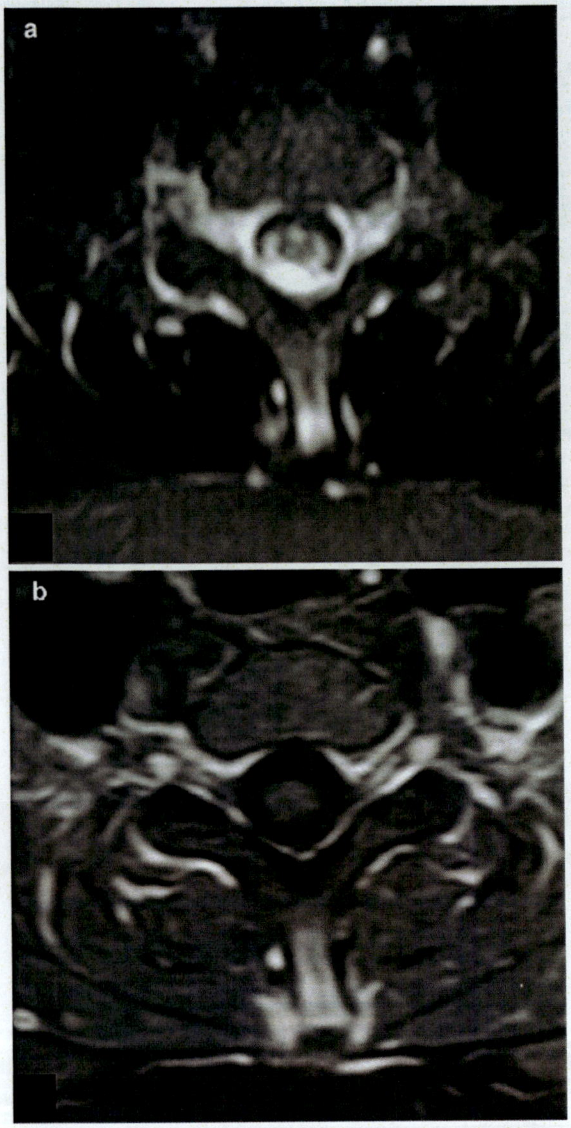

Fig. 12 Stress injury in the cervicothoracic spine in a 14-year-old female synchronized swimming athlete. The axial STIR (**a**) and fat-suppressed contrast-enhanced T1-w (**b**) MR images show bone marrow edema and enhancement within the spinous process and the surrounding soft tissues

at risk. As a result, severe cervical spine injuries, with or without spinal cord involvement, are usually seen during summer months. "Feet first-first time" programs have reduced the incidence of diving injuries in controlled and supervised areas.

Any dive can result in death or severe disability throughout lifetime. Diving injuries are more disabling than those from motor vehicle accidents or falls, as nearly all involve the cervical region. In the majority of cases, C5 and C6 are the levels most commonly involved with fractures and neurological injuries (Bailes et al. 1990). Few injuries may involve the thoracolumbar region. CT and MRI are the methods of choice for assessing osseous and cord injuries, respectively.

Few data exist on competitive diving as well as on bungee jumping regarding the immature skeleton. According to one study, spinal cord injury and in general diving-related trauma is very common in children aged 6–15 (Blanksby et al. 1997). In our database, 13 spinal cord injuries with permanent disability were recorded in the last 5 years in recreational divers, all young adults. This may reflect that supervision on adolescents both in the Greek family and among tourists is an effective and thus advisable preventive act of such injuries.

3 Sports Under the Water

Free diving or *scuba diving* is very popular in the tourist destinations. Fatalities are quite common and have been associated with preexisting medical conditions such as ischemic heart disease (Sykes 1995). No injury related to free diving or scuba diving was recorded in the adolescent age team in our health area. The rate of participation of young athletes in sports under water normally should be quite low.

4 Sports on the Water

4.1 Personal watercrafts injuries

Personal watercrafts, also known as *Jet Ski* crafts, are powered by a water jet. It has been shown that 9–30% of the injured patients are younger than 16 years (Hamman et al. 1993). The wide availability, easy accessibility, and lack of previous experience are the main causes of serious Jet Ski–related injuries. Most accidents involve collision between two vessels. Head/face and neck followed by spine and extremities are the most common locations of these injuries (Rubin et al. 2003; Carmel et al. 2004). Lower extremity injuries include hip and femoral fractures. The primary cause of death is blunt trauma and, more particularly, injury to the central nervous system (Branche et al. 1997; Kim et al. 2003). About one third of the injuries requiring care at a trauma center involve riders younger than 15 years (Hamman et al. 1993; Kim et al. 2003).

Safety recommendations include minimum age of 16, operator training, operating regulations, and required helmet use. CT is the method of first choice for all serious injuries followed by MR imaging of the spine whenever neurological deficits exist. Jet skiing is not allowed for children and adolescents by law. The few head injuries and femoral and rib fractures in our database were related to illegal use of a craft by a non-trained person in late adolescence.

4.2 Wind and Kite Surfing

Windsurfing is a popular sport and is practiced by using a board, a mast, and a sail using the wind for propulsion. Most of the injuries are acute due to impact with equipment (Neville and Folland 2009). Overall, the injury incidence is low (1.5/person/year) including routinely muscle/tendon strains and ligament sprains (Dyson et al. 2006). Different injuries occur depending upon the age and expertise of the athlete. Preadolescent and adolescent athletes present with injuries due to insufficient training and/or warming-up. They most commonly sustain skin and muscle wounds caused by the cutting edge of the keel fin. Beginners suffer from low back pain as they do not take sufficient advantage of the wind power (Fig. 13). Stress reaction and spondylolysis may occur. Beginners may also present with iliotibial band friction syndrome due to poor technique, which results in increased loading of the knee joints (Fig. 14). In athletes with moderate experience, low back pain results when light wind conditions create prolonged lordosis of the spine while pumping. In addition, lumbar compression occurs when sailing without the use of a harness, which attenuates the force transmitted through the spine. At this level of expertise, more severe injuries include rib fractures following fall on the boom and fracture/dislocation of the elbow, following fall on the mast while hand is firmly attached to the boom, and thus hyperextension occurs. Posterior impingement with "os trigonum" syndrome may occur following repetitive attempts for water start during which the posterior ankle is used to raise the whole body weight with the help of the blowing wind (Fig. 15). With the same mechanism, a focal stress reaction may appear in the posterosuperior calcaneus (Fig. 16). In experienced athletes, fractures, osteochondral injuries, shoulder dislocation, stress reactions, and labral tears may also occur. CT, MRI, and MR arthrography may be applied for diagnosing the lesions (Figs. 17–19). More severe injuries in the head and spinal cord may also occur in the elite level but are rare in the young age range (Kalogeromitros et al. 2002).

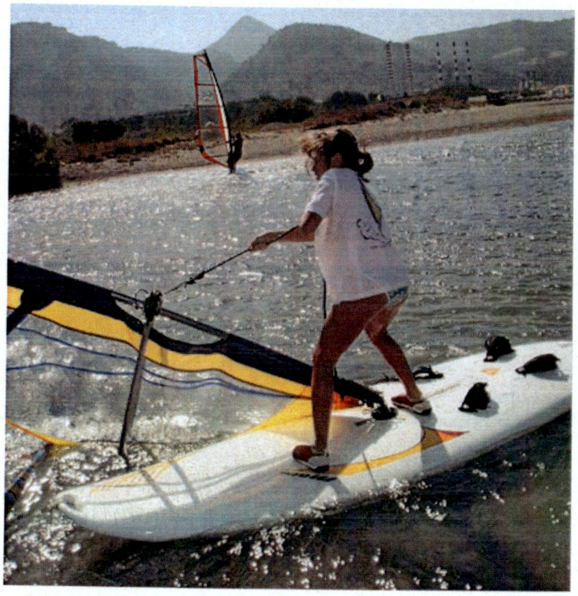

Fig. 13 A 12-year-old elite swimmer and beginner in windsurfing with persistent low back pain. Lifting of the mast and sail induces forces to biceps, back, thighs, and knees

Kitesurfing is a water sport where a rider is on a surfboard, powered by a power kite and is reported to show 7 injuries per 1,000 h of practice (Nickel et al. 2004). In the early phase of learning, major injuries, such as those in head, neck, spine, and chest, may occur. Adolescent athletes are rarely involved in this sport. Foot and ankle injuries usually occur during the jump (Fig. 20). Traumatic injuries in the knees may occur in collision with hard surfaces (Fig. 21). The use of helmet and the use of a quick release system, which enables the surfers to detach the kite in emergency situations, will further reduce injuries (Zantop and Zernial 2005). In elite athletes who practice without breaks, painful syndromes in the ankle and foot include stress reactions and painful "os naviculare" (Figs. 22 and 23).

4.3 Water Ski-Wakeboarding

Water skiing is using skis to slide over the water while being pulled by a boat or other device. The usual bat

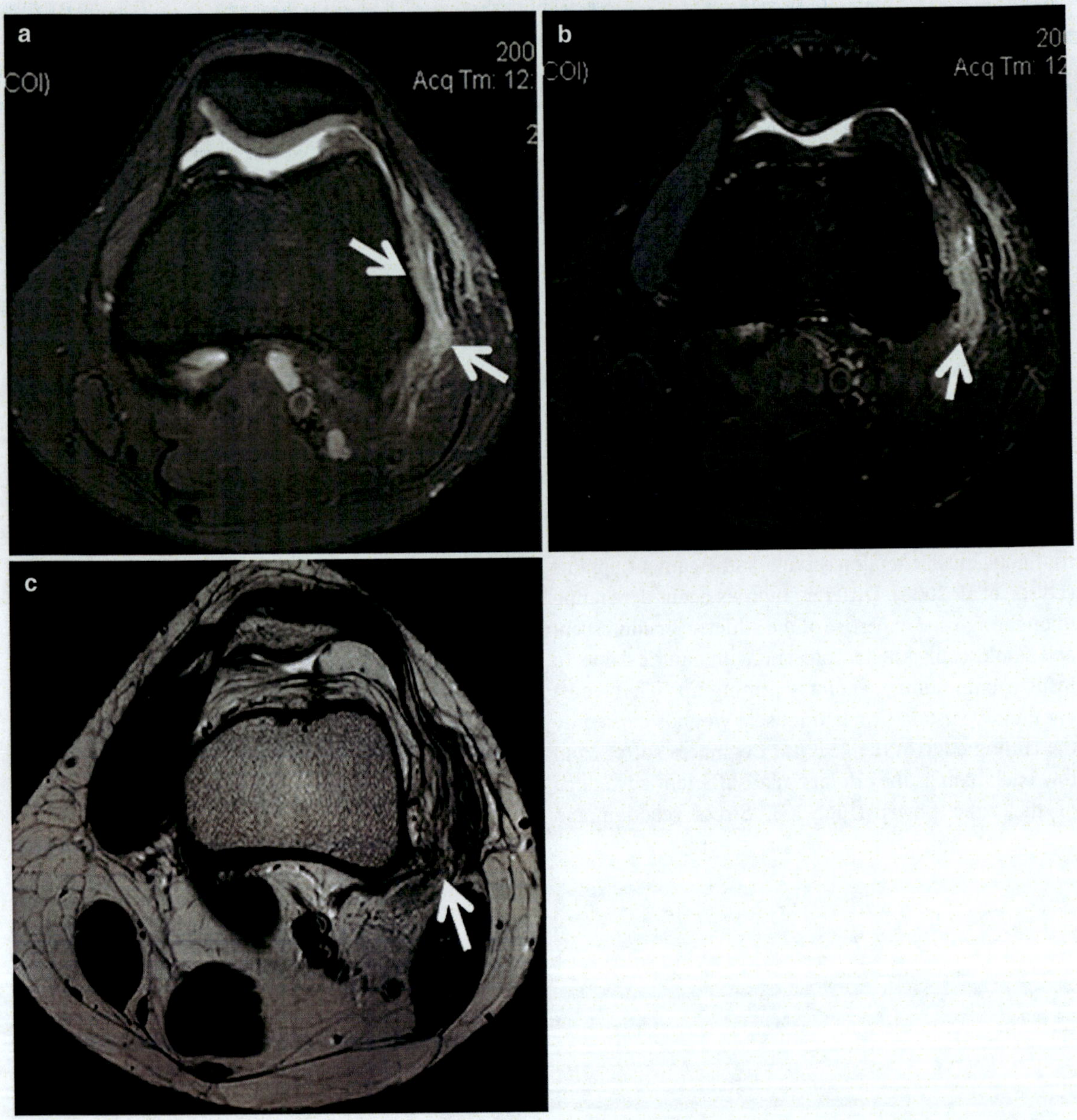

Fig. 14 A 16-year-pld female windsurfer with pain and tenderness in the lateral aspect of the knee joint. The fat-suppressed PD-w (**a**, **b**) and T2-w (**c**) axial MR images show edema in the soft tissues between the iliotibial band and the lateral femoral condyle (*arrows*) in keeping with iliotibial band friction syndrome

speed used for slalom water skiing can reach 30–35 mph in certain competitions. Water skiing-related injuries depend upon the level of experience with novices injured during take-off and experts injured during high speed falling involving knees, spine, or shoulder. These injuries peak during young adulthood and middle age, mostly in men, and include strains or sprains of the lower extremity (Hostetler et al. 2005). In adolescent skiers, minor and moderate ankle sprains were mostly recorded in our database (Fig. 24). On the other hand, wakeboarding-related injuries peak during adolescence, mostly among males (Hostetler et al. 2005). *Wakeboarding* is similar to water skiing but using only one board attached to the feet. This sport is named after the fact that the rider jumps after the wake of the boat. The jumps can

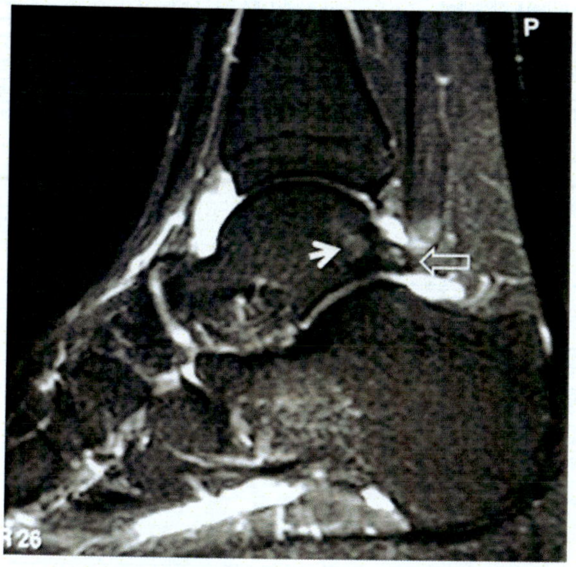

Fig. 15 A 16-year-old female windsurfer with clinical findings of posterior impingement syndrome in the ankle. The sagittal STIR MR image shows the os trigonum with bone marrow edema within it (*open arrow*), reactive changes in the talus (*arrow*), and soft-tissue edema surrounding the os. The findings suggest "os trigonum" syndrome. There is also effusion in the ankle joint

be as high as 7 m, and significant forces can be generated as the athlete falls or lands hard on the water. The usual boat speed for wakeboarding is between 18 and 23 mph, which allows the rider to jump a larger boat wake, go higher into the air, and thus better enables the rider to perform the various flips, spins, and other aerials. The most common injuries include anterior cruciate ligament tears, fractures (of thoracic-lumbar spine, femur, tibia, calcaneus and ribs), shoulder dislocations, and ankle sprains (Carson 2004). Osteochondral lesions following sprains may be seen (Fig. 25). Overuse injuries in the bone marrow of the foot may also occur (Fig. 26). Head and face are injured 6.7 times more likely than in water skiing according to data from emergency departments (Hostetler et al. 2005). Interestingly, it seems that no correlation exists between injuries and level of expertise, frequency of riding, length of practice or strength training (Carson 2004). A relation of injuries to certain tricks such as inversion exists, and most injuries occur by direct twisting contact with the water rather than by collision (Fig. 27).

4.4 Water Parks

Water park injuries, becoming more common in recent years, include those occurring in waterslides, pools and slipping, and falling on wet surfaces. The most common injuries in children are located on the

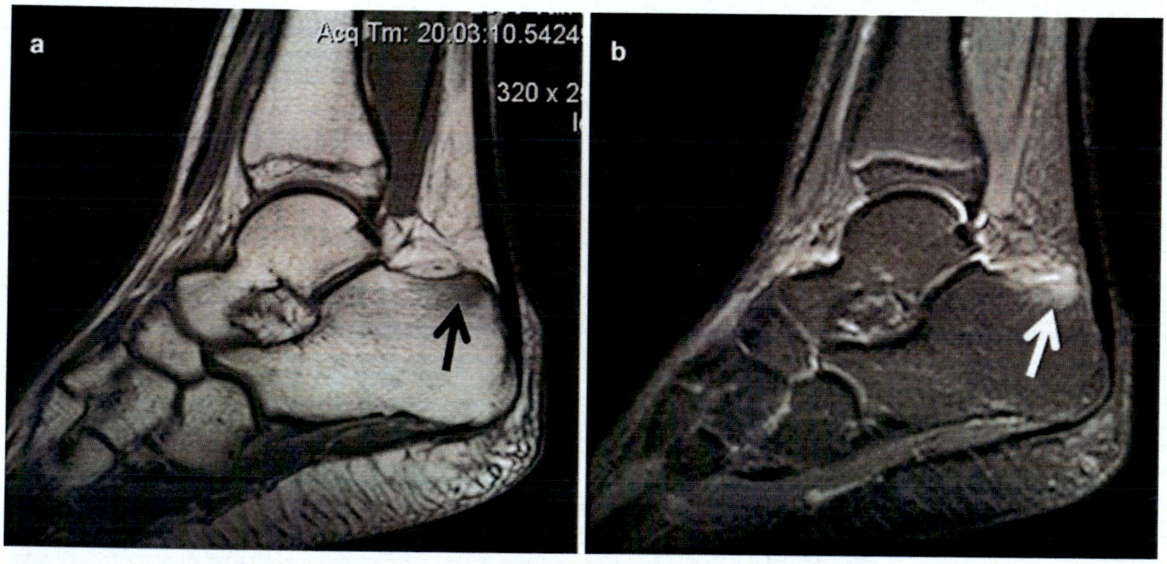

Fig. 16 A beginner 12-year-old female windsurfer with posterior foot pain following repetitive attempts for water start, which requires pressure of the heel over the board. The T1-w (**a**) and STIR (**b**) MR images show bone marrow edema in the posterosuperior calcaneal bone (*arrows*) in keeping with stress reaction

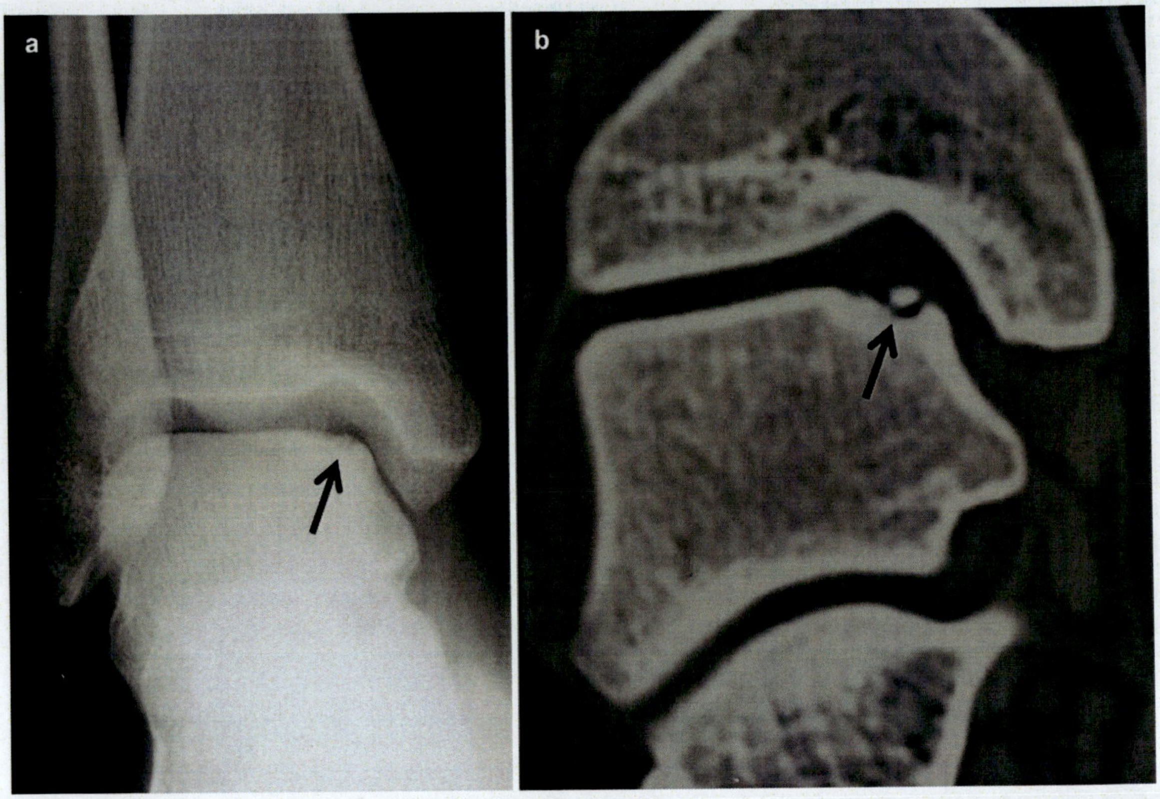

Fig. 17 Unstable osteochondral lesion in a 15-year-old female windsurfer with a history of painful ankle following a severe sprain 3 years before imaging. The plain AP radiograph (**a**) and the coronal CT reconstruction (**b**) show a small osteochondral injury in the medial aspect of the talar dome (*arrows*). The presence of air between the lesion and the talus in (b) suggests instability

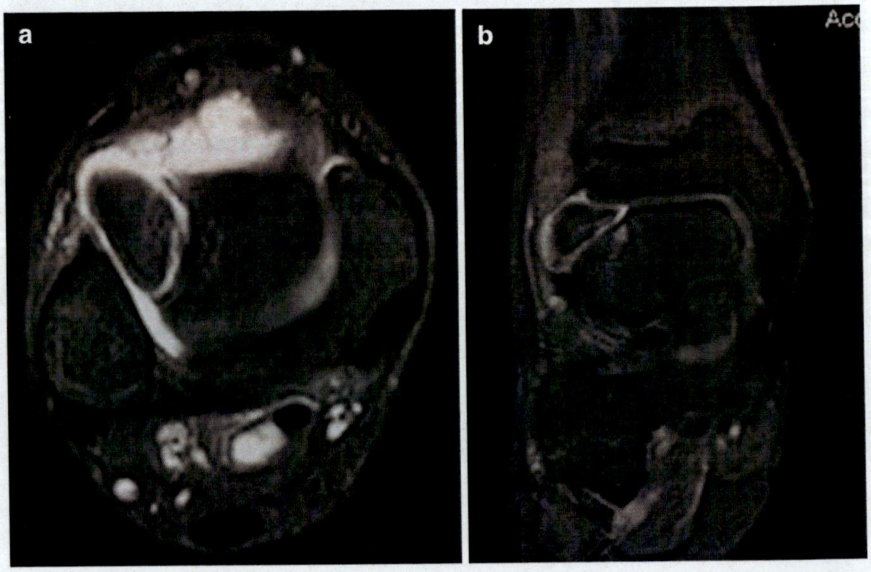

Fig. 18 Osteochondral injury Grade IV in 14-year-old male windsurf athlete. The axial (**a**) and coronal (**b**) fat-suppressed PD-w as well as the sagittal 3D-water excitation gradient echo (**c**) MR images show the lateral talar dome lesion which is completely detached but not displaced. The articular fluid surrounds the lesion, and thus there is no need for arthrography to assess instability

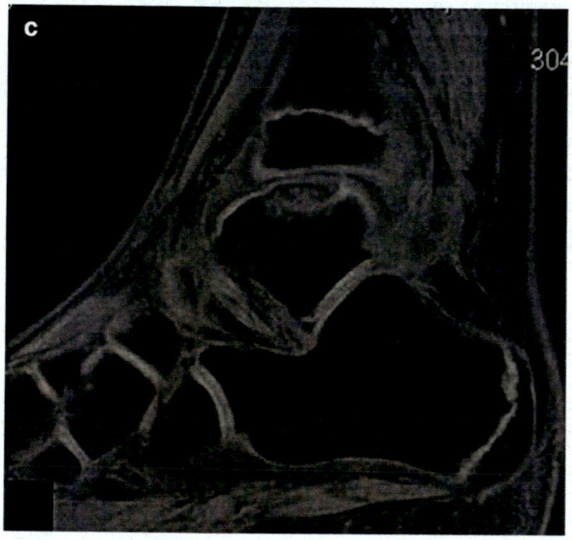

Fig. 18 (continued)

face and head (Soyuncu et al. 2009). CT is the method of choice for investigating all serious injuries. Soft-tissue hematomas may occur after contacting hard surfaces (Fig. 28). Obese or adolescents lacking regular exercise may sustain various injuries such as muscle strains and stress reactions and fractures (Figs. 29–31).

4.5 Skimboarding

Skimboarding is the sport of riding a skimboard over shallow water on a beach and into oncoming waves close to shore. The board is usually tossed ahead and jumped on after a running approach. This sport is quite popular among adolescents and is practiced in windy areas providing high waves. All the north part of Crete and all Greek islands during summertime are suited for this until recently unknown activity. Skimboarding-related injuries occur by the sudden deceleration of the board as it transitions from water to land or from falls into shallow water (Merriman et al. 2008). Fractures of the distal radius and the ankle are the commonest injuries (Sciarretta et al. 2009) (Figs. 32 and 33). Hyperdorsiflexion-related injuries of the 1st and 2nd metatarsophalangeal joints, not recorded in our series, have been reported (Donnelly et al. 2005). Extreme aerial maneuvers may result in spinal cord injuries (Collier et al. 2010).

4.6 Rowing Injuries

Rowing-related injuries in young athletes include overuse (74%) and single traumas (26%) with a slight female predilection (Smoljanovic et al. 2009). The injuries are most commonly located in

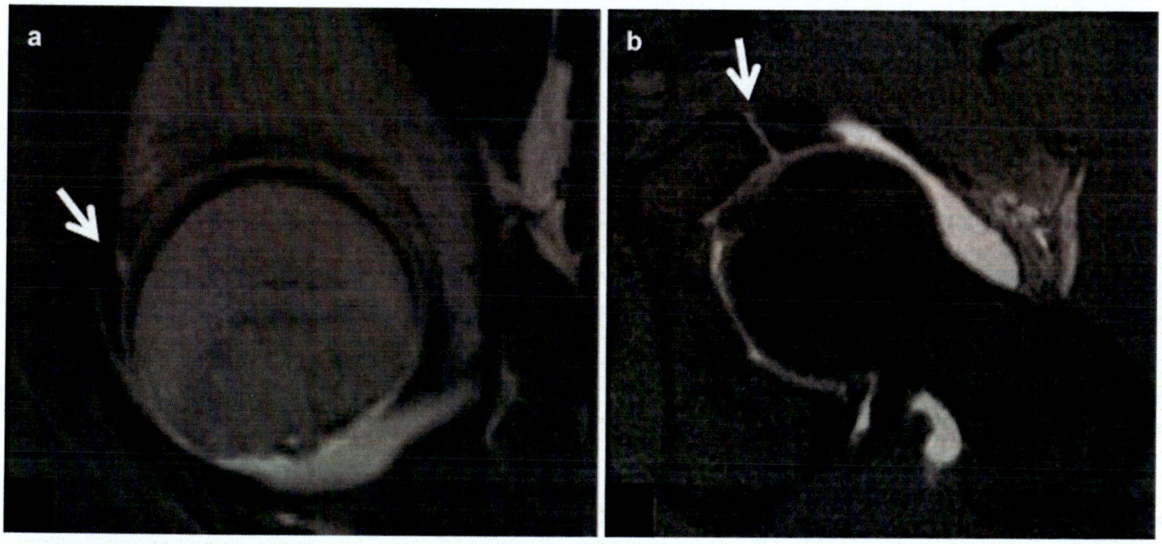

Fig. 19 Anterolateral labral tear grade IIIA in an elite windsurfer 16-year-old who reports pain, a clicking sound, and inability to surf following a bad fall one year before imaging. The sagittal T1-w (**a**) and oblique axial fat-suppressed T1-w (**b**) MR arthrographic images show the tear in the base of the labrum (*arrows*)

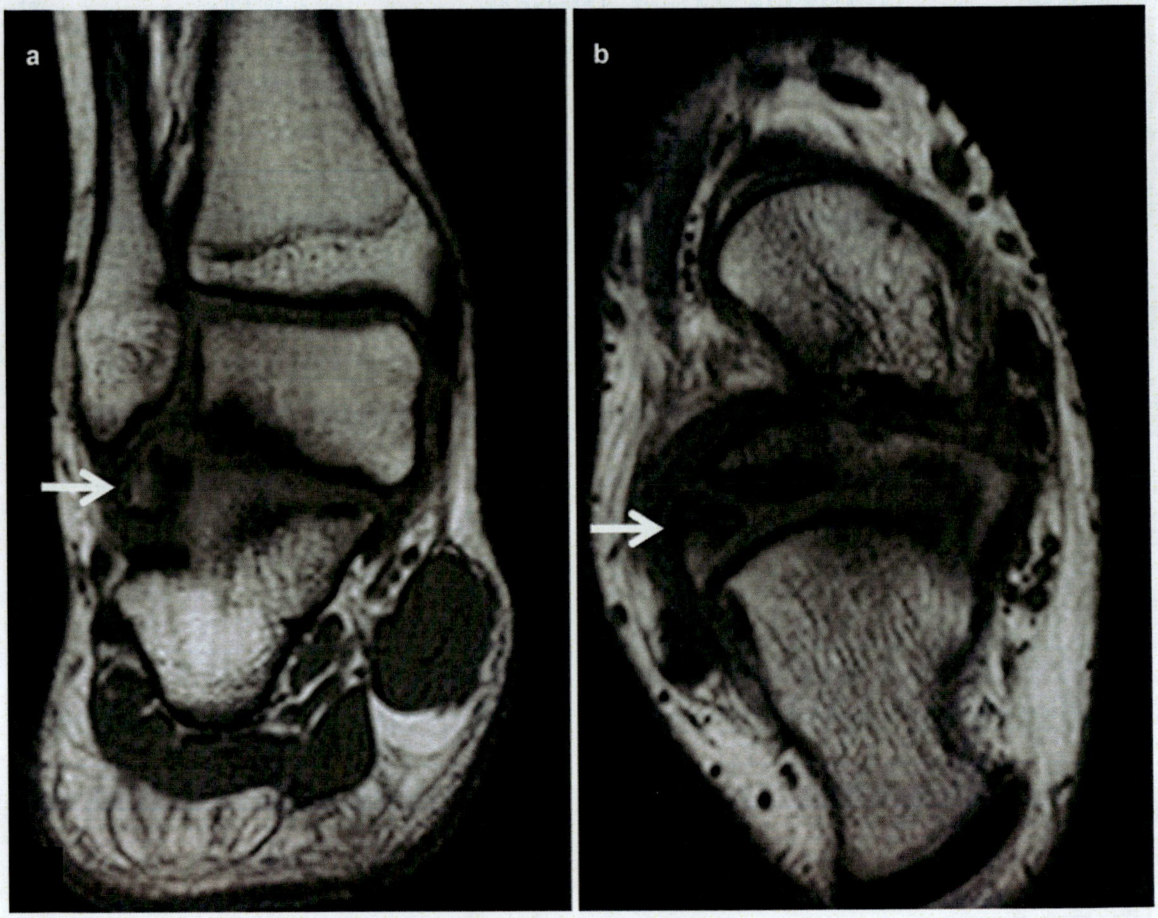

Fig. 20 A 15-year-old male kitesurfer with an osteochondral lesion of the inferior aspect of the talus, stage IV. The coronal (**a**) and axial (**b**) T1-w MR images show the detached osteochondral fragment (*arrows*)

the lower lumbar spine (spondylolysis, sacroiliac joint dysfunction, and disc herniation), knees (patellar maltracking, iliotibial band friction syndrome), and forearm/wrist (deQuervain's tenosynovitis, exertional compartment syndrome, lateral epicondylitis, intersection syndrome) (Rumball et al. 2005) (Fig. 34). The injuries seem to relate to the level of experience. Rib stress fractures may occur in elite athletes in late adolescence (Dragoni et al. 2007). Low back pain is common in adolescent female rowers (Perich et al. 2010). Costochondritis, costovertebral joint subluxation, and intercostal muscle strains may be seen in the anterior chest wall (Rumball et al. 2005). In general, rowing injuries are so typical that they can be diagnosed without any imaging (McNally et al. 2005).

4.7 Sailing

The objective of the novice sailor is skill development rather than increasing performance. Injuries are thus mild and include contusions and bruises, abrasions, and cuts (Neville and Folland 2009). The upper limb is the most injured body region in novice sailors. At particular risk are the hands and fingers and the head as a result of impact with and use of equipment usually during maneuvers such as tacking and jibing (Fig. 35). Loading of the lumbar spine can result in stress reaction (Fig. 36).

4.8 Various

"*Banana*" *boats* have become a popular activity among tourists throughout the world. They are cylindrical

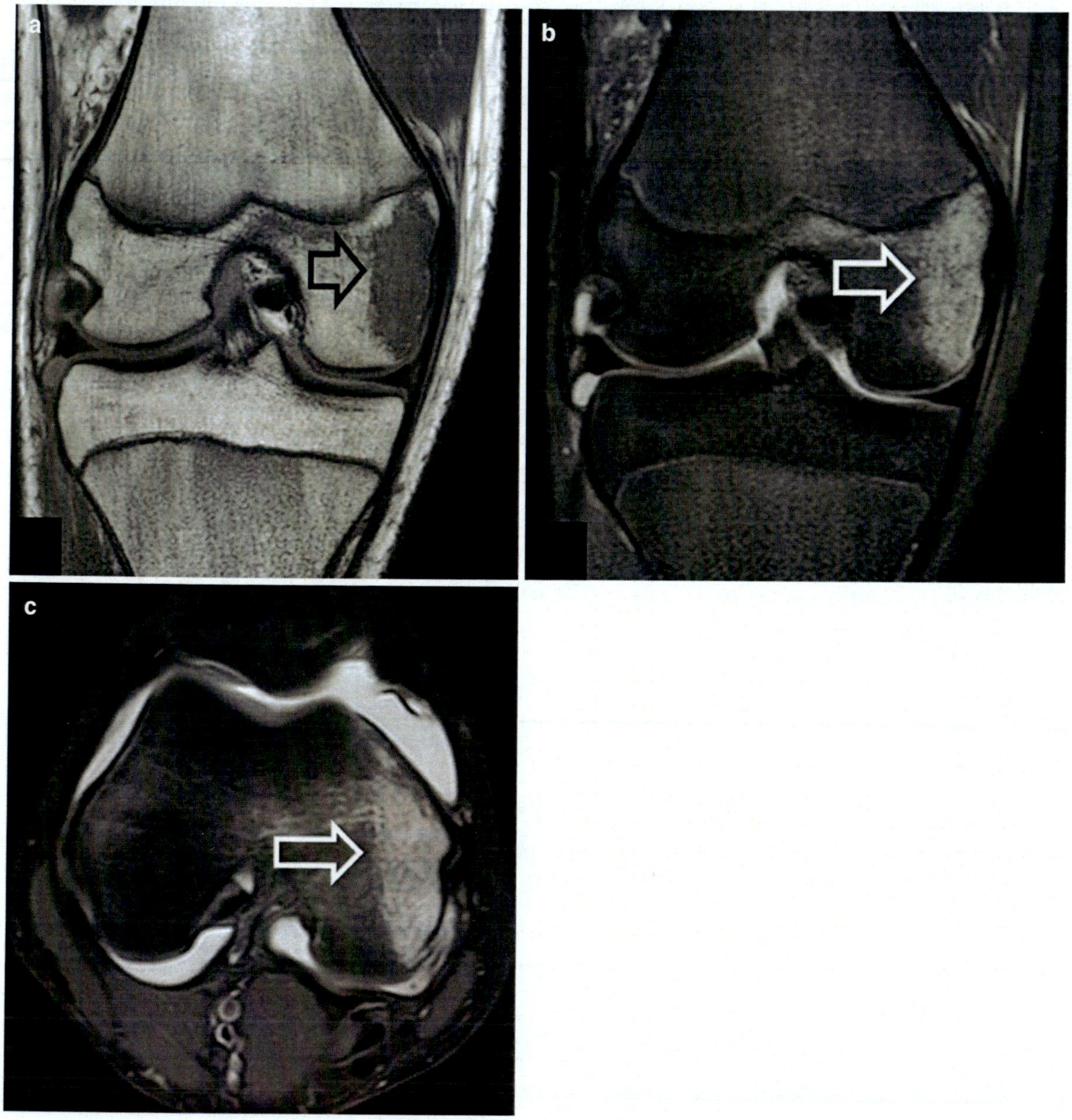

Fig. 21 A 16-year-old male kitesurfer with a fall on hard surface during jumping. The coronal PD-w (**a**), fat-suppressed PD-w (**b**), and axial fat-suppressed PD-w (**c**) MR images show bone marrow edema in keeping with bone bruise *(arrows)*. A moderate joint effusion is also seen

plastic inflatable boats. Up to eight passengers may be seated, each with their own seat and handlebar and towed at high speed behind a powerboat. Lifejackets are normally worn but helmets only occasionally. The tight turn at the end of the ride results in all passengers being thrown off into the sea. When passengers are towed at speeds greater than those recommended by manufacturers, there is a risk for severe injury. The mechanism most commonly implicated is an accidental blow from the flailing limb of a fellow passenger during group's ejection from the boat. Head fractures and dislocations of the shoulder area are the most common injuries according to one report (Hawthorn et al. 1995). Same kind of injuries occurs with "*Water tubing.*"

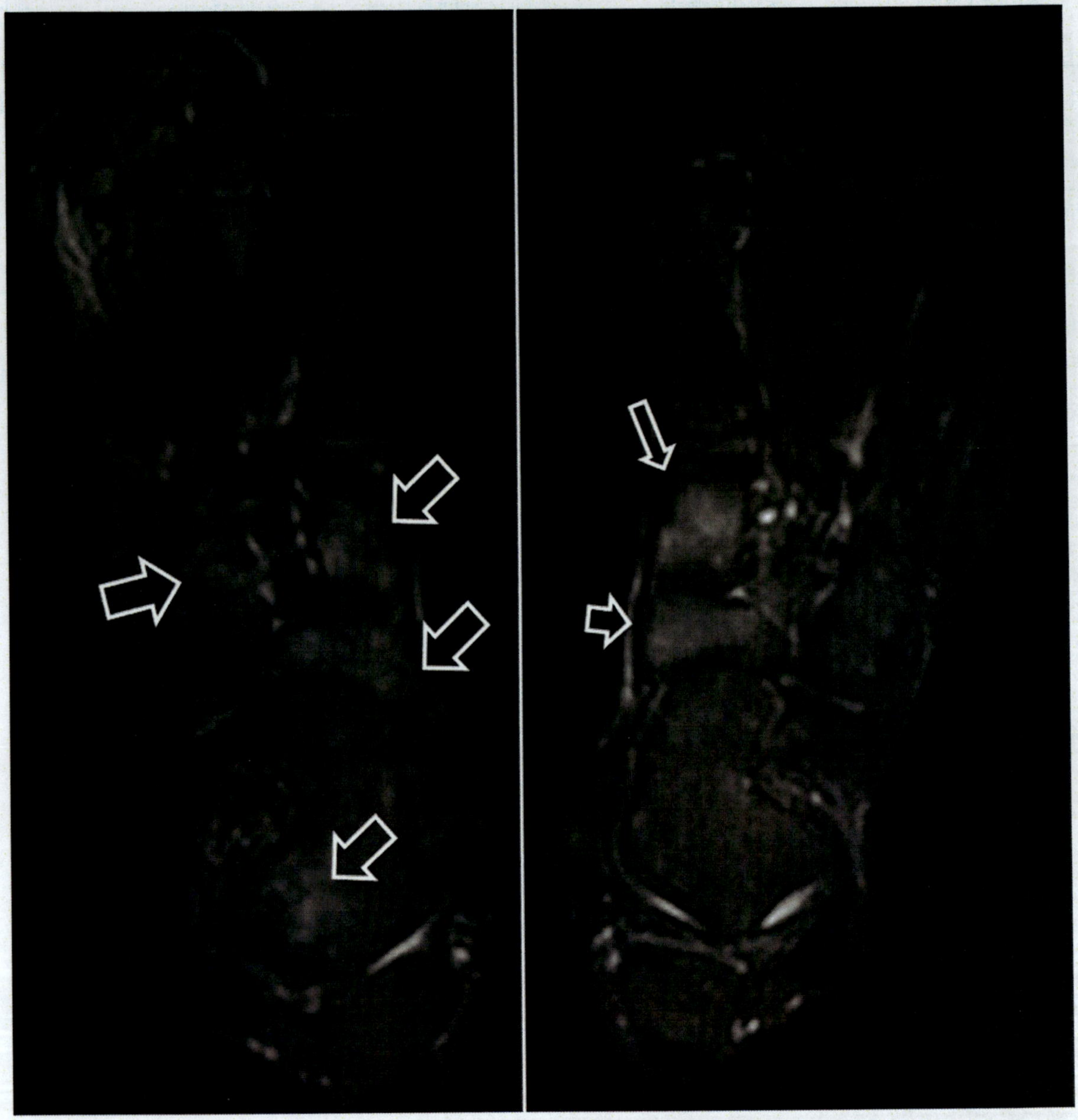

Fig. 22 A 14-year-old male kitesurfer with stress reaction in both feet. The oblique axial fat-suppressed PD-w MR images show bone marrow edema in calcaneus, navicular, medial and lateral cuneiforms on the right and navicular and medial cuneiform bones on the left (*arrows*)

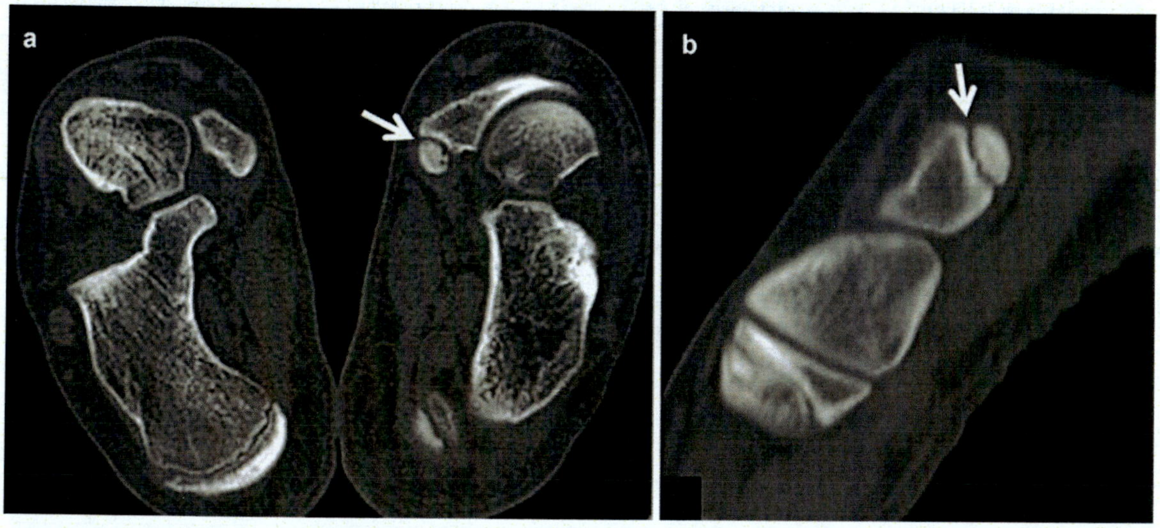

Fig. 23 A 14-year-old male kitesurfer with painful os naviculare syndrome. The axial CT (**a**) and the sagittal reconstruction (**b**) show the irregular synchondrosis of a large os naviculare (type II) with the navicular bone (*arrows*)

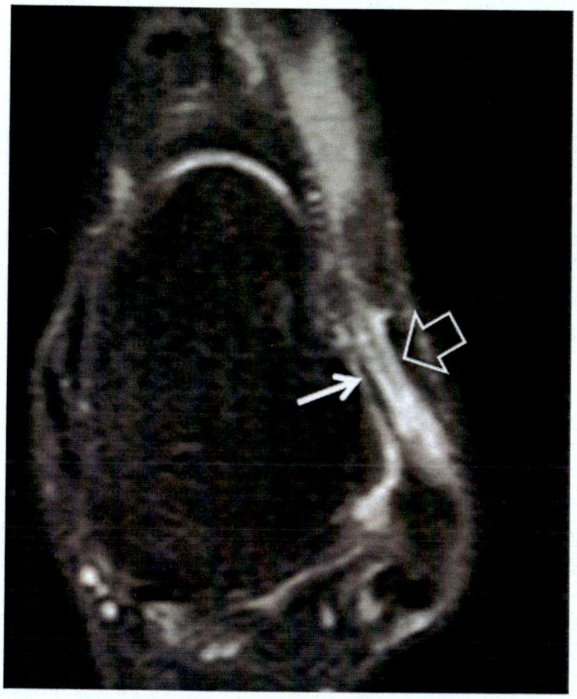

Fig. 24 A 13-year-old female with pain in the anterolateral aspect of the ankle. During summer holidays, intense training in water skiing resulted in many falls and injuries in the ankles. The axial fat-suppressed PD-w MR image shows attenuation of the anterior talofibular ligament (*arrow*) in keeping with partial tear. Edema is also seen in the surrounding soft tissues (*open arrow*)

Parasailing, also known as *parascending*, is a recreational activity where a person is towed behind a vehicle (usually a boat) while attached to a specially designed parachute, known as a parasail. The boat then drives off, carrying the parascender into the air. If the boat is powerful enough, two or three people can parasail behind it at the same time. The parascender has little or no control over the parachute. No injuries have been recorded with this kind of activity.

Canoeing and *Kayaking* are not popular in Mediterranean islands. In Greece, these sports are practiced in rivers located north. Close supervision and strict rules imposed by specific clubs and professional trainers regarding participation have resulted in practically absence of severe injuries. Extremely rare among adolescent athletes are *skurfing* where the athlete "skurfs" behind a boat on a surfboard, *bodyboarding* with the athlete lying on a smaller board, *sit-down hydrofoiling*, *surfing* downhill on ocean waves and *barefoot water skiing*.

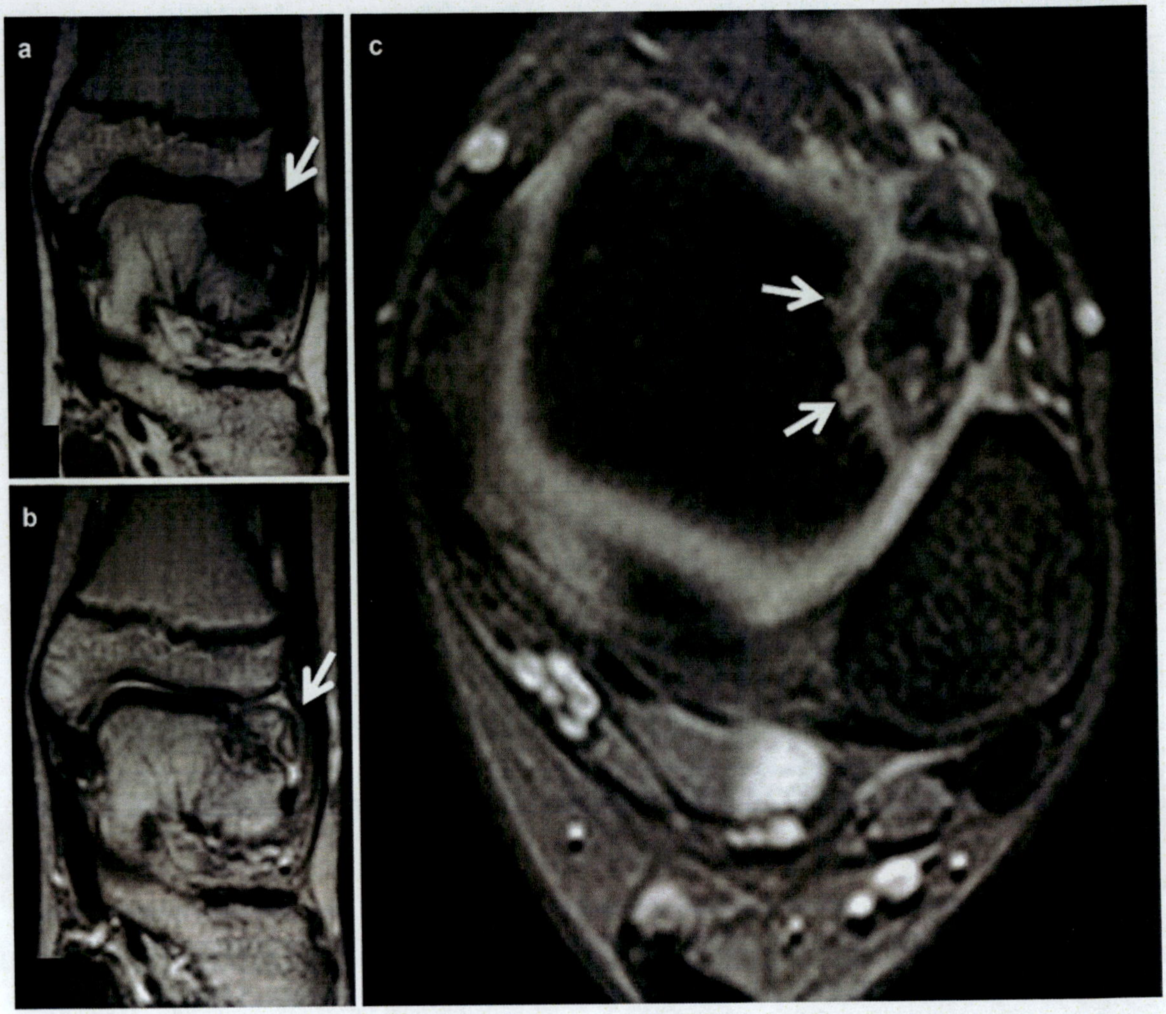

Fig. 25 Osteochondral lesion of the talus in a 12-year-old male wakeboarder with a history of severe ankle sprain during training. The coronal T1-w (**a**), coronal T2-w (**b**), and axial fat-suppressed PD-w (**c**) MR images show a completely detached osteochondral lesion with displacement and fragmentation (*arrows*)

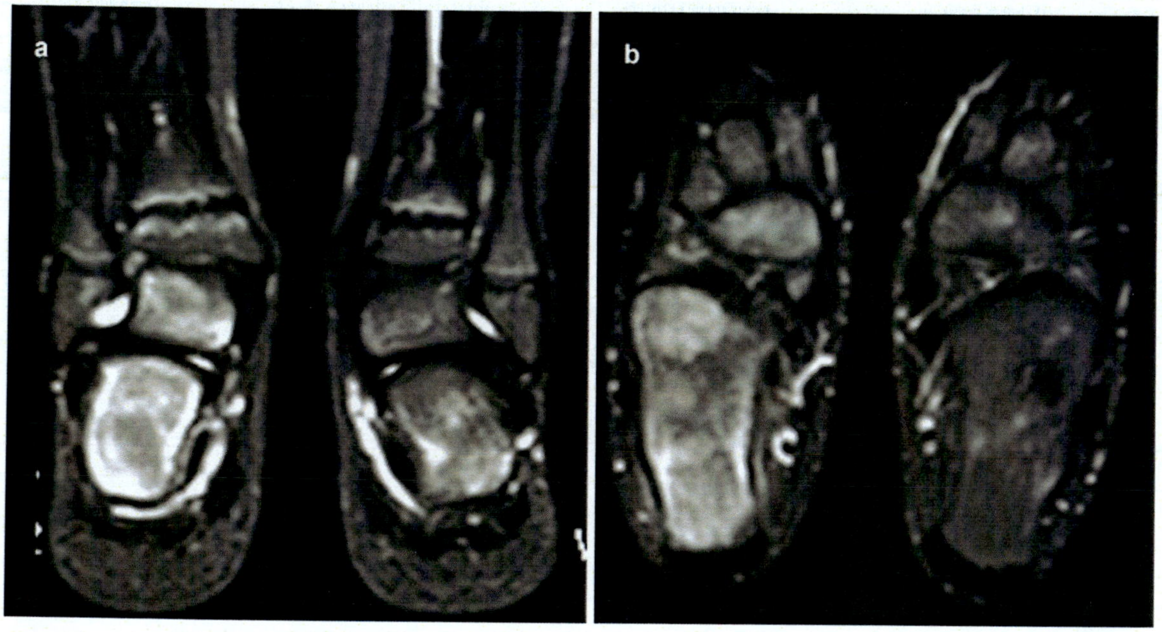

Fig. 26 A 11-year-old male with stress reaction injuries in the end of extensive summer holidays with intense wakeboarding training. The coronal (**a**) and axial (**b**) STIR MR images show bone marrow edema in the calcaneal, talus, navicular, and cuneiform bones

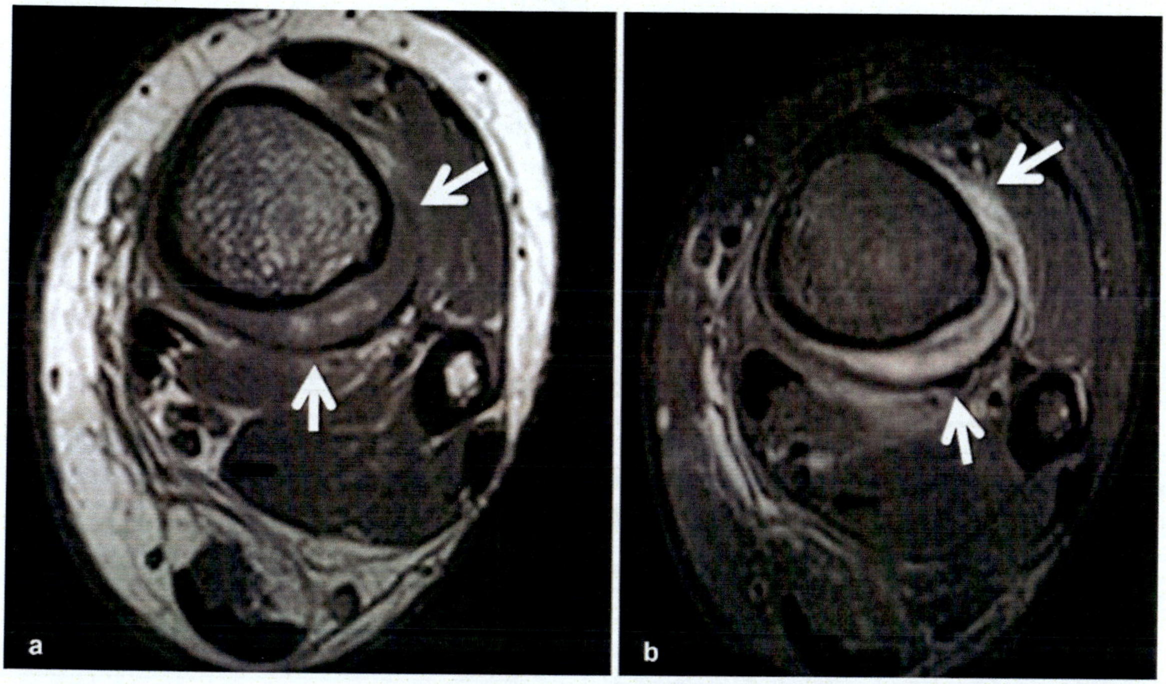

Fig. 27 A 12-year-old female wakeboarder with a Salter-Harris I injury in the distal tibia following a twisting injury. The axial T1-w (**a**) and fat suppressed PD-w (**b**) MR images show a subperiosteal hematoma (arrows). The sagittal T1-w (**c**) and fat-suppressed PD-w (**d**) MR images show the subperiosteal hematoma extending cranially (*arrows*). A Salter-Harris I injury of the growth plate is also seen (*open arrows*)

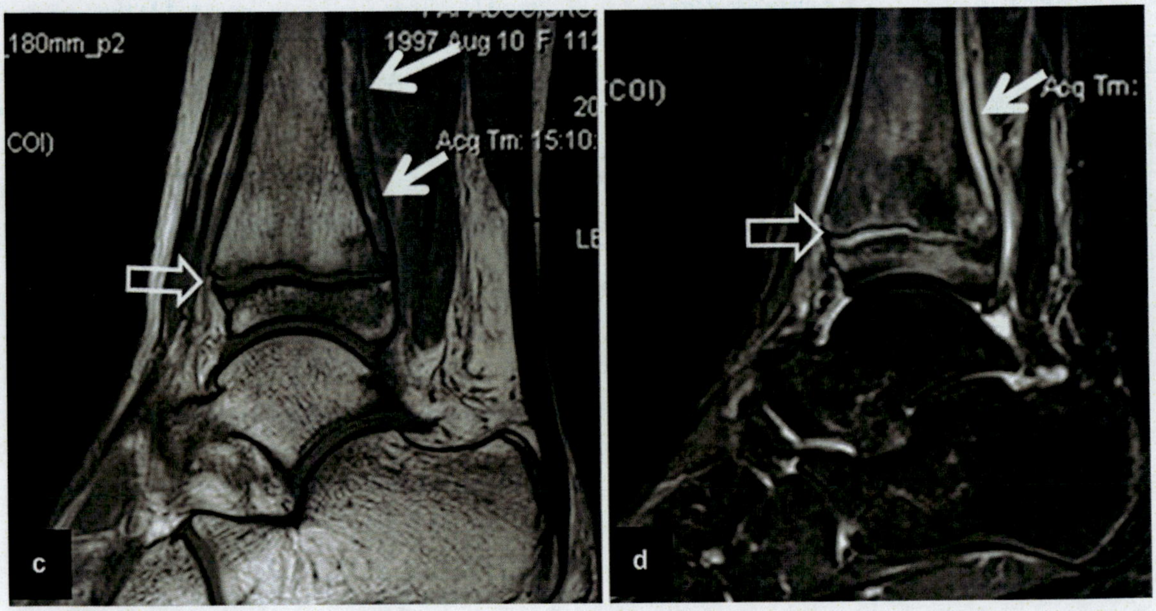

Fig. 27 (continued)

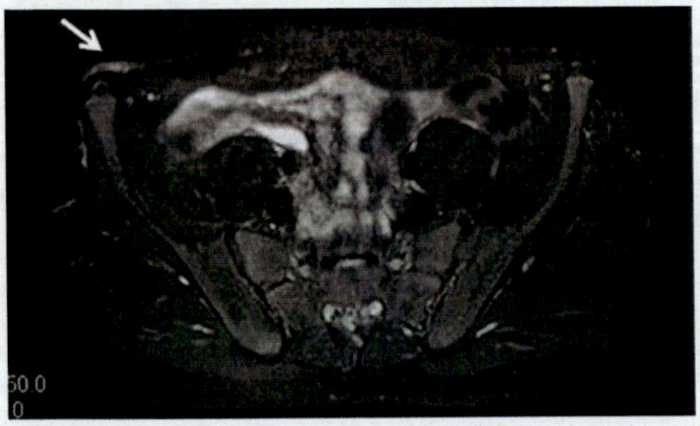

Fig. 28 The axial STIR MR image in a 14-year-old male shows a small hematoma in the anterolateral lower abdominal wall (*arrow*)

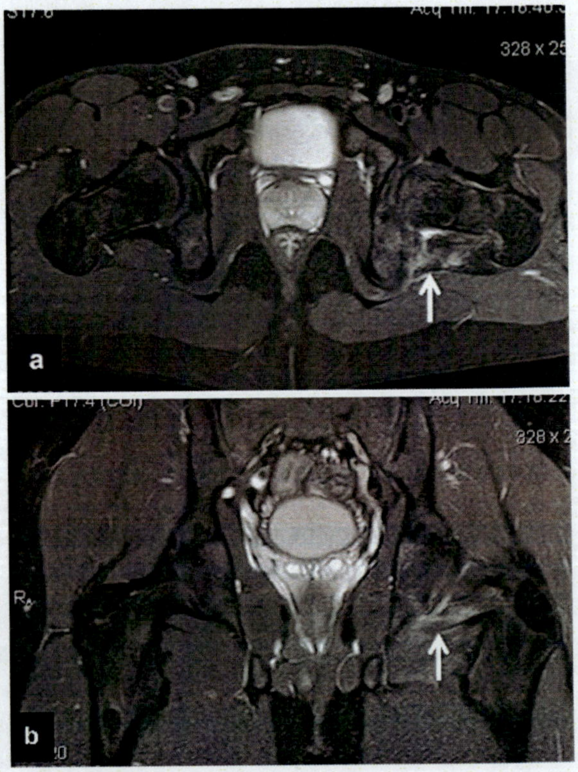

Fig. 29 A 16-year-old male with a quadratus femoris muscle strain following an injury in a waterslide. The axial (**a**) and coronal (**b**) fat-suppressed PD-w MR images show edema and swelling in the left quadratus femoris muscle (*arrows*)

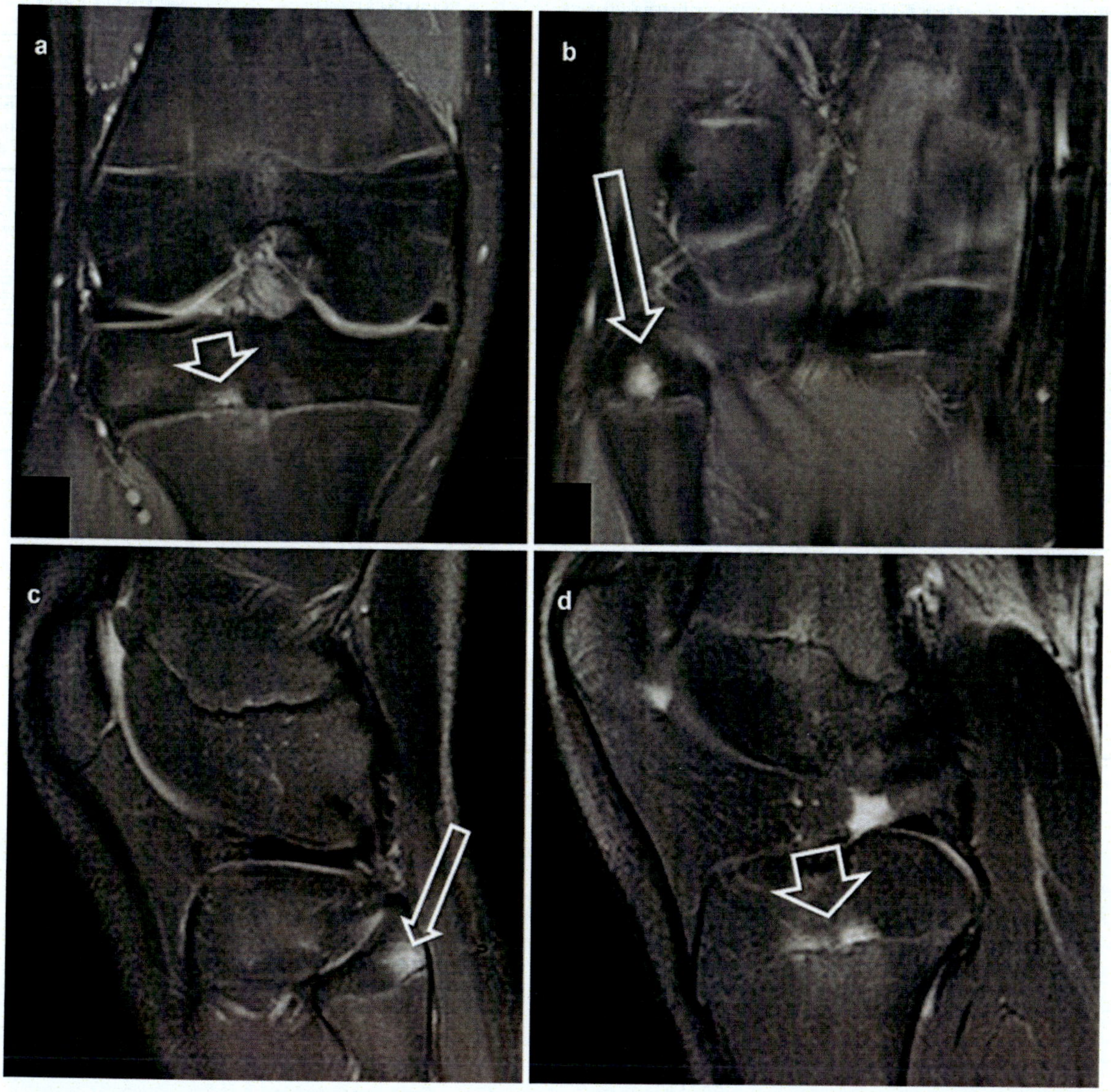

Fig. 30 A 14-year-old male, previously unfit, with pain in the knee following a 8-h play in a water park. The coronal (**a**, **b**) and sagittal (**c**, **d**) fat-suppressed MR images show stress reaction in the fibular head (*long arrows*) and a focal tibial growth plate injury (*short arrows*). A discoid lateral meniscus is also seen

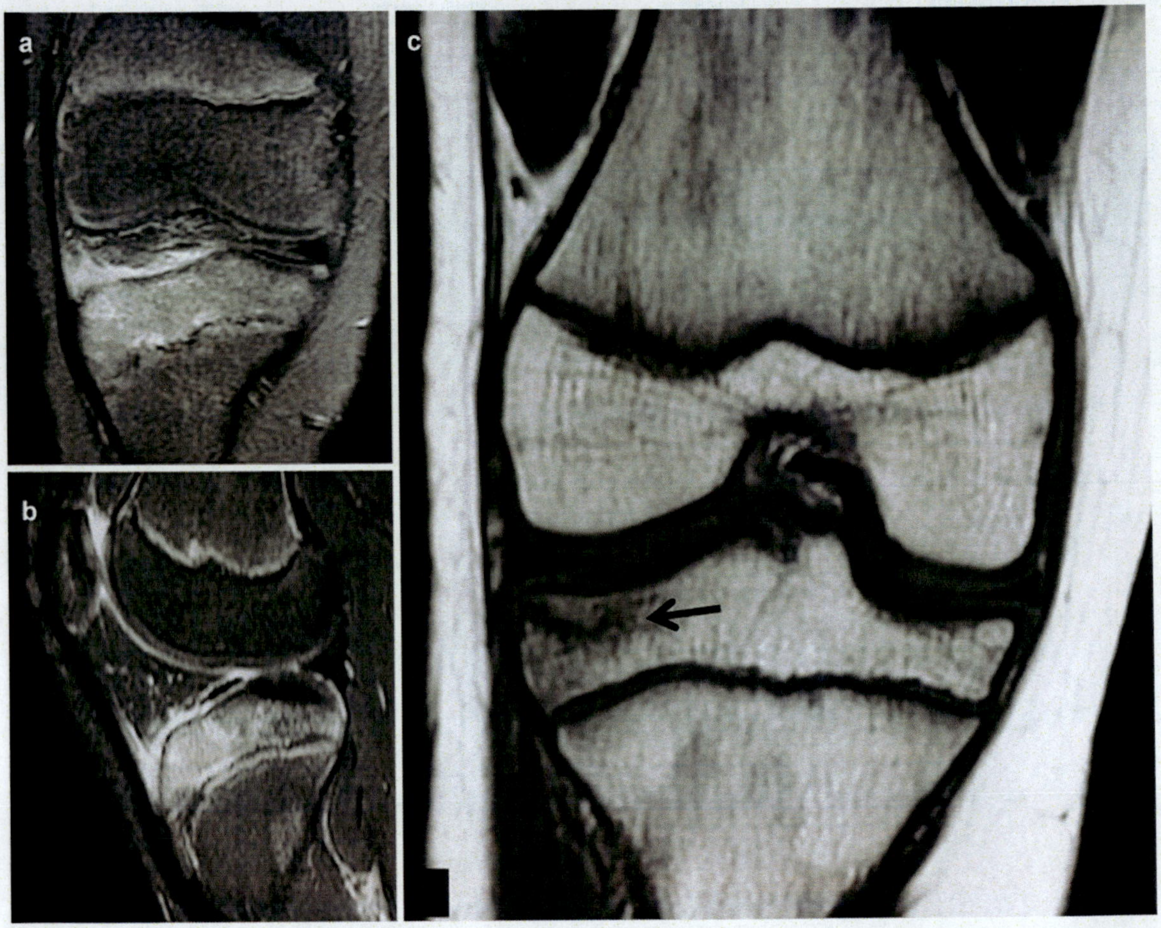

Fig. 31 A 12-year-old male, previously unfit, with pain in the knee following a four consecutive days play in a water park. The coronal (**a**) and sagittal (**b**) fat-suppressed PD-w MR images show extensive bone marrow edema in the proximal tibial epiphysis. (**c**) The coronal T1-w MR image shows a low signal intensity stress fracture in the subchondral area (*arrow*)

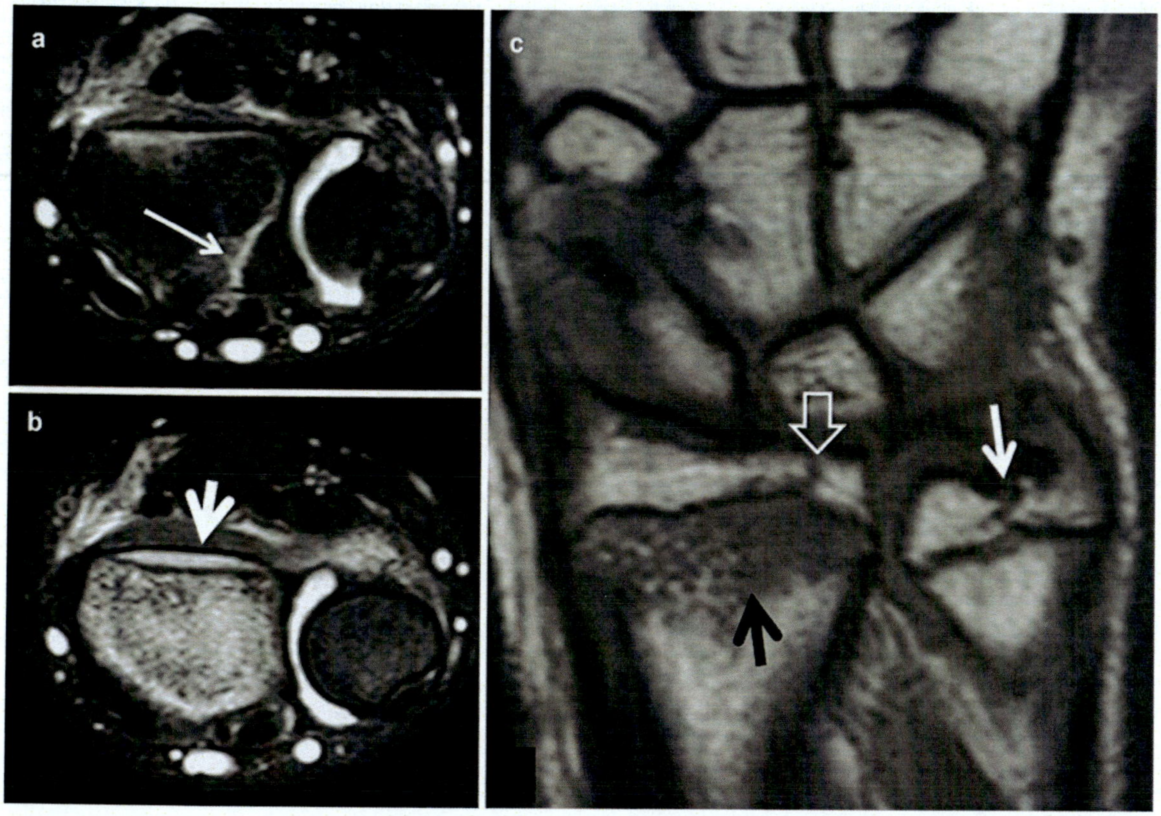

Fig. 32 A 16-year-old male skimboarder with a history of fall on the outstreched hand. The axial fat-suppressed PD-w MR images (**a**, **b**) show a fracture of the radius (*arrow*), bone marrow edema, effusion within the distal radioulnar joint, and a subperiosteral hematoma (*thick arrow*). (**c**) The coronal T1-w MR image shows bone bruise in the distal radial metaphysis (*black arrow*), the radial fracture (*open arrow*), and a fracture of the distal ulna (*white arrow*)

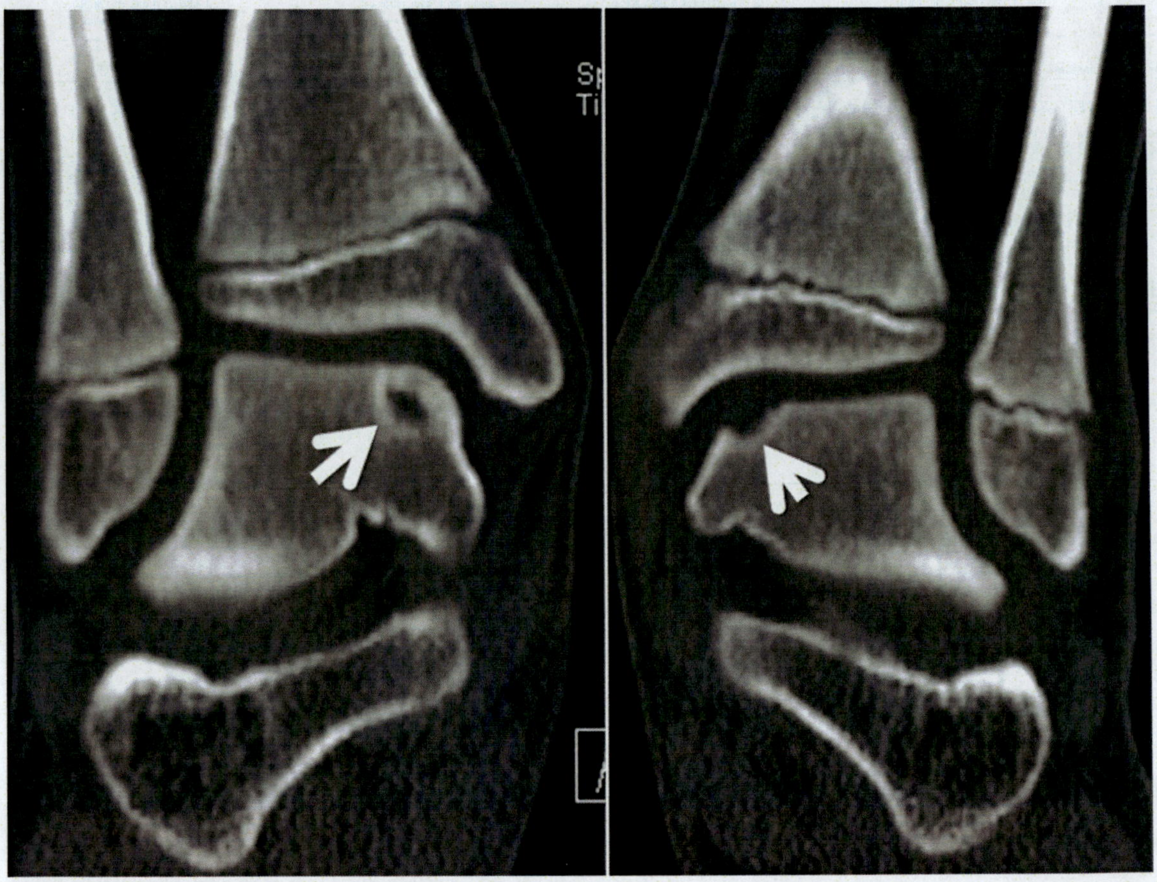

Fig. 33 A 11-year-old male athlete with ankle pain following intense skimboarding training. The coronal CT reconstructions show bilateral osteochondral lesions located in the medial talar dome (*arrows*)

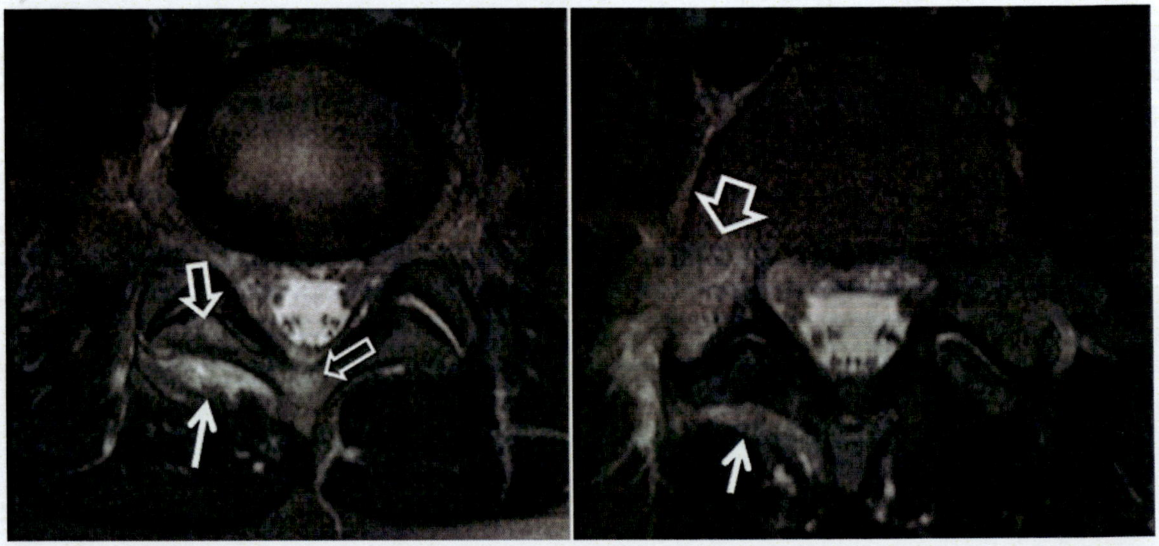

Fig. 34 A 12-year-old male rower with intense low back pain. The axial T2-w MR images show soft-tissue edema (*thin arrows*) and bone marrow edema (*open arrows*) in keeping with stress reaction

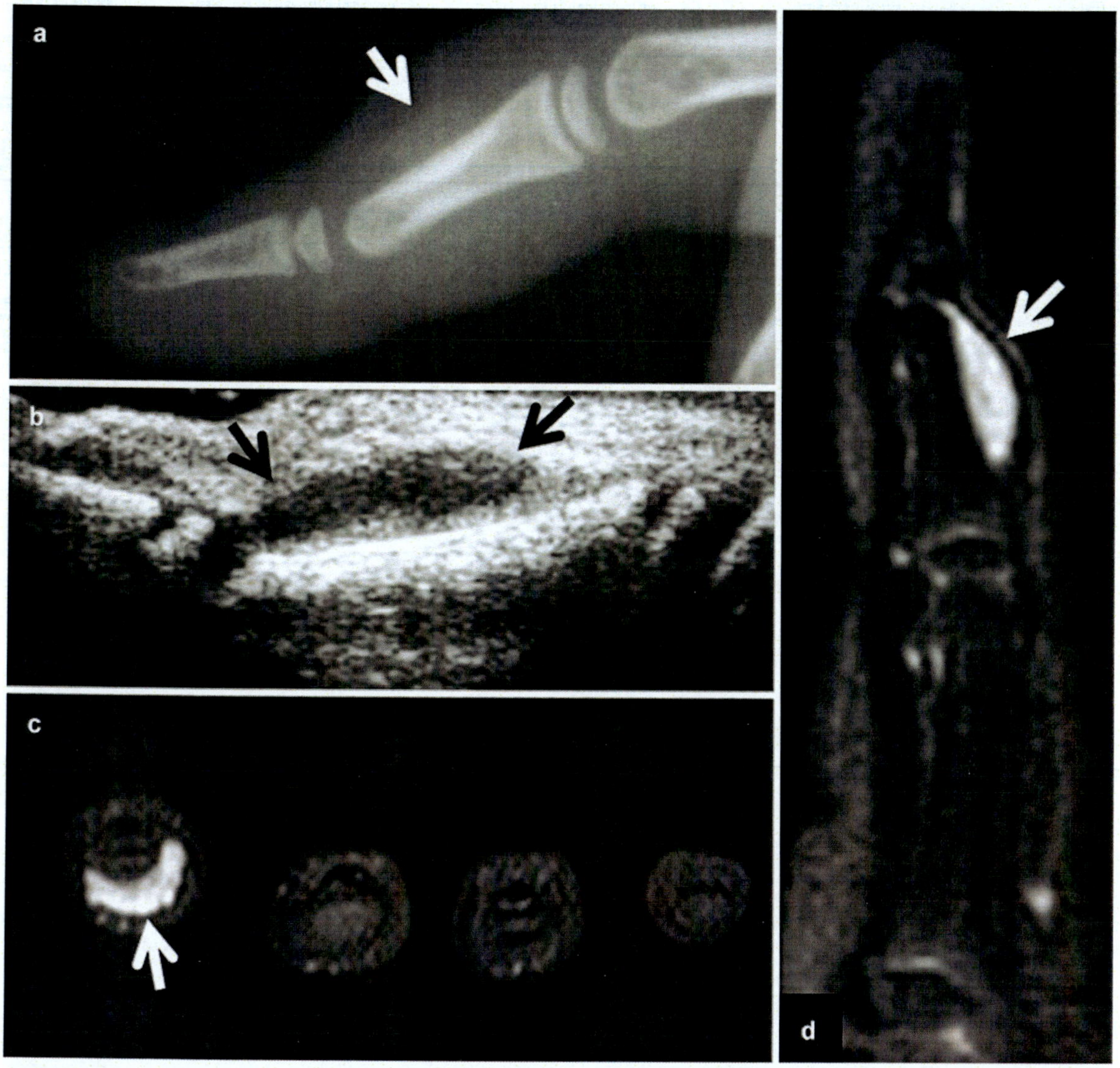

Fig. 35 A 9-year-old female athlete with a history of injury (contact with equipment) 1 year before imaging during sailing and a persistent swelling in the dorsal part of the middle phalanx. The plain radiograph (**a**) shows increased opacity without any cortical disruption (*arrow*). The longitudinal ultrasonogram (**b**) shows a hypoechoic area suggesting effusion (*arrows*). The transverse (**c**) and sagittal (**d**) STIR MR images confirm the presence of effusion. Surgery confirmed the presence of a chronic hematoma

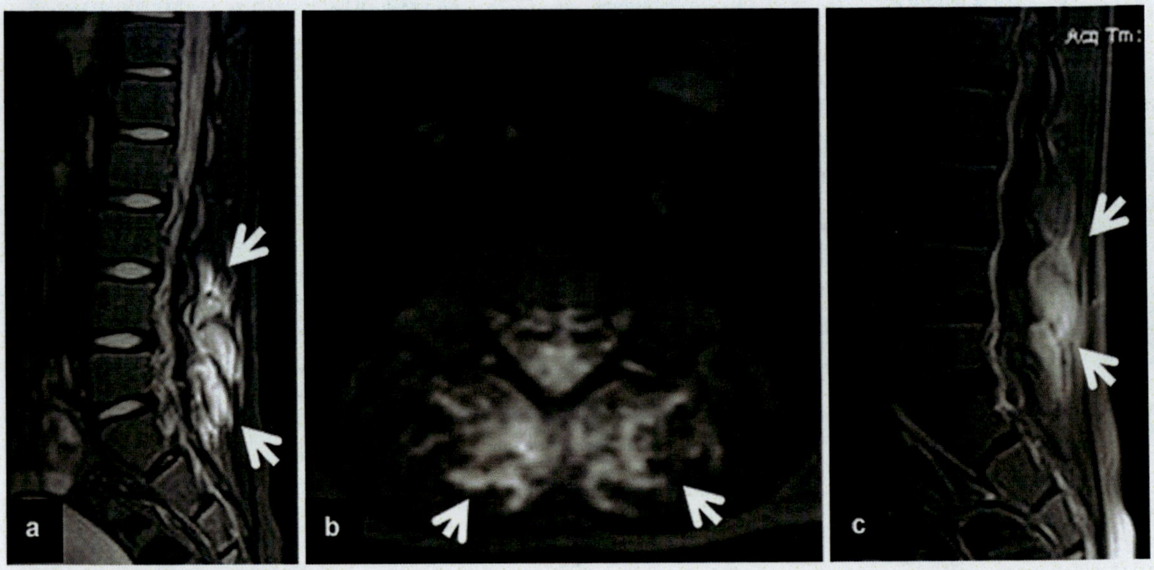

Fig. 36 A previously non-athletic 9-year-old male was hospitalized because of severe back pain following one week of intense practice on sailing. The sagittal STIR (**a**), axial STIR (**b**), and contrast-enhanced fat-suppressed T1-w (**c**) MR images show extensive intramuscular edema (*arrows*) suggesting severe muscle strain

5 Conclusions

Water sports–related injuries cannot be easily classified due to the variability of the involvement of each individual. These injuries may result from lack of general fitness, overuse, overtraining, or macro-traumatic accidents. Some of the sports cannot be performed within the age range of childhood and adolescence. Others, such as diving, induce major consequences to patients, families, and society and could be prevented with appropriate supervision. Radiology plays a crucial role in early diagnosis and estimation of prognosis in water sports–related injuries.

References

Aito S, D'Andrea M, Werhagen L (2005) Spinal cord injuries due to diving accidents. Spinal Cord 43:109–116

Bailes JE, Herman JM, Quigley MR et al (1990) Diving injuries of the cervical spine. Surg Neurol 34:155–158

Barss P, Djerrari H, Leduc BE, Lepage Y, Clermont ED (2008) Risk factors and prevention for spinal cord injury from diving in swimming pools and natural sites in Quebec, Canada: A 44-year study. Acc Anal Prevent 40:787–797

Blanksby BA, Wearne FK, Elliott BC, Blitvich JD (1997) Aetiology and occurrence of diving injuries. A review of diving safety. Sports Med 23:228–246

Branche CM, Conn JM, Annest JL (1997) Personal watercraft-related injuries: A growing public health concern. JAMA 278:663–665

Cain EL, Dugas JR, Wolf RS, Andrews JR (2003) Elbow injuries in throwing athletes: a current concepts review. Am J Sports Med 31:621–635

Carmel A, Drescher MJ, Leitner Y, Gepstein R (2004) Thoracolumbar fractures associated with the use of personal watercraft. J Trauma 57:1308–1310

Carson WG Jr (2004) Wakeboarding injuries. Am J Sports Med 32:164–173

Collier TR, Jones ML, Murray HH (2010) Skimboarding: a new cause of water sport spinal cord injury. Spinal Cord 48: 349–351

Colville JM, Markman BS (1999) Competitive water polo upper extremity injuries. Clin Sports Med 18:305–312

DeVivo MJ (1997) Causes and costs of spinal cord injury in the United States. Spinal Cord 35:809–813

Donnelly LF, Betts JB, Fricke BL (2005) Skimboarder's toe: findings on high-field MRI. AJR Am J Roentgenol 184:1481–1485

Dragoni S, Giombini A, Di Cesare A, Ripani M, Magliani G (2007) Stress fractures of the ribs in elite competitive rowers: a report of nine cases. Skeletal Radiol 36:951–954

Dyson R, Buchanan M, Hale T (2006) Incidence of sports injuries in elite competitive and recreational windsurfers. Br J Sports Med 40:346–350

Franić M, Ivković A, Rudić R (2007) Injuries in water polo. Croat Med J 48:281–288

Hamman BL, Miller FB, Fallat ME, Richardson JD (1993) Injuries from motorized personal watercraft. J Pediat Surg 28:920–922
Hawthorn IE, Monaghan AM, Mason PF, Howell GP (1995) How safe the "banana" boat? Injury 26:265–266
Hostetler SG, Hostetler TL, Smith GA, Xiang H (2005) Characteristics of water skiing-related and wakeboarding-related injuries treated in emergency departments in the United States, 2001–2003. Am J Sports Med 33:1065–1070
Hutchinson M, Tansey J (2003) Sideline management of fractures. Curr Sports Med Rep 2:125–135
Jobe CM, Coen MJ, Screnar P (2000) Evaluation of impingement syndromes in the overhead-throwing athlete. J Athl Train 35:293–299
Johnson JN, Houchin G (2006) Adolescent athlete's shoulder. A case series of proximal humeral epiphysiolysis in nonthrowing athletes. Clin J Sport Med 16:84–86
Kalogeromitros A, Tsnagaris H, Bilais D, Karabinis A (2002) Severe accidents due to windsurfing in the Aegean Sea. Eur J Emerg Med 9:149–154
Kenal KA, Knapp LD (1996) Rehabilitation of injuries in competitive swimmers. Sports Med 22:337–347
Kim CW, Smith JM, Lee A, Hoyt DB, Kennedy F (2003) Personal watercraft injuries. J Orthop Trauma 17:571–573
Korres DS, Benetos IS, Themistocleous GS et al (2006) Diving injuries of the cervical spine in amateur divers. Spine J 6:44–49
McMaster WC, Troup J (1993) A survey of interfering shoulder pain inUnited States competitive swimmers. Am J Sports Med 21:67–70
McNally E, Wilson D, Seiler S (2005) Rowing injuries. Semin Musculoskelet Radiol 9:379–396
Merriman D, Carmichael K, Battle SC (2008) Skimboard injuries. J Trauma 65:487–490
Mountjoy M (1999) The basics of synchronized swimming and its injuries. Clin Sports Med 18:321–336
Neville V, Folland JP (2009) The epidemiology and aetiology of injuries in sailing. Sports Med 39:129–145
Nickel C, Zernial O, Musahl V, Hansen U, Zantop T, Petersen W (2004) A prospective study of kitesurfing injuries. Am J Sports Med 32:921–927
Ouzky M (2002) Towards concerted efforts for treating and curing spinal cord injury. Parliamentary Assembly, Council of Europe. Social, Health and Family Affairs Committee. http:/assembly.coe.int/Documents/WorkingDocs/doc02/EDOC9401.htm
Perich D, Burnett A, O'Sullivan P, Perkin C (2010) Low back pain in adolescent female rowers: a multi-dimensional intervention study. Knee Surg Sports Traumatol Arthrosc. doi: 10.1007/s00167–010–1173–6
Rettig AC (2003) Athletic injuries of the wrist and hand. Part I: traumatic injuries of the wrist. Am J Sports Med 31: 1038–1048
Richardson AB (1999) Thoracic outlet syndrome in aquatic athletes. Clin Sports Med 18:361–378
Richardson AB, Jobe FW, Collins HR (1980) The shoulder in competitive swimming. Am J Sports Med 8:159–163
Rubin LE, Stein PB, DiScala C, Grottkau BE (2003) Pediatric trauma caused by personal watercraft: a ten-year retrospective. J Pediatr Surg 38:1525–1529
Rumball JS, Lebrun CM, Di Ciacca SR, Orlando K (2005) Rowing injuries. Sports Med 35:537–555
Sciarretta KH, McKenna MJ, Riccio AI (2009) Orthopaedic injuries associated with skimboarding. Am J Sports Med 37:1425–1428
Smoljanovic T, Bojanic I, Hannafin JA, Hren D, Delimar D, Pecina M (2009) Traumatic and overuse injuries among international elite junior rowers. Am J Sports Med 37:1193–1199
Soyuncu S, Yigit O, Eken C, Bektas F, Akcimen M (2009) Water park injuries. Ulus Travma Acil Cerrahi Derg 15:500–504
Swischuk LE, John SD, Allbery S (1998) Disk degenerative disease in childhood: Scheuermann's disease, Schmorl's nodes, and the limbus vertebra: MRI findings in 12 patients. Pediatr Radiol 28:334–338
Sykes JJW (1995) Medical aspects of scuba diving. Br Med J 308:1483–1488
Webster MJ, Morris ME, Galna B (2009) Shoulder pain in water polo: a systematic review of the literature. J Sci Med Sport 12:3–11
Weiberg S (1986) Medical aspects of synchronized swimming. Clin Sports Med 5:159–167
Zantop T, Zernial O (2005) Kitesurfing injuries. A trendy youth sport. Orthopäde 34:419–425

Common Injuries in Tennis

Jan L. Gielen, Filip M. Vanhoenacker, and Pieter Van Dyck

Contents

Key Points

- Tennis has a unique profile of injuries
- Overall risk injury in children and adolescents is low compared to adults
- In children acute lesions are related to a fall on the outstreched hand and are more frequent compared to overuse lesions
- Overuse lesions are more frequent in adolescent players and are predominant at the lower extremity

1 Introduction

Like many other sports, playing tennis – at either a recreational, collegiate, or high level – places children and adolescents at risk of injury. Though many injuries that occur in tennis are common to other sports, tennis does have a unique profile of injuries. Tennis places acute physical demands on players, requiring them to move quickly in all directions, change directions often, stop and start, while maintaining sufficient balance, control, and upper body strength to hit the ball effectively (Chandler 1995).

There are only a few population-based studies that accurately show the incidence of injuries in tennis players (Kibler 1994; Pluim et al. 2006). Most studies are small and the populations closely defined, so

J.L. Gielen (✉)
Department of Radiology and SPORTS medicine, Antwerp University Hospital, Wilrijkstraat 10, 2650, Edegem Belgium and Department of Morphology, Antwerp University, Belgium
e-mail: jan.gielen@uza.be

F.M. Vanhoenacker
Department of Radiology, University Hospital Antwerp, Wilrijkstraat, 10, 2650, Edegem, Belgium
Department of Radiology, General Hospital Sint-Maarten Duffel-Mechelen, Rooienberg, 25, 2570 Duffel, Belgium
e-mail: filip.vanhoenacker@telenet.be

P. Van Dyck
Department of Radiology, Antwerp University Hospital

A.H. Karantanas (ed.), *Sports Injuries in Children and Adolescents*,
Med Radiol Diagn Imaging, DOI: 10.1007/174_2010_9,

the injury rates and risks cannot be generalized to larger or different populations of tennis players. Information comparing competitive and recreational players is not readily available (Pluim et al. 2006). Much of the published research and commentary has been devoted to tennis elbow.

Overall injury risk in tennis is low in children and adolescents compared to adults; it has been shown to gradually increase with age, from 0.01 injuries per player per year in the 6–12-year age group to 0.5 injuries per player per year in those over 75 years of age. In the younger age group the injuries are generally acute. Tennis injury among children (aged <15 years) accounts for 2% of all sports injury (Chandler 1995). Forty percent of injuries to children occur during formal competition (Ellenbecker et al. 2009). Most acute injuries occur in the upper extremities, whereas most chronic injuries are located in the lower extremities. Falls are the most common cause of injury to children during formal tennis play, accounting for 31% of all injuries. Children are probably more prone to fall injury than adults. Their skills, technique, and coordination are less well-developed which causes loss of balance and falls, commonly onto an outstretched arm. The most common orthopedic lesions are cramps (51.8%), strains (35.5%), and sprains (25.5%). More severe injuries like meniscal lesions or ruptures of the cruciate- and ankle-ligaments or the achilles tendon are found in 2–4%. Most of the injuries and complaints are treated conservatively with good results. Only 3.3% of all acute and 2.2% of the chronic lesions need surgical intervention (Kühne et al. 2004).

Physicians involved in elite sports players use a low threshold in their use of radiological imaging. Up to date, high resolution ultrasound and magnetic resonance imaging are able to demonstrate lesions with a remarkable definition. Because of these conditions, subtle lesions are encountered in a growing number of patients involved in elite sports. As sports performance may be influenced by these subtle lesions, their documentation may be of more interest compared to the general population. This chapter focuses on less frequent lesions encountered in tennis players and particularly those conditions that may influence sports performance. A typical example is bone bruise and fatigue reaction that may be encountered in tennis players at very specific sites.

2 Acute Injuries

Accidental factors, such as tripping on court, are prominent causes of acute injuries where strains and sprains are the most common type of injury accounting for 71% of all injuries. Upper limb injuries are more common than lower limb injuries among children. Forty-five percent of all tennis injuries in children are located at the upper limbs, particularly fractures of the radius/ulna (7% of all injuries) and sprain/strains of the wrist (4%). Thirty-one percent of injuries affect the lower limbs, particularly ankle sprains/strains (28% of all injuries) and sprains/strains of the knee (24%) (Pluim et al. 2006). The vast majority of ligamentous sprain injuries (88%) are located at the knee and ankle. Nine percent of injuries are to the head and face (Pluim et al. 2006). The most common anatomic site of injury in junior elite tennis players is the back (16% of all injuries) (Ellenbecker et al. 2009). Rupture of the latissimus dorsi muscle in an athlete is rare. A case report presents a case of rupture of the latissimus dorsi muscle that occurred during a tennis sports activity (Park et al. 2008). The muscle ruptures at the musculotendinous junction during forceful resisted arm adduction or extension. The latissimus dorsi muscle is not a critical muscle for activities of daily living; however, the significance of the muscle is increased in professional or elite athletes.

2.1 Topographic Discussion

Extensive discussion of lesion pathophysiology and radiological imaging encountered in young tennis players is beyond the scope of this chapter. An overview of topographic distribution and type of lesions is discussed in Table 1.

3 Overuse Injuries

Although overuse injuries are less common, the majority of elite adolescent tennis players will have their playing temporarily interrupted by an overuse injury, with lower extremity problems predominating. Overuse

Table 1 Acute injuries

Region	Location	Type and mechanism	Imaging	Age (years)
Axial skeleton	Orbita	*Blow-out fracture of the floor, associated ocular injury in 30%* *Ball hits the eye*	CT	
		Blow-in fracture of the floor *Ball hits the inferior margin of the orbit*	CT	
		Fracture of the medial wall (lamina papyracea) association with blow-out and blow-in fracture (cfr supra)	CT	
	Mandible	*Fracture of the body* *Slip and anterior fall*	XR, CT	
	Cervical spine	*Intervertebral disc injury*	MRI	
	Brachial Plexus, C5, C6 roots, and axillary and suprascapular nerves	*Acute brachial neuropathy, Parsonage–Turner syndrome*	EMG MRI	
	Lumbar spine	*Intervertebral disc injury*	MRI	
Chest and abdomen	Abdominal wall muscles	Internal and external oblique, rectus abdominis muscle strain Serve or resisted abdominal rotation	US (Fig. 1) MRI	
Shoulder girdle	Lattisimus dorsi	*Muscle strain* *Serve*	MRI US (Fig. 2)	
	Clavicle	Middle third greenstick fracture, bowing fracture Fall on shoulder, FOOSH	XR	
		Medial apophyseal avulsion fracture	XR	
	Acromio-clavicular Joint	*Sprain*	XR	>16
	Glenohumeral joint	*Anterior dislocation*	XR MRA	
	Proximal humerus	*SH I or II* *Fall on outstretched arm of direct blow to the shoulder*	XR	10–15
Elbow and upper arm	Distal humerus	Supracondylar fracture, torus, greenstick, or complete(transcondylar fracture) Elbow hyperextension due to FOOSH	XRCT	
		Lateral condyle SH type IV FOOSH with forearm supinated and elbow varus	XR CT	4–10
		Epiphysiolysis (SH type I) or SH II *FOOSH*	XR (Fig. 3) CT	<5
		Apophysiolysis medial epicondyle Valgus stress during FOOSH	XR (Fig. 4) CT	
		Apophysiolysis medial epicondyle with intra-articular entrapment *Valgus stress during FOOSH*	XR CT	
	Elbow joint	Osteochondral fracture	XR MRI	
		Dislocation, posterior, or posterior lateral Exclude associated medial epicondyle apophysiolysis and radial neck fracture Elbow hyperextension due to fall on outstretched arm	XR MRI	
	Proximal radius	Radius neck fracture, SH II Exclude associated olecranon fracture	XR CT	
Forearm, wrist and hand	Diaphysis radius and ulna	Fractures Greenstick, bowing FOOSH	XR	2–14
	Diaphysis ulna, proximal third	Fractures greenstick and bowing Cave-associated anterior or lateral radius head dislocation (Monteggia) FOOSH with forearm pronation	XR	5–9

(continued)

Table 1 (continued)

Region	Location	Type and mechanism	Imaging	Age (years)
	Distal radius and ulna	Epiphyseal fractures or apophyseal epiphyseal avulsion fracture (SH type I) Fall on outstretched hyperextended hand Metaphyseal fractures Torus, lead pipe Fall on outstretched hyperextended hand SH type II Fall on outstretched hyperextended hand	XR (Fig. 5) XR XR	<5 6–10 10–16 Girls 8–13 Boys 11–14
	Scaphoid	*Fracture of the distal third* *Fall on outstretched hyperextended hand*	XR (Fig. 6) MRI (Fig. 7)	>11
	Triquetrum	*Avulsion dorsal surface* *Fall on outstretched hyperextended hand*	XR	
	Hamate	Fracture of the hook Result of direct blow or swinging of the racket with butt end of racket against hook	CT (Fig. 8) MRI (Figs. 8 and 9)	
	Pisiform	*Vertical fracture* *Fall on outstretched hyperextended hand*	XR (Fig. 9)	
	Wrist	Scapholunate ligament sprain Fall on outstretched, radial deviated hand TFCC tear Axial loading with pronation	MRI (Fig. 10) MRI (Fig. 11)	
	Phalanx	SH, most often type II, rare type III Third phalanx lesions most frequent Fall Epiphysiolysis (SH type I)	XR XR	10–16 <5
	MCP 1	Ulnar collateral ligament lesion (sprain or avulsive fracture proximal phalanx). In case of ligament sprain grade III cave-luxated ligament superficially to adductor pollicis (Stener's lesion) Forceful radial deviation of the thumb	XR US	
Pelvic girdle and hip	Ischium	*Apophysiolysis or avulsive fracture* *Pull of hamstring muscles*	XR MRI	Adolescents
	Anterior superior iliac spine	*Apophysiolysis* *Pull of sartorius muscle*	XR US-MRI CT	Adolescents
	Anterior inferior iliac spine	*Apophysiolysis* *Pull of rectus femoris muscle*	XR US-MRI CT (Fig. 12)	<16
	Iliac crest	Apophysiolysis Pull of abdominal wall muscles	XR MRI CT (Fig. 13)	Adolescents
	Adductor tubercle	*Apophysiolysis*	XR MRI	
	Hip joint	*Dislocation (posterior)* *Fall, trivial trauma*	XR, CT MRI	4–15
	Proximal femur	*Salter Harris lesion Epiphysiolysis (SH type I)* *Lesser tuberosity avulsive fracture or apophysiolysis* *Resisted hip flexion*	XR, MRI XR MRI	
Upper leg and knee	Distal femur	*SH type II, V* *Valgus stress, clipping injury Varus stress*	XR	10–17
	Knee joint	*Avulsion anterior tibial spine (ACL insertion)* *Knee hyperextension* Lateral patellar dislocation "Cutting maneuver": flexed knee with fixed foot, valgus position, internally rotated femur, quadriceps contraction Meniscal lesion Rotatory stress *Ligament lesion* *Varus or valgus stress*	XR MRI XR MRI MRI MRI	<17 >11 Girls! Adolescents

Table 1 (continued)

	Proximal tibia	SH type I or II *SH type V exclude associated fracture of femur or tibia-fibula* Valgus stress, clipping injury	XR MRI (Fig. 14)	12–16
Lower leg, ankle and foot	Distal tibia	SH type II with lateral displacement of the epiphysis Associated fracture of the distal fibular diaphysis *Epiphysiolysis (SH type I)* Abduction injury in pronated foot	XR CT	<12
		SH type II medial malleolus with medial displacement of the epiphysis 50% associated fibula lesion Adduction injury in pronated foot	XR CT	<12
		SH II with posterior displacement of the epiphysis External rotation with plantar flexion of the foot	XR CT	<12
		SH type II with posterior lateral metaphyseal fragment External rotation in supinated foot	XR CT	<12
		SH type III, lateral half or anterior part of lateral half of the epiphysis (juvenile Tillaux fx) External rotation in supinated foot	XR CT	10–15
		SH type III, medial malleolus50% associated fibula lesion Adduction (inversion or varus) injury in supinated foot	XR CT	10–15
		SH type IV medial malleolus50% associated fibula lesion *Adduction injury*	XR CT	
	Distal fibula	SH type I, cave-associated distal fibular greenstick fracture Adduction (inversion or varus) injury in supinated foot	XR	<16
		Greenstick Cave-associated distal tibial epiphysis separation (SH I, II). Abduction injury	XR	<16
		SH Type II, posterior located metaphyseal component External rotation in supinated or pronated foot	XR	<16
	Calcaneus	Sustentaculum tali fracture	XR CT	
		Anterior margin compression fracture (nutcracker fracture) Cave-associated cuboid compression fracture Abduction of forefoot	XR CT US	
		Anterior lateral process fracture Pull of bifurcate ligament: Inversion trauma with adduction of forefoot with foot in equinus position Dorsiflexion compression	XR CT US	
	Os peroneum	*Fracture with associated peroneus longus tear* *Plantar flexion and inversion ankle injury*	XR CT US	
	First MTP	Sprain or avulsive fracture at plantar side of metatarsal neck with or without dorsal dislocation (turf toe) Dorsiflexion, hyperextension	XR US	
	Fifth metatarsal	Apophysiolysis of the tuberosity with or without transverse fracture Inversion trauma of the foot	XR US	
		Proximal metaphyseal transverse fracture: Jones' fracture Inversion trauma of the foot	XR	

Overview of acute lesions encountered in youth tennis players. Different parameters such as location, mechanism of trauma, age, and preferred (imaging) technique are emphasized. Rare lesions are in italics. *SH* Salter–Harris; *XR* radiography; *CT* computed tomography; *MRI* magnetic resonance imaging; *MRA* magnetic resonance arthrography; *US* ultrasound; *EMG* electromyography; *FOOSH* fall on outstretched hand; *TFCC* triangular fibrocartilage complex

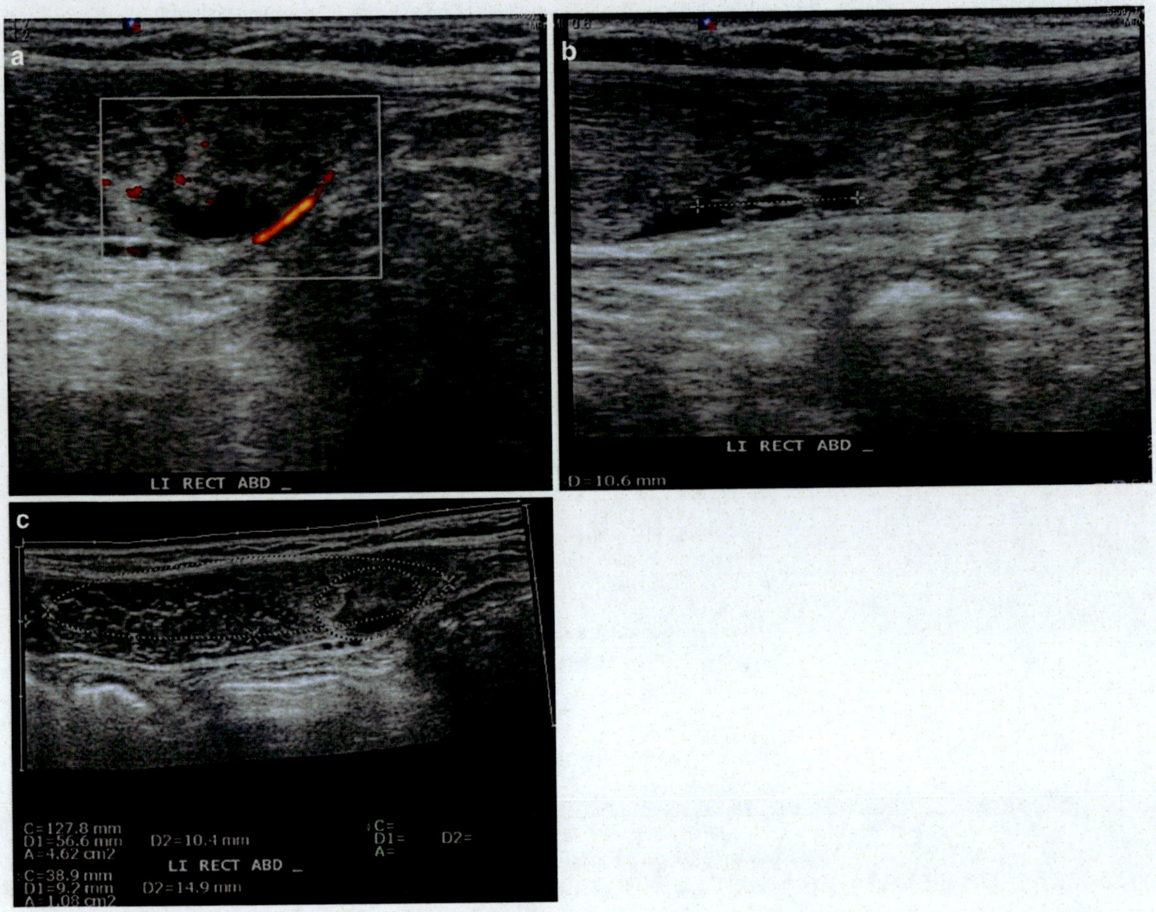

Fig. 1 Rectus abdominis grade II muscle strain in a 17-year-old girl with sudden snap and pain during serve 1 week ago at the left rectus abdominis muscle region. Ultrasound demonstration or fluid-filled area (*arrows*) in the neighborhood of tendinous intersection involving 15% of the transverse surface of the muscle. (**a**) Transverse section with power Doppler, fluid-filled sonolucent area without hypervascularity. (**b**) Longitudinal section. (**c**) Panoramic transverse section with documentation of the relative involved area. Calculation of the percentage of involved muscle, i.e., the surface of the abnormal area relative to the overall transverse surface of the muscle

injuries are found to increase with the standard and duration of play. The highest injury incidence is in those practicing for 16–20 h a week. "Training error" is the most common cause attributed to chronic injuries (Ellenbecker et al. 2009). Although upper extremity injuries occur less frequently, they tend to be more troublesome. Injuries include "King Kong" arm, slipped capital humeral epiphysis, "Osgood–Schlatter disease" of the shoulder, tennis elbow, stress synovitis and elbow flexion contracture, and friction burns and collagen stress fractures of the rotator cuff (Gregg and Torg 1988). The chronic overuse problems seen in older players, such as patellar tendinosis and tennis elbow, are less common in younger players.

3.1 Fatigue Reactions and Fractures and Insufficiency Fractures

Fatigue reactions and fatigue fractures generally occur as a result of repetitive muscle activity (distraction fatigue fracture type) or repetitive bone compression (compression fatigue fracture type) that exceeds the intrinsic repair ability of the bone. Minimal traumatic fractures are not common in children and adolescents. More commonly seen are the insufficiency fractures in preexisting systemic bone disease (i.e., rickets, osteogenesis imperfect, disuse osteopenia) and the pathological fractures occurring in preexisting focal bone disease (i.e., tumor, fibrous dysplasia, non ossifying fibroma).

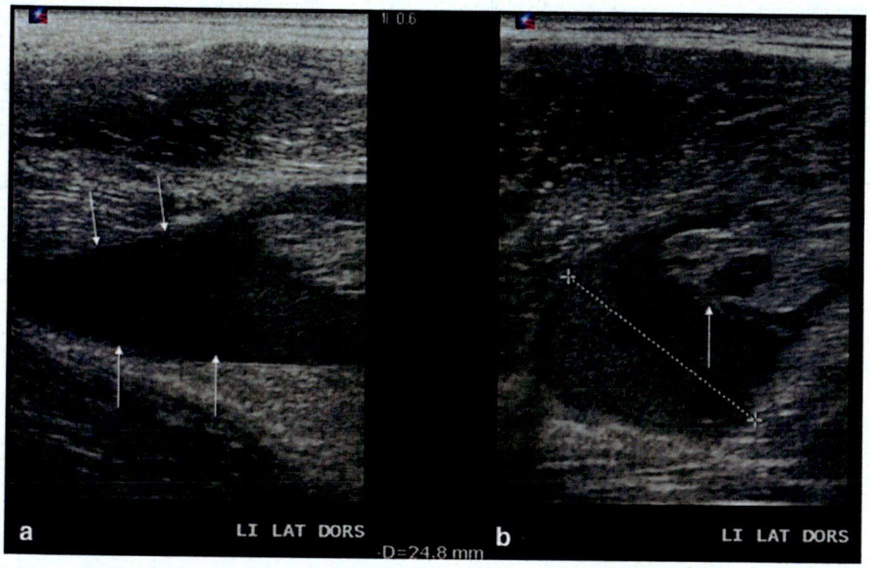

Fig. 2 Tear musculotendinous junction of the latissimus dorsi. Rupture of the latissimus dorsi muscle in an athlete is rare. A case report presents a case of rupture of the latissimus dorsi muscle that occurred during a tennis sports activity (Park et al. 2008). The muscle ruptures at the musculotendinous junction during forceful resisted arm adduction or extension. The latissimus dorsi muscle is not a critical muscle for activities of daily living; however, the significance of the muscle is increased in professional or elite athletes. (**a**) Ultrasound anterior longitudinal view. A fluid collection surrounding the retracted latissimus dorsi muscle is seen (*arrows*). (**b**) Ultrasound anterior axial view. The retracted latissimus dorsi muscle is seen (*arrow*).The humeral insertion of the latissimus dorsi muscle is located distal to the minor tubercle of the humerus and in-between the superficial located humeral insertion of the pectoralis major and the deep located humeral insertion of the teres major. Teres major muscle has a similar distal trajectory running distal, medial and posterior, whereas the superficial pectoralis major is running anteriorly in a more horizontal plane. Fluid collection and retracted tendon in strain grade II or III is located superficially to the teres major muscle and in its distal region deep to the pectoralis major tendon

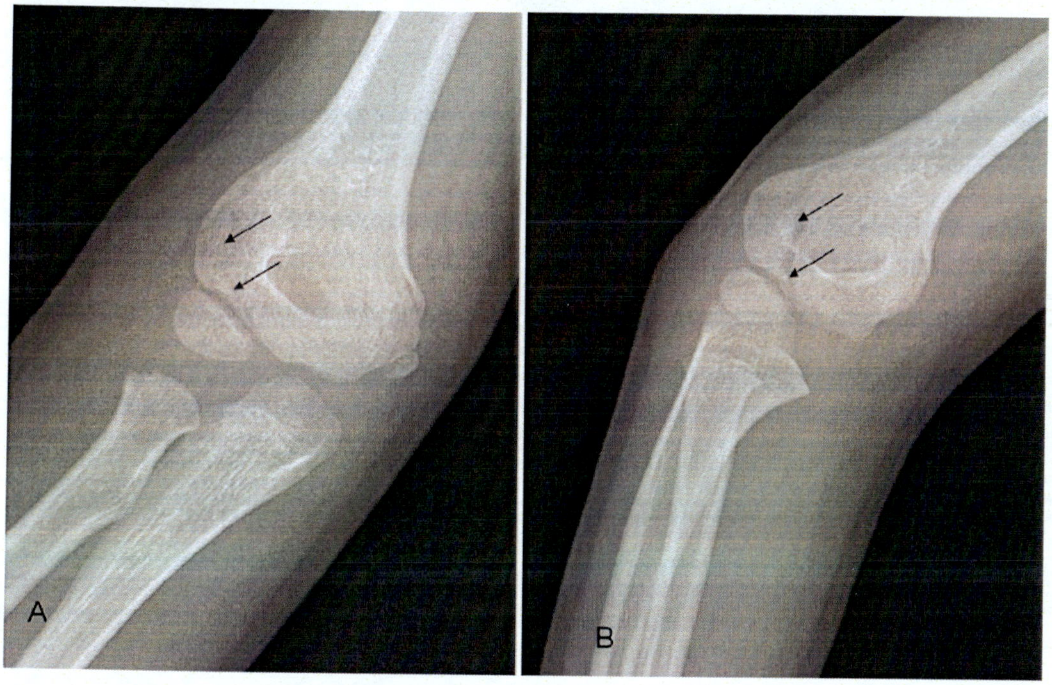

Fig. 3 Elbow SH II fracture lateral epicondyle in a 6-year-old boy with fall on right outstretched hand. Nondisplaced Salter Harris II fracture of the lateral epicondyle (*arrows*) is best documented on internally rotated images. (**a**) Anteroposterior view. (**b**) Internally rotated view

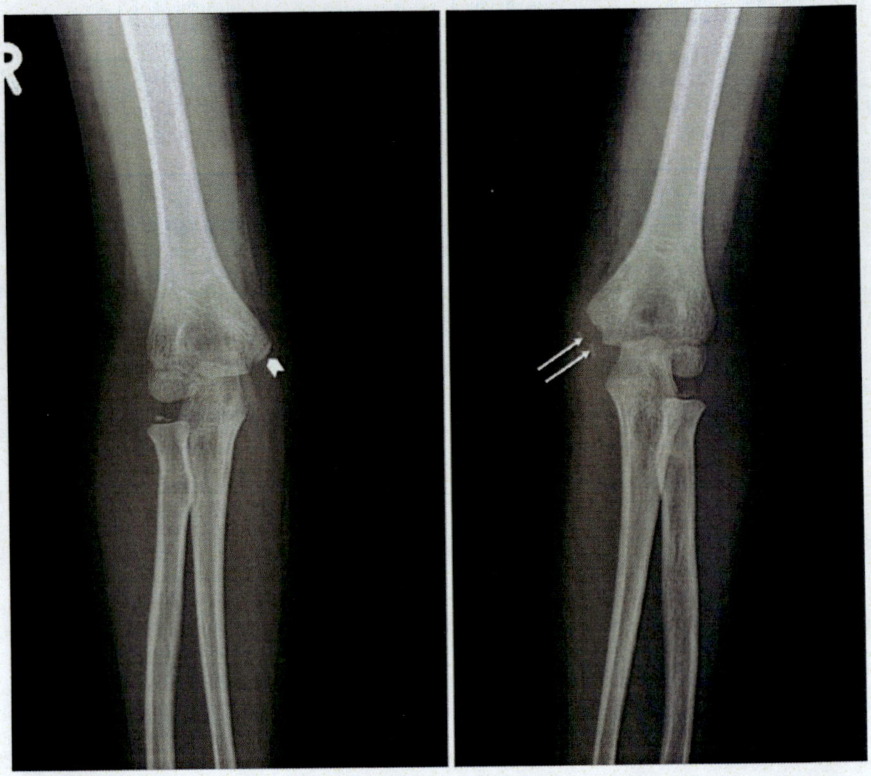

Fig. 4 Acute apophyseal or avulsion fracture of the medial epicondyle of the humerus in a 7-year-old boy with fall on outstretched hand and elbow valgus. Anteroposterior radiographs of left elbow and right elbow for comparison. Soft tissue ossifications (*arrows*) at the level of the left epicondylus medialis representing a fragmented and displaced apophysis of the medial epicondyle. Note the normal appearance at the right side (*arrowhead*)

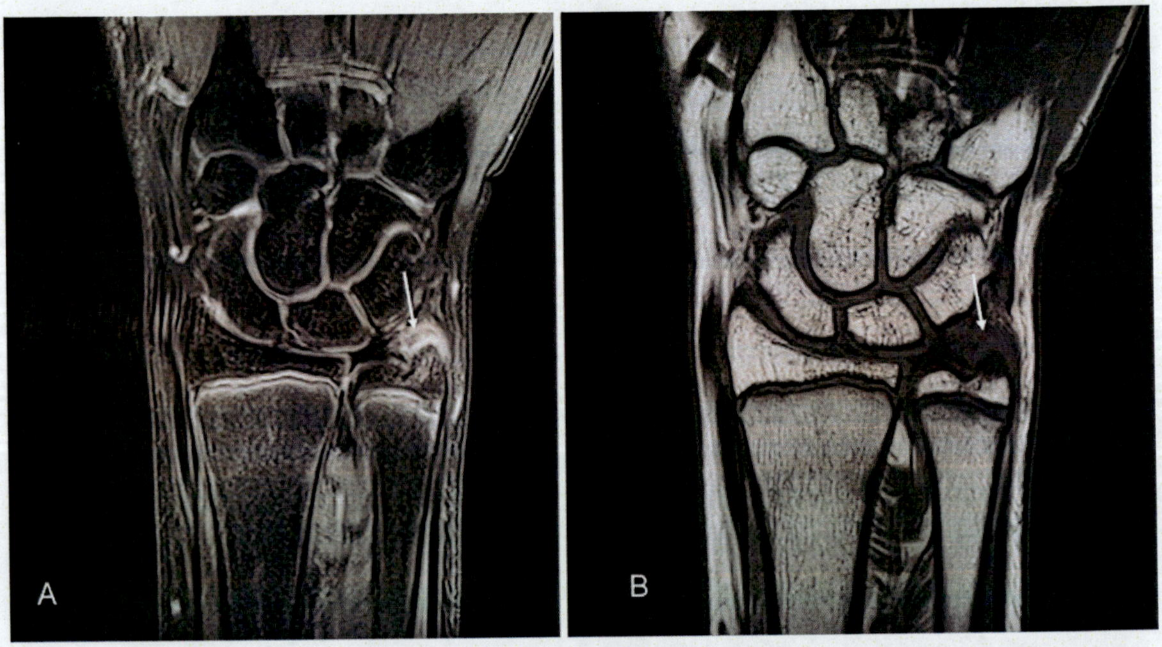

Fig. 5 Avulsive fracture of the ulnar styloid process. Loose fragment (*arrows*) at the apex of the ulnar styloid process is seen with high SI of the trabecular bone on coronal fat-suppressed T2-w (**a**) and low SI on T1-w (**b**) MR images. The disruption of the cortical lining is best documented on T1-w images

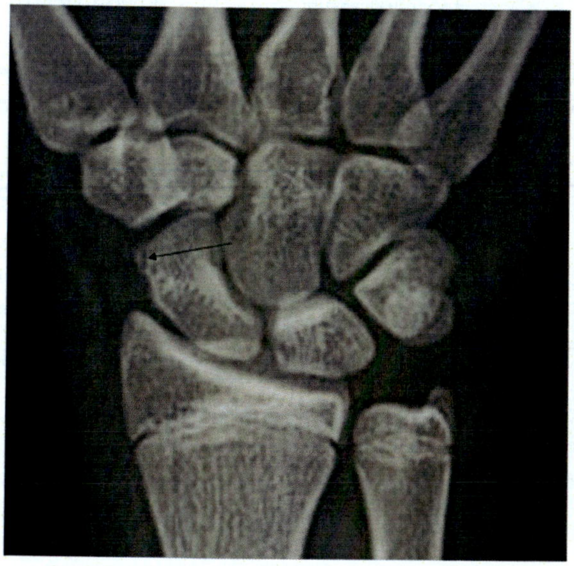

Fig. 6 Scaphoid fracture at the distal third in a 16-year-old boy with fall on the right outstretched hand. The radiograph of the right wrist shows the fracture at the distal radial lining of the scaphoid bone (*arrow*). Differentiation with accessory center of ossification with bone scintigraphy

Radiological imaging has an important role in the exclusion of preexisting focal bone disease in these patients.

Fatigue reactions and fractures are reported in adolescents participating in high standard sports and they are associated with specific sites for fatigue (Bylak and Hutchinson 1998). Compression fractures are more common in young children compared to distraction fatigue fractures. In children as well as adults, compression fatigue fractures are most frequent at the lower extremities. Preadolescent and adolescent players have open growth plates with distraction type of fatigue resulting in physeal or growth plate lesions, with widening and blurring of the growth plate. The traction apophysitides Osgood–Schlatter and Sinding–Larssen–Johansson, are not common in tennis players.

3.2 Radiological Investigation of Fatigue Fractures and Reactions

Radiographs should be obtained in the initial workup of suspected fatigue fractures and fatigue reactions. They

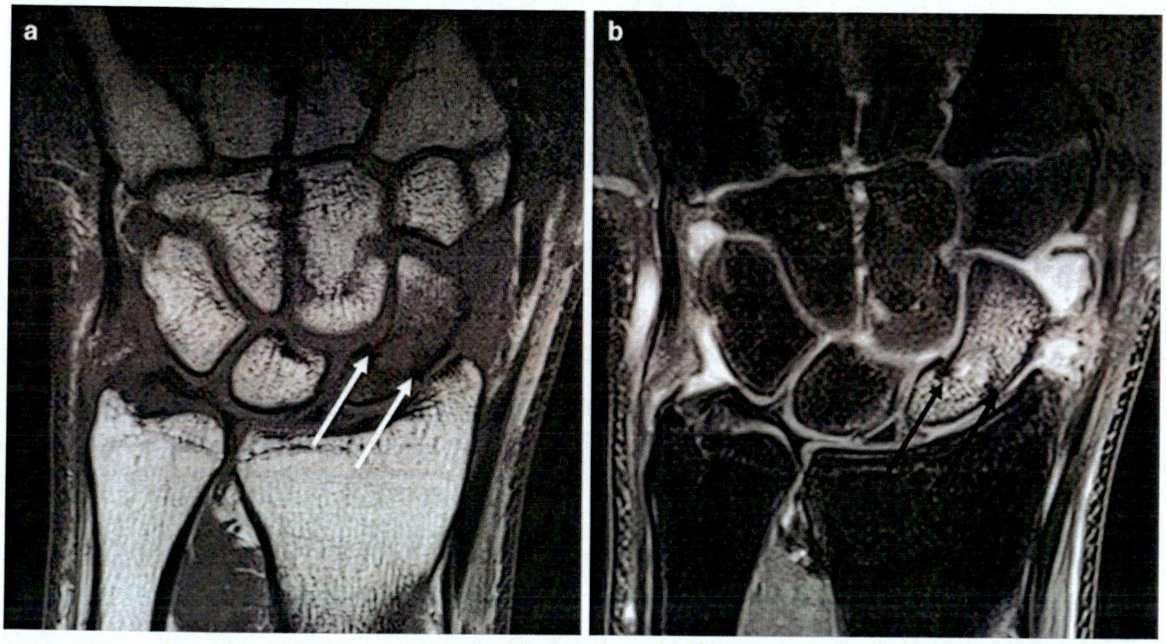

Fig. 7 Scaphoid fracture in a 17-year-old boy. The coronal T1-w (**a**) and fat-suppressed T2-w (**b**) MR images show the cortical disruption and fracture line at the middle third of the scaphoid bone (*arrows*) with diffuse bone marrow edema exhibiting low SI on T1-w and high SI on fat-suppressed T2-w MR images

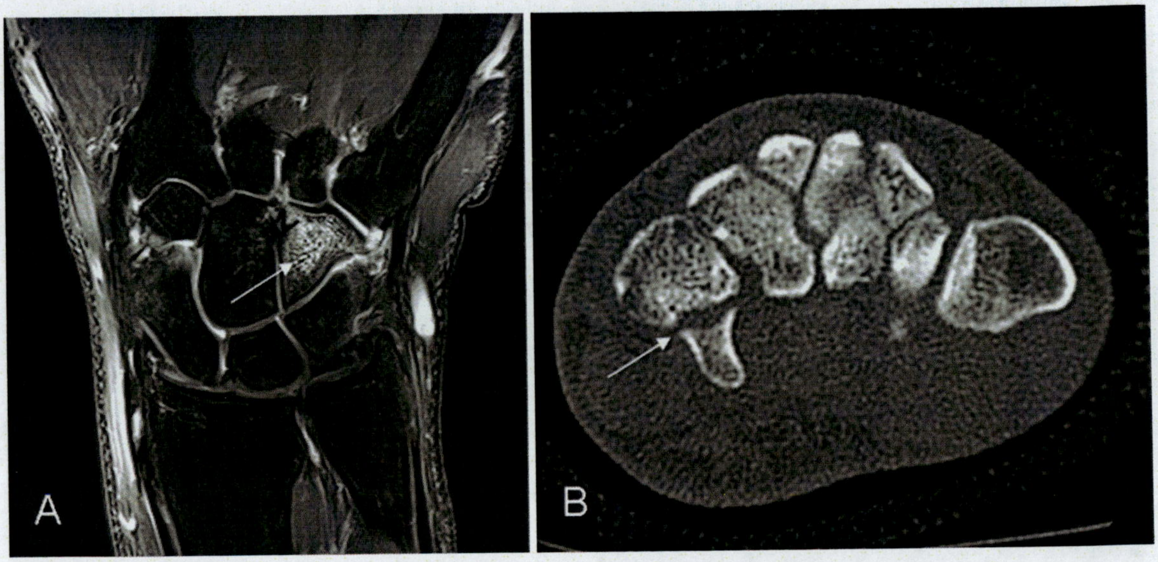

Fig. 8 Fracture hamulus hamatum in a 19-year-old male with a history of a recent fall on the left outstretched hand. Clinically, there was pain at the ulnar and ventral aspect of the wrist. (**a**) The coronal fat-suppressed T2-w MR image shows bone marrow edema at the os hamatum (*arrow*). (**b**) The axial CT scan shows the fracture line at the base of the hamulus of the hamatum (*arrow*). Because of direct visualization of calcified structures, CT is superior to MRI to detect fractures. MRI with the use of fat-suppressed T2-w or STIR is the only radiological imaging modality to detect bone marrow edema

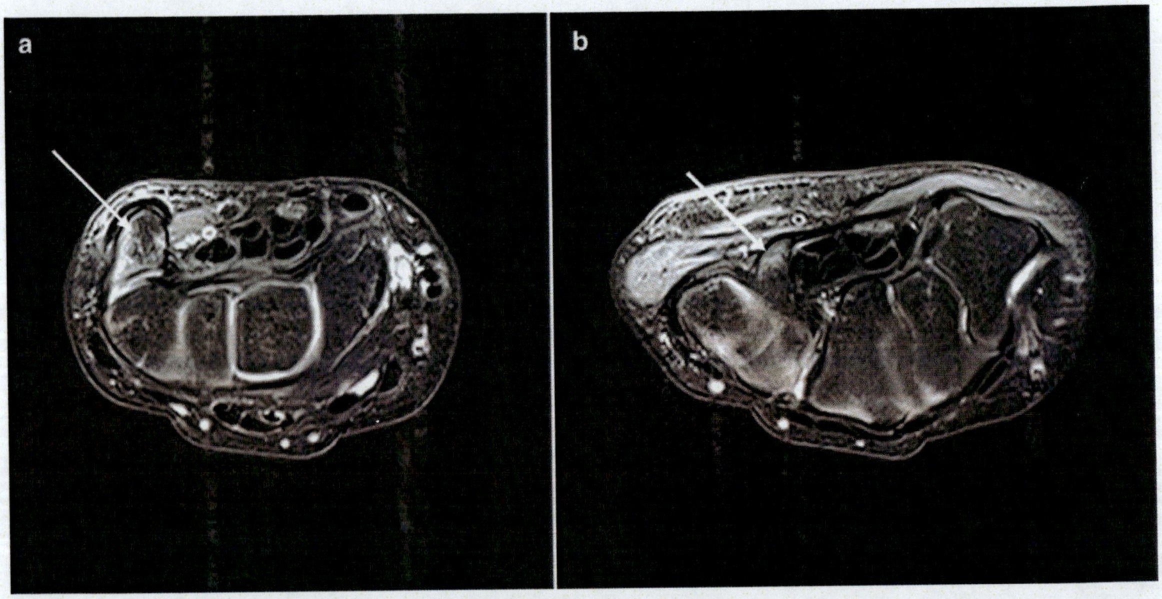

Fig. 9 Hamulus hamatum and os pisiforme bone contusion in an 11-year-old girl with fall on outstretched hand. Bone marrow edema (*arrows*) at the os pisiforme (**a**) and the hamulus of hamatum (**b**) without any fracture line are seen with high signal intensity on fat-suppressed T2-w MR images

often do not reveal a fatigue fracture soon after the symptom onset, but are essential to exclude preexisting bone disease. Evidence of a fracture may never appear (50% of cases) on plain radiographs or may not appear until several weeks or months after the onset of symptoms (Nielsen et al. 1991). Initially, osteoclastic bone resorption occurs 5–14 days after the onset of symptoms. The cortical tunneling that may be present in this early phase

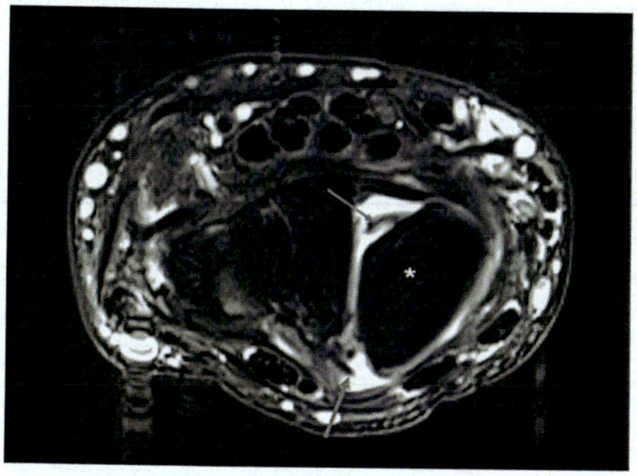

Fig. 10 Scapholunate ligament tear in a 17-year-old male with fall on outstretched hand 6 weeks before imaging. The axial fat-suppressed T2-w MR image shows a tear of the dorsal and palmar aspect of the intrinsic scapholunate ligaments (*arrows*) The bone marrow is normal (*asterisk*)

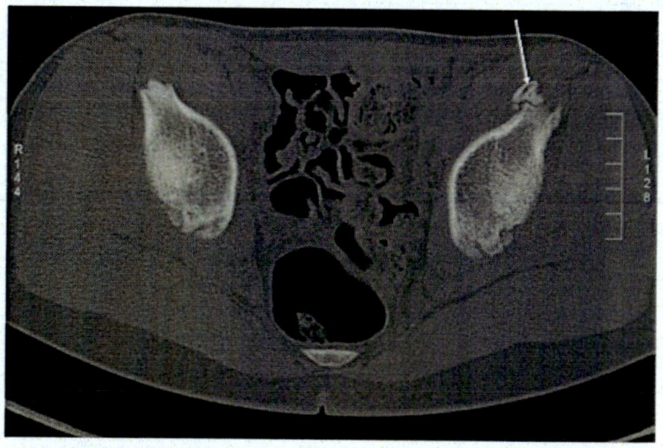

Fig. 12 Acute apophysiolysis or avulsion fracture of the anterior inferior iliac spine in a 13-year-old boy with sudden snap at the left groin region. The axial CT scan, 4 weeks postinjury, shows hypertrophic ossification (*arrow*) at the left spina iliaca anterior inferior apophysis without bony fusion to the pelvic bone

is often overlooked on radiographs, whereas the subtle blurring of cancellous bone is not detected on radiographs. This is followed by endosteal and periosteal callus formation in phases 2 and 3. With continued activity, a true fracture occurs in phase 4. Most of the fractures are at the cancellous bone (72%) and 23% are cortical. In the osteoclastic phase, cortical fractures are easily detected on radiographs. The late sclerotic aspect that is present in the phase 2 and 3 of endosteal callus formation reveals the cancellous fatigue fracture on radiographs. Early in the clinical course, i.e., as early as 24 h after the onset of symptoms, bone scintigraphy and MRI are more sensitive than radiographs in the detection of fatigue fractures. MRI is the first choice in the secondary workup because of its higher specificity to characterize the findings related to fatigue fractures compared to bone

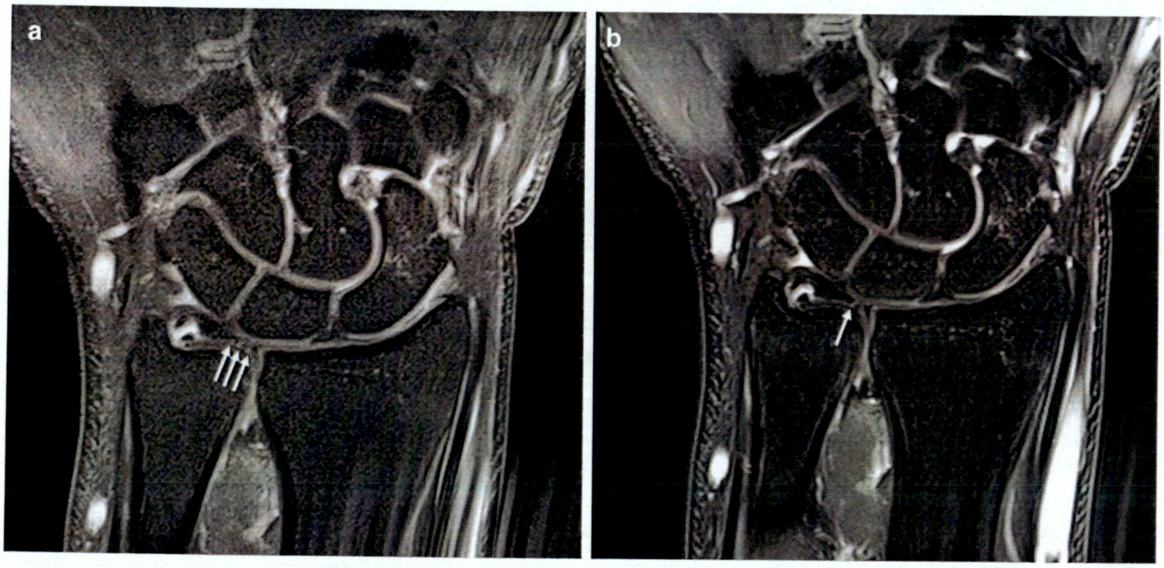

Fig. 11 Palmer IA Lesion in a 16-year-old male with a history of fall on the outstretched hand presenting with pain at the ulnar aspect of the wrist. The coronal fat-suppressed contrast-enhanced (indirect arthrogram) T1-w (**a**) and fat-suppressed T2-w (**b**) MR images show the abnormal signal throughout radial aspect of the triangular fibrocartilage (*arrows*)

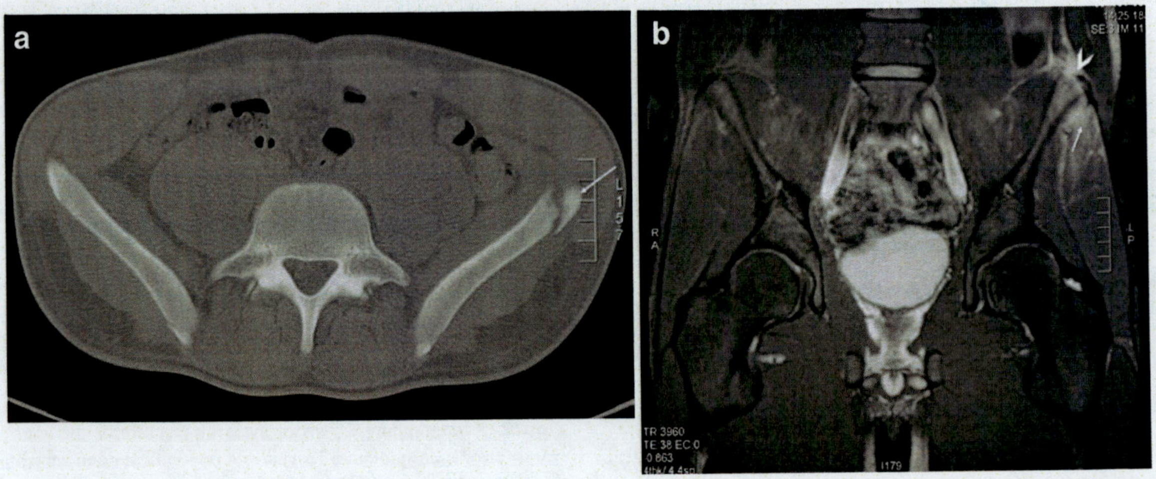

Fig. 13 Acute apophysiolysis or avulsion fracture of the iliac crest in a 17-year-old boy with acute pain following a rotational injury of the abdomen. (**a**) The axial CT image shows separation and dissociation of the left spina iliaca anterior superior (*arrow*). (**b**) The coronal fat-suppressed PD-w MR image of the pelvis shows separation and caudal displacement of the left spina iliaca anterior superior (*arrowhead*). There is also increased signal due to edema at the origin of the musculus tensor fascia latae (*arrow*)

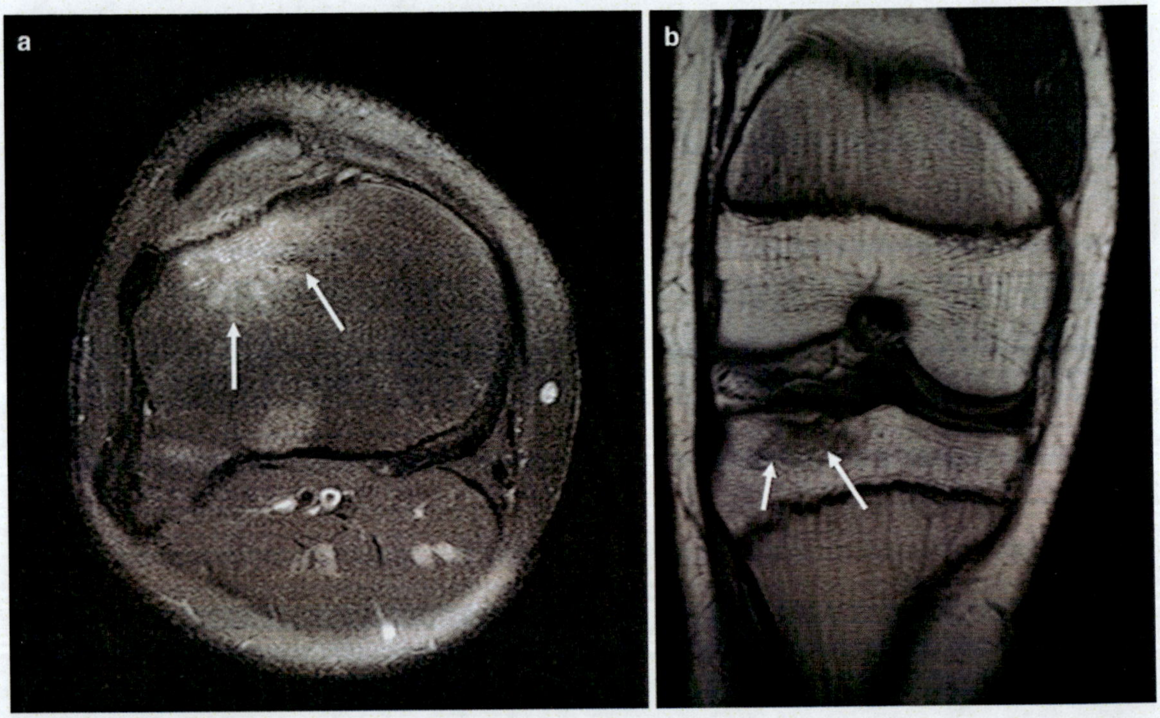

Fig. 14 The axial fat-suppressed T2-w (**a**) and the coronal T1-w (**b**) MR images show bone contusion at the anterior lateral aspect of the tibia epiphysis (*arrows*) in this13-year-old girl with a history of fall on the knee

scintigraphy. Especially fluid-sensitive sequences, T2-w with fat-suppression or short tau inversion recovery (STIR), are needed to detect bone marrow-, periosteal and even muscle edema and the fluid signal in the cortical tunneling and resorption cavities related to the early destructive phase of fatigue fractures. The fracture line that is present in the late phases is of low SI on T2-w and T1-w MR images. The imaging planes should be planned perpendicular to the expected fracture line, i.e., coronal and/or sagittal. Ultrasonography and CT scan are not recommended for the routine workup of fatigue fractures. CT is well-suited at the tarsal bones, in spondylolysis, and sacral fatigue fractures. These types of fatigue fractures are not described in tennis players at child or adolescent age. In fatigue reaction, plain radiographs are negative, the bone scan is positive, and the MR imaging findings include bone marrow edema without any detectable fracture line.

3.3 Topographic Discussion of Fatigue Fractures and Apophysitis

Fatigue fractures of the femoral bone in racquet sports represent a small subset of lower extremity fatigue injuries, but can have significant consequences if complicated with displacement. Bilateral supracondylar femoral bone fatigue fractures have been described in an otherwise healthy 15-year-old male athlete, which required intramedullary nailing due to unilateral displacement (Hutchinson et al. 2008).

In children, a common location for fatigue fractures is the anterior proximal third of the tibia. In adolescents the clinical differential diagnosis includes "anteromedial shin splints" (periostitis) and anterior compartment syndrome. Another location of such injuries in children (approximately 20%) is the fibula, more commonly in the distal third.

The "Jumper's" knee is often found in basketball, volleyball, and adult tennis playing athletes; it is not common in children. Overuse of extension apparatus before skeletal maturity is more likely to cause traction apophysitis lesions. The younger age group, around 11 year of age, has a predominant traction apophysitis at the patellar apex, also known as Sinding–Larsen–Johannson disease. The older age group around 15–16 year of age has a predominant location at the tuberositas tibiae apophysis, better known as Osgood–Schlatter disease.

Jone's fatigue fracture at the fifth metatarsal bone has also been described in tennis players.

Concerning upper extremity lesions, distraction humeral shaft fatigue fractures are only reported in adult tennis players, but not in children. The forces placed on the upper extremity in the forearm stroke and the serve are very similar to those characteristic of baseball pitching with possible distraction fatigue fracture of the proximal humeral epiphysis in children and adolescents. Recurrent posterior subluxations of the shoulder (RPS) is caused by the precarious position of the follow-through of overhead position in tennis serve and the take away phase of the backhand stroke in tennis. It is well-known in adults, may be found in adolescents, but is rare in children. Repetitive microtrauma to the posterior static restraints shifts the load to the dynamic muscular restraints that fatigue over time allowing RPS.

Distraction fatigue reaction and fracture may also occur at the olecranon in relation to repetitive triceps muscle action. Ulnar diaphysis fatigue fracture that is located at the nondominant arm using a double-handed backhand stroke is not described in children. A special case of fatigue reaction is posteromedial elbow impingement with compression fatigue fracture or fatigue reaction at the medial tip of the olecranon. A single case report described a pseudarthrosis of the first rib in an adult competitive tennis player at international level, but this injury was never described in children (Trieb et al. 2008) (Table 2).

Table 2 Overuse lesions

Region	Location	Type and mechanism	Imaging	Age (years)
Axial skeleton	Lumbar spine	*Spondylolysis and -olisthesis* *Hyperextension*	XR (Fig. 15) CT (Fig. 15) SPECT–CT MRI (Fig. 15)	9–14
Shoulder girdle	Glenohumeral joint	*Anterior shoulder instability* *Anterior shoulder dislocation*	MRA	
		Posterior shoulder instability, recurrent posterior subluxations (RPS) *Backhand stroke*	MRA	
		Slap *Serve*	MRA	
		Posterior superior glenoid impingement (internal impingement): rotator cuff articular surface impingement, with possible tear, between posterosuperior glenoid (with possible tear) and posterior greater tubercle (with possible bony contusion and chondral lesion) *Serve*	MRA	
	Suprascapular nerve	Traction Late cocking phase of serve	EMG MRI	
	Proximal humerus	Physeal stress injury at the lateral margin	XR	
Elbow and upper arm	Capitellum	Osteochondral fracture, osteochondritis dissecans Valgus stress	XR MRI	>11
		Osteochondrosis (Panner's disease) Valgus stress	XR	7–11
	Olecranon	Impingement apophyseal tip Forced extension	MRI (Figs. 16 and 17)	
	Olecranon	Traction apophysitis Serve stress	XR	<15
		Stress fracture Serve stress	XR (Fig. 18) Bone scan	>15
	Ulna diaphysis	Stress fracture	XR MRI bone scan	
	Medial epicondyle	Medial elbow tension stress syndrome (Little League Elbow) Medial traction apophysitis, association with capitellum or radial head osteochondrosis	XR	9–12
		Valgus extension overload, medial collateral ligament laxity, capitellum and radial head chondromalacia, or osteochondritis dissecans Valgus force during the act of hitting the tennisball with the racquet	MRI	>12
		Medial tennis elbow: tendinosis pronator tibia-fibula carpi radialis	MRI	
	Lateral epicondyle	*Tennis elbow, tendinosis common extensor origin*	US	
Forearm, wrist and hand	Distal radius and ulna	*Physeal stress injury*	XR	
	Wrist	De Quervain tenovaginitis Forceful gripping in ulnar deviation	US	

Table 2 (continued)

		Sprain extensor retinaculum, grade III: luxation ECU Double-handed backhand	US MRI (Fig. 19)	
		Ulnar nerve compression at Guyon's canal Repetitive compression	US	
		Carpal fatigue reaction	MRI (Fig. 20)	
Pelvic girdle and hip	Spina iliaca anterior superior and inferior	*Apophysitis*	XR US	
	Pubic ramus	Ischiopubic synchondrotic fatigue	XR (Fig. 21)	
	Femur diaphysis	*Fatigue fracture*	XR	
	Distal femur	Physeal fatigue injury, lateral condylar portion	XR	
Upper leg and knee	Medial femur condyle	Osteochondritis dissecans (lateral margin of medial condyle)	XR MRI	
	Patella	Traction apophysitis apex of the patella, Sinding–Larsen–Johansson	XR US	
		Fatigue fracture	XR MRI (Fig. 22)	
	Proximal tibia	Physeal fatigue injury	XR	
		Metaphyseal fatigue fracture	XR (Fig. 23) Bone scan MRI (Fig. 23)	
	Tuberositas tibiae	*Traction apophysitis, Osgood-Schlatter*	XR US (Fig. 24)	
	Fibula proximal diaphysis	Fatigue fracture	XR Bone scan MRI	
	Tibia proximal diaphysis	Fatigue fracture	XR Bone scan MRI (Fig. 25)	
Lower leg, ankle and foot	Fibula Distal diaphysis	Fatigue fracture	XR Bone scan MRI	
	Tibia distal diaphysis	Fatigue fracture-reaction	XR Bone scan MRI (Fig. 26)	
	Achilles tendon	Tendinopathy, bursitis	US (Fig. 27)	
	Navicular bone	Fatigue fracture, sagittal	XR Bone scan MRI	
		Fatigue at accessory navicular synchondrosis	XR MRI	Adolescent
	Muscle compartments	*Anterior tibial compartment muscle herniation*	US MRI (Fig. 28)	Adolescent
	Metatarsals	Fatigue fracture (2-3-4)	XR (Fig. 29) MRI (Fig. 30)	

Summary of overuse and chronic lesions sorted by region and anatomical structure encountered in tennis players. The type of lesion is defined with mechanism of injury. Best-suited imaging procedure is mentioned in appropriate order. Age distribution is given if epidemiologic evidence is available

Italics rare lesions; *XR* radiography; *CT* computed tomography; *MRI* magnetic resonance imaging; *MRA* magnetic resonance arthrography; *US* ultrasound

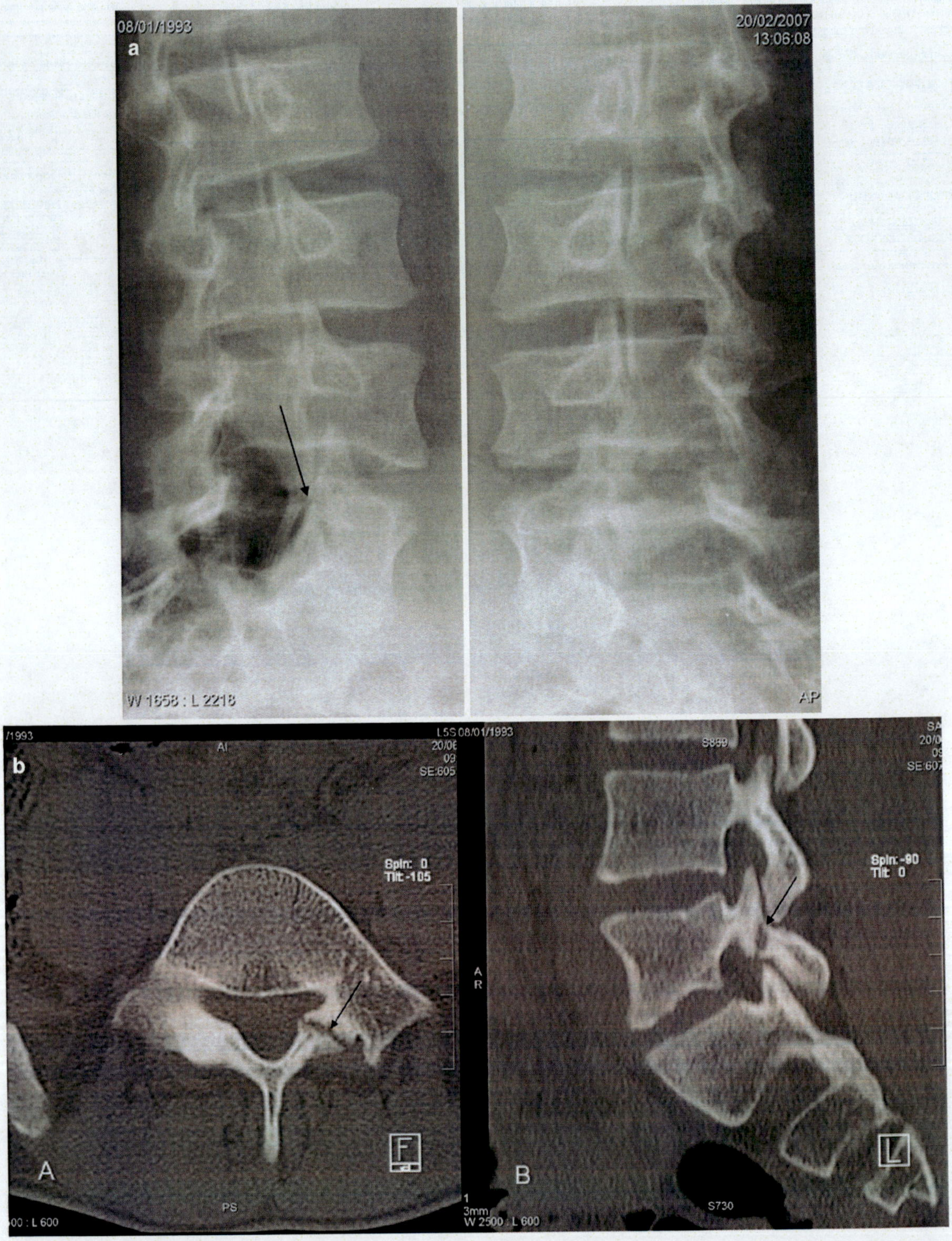

Fig. 15 Unilateral spondylolysis in a 15-year-old male with unilateral left-sided defect of the isthmus of L5 (*arrows*) demonstrated with 3/4th radiographic view (**a**), sagittal reconstruction with CT (**b**) and sagittal T2-w images (**c**), which also shows the high signal of the bone marrow edema at the isthmus adjacent to the fracture line

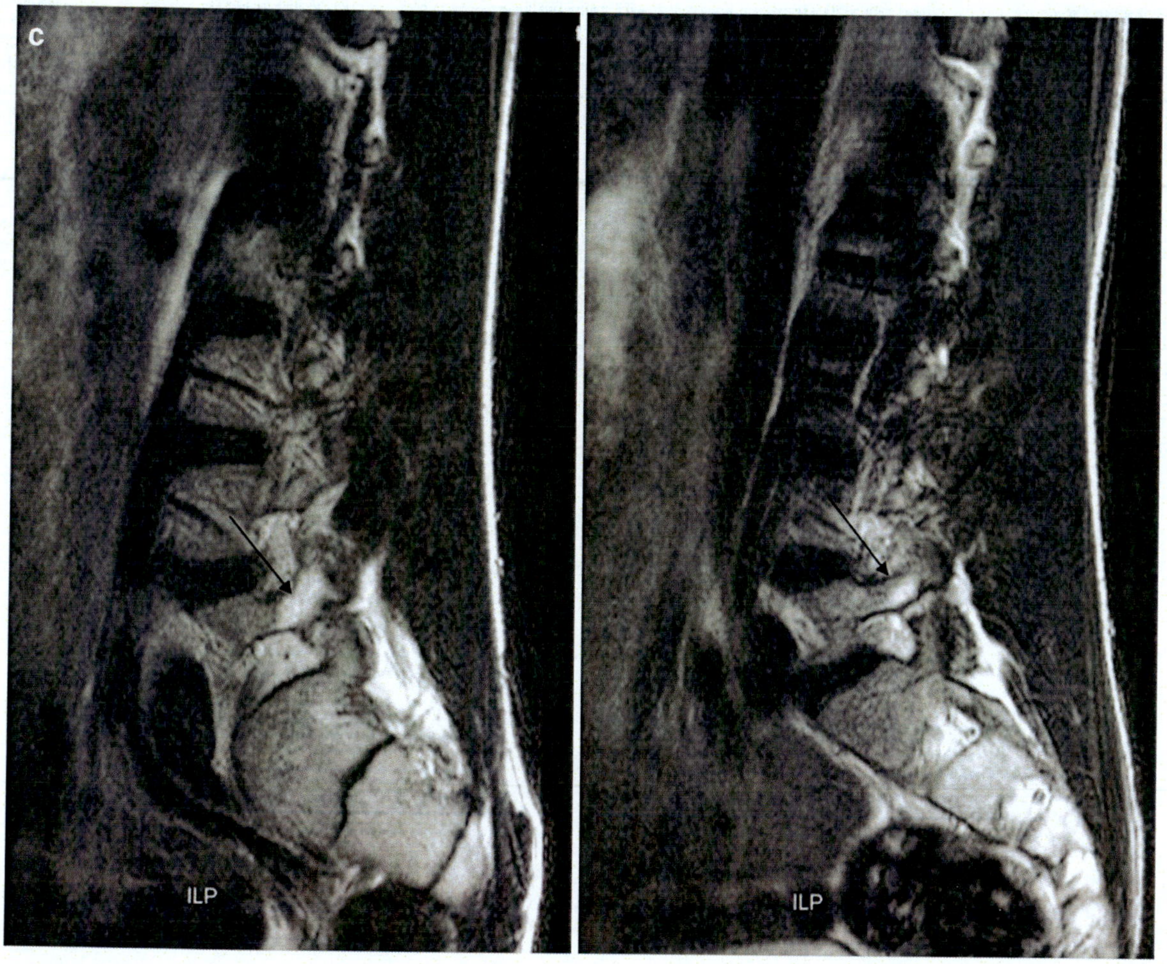

Fig. 15 (continued)

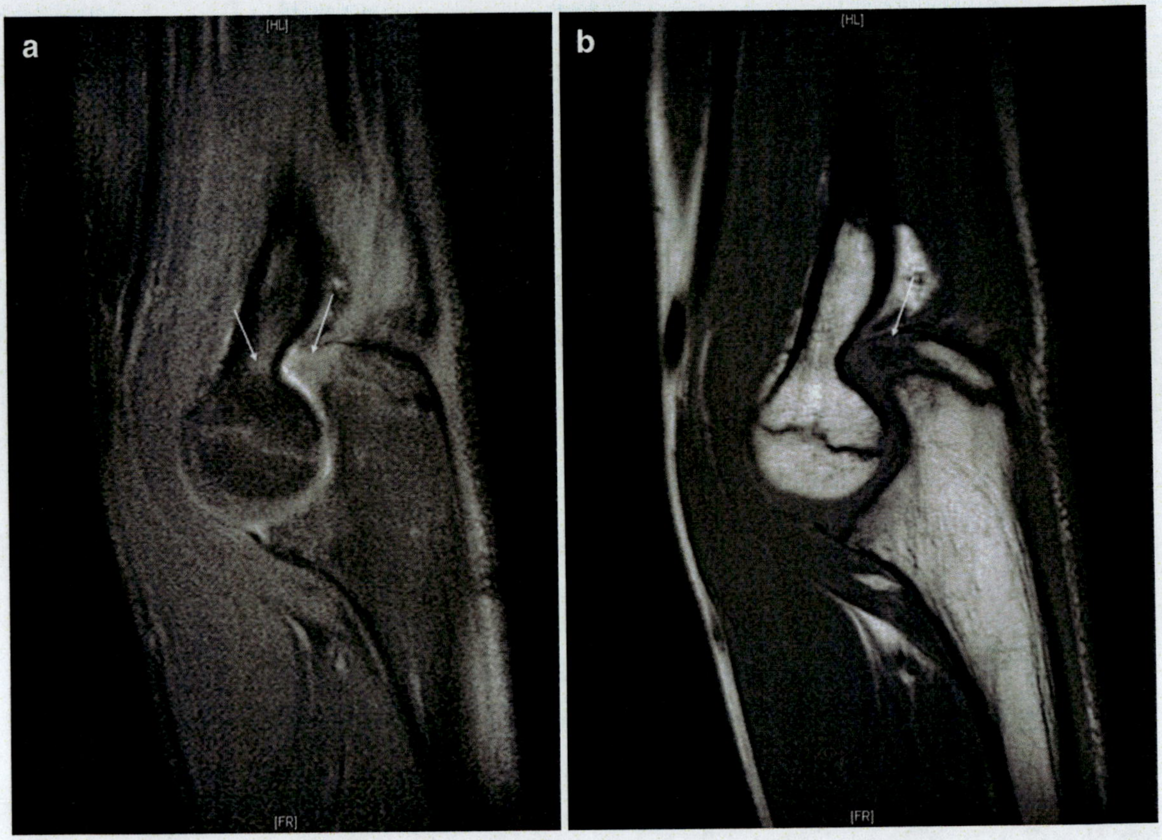

Fig. 16 Olecranon impingement (compression fatigue reaction) at the right elbow in a 13-year-old male right-handed tennis player with chronic pain during serve at the fossa olecrani. Clinical examination showed pain during passive extension with terminal block and no pain during active extension. The sagittal fat-suppressed PD-w (**a**) and T1-w (**b**) MR images show bone marrow edema at the tip of the elecranon and faint bone marrow edema at the fossa olecrani (*arrows*)

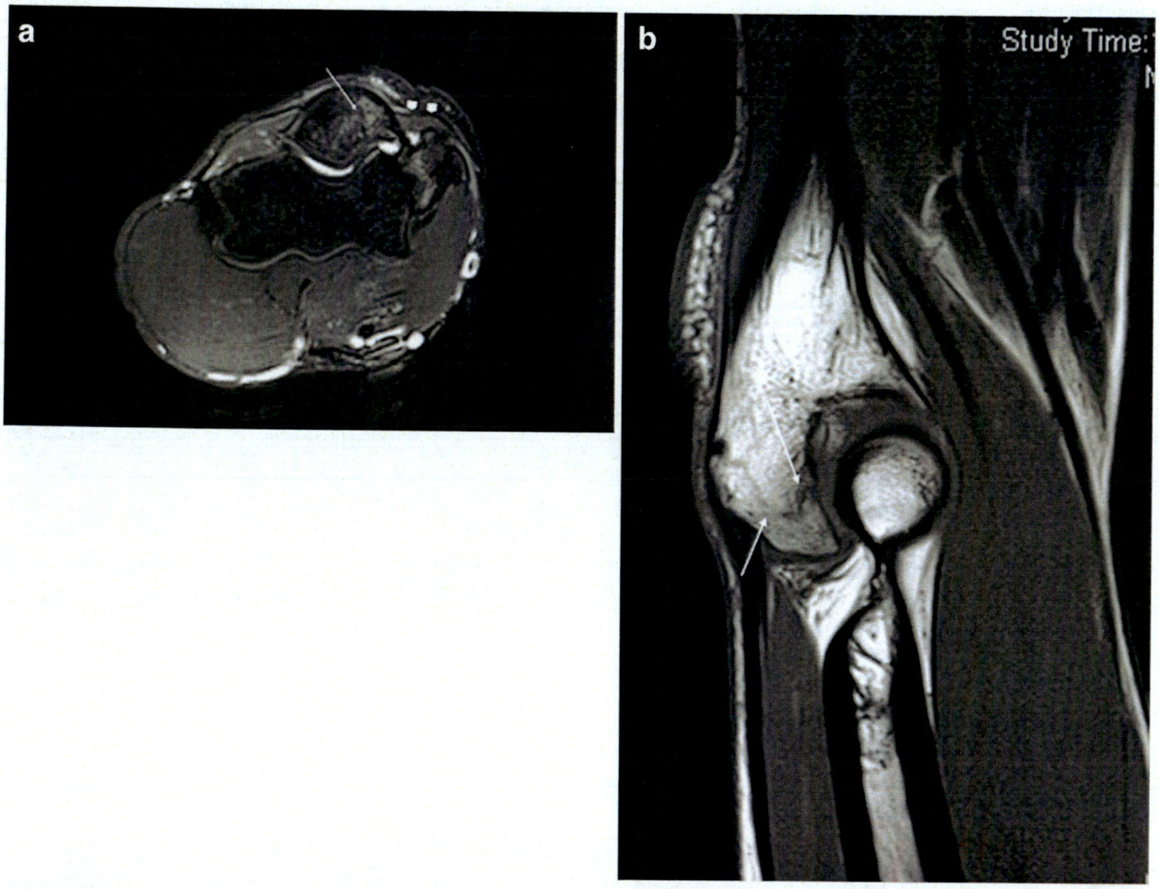

Fig. 17 Olecranon impingement with fatigue fracture at the right elbow in a 15-year-old male right-handed tennis player with chronic pain during serve at the olecranon. The axial fat-suppressed PD-w (**a**) MR image shows marked bone marrow edema at the medial part of the tip of the olecranon (*arrow*). Note also a small musculus anconeus epitrochlearis, not related to the clinical complaints (*arrowheads*). (**b**) The sagittal T1-w MR image show a low signal intensity fracture line at the tip of the olecranon (*arrows*) surrounded by decreased signal intensity bone marrow edema

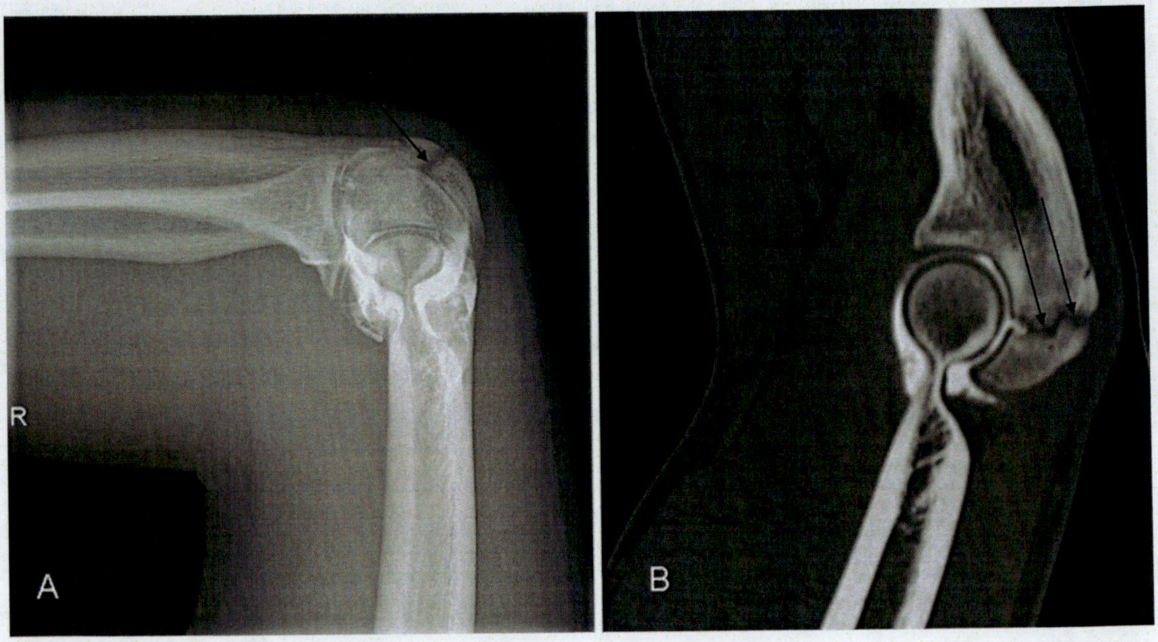

Fig. 18 Fatigue distraction fracture of the olecranon in a 15-year-old boy with long-standing pain during serve and play at the posterior aspect of the elbow. The lateral view conventional arthrogram (**a**) and the sagittal reconstruction of the CT arthrogram show the fracture line with sclerotic margins (*arrows*). Contrast extending within the fracture line subchondrally is better depicted with CT

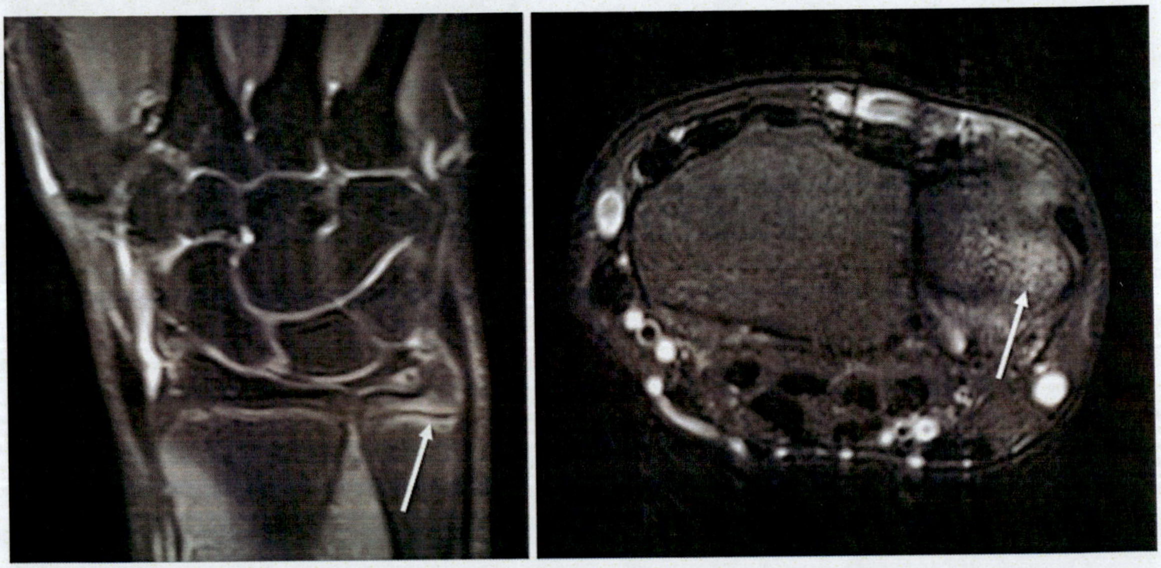

Fig. 19 Fatigue reaction at the distal ulna in a 15-year-old girl with chronic pain at the ulnar side that increases during dorsiflexion and ulnar deviation of the wrist. The fat-suppressed coronal (**a**) and axial (**b**) T2-w MR images show the high signal intensity bone marrow edema at the ulnar styloid process and the adjacent metaphyseal growth plate (*arrows*). The lesion is related to chronic traction on the extensor retinaculum at the level of the ulnar insertion due to ulnar and dorsal strain on the extensor carpi ulnaris tendon during double-handed backhand stroke. Ulnar dislocation of the extensor carpi ulnaris tendon is also shown

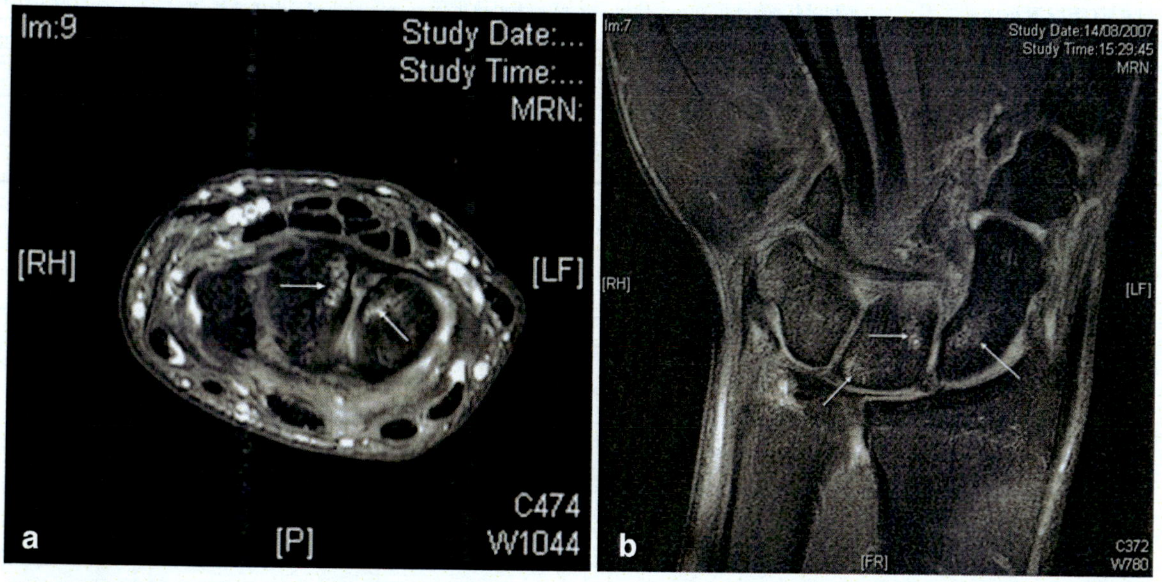

Fig. 20 Fatigue reaction in an 18-year-old right-handed player with chronic pain sensation at the carpus. The axial fat-suppressed PD-w (**a**) and coronal contrast-enhanced fat-suppressed (indirect arthrogram) T1-w (**b**) MR images show bone marrow edema at the opposing right lunate and scaphoid bones (*arrows*)

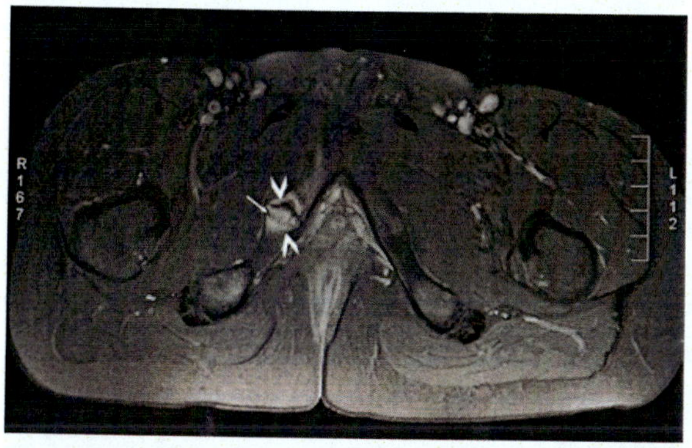

Fig. 21 Ischiopubic synchondrosis stress injury in an 11-year-old boy. The axial constrast-enhanced fat-suppressed T1-w MR image shows enhancement at the central cartilaginous area (*arrow*) and on both sides of the subchondral bone (*arrowheads*)

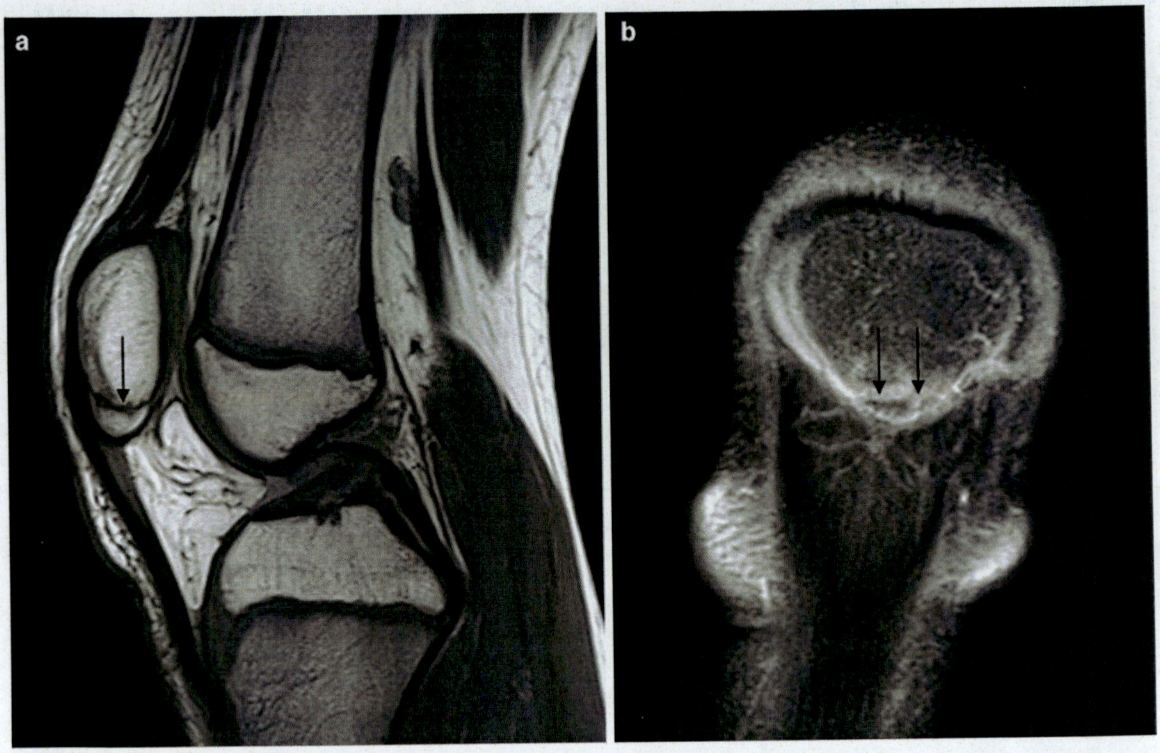

Fig. 22 Fatigue distraction fracture of the apex of the patella in a 12-year-old boy with anterior knee pain. The sagittal PD-w (**a**) and the fat-suppressed coronal T2-w (**b**) MR images show the low signal intensity horizontal line which corresponds to a fatigue fracture (*arrows*)

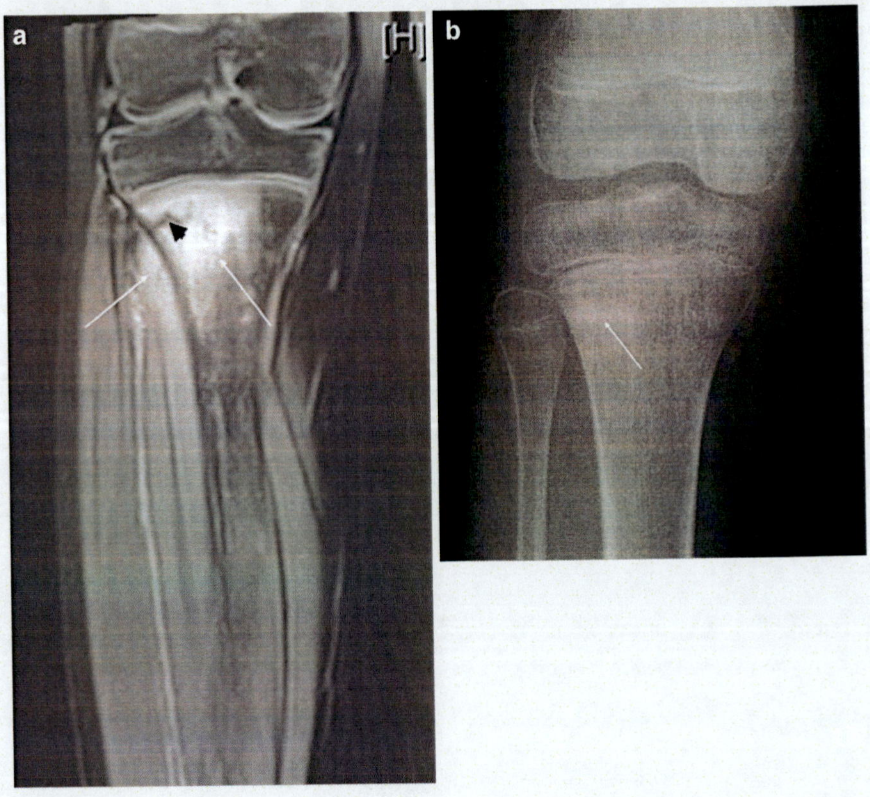

Fig. 23 Fatigue fracture at the proximal lateral tibia metaphysis in an 8-year-old female with history of tibial shaft fracture 6 months earlier which was complicated with disuse osteopenia. Following fracture healing, the patient reported a gradually increasing pain at the posterior and lateral aspect of the right knee during and after sports activity. (**a**) The coronal fat-suppressed PD-w MR image shows high signal intensity edema at the cancellous bone of the proximal and lateral aspect of the tibial metaphysis and edema at the adjacent soft tissues (*arrows*). A low signal intensity irregular fracture line is also obvious (*arrowhead*). The AP radiograph of the right knee performed 1 month later shows osteoblastic endosteal callous at the lateral metaphyseal area of the tibia (*arrow*)

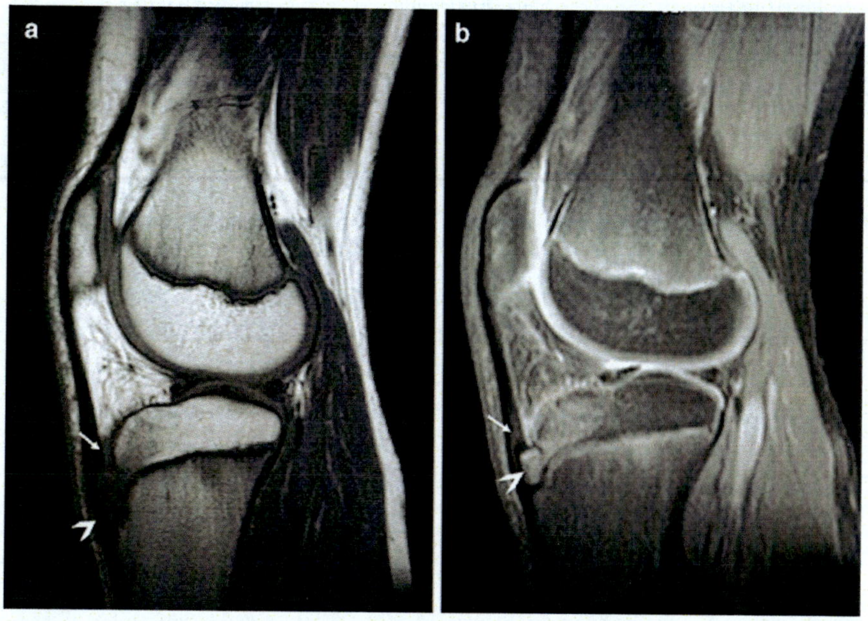

Fig. 24 Osgood–Schlatter in a 14-year-old boy. (**a**) The sagittal T1-w MR image shows thickening of the tuberositas tibiae apophysis (*arrowhead*) with some widening of the bursa infrapatellaris profunda (*arrow*). (**b**) The fat-suppressed PD-w MR image in the sagittal plane shows edema at the tuberositas tibiae apophysis (*arrowhead*) and the deep infrapatellar bursa. Minor prolonged T2 at the distal third of the patellar tendon with some associated thickening, in keeping with tendonitis is also seen (*arrow*)

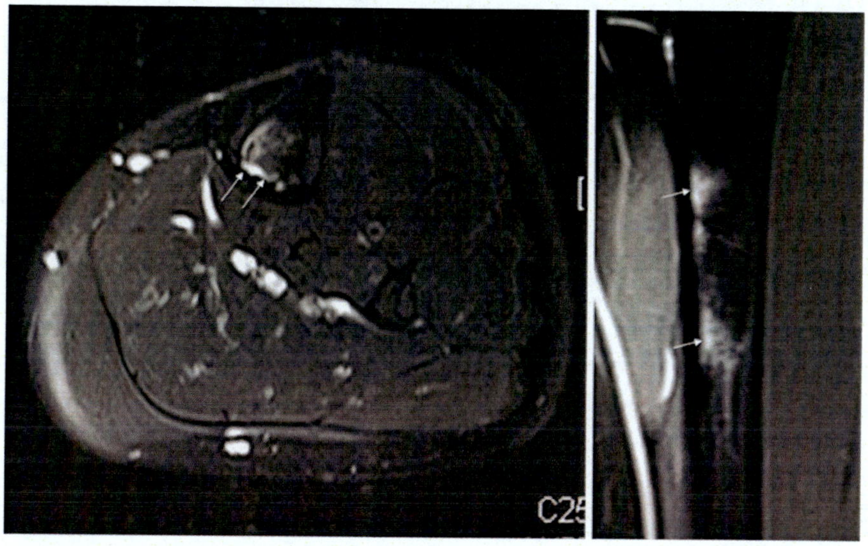

Fig. 25 Fatigue reaction at the left tibial diaphysis in a 19-year-old male presenting with local stress-induced pain. The axial and sagittal fat-suppressed MR images show bone marrow edema most pronounced at the endosteal side of the middle third of the left tibia diaphysis (*arrows*)

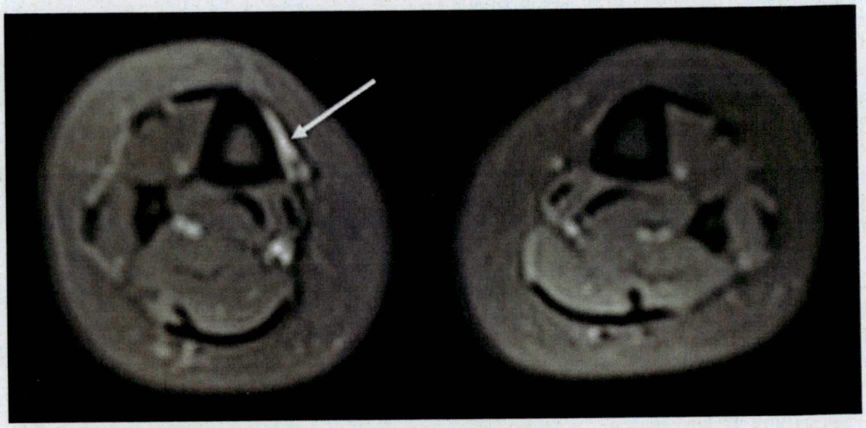

Fig. 26 Shin Splint in a 17-year-old female with chronic pain during and following the game at the anteromedial aspect of the right distal tibia. Note thickening and edema of the periosteum (*arrow*) at the right side on axial fat-suppressed MRI with intermediate TE

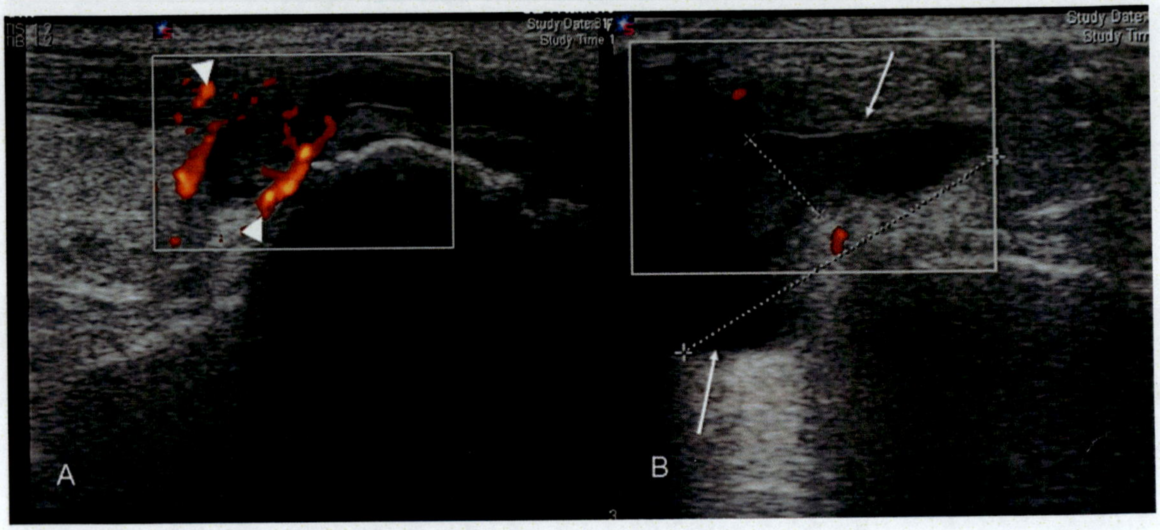

Fig. 27 Achilles tendinopathy with retrocalcaneal bursitis in a10-year-old boy with long-standing pain at the right retrocalcaneal region. Ultrasound with power Doppler examination (*arrowheads*) reveals hypervascularity of the Achilles tendon and paratenon at the retrocalcaneal region with hypoechoic aspect and irregular anterior lining of the tendon. There is also marked thickening and expansion with fluid at the deep retrocalcaneal bursa (*arrows*). (**a**) longitudinal imaging plane, (**b**) transaxial imaging plane

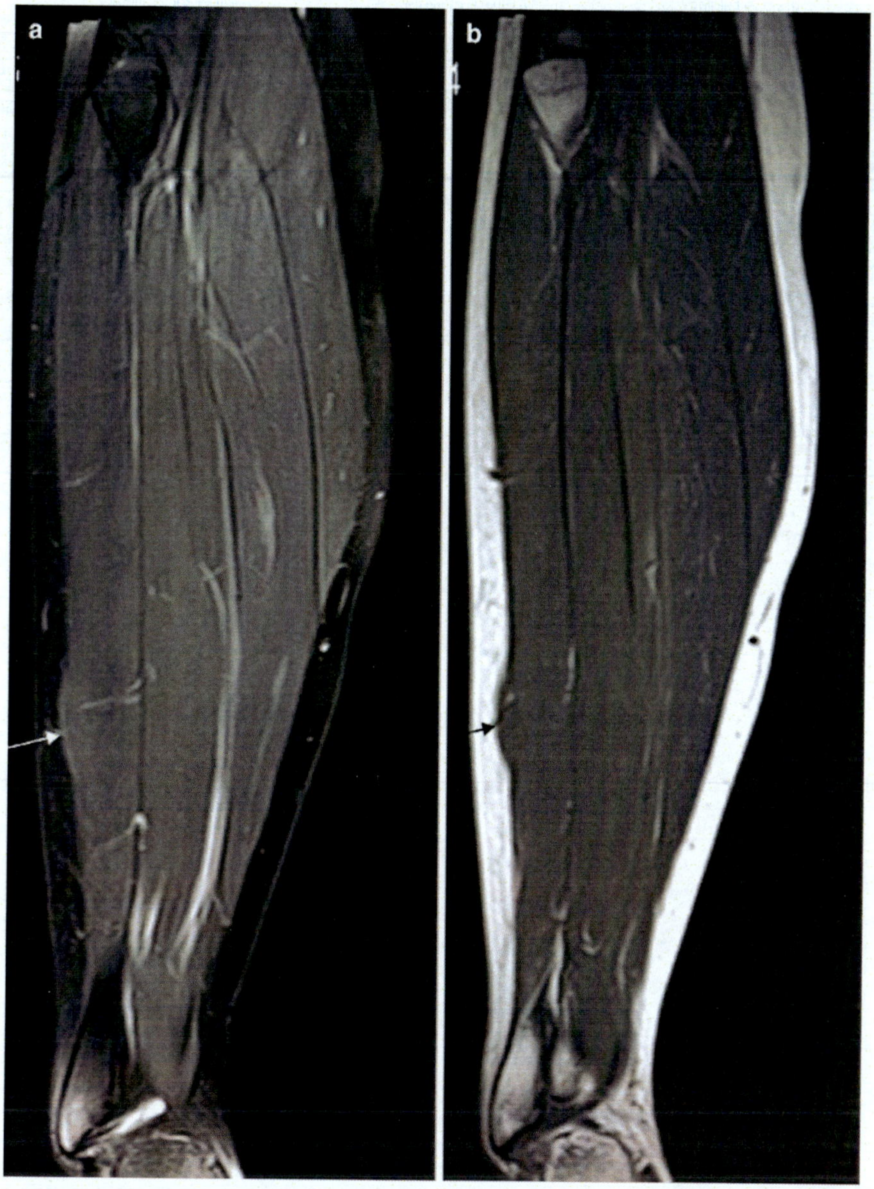

Fig. 28 Muscle herniation in the peroneal compartment of an 18-year-old female who sustained a blunt direct trauma to the lateral side of the right lower leg. Pain and swelling were persistent for weeks following trauma. The coronal fat-suppressed PD-w (**a**) and T1-w (**b**) MR images, obtained at rest, reveal a local extrusion (*arrows*) of the distal peroneal muscle in the subcutaneous tissue at site of local weakening of the superficial muscle fascia. There is also a slightly increased signal intensity within the herniation on the fat-suppressed image

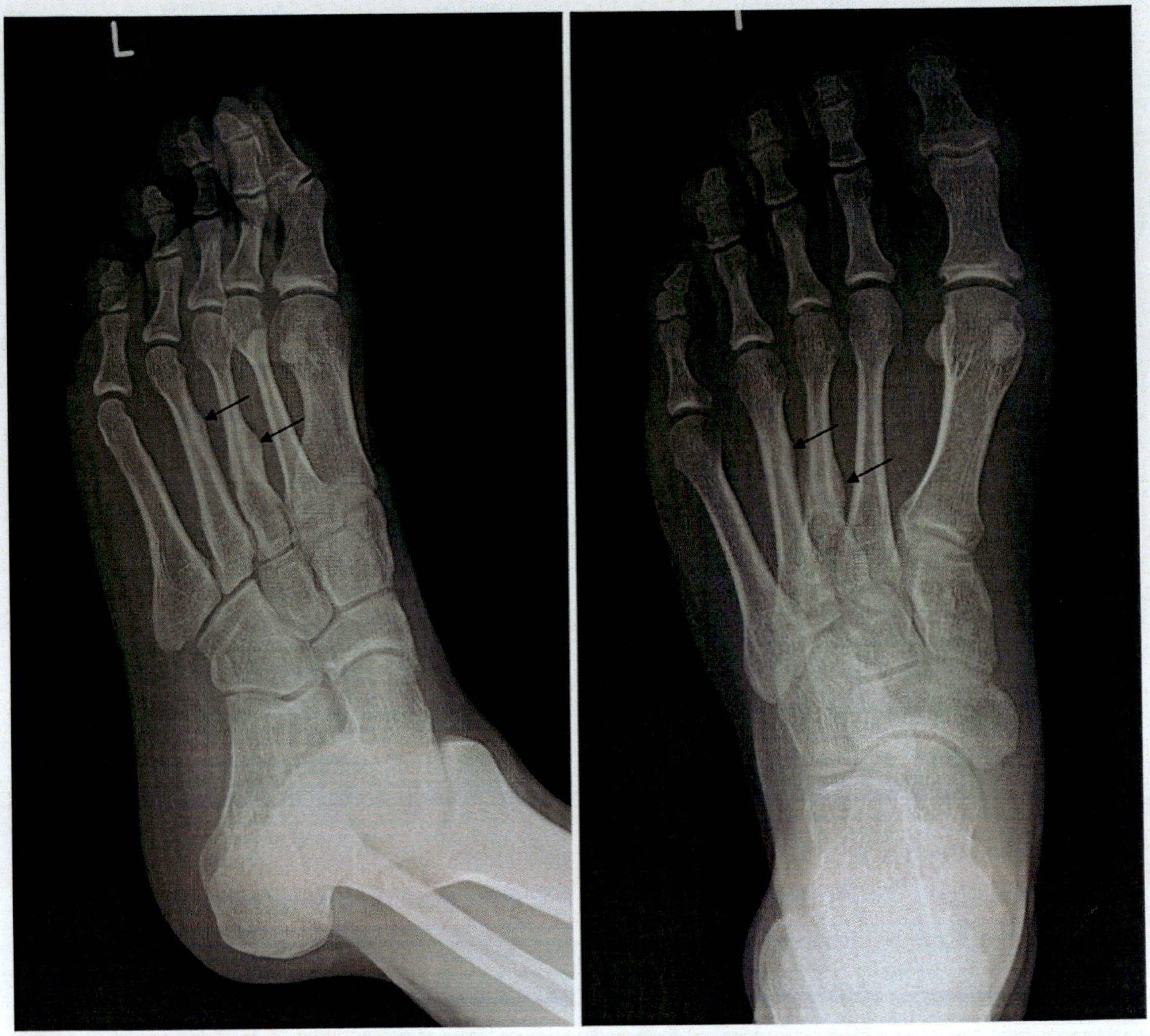

Fig. 29 Stress reaction at the third and fourth metatarsal bones in a 17-year-old male with long-standing forefoot pain. A solid periosteal reaction is seen at the third and fourth metatarsal bones (*arrows*)

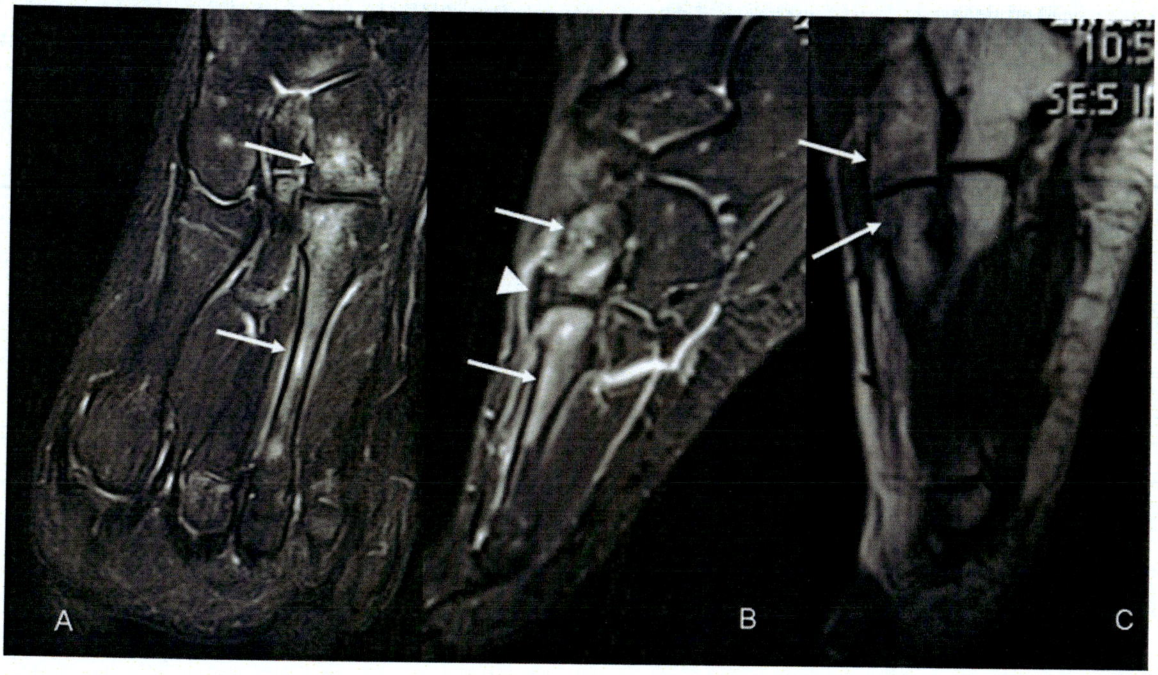

Fig. 30 Fatigue reaction at the Lisfranc region and third metatarsal row. The axial (**a**) and sagittal (**b**) fat-suppressed PD-w as well as the sagittal T1-w (**c**) MR images show bone marrow edema at the level of the proximal two third of the third metatarsal bone and the cuboid (*arrows*) and a thickened dorsal capsule of the Lisfranc joint (*arrowhead*)

References

Bylak J, Hutchinson MR (1998) Common sports injuries in young tennis players. Sports Med 26:119–132

Chandler TJ (1995) Exercise training for tennis. Clin Sports Med 14:33–46

Ellenbecker TS, Pluim B, Vivier S, Sniteman C (2009) Common injuries in tennis players: exercises to address muscular imbalances and reduce injury risk. J Strength Cond Res 31:50–58

Gregg JR, Torg E (1988) Upper extremity injuries in adolescent tennis players. Clin Sports Med 7:371–385

Hutchinson PH, Stieber J, Flynn J, Ganley T (2008) Complete and incomplete femoral stress fractures in the adolescent athlete. Orthopedics 31:604

Kibler WB (1994) Clinical biomechanics of the elbow in tennis: implications for evaluation and diagnosis. Med Sci Sports Exerc 26:1203–1206

Kühne CA, Zettl RP, Nast-Kolb D (2004) Injuries- and frequency of complaints in competitive tennis- and leisure sports. Sportverletz Sportschaden 18:85–89

Nielsen MB, Hansen K, Hølmer P, Dyrbye M (1991) Tibial periosteal reactions in soldiers. A scintigraphic study of 29 cases of lower leg pain. Acta Orthop Scand 62:531–534

Park JY, Lhee SH, Keum JS (2008) Rupture of latissimus dorsi muscle in a tennis player. Orthopedics 31; 10

Pluim BM, Staal JB, Windler GE, Jayanthi N (2006) Tennis injuries: occurrence, aetiology, and prevention. Br J Sports Med 40:415–423

Trieb K, Huber W, Kainberger F (2008) A rare reason for the end of a career in competitive tennis. J Sports Med Phys Fitness 48:120–122

Common Injuries in Gymnasts

Maaike P. Terra, Mario Maas, Charlotte M. Nusman, Ana Navas-Canete, and Milko C. de Jonge

Contents

M.P. Terra, M. Maas (✉), C.M. Nusman, A. Navas-Canete, and M.C. de Jonge
Department of Radiology, Academic Medical Center, Meibergdreef 9, 1105 AZ Amsterdam, The Netherlands
e-mail: m.maas@amc.uva.nl

Key Points

- Both acute injuries as well as chronic overuse injuries should be considered when evaluating examinations of elite gymnastic athletes.
- Injuries of the growing skeleton are typically seen in gymnasts.
- Imaging in gymnasts comprises mainly conventional radiographs, MR imaging and CT.
- There is an important additional role for Multi detector Helical CT when MR imaging is suggestive of disease: CT will better delineate extend of lesion especially in the osseous structures.
- Correlation between imaging findings and clinical situation is mandatory. Therefore close interaction between radiologist and treating physician is essential.

1 Introduction

Participation in gymnastics has undergone rapid growth in past decades, especially in the female population (Backx et al. 1989; Caine and Nassar 2005). A recent study demonstrated that gymnastics has one of the highest injury rates of all girl-sports (Singh et al. 2008). Children are entering this sport when they are very young, and many elite gymnasts start with training and specialization as early as 6 or 7 years of age (Caine and Nassar 2005; Sands 2000). Gymnastics is a very demanding sport in which the musculoskeletal system is subjected to extensive loads. The high intensity and volume of training required to be competitive make young gymnasts with an immature skeleton extremely vulnerable to injury during their training

A.H. Karantanas (ed.), *Sports Injuries in Children and Adolescents*,
Med Radiol Diagn Imaging, DOI: 10.1007/174_2010_6, © Springer-Verlag Berlin Heidelberg 2011

and competition years. Physicians should be alert to recognize the typical injuries of the growing skeleton, which can especially be found at the epiphysis and apophysis (Kerssemakers et al. 2009).

Gymnastics-related injuries can roughly be divided in two main categories, acute injuries and chronic overuse problems. Acute injuries, usually resulting from a fall or faulty landing, comprise primarily of fractures, dislocations, sprains and strains. Chronic overuse problems result from chronic repetitive injury over an extended period of time leading to e.g., stress fractures and osteochondral injuries. Caine and Nassar revealed in a recent review of the literature that the majority of injuries in gymnastics were of sudden onset in nature (range = 52–83.4%) (Caine and Nassar 2005). They also showed that the pattern of injuries varies according to the competition level, with more chronic injuries found in elite compared to nonelite gymnasts. Injuries also vary by location. The ankle injuries are mainly due to an acute trauma whereas wrist and low back injuries are generally due to chronic overuse.

In this chapter an overview is given of typical gymnastics-related injuries of the upper extremities, lower extremities and the axial skeleton in elite gymnasts. To prevent overlap with other chapters we have focused per category only on the most common injuries and their radiological features as seen in our institution.

2 Upper Extremity Injuries

During gymnastic activities the upper extremity is generally used to support body weight and is subjected to many different types of stress, including repetitive motion, high impact loading and axial compression. A review of upper extremity injuries in gymnasts showed that the highest incidence occurs in the wrist in females and the shoulder in male gymnasts (Caine and Nassar 2005).

2.1 Wrist

2.1.1 Growth Plate Injury

In the immature skeleton, the growth plates of the wrist are at risk for injury. Because most of the load applied to the wrist in dorsal flexion is applied to the distal radius, most of the overuse injuries are found in the distal radial physis with prevalence rates ranging from 10 to 85% (Caine and Nassar 2005). Conventional radiographs in advanced stages show widening of the growth plate, cystic changes of the metaphyseal aspect of the growth plate, a beaked appearance of the distal aspect of the epiphysis, and haziness within the normally radiolucent area of the growth plate (DiFiori et al. 2006; Roy et al. 1985) (Fig. 1). Early growth plate injury will often not be revealed on radiographs (DiFiori et al. 2006). With MR imaging a more accurate diagnosis can be achieved (Koh et al. 2007; Shih et al. 1995). MR imaging features include horizontal fractures, vertical fractures, widened growth plate, transphyseal linear striations and metaphyseal bone bruise (Fig. 2). Physeal cartilage extension into the metaphysis is reported to be a sign representing healing (Shih et al. 1995). A relation between premature growth plate closure due to repetitive physeal injury and subsequent positive ulnar variance has been reported, but prospective data concerning the relations between

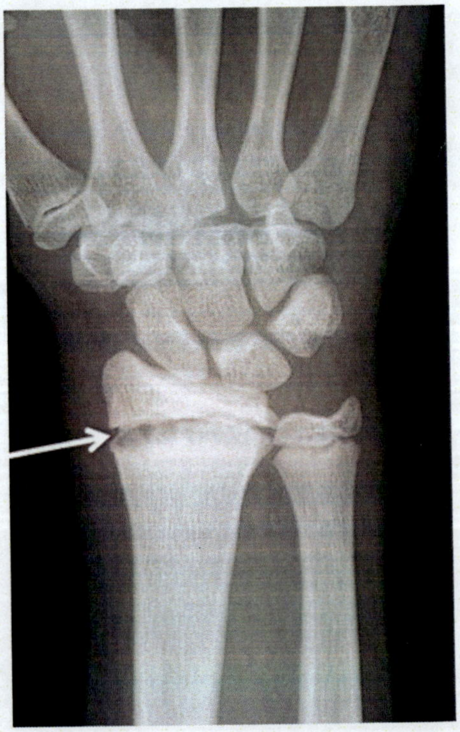

Fig. 1 The PA radiograph of the right wrist in a 14-year-old female gymnast, demonstrates widening of the growth plate of the distal radius with lucent areas mainly at the metaphyseal aspect of the growth plate (*white arrow*)

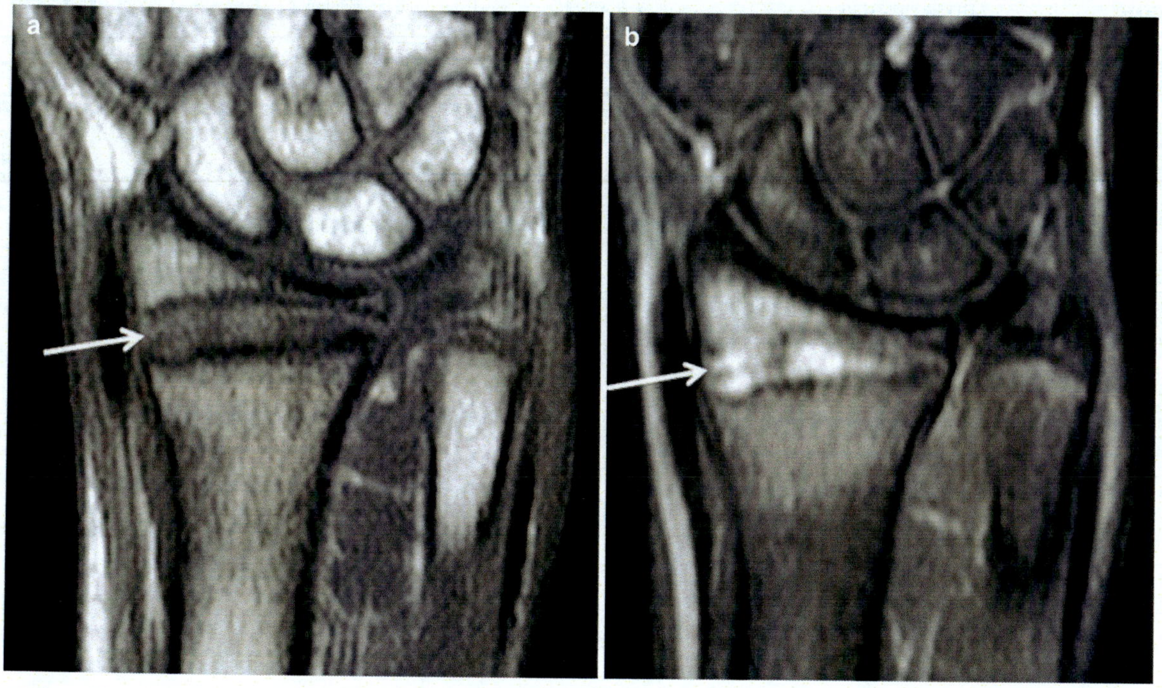

Fig. 2 Coronal T1-w (**a**) and STIR (**b**) MR images from the same patient as Fig. 1. Widening of the growth plate with an irregular surface of the metaphyseal aspect of the growth plate and vertical fractures is best seen at the T1-w image (*white arrow*), while the hyperintense signal of the widened physeal plate with the associated epiphyseal and metaphyseal bone marrow edema is best visualized at the STIR image (*white arrow*)

these items, skeletal maturation and wrist pain are lacking (DiFiori et al. 2006).

2.1.2 Fracture

The most frequent, and also the most problematical fracture, in the wrist of gymnasts is that of the scaphoid. Scaphoid fractures in general account for approximately 60% of all carpal fractures. They occur primarily during a fall on the outstretched hand. However, in gymnastics, extreme dorsiflexion drives the scaphoid volarly and repetitive forces applied to it may lead to a stress fracture. Both acute and stress fractures occur most commonly at the waist (70–80%), the weakest point in the scaphoid, but the fracture line can also be located in the tuberosity, the distal pole (5–10%) or the proximal pole (15–20%).

Posteroanterior and lateral radiographs of the wrist together with scaphoid-specific views usually suffice to detect the fracture line in acute injuries. However, initial radiographs may be negative and in these cases MR imaging or multi-detector CT can be considered (Karantanas et al. 2007). Both techniques have proved to be accurate in depicting scaphoid fractures (Ring and Lozano-Calderon 2008). We advocate the use of MR imaging with a protocol including coronal STIR or fat suppressed T2-w and T1-w sequences to allow demonstration of subtle fractures, stress related response or alternative diagnosis (Fig. 3). In gymnasts with a scaphoid stress fracture, radiographs may initially show sclerosis at the waist and later a discrete fracture line.

2.2 Elbow

2.2.1 Osteochondritis Dissecans

Osteochonditis dissecans (OD) is a form of osteochondrosis of the articular epiphysis. In the elbow of the gymnasts this condition is frequently seen at the humeral capitellum and trochlea, mainly in females (Bradley and Petrie 2001). OD lesions generally tend to occur in patients 11–15 years of age (Banks et al. 2005). Repeated microtrauma due to compression and shearing

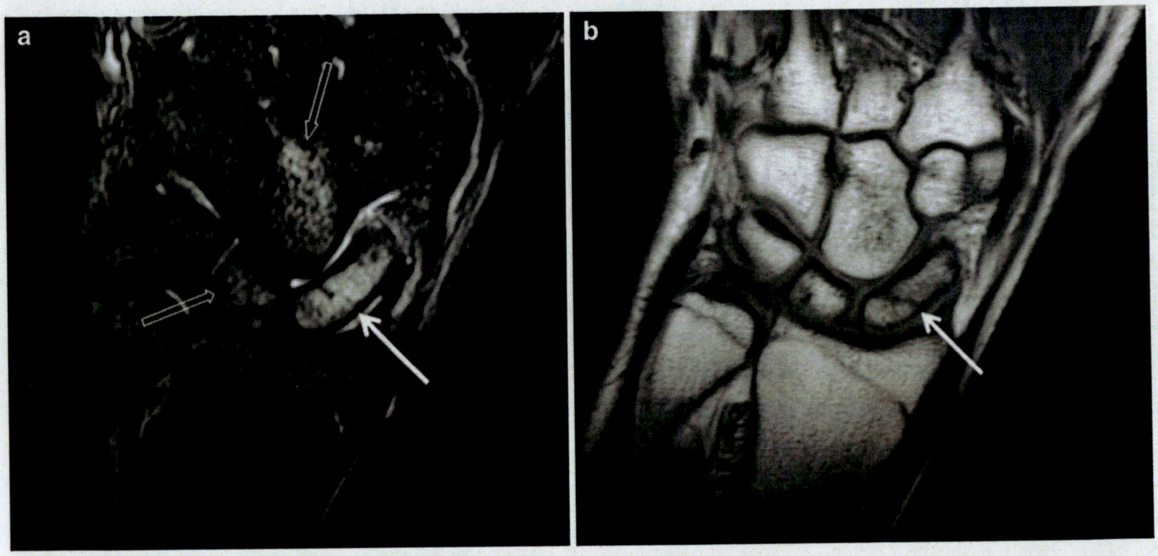

Fig. 3 The coronal STIR (**a**) and T1-w (**b**) MR images in a 16-year-old female patient who sustained a fall during training, demonstrate bone marrow edema of the scaphoid (**a**, *white arrow*) with a proximal pole fracture (**b**, *white arrow*). Also bone marrow edema (bone bruise) in the absence of a fracture is shown in the capitate and lunate (**a**, *open white arrows*)

forces are believed to play a major role in the pathogenesis. An OD lesion is illustrated by separation of a segment of articular cartilage and subchondral bone and it typically progresses through four stages (Bradley and Petrie 2001). In the first stage only a small area of compression of subchondral bone is observed, while in the final stage a loose body, a detached fragment displaced from the underlying crater bed, is found. The earliest sign at radiographs is flattening of the normal capitellar and trochlear contour. Later on, patchy sclerosis, fragmentation, intra-articular loose bodies and finally radiohumeral joint degeneration can be detected. Early findings are best evaluated by multi-detector CT and MR imaging. Multi-detector CT can demonstrate the extent of the osteochondral lesion and may show a lucent zone separating the parent bone and the loose fragment (Fig. 4).

MR imaging can be used to evaluate the status of the cartilage on T2*-w gradient-echo images (Fig. 5a). A hypointense signal within the fragment on T1-w and a hyperintense fluid rim surrounding loose fragments on STIR images can be seen (Fig. 5b) (Banks et al. 2005). Joint effusion, detached intra-articular fragments and subchondral cystic lesions can also be observed. When evaluating the presence of osteochondritis of the elbow it is important to be aware of the normal "pseudodefect of the capitellum" (Rosenberg et al. 1994). This pseudodefect is located at the posteroinferior junction of the articular and nonarticular portions of the capitellum. The absence of associated marrow edema or subchondral cystic changes enables the right diagnosis.

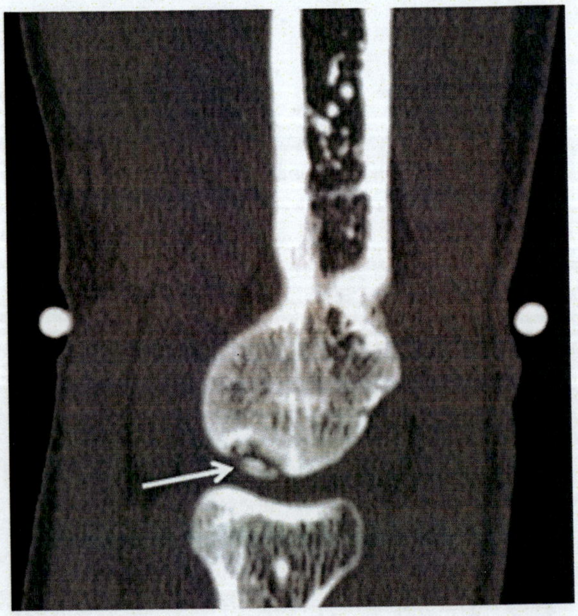

Fig. 4 Sagittal CT MPR image showing an osteochondral lesion with a loose bone fragment of the capitellum (*arrow*) in a 15-year-old female gymnast

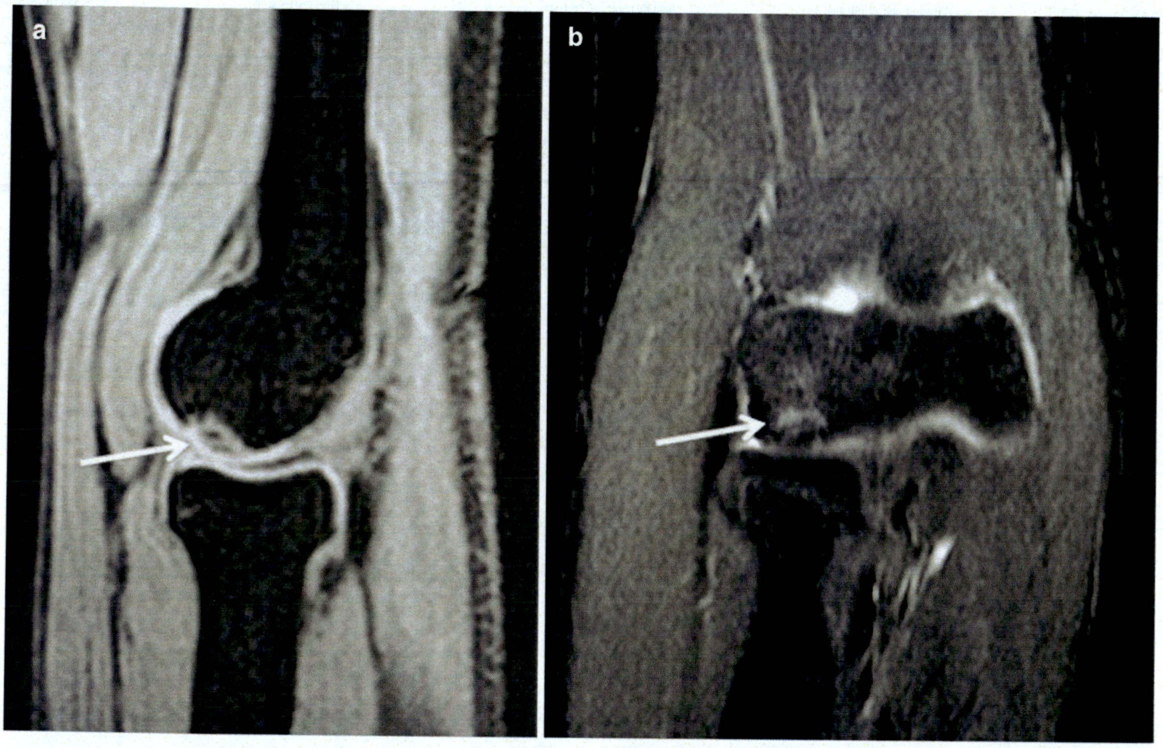

Fig. 5 Sagittal gradient-echo (**a**) and coronal STIR (**b**) MR images obtained in the same patient as Fig. 4. The gradient-echo image demonstrates the osteochondral lesion with the loose fragment and irregularity of the overlying cartilage. The bone marrow edema in the capitellum and the hyperintense fluid rim surrounding the loose fragment are shown on the STIR image

2.2.2 Growth Plate Injury

Traction apophysitis, also known as "little league elbow," is a growth plate injury of the medial epicondylar apophysis. This kind of stress injury is particularly seen in throwing athletes, but as the underlying mechanism is excessive valgus stress at the elbow it affects also gymnasts (Banks et al. 2005). Anteroposterior radiographs and multi-detector CT may show widening or avulsion of the medial epicondyle (Fig. 6). MR imaging findings include low signal in the apophysis on T1-w and depending on the presence of sclerosis or marrow edema, either low or high signal on fat suppressed T2-w images respectively (Banks et al. 2005) (Fig. 7). Edema may be also seen in the ulnar collateral ligament itself on fat suppressed MR images.

2.2.3 Lateral Epicondylitis

Lateral elbow pain in gymnasts due to an overuse injury involving the extensor tendons inserting on the lateral distal humeral epicondyle resemble tennis elbow (lateral epicondylitis). The extensor carpi radialis brevis is primarily affected, followed by the extensor digitorum communis. MR imaging may show various abnormalities, ranging from degenerative tendinosis with thickening and increased signal of the tendon to complete tendon disruption with a fluid-filled gap separating the tendon from its normal osseous origin (Banks et al. 2005) (Fig. 8).

2.3 Shoulder

2.3.1 Rotator Cuff Injury

Rotator cuff injuries in gymnasts are thought to be related to tensile failure rather than to subacromial impingement. The excessive load applied to the tendon exceeds the tensile limit of the tendon's collagenous structure with consequent tendinopathy that may progress into a partial or full-thickness tear

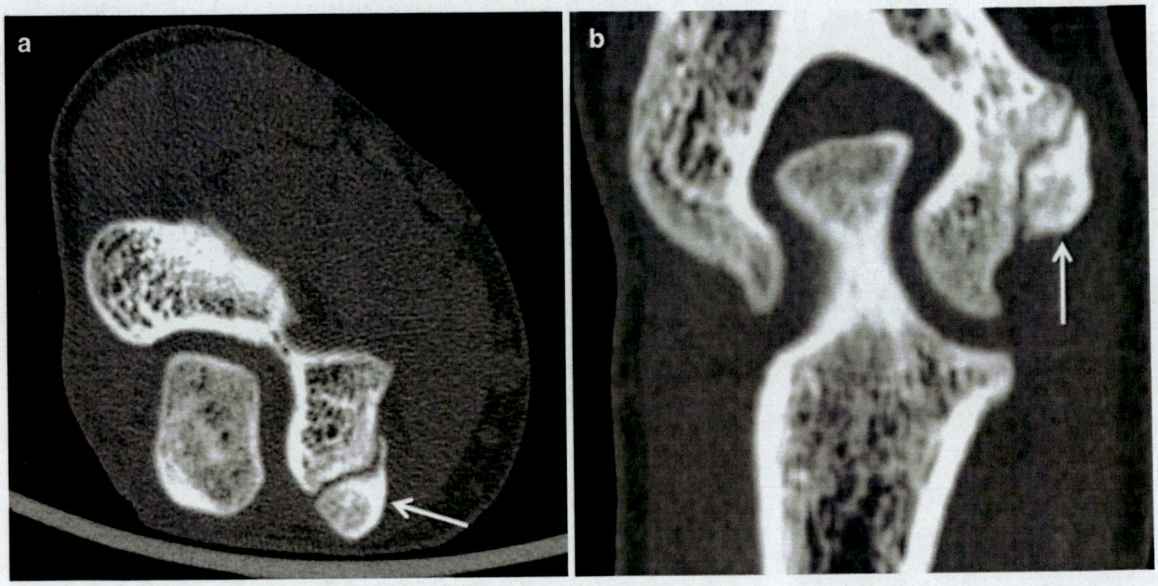

Fig. 6 Avulsion of the medial epicondyle is shown on axial (**a**) and coronal MPR (**b**) CT images in a 17-year-old female gymnast with chronic elbow pain (*arrows*)

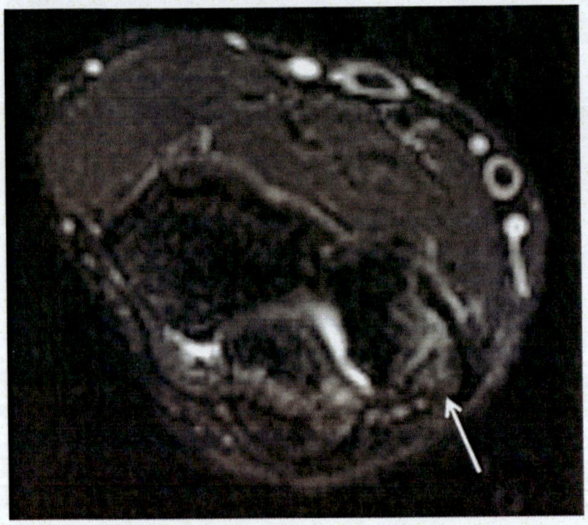

Fig. 7 The axial fat suppressedT2-w MR image obtained in the same patient as Fig. 6, shows bone marrow edema and loose fragment (*arrow*)

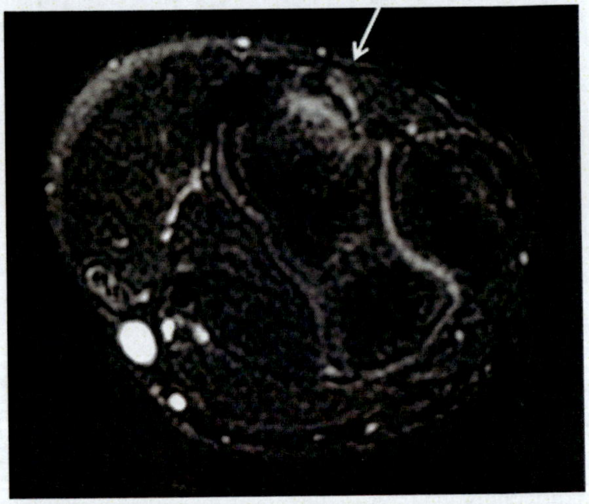

Fig. 8 Axial STIR MR image obtained in a 13-year-old patient with left lateral elbow pain aggravating during training. Edema in the lateral epicondyle and at the insertion of the tendon is demonstrated supporting the clinical diagnosis of lateral epicondylitis (*arrow*)

(Banks et al. 2005). Ultrasound, MR imaging and MR arthrography can all be used to evaluate the presence of rotator cuff pathology. Tendinosis at ultrasound manifests as a thickened tendon with decreased echogenicity and at MR imaging as a thickened inhomogeneous tendon with mildly increased signal intensity on T2-w and PD-w sequences (Fig. 9). A recent meta-analysis of the literature showed that MR imaging and US have a comparable accuracy for the depiction of full-thickness tears, although MR arthrography and ultrasound might be more accurate for the detection of partial-thickness tears compared to conventional MR imaging (Shahabpour et al. 2008). Partial tears are recognized at sonography by thinning and a focally decreased echogenicity and at MR imaging by a focal hyperintensity filling a gap within the tendon on T2-w images. A complete tear manifests as focal tendon

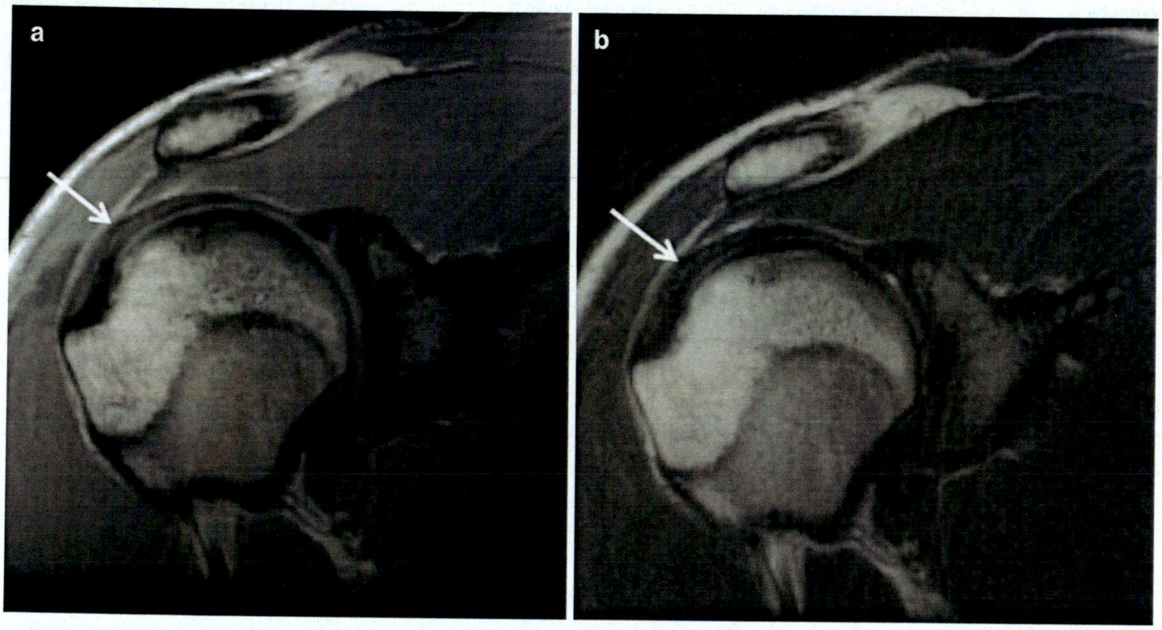

Fig. 9 Tendinopathy of the infraspinatus tendon in a 19-year-old male gymnast. The oblique coronal proton density (PD) (**a**) and T2-w (**b**) MR images show inhomogeneous tendon with mildly increased signal intensity on both sequences (*arrows*)

interruption with hypoechogenic gap and as a hyperintense T2-w signal extending through the full thickness of the tendon at ultrasound and MR imaging respectively.

2.3.2 Internal Impingement

Internal impingement can be seen in gymnasts due to the performance of repetitive overhead motions. During these motions impingement of the soft tissues of the rotator cuff and joint capsule on the glenoid or between the glenoid and the humerus can occur. MR imaging is the method of choice to evaluate internal shoulder impingement and may reveal rotator cuff tears, especially partial ones located in the undersurface of the supraspinatus and perhaps the infraspinatus tendons. Additional ABER (abduction and external rotation) views are helpful. Additional findings include fraying or tear of the posterior-superior labrum and degenerative changes of the humerus (Grainger 2008).

2.3.3 Slap Tear

Gymnasts are vulnerable to labral injuries of the shoulder. A superior labrum anterior to posterior (SLAP) tear involves the superior labrum. A SLAP tear is classified depending on its morphology and the associated biceps anchor involvement. MR arthrography with coronal, sagittal and axial images of the biceps labral complex is the best technique to demonstrate the several types of SLAP tears. SLAP tears are recognized as hyperintense linear fluid signal within the superior labrum at fat suppressed PD/T2-w images (Fig. 10) (Koh et al. 2007).

3 Lower Extremity Injuries

The extreme physical forces experienced by gymnasts during training, mainly at landing, make the lower extremity at risk for injury. The ankle is the most frequent site of injury, followed by the knee and hip (Caine and Nassar 2005).

3.1 Ankle/Foot

3.1.1 Fractures

Several kinds of acute fractures can be seen in the ankle and foot of elite gymnasts, depending on the injury

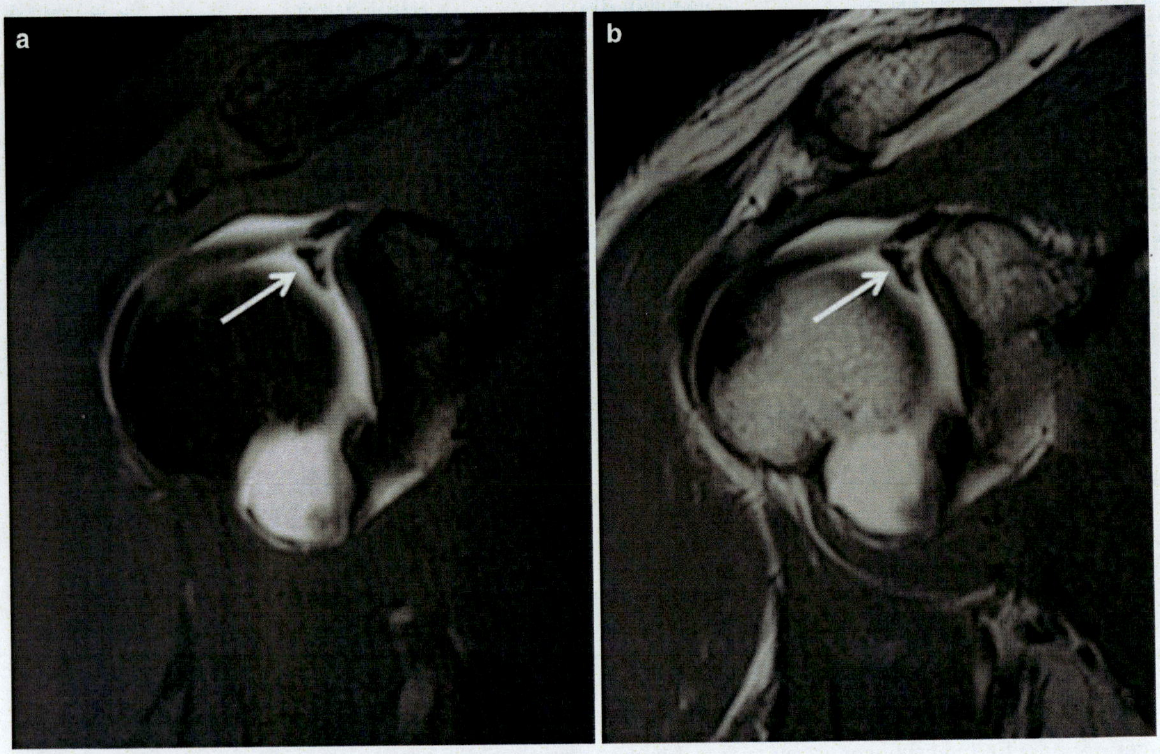

Fig. 10 MR arthrography of the right shoulder in a male gymnast. A SLAP type III lesion is demonstrated both on the coronal oblique fat suppressed T1-w (**a**, *arrow*) and on the PD (**b**, *white arrow*) MR images

mechanism. In addition to fractures of the distal tibia and fibula, the tarsal, metatarsal, phalangeal and even the sessamoid bones can be affected. Stress fractures of the tarsus are mainly found in the navicular bone, but they are sometimes also seen in the other tarsal bones (Berger et al. 2007). Other common sites for stress fractures in the ankle and foot comprise the medial malleolus, metatarsal bones and sesamoid bones. In acute fractures it is often important to evaluate their extension. In this respect, multi-detector CT may have a complementary role to radiographs (Figs. 11 and 12).

Contrary to acute fractures, stress fractures are often difficult to diagnose or may not be obvious on conventional radiographs (Berger et al. 2007). Features of stress fractures in primarily cortical bone (e.g., navicular bone) include: endosteal or periosteal callus formation without a fracture line, circumferential periosteal reaction with a fracture line through one cortex and a distinct fracture (Berger et al. 2007). Fractures in primarily cancellous bone (e.g., calcaneus) are more difficult to depict and may present as flake-like patches of new bone formation, cloudlike areas of mineralized bone or a focal linear area of sclerosis (Berger et al. 2007). MR imaging with STIR, T1-w and fat suppressed PD/T2-w sequences is the ideal imaging method to evaluate stress responses and fractures (Fig. 13). Based on several MR imaging characteristics, stress fractures can be graded in the following stages; grade 1 with mild to moderate periosteal edema on STIR and no marrow changes, grade 2 with moderate to severe periosteal edema on STIR and marrow changes on T2-w images, grade 3 with moderate to severe periosteal edema on STIR and marrow changes on T2-w and T1-w images and finally grade 4 with a visible fracture line.

3.1.2 Calcaneal Apophysitis

Calcaneal apophysitis, also known as Sever's disease, is a relatively common well known clinically diagnosed overuse disorder in the growing gymnast (Lau et al. 2008). It is caused by repetitive trauma to the calcaneal apophysis by the pull of the Achilles tendon on its insertion. Plain radiographs may show increased sclerosis and fragmentation of the calcaneal apophysis. On MR imaging, fragmentation of the apohysis accompanied by bone marrow edema can be seen

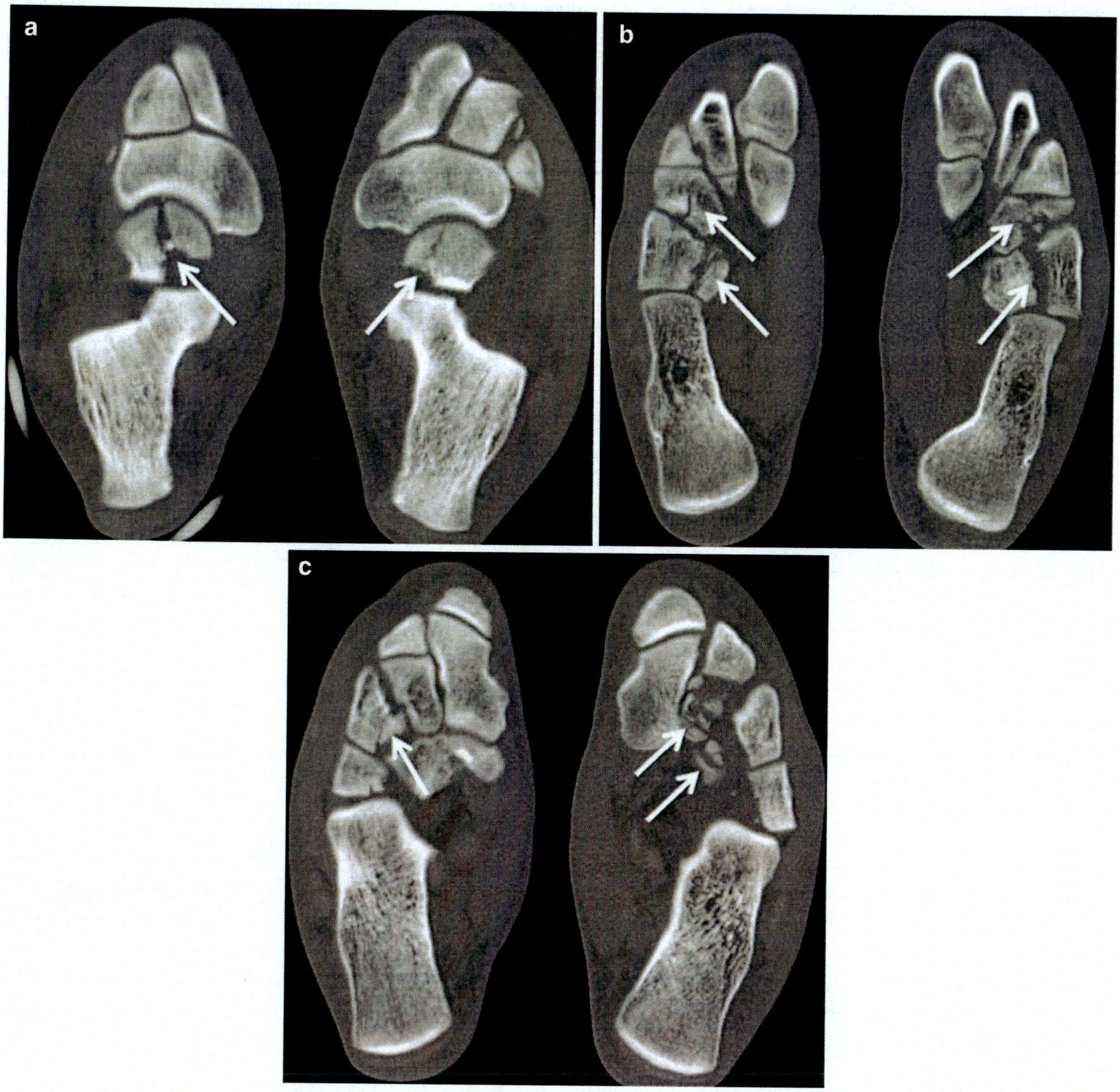

Fig. 11 Three axial CT images in a 18-year-old male patient who had a serious injury of both feet during landing. A longitudinal fracture of the talus on both sides with a discrete dislocation on the right side and some loose bodies at both sides (**a**), a fracture of the cuboid and the lateral cuneiform bone with dislocation and loose fragments bilaterally (**b**) and a fragmented intermediate and medial cuneiform bone on the left side are demonstrated (**b**, **c**) (*arrows*)

(Fig. 14). The major benefit of using imaging techniques in this clinical diagnosis is to exclude other pathologies like a fracture, osteomyelitis or an achilles tendon rupture.

3.1.3 Osteochondral Lesion

Osteochondral lesions in the ankle are mainly found in the talus and result primarily from direct or repetitive inversion injury to the ankle (Lau et al. 2008). The talus is prone to osteochondral changes because of its blood supply and the convex surface of the joint. With conventional imaging it is often not easy to diagnose an osteochondral lesion and no accurate assessment of the articular cartilage can be made. Both multi-detector CT and MR imaging are useful in identifying and localizing osteochondral lesions. MR imaging is highly accurate both in excluding the presence of an osteochondral lesion and in assessing the integrity of the articular cartilage (Verhagen et al. 2005). Multi-detector CT can better appreciate the extent of the lesion (Figs. 15 and 16).

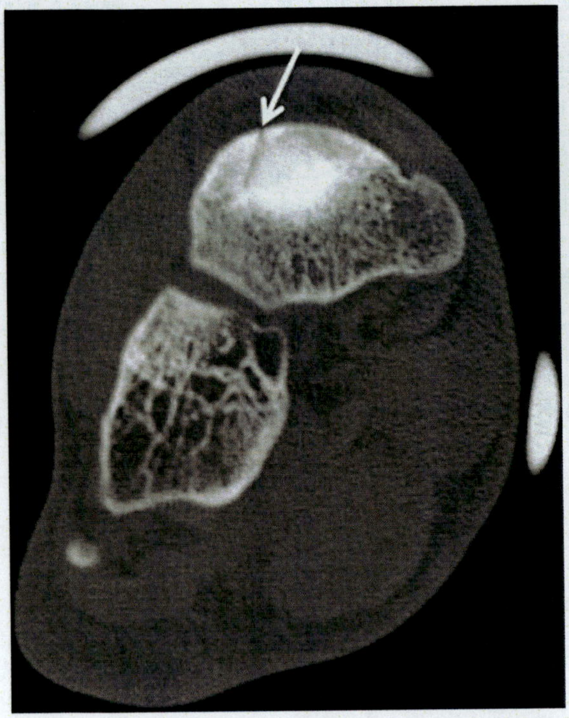

Fig. 12 Axial CT image in a 17-year-old patient demonstrating a linear lucent line surrounded by sclerosis at the anterolateral part of the navicular bone of the right foot representing a stress fracture (*white arrow*)

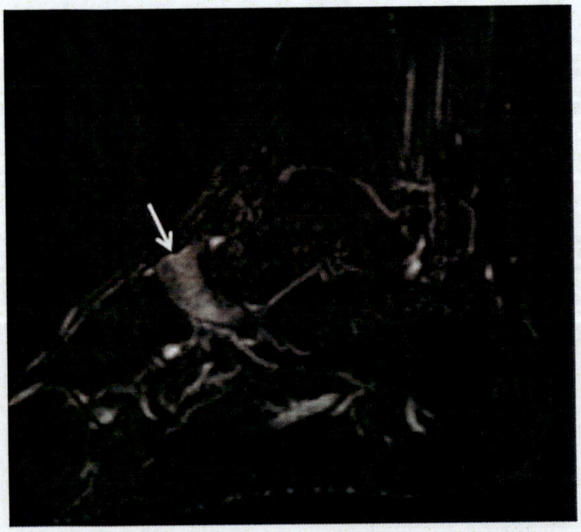

Fig. 13 Sagittal STIR MR image obtained in the same patient as Fig. 12 showing diffuse edema in the navicular bone (*white arrow*)

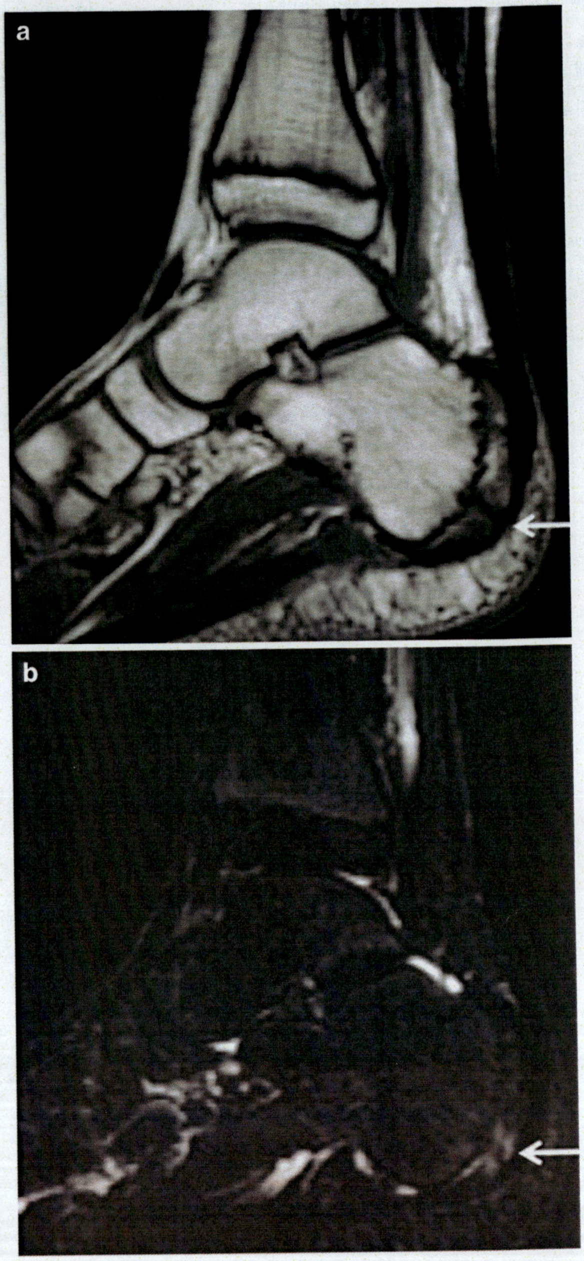

Fig. 14 Sagittal T1-w (**a**) and STIR (**b**) MR images of the left foot obtained in an 11-year-old female gymnast demonstrating fragmentation (**a**, *arrow*) and edema (**b**, *arrow*) of the calcaneal apophysis

3.1.4 Ligament Sprain or Injury

Ankle sprain in gymnasts are principally the result of violent excessive inversion trauma leading to injury of

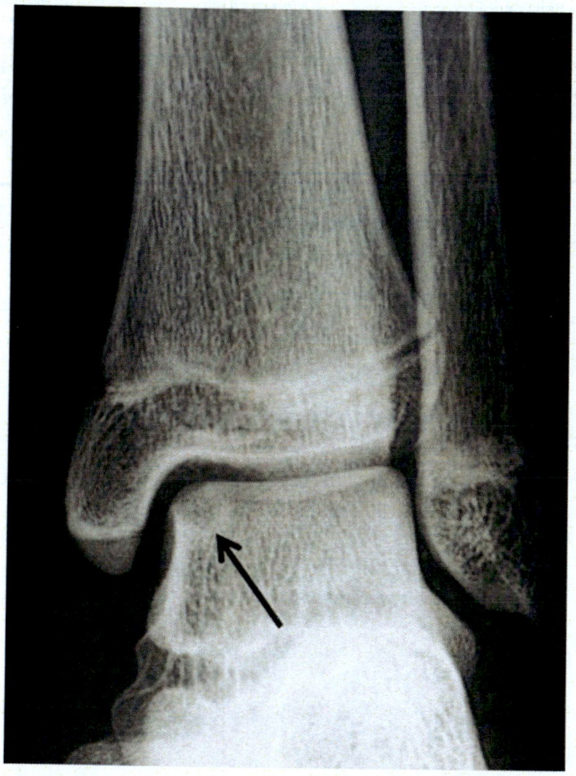

Fig. 15 Anteroposterior mortise weight-bearing radiograph of the left ankle showing an osteochondral lesion of the medial aspect of the talus (*arrow*) in an 11-year-old female gymnast

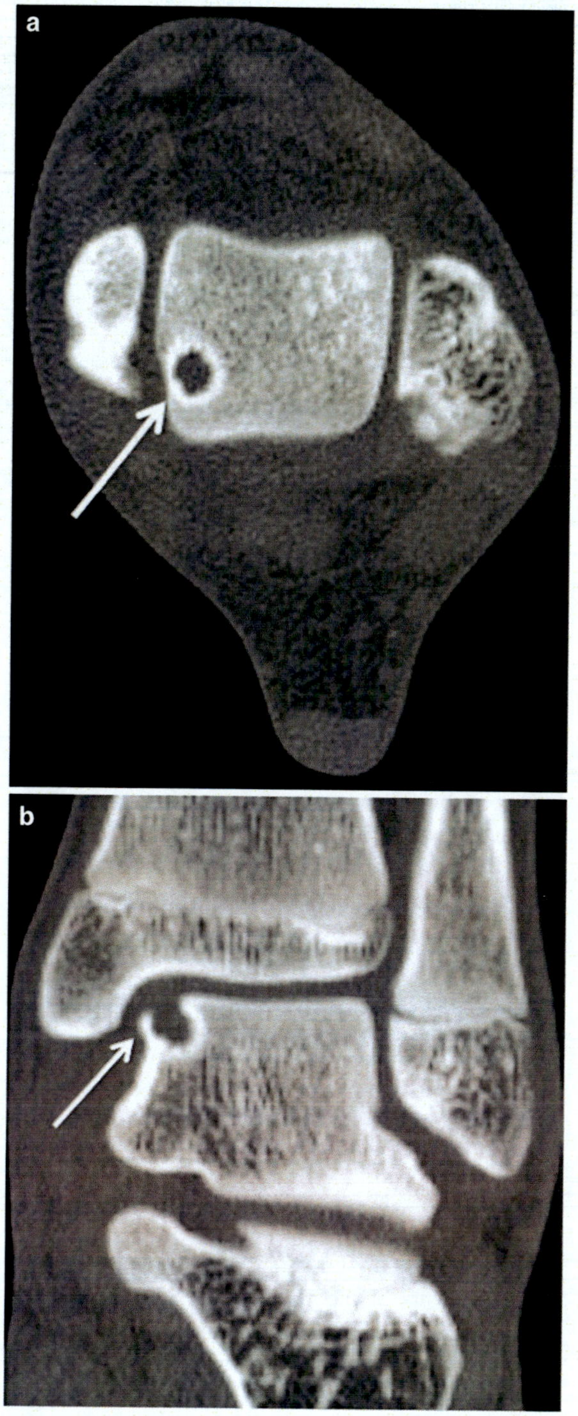

Fig. 16 Axial (**a**) and coronal (**b**) CT image obtained in the same female gymnast as in Fig. 15 showing an osteochondral lesion with a sclerotic margin of the posteromedial aspect of the talus (*arrow*)

the lateral collateral ligaments (i.e., anterior talofibular ligament, posterior talofibular ligament, calcaneofibular ligament). Less frequent sprains of the medial collateral (deltoid) ligaments (i.e., superficial and deep components) are seen. MR imaging protocols require T1-w and PD/T2-w images, especially in the axial plane. Typical findings include obliteration of the interligamentous fat, loss of normal ligament morphology and/or continuity. Bone marrow edema at the insertion and surrounding soft tissue edema may be associated features (Fig. 17).

3.2 Knee/Lower Leg

3.2.1 Traction Apophysitis

Osgood–Schlatter disease and Sinding–Larsen–Johansson disease are both clinically diagnosed overuse

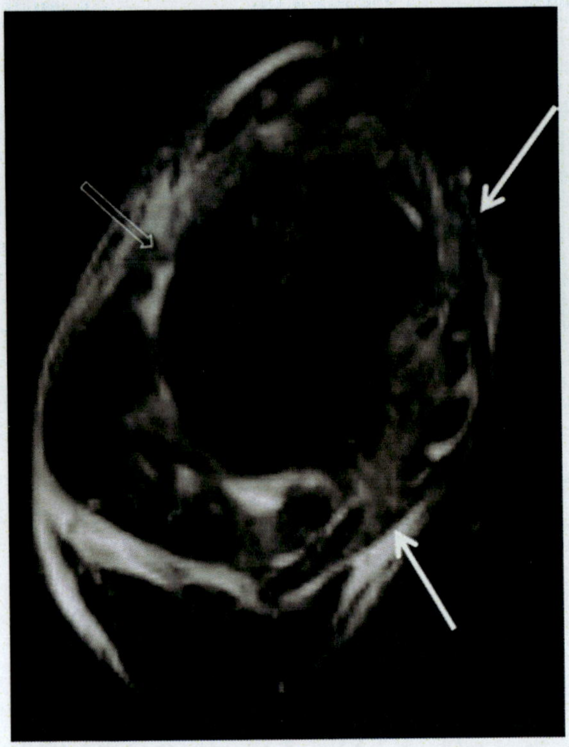

Fig. 17 Diffuse soft tissue edema of the right ankle (*arrows*) in a female gymnast with a disruption of the anterior talofibular ligament (*open arrow*) on an axial fat suppressed T2-w MR image

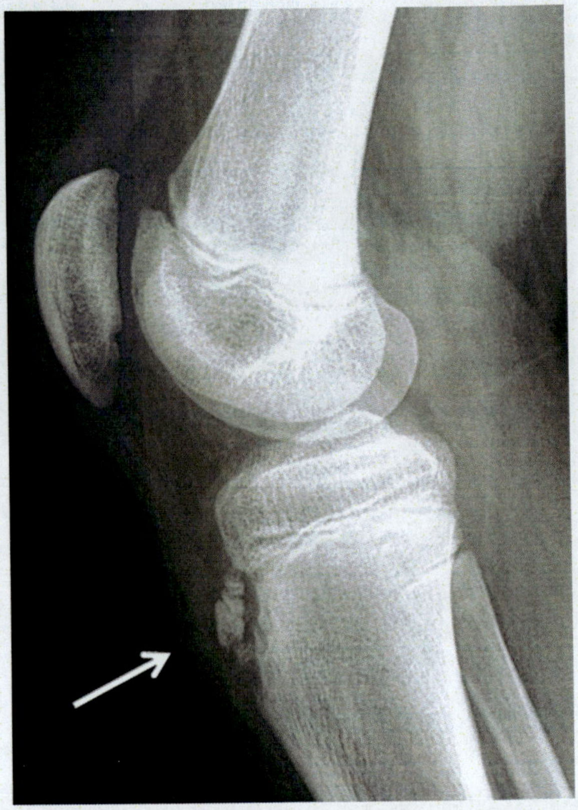

Fig. 18 Lateral radiograph of the left knee showing soft tissue swelling and fragmented appearance of the tibial tubercle (*white arrow*) in a symptomatic 12-year-old male gymnast

syndromes which can be encountered in the skeletally immature gymnast. Osgood–Schlatter disease is traction apohysitis of the patellar ligament insertion on the tibial tubercle, while Sinding–Larsen–Johansson is a traction apohysitis of the patellar ligament insertion on the inferior pole of the patella (Lau et al. 2008). Plain films in Osgood–Schlatter disease may show soft tissue swelling and fragmented appearance of the tibial tubercle (Fig. 18). MR imaging may demonstrate thickening of the distal patellar tendon and edema. The presence of soft tissue swelling and pain are important in Osgood–Schlatter disease to make the diagnosis as several ossification centers at the tibial apophysis can be seen normally. In Sinding–Larsen–Johansson fragmentation of the inferior pole with bone marrow edema, proximal patellar tendinopathy and infiltration of Hoffa's fat pad can be observed (Figs. 19–21).

3.2.2 Fractures

In gymnasts acute fractures in the knee occur mainly in the tibia plateau. Acute fractures result from high-energy axial loading, but low-energy rotation forces might also play a role. Fat suppressed MR images, are able to depict bone marrow edema and hemorrhage secondary to trabecular microfractures (Fig. 22). Multidetector CT in addition to radiographs is necessary to evaluate the extent of the fracture and the depression of the fragments (Fig. 23). The tibial plateau is a common location of stress responses/fractures, but these can also be observed in femoral condyles. The imaging characteristics of stress fractures have been described in the ankle/foot section.

3.3 *Pelvis/Hip*

3.3.1 Traction Apophysitis

Traction apophysitis can occur at different sites of the pelvis in young gymnasts. The three most common

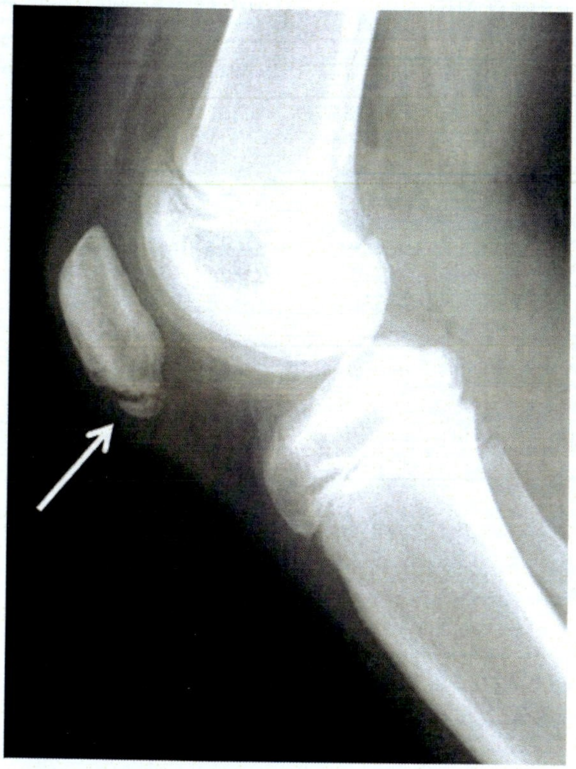

Fig. 19 Lateral radiograph of the left knee in an 11-year-old female gymnast with pain at the inferior pole of the patella. Fragmentation of the inferior patellar pole (*white arrow*) is shown

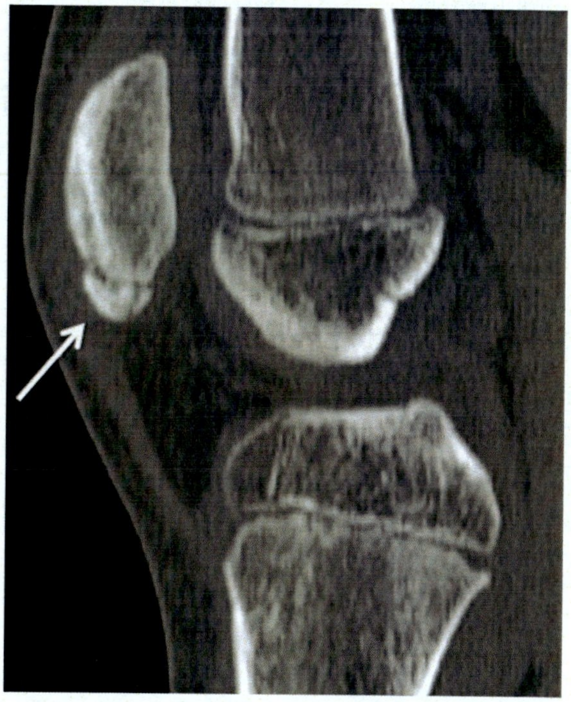

Fig. 20 Sagittal CT MPR of the left knee obtained in the same patient as in Fig. 19 demonstrating fragmentation of the inferior patellar pole (*arrow*)

sites of injury include the ischial tuberosity, the anterior inferior iliac spine and the anterior superior iliac spine. The lesions are mainly the consequence of exaggerated forces applied to the muscle-tendon unit. Radiographs may reveal irregularity of the apophysis in patients with chronic injury and an avulsed piece of bone in patients with an acute injury (Fig. 24).

In nonconclusive X-rays, multi-detector CT may demonstrate the cortical irregularity or the avulsion. MR imaging is mainly helpful to show marrow edema and to evaluate the status of the musculotendinous unit (Fig. 25). It is less sensitive in depicting the avulsed fragment.

3.3.2 Tendinopathy

In elite gymnasts, tendinopathy in the pelvic region occurs mainly at the proximal conjoined tendons of the common hamstring group (i.e., biceps femoris, semimembranosus and semitendinosus) (Bencardino and Mellado 2005). It is generally a result of chronic repetitive microtrauma. MR imaging findings comprise thickening of the tendon with increased signal on fat suppressed MR images corresponding to edema within and also parallel to the tendon. Sometimes edema of the adjacent ischial tuberosity is seen.

3.3.3 Muscle Strain

Muscle strain injuries are often the result of excessive stretch or stretch while the muscle is being eccentrically loaded. The tear is usually located at the musculotendinous junction (Garrett 1996). In gymnasts typical strains of the pelvis region include the quadratus femoris muscle, the hamstring muscle, the gluteus medius muscle and the adductor magnus muscle. MR imaging is the method of choice to demonstrate these injuries (Fig. 26). Intramuscular edema is the most important finding. Muscle strains at MR imaging can be classified in three stages based on the extent of disruption. Grade one indicates a minor degree of fiber disruption with edema and hemorrhage at the musculotendinous junction. Grade two represents a partial tear, while grade three indicates a complete tear with or without retraction (Bencardino and Mellado 2005).

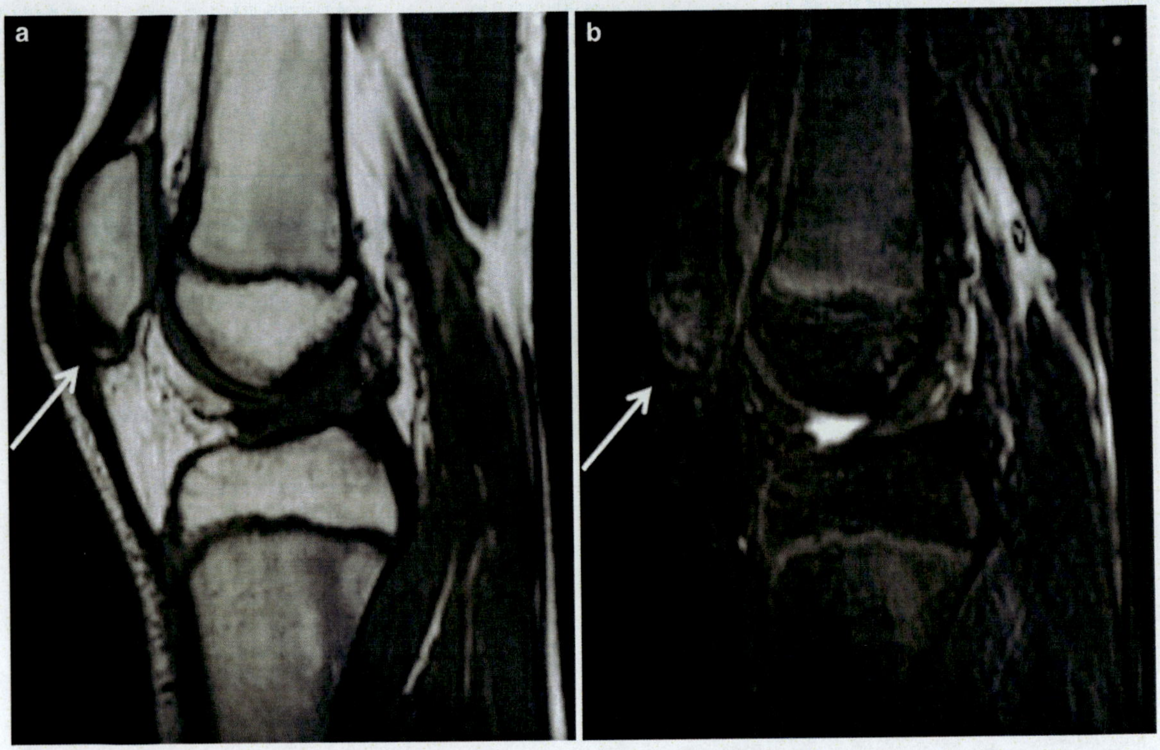

Fig. 21 Sagittal T1-w (**a**) and STIR (**b**) MR images of the left knee obtained in the same patient as in Fig. 19 showing fragmentation of the inferior patellar pole (**a**, *arrow*) with bone marrow-edema (**b**, *arrow*) of the fragment and inferior patellar pole

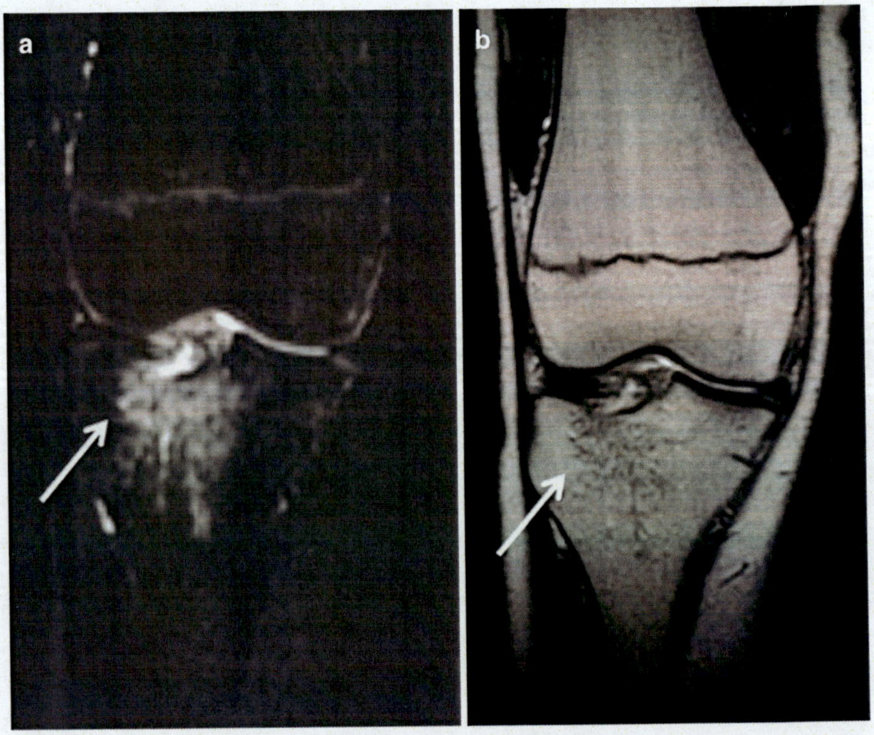

Fig. 22 Coronal STIR (**a**) and T1-w (**b**) MR images of the right knee obtained in a 16-year-old female gymnast showing extensive bone marrow edema in the tibial epiphysis and metaphysis (*arrows*) corresponding to trabecular micro-fractures

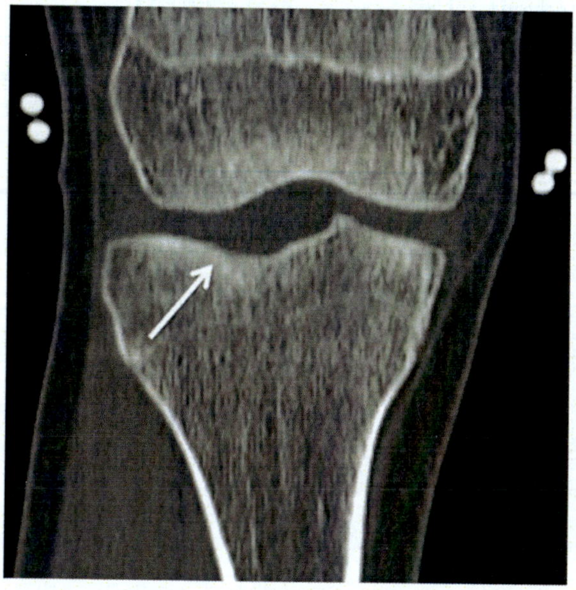

Fig. 23 The coronal CT MPR image of the right knee was obtained in the same patient as in Fig. 22 to assess the integrity of the tibial plateau. No cortical involvement is seen (*white arrow*)

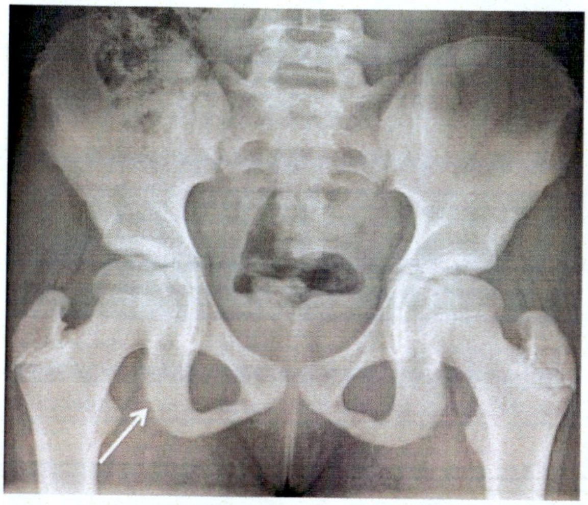

Fig. 24 Anteroposterior radiograph of the pelvis in a 12-year-old female gymnast demonstrating cortical irregularity and minor bony apposition at the right ischial tuberosity (*white arrow*)

4 Axial Skeleton

During gymnastics diverse and intense dynamic forces, like repetitive flexion, hyperextension, rotation, and compressive loading forces are applied across the spine. The lumbar spine is the most commonly injured part of the axial skeleton. Several authors reported significantly

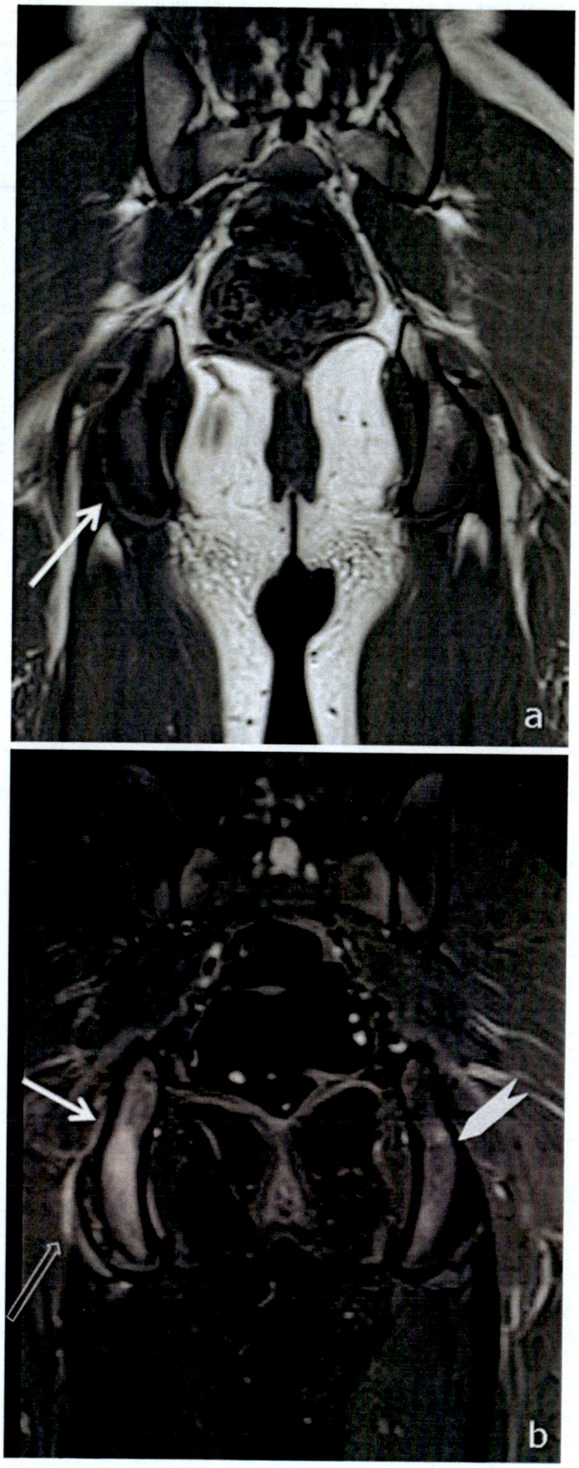

Fig. 25 Coronal T1-w (**a**) and STIR (**b**) MR images obtained in the same patient as in Fig. 24 showing irregularity of the apophysis (**a**, *arrow*) with extensive edema of the right ischial tuberosity (**b**, *white arrow*). Edema parallel to the right hamstring tendon insertion is also observed (**b**, *open arrow*). Minor bone marrow edema is seen at the left side (**b**, *thick arrow*)

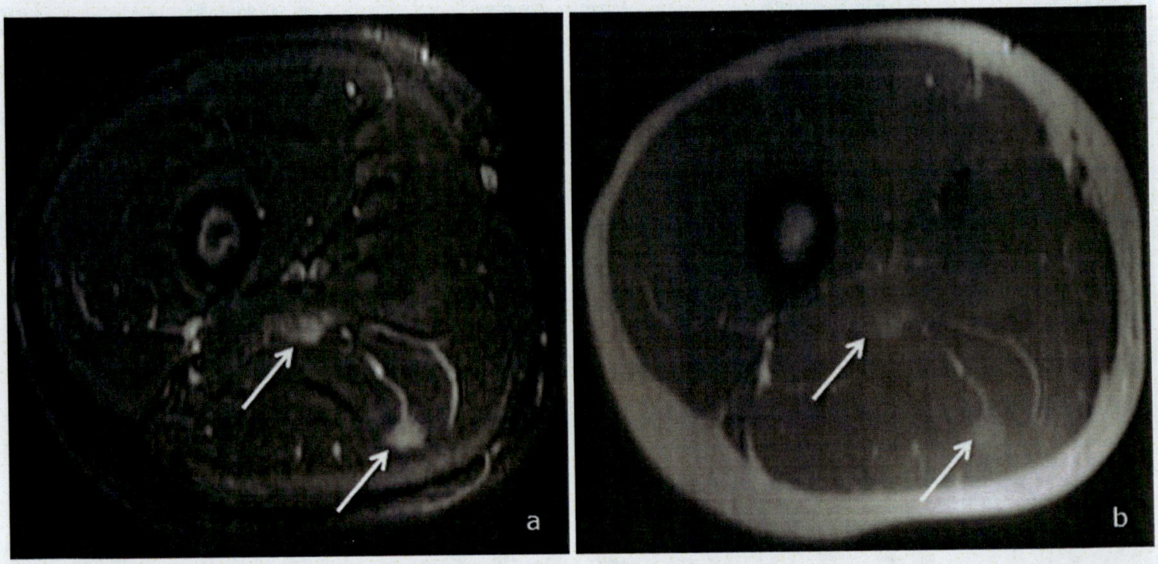

Fig. 26 The axial fat suppressed T2-w (**a**) and PD-w (**b**) MR images obtained in a 13-year-old female gymnast, demonstrate a strain injury of the right adductor magnus muscle with intramuscular edema (*arrows*)

higher rates of low-back pain in elite gymnasts compared to controls and other athletes (Bono 2004; Caine and Nassar 2005).

4.1 Stress Fractures

Gymnastics require complex movements of the spine, like hyperextension, extension and rotation. Thus, there is increased risk for the development of a stress fracture, also known as spondylolysis, with a reported prevalence of 17% in gymnasts (Soler and Calderon 2000). Spondylolysis can develop at various sites, but most commonly is located in the pars interarticularis. The vast majority of injuries are seen at level L5 (84%), followed by level L4 (12%) (Soler and Calderon 2000). Spondylolysis may be accompanied by spondylolisthesis, a forward translation of one vertebra relative to another. Lateral and oblique lumbar radiographs are useful to depict spondylolysis and the degree of spondylolisthesis. Multi-detector CT is valuable in demonstrating profound sclerosis and the extent of the fracture line (Fig. 27). MR imaging may show bone marrow edema and a hypointense fracture line (Fig. 28). Bilateral pedicle bone-marrow edema is reported to be a precursor of spondylolysis and if treated adequately it possibly prevent further development to spondylolisthesis (Stabler et al. 2000). The sacrum is another common site for stress fractures in gymnasts. Since plain radiographs are usually normal, when clinically suspected,

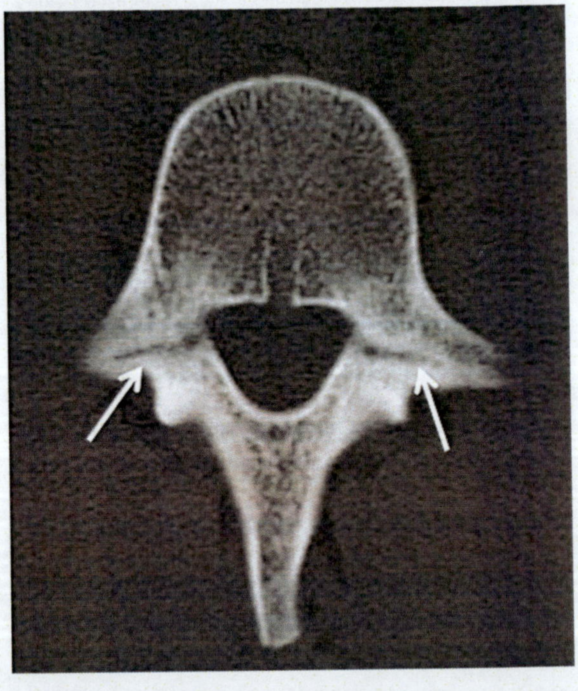

Fig. 27 Axial CT of the fourth lumbar vertebra in an 18-year-old male gymnast showing a bilateral stress fracture (*arrows*)

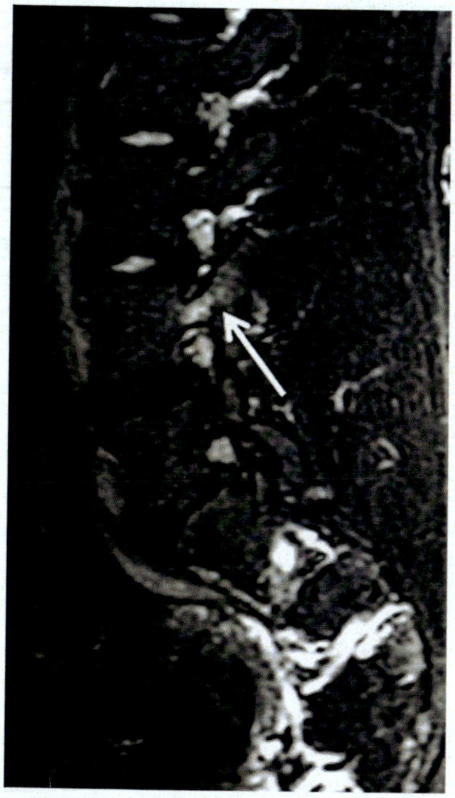

Fig. 28 The sagittal STIR MR image obtained in the same patient as in Fig. 27, demonstrates pedicle bone marrow edema (*white arrow*)

such a fracture should be confirmed or ruled out with MR imaging.

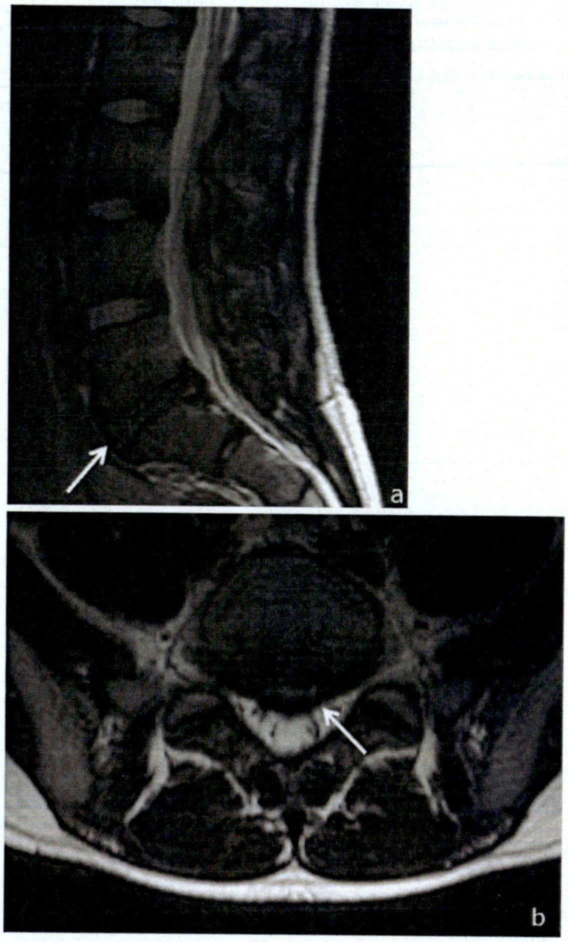

Fig. 29 The sagittal T2-w (**a**) and axial T2-w (**b**) MR images in a 15-year-old female gymnast show reduced disc-space height with decreased disc signal intensity (**a**, *arrow*) at level L5-S1. Posterior disc herniation is also observed (**b**, *arrow*)

4.2 Degenerative Disease

Degenerative changes of the lumbar spine are more frequently seen in gymnasts compared to nonathletes (Sward et al. 1991). MR imaging may show a decrease in disc-space height and decreased disc signal intensity on T2-w images (Fig. 29a). The level L5-S1 is most commonly affected. In addition to changes in disc signal intensities, bulging or focal herniation of the disc, with or without compression on the thecal sac, can occur (Fig. 29b). Degenerative changes, like osteophyte formation, will compensate for the diminished capacity of the disc to sustain loads.

4.3 Scheuermann's Disease

In gymnastics, the repetitive flexion can cause injuries to the vertebral endplates, mainly at the thoracolumbar junction, leading to Scheuermann's disease (Kruse and Lemmen 2009). In Scheuermann's disease, Schmorl's nodes, irregularities of the end plates and anterior wedging of the vertebral body are seen, resulting in a kyphotic deformity. These findings can be seen with plain radiographs. MR imaging can show the bone marrow edema adjacent to the endplates resulting from acute Schmorl's nodes, which is associated with the back pain (Fig. 30).

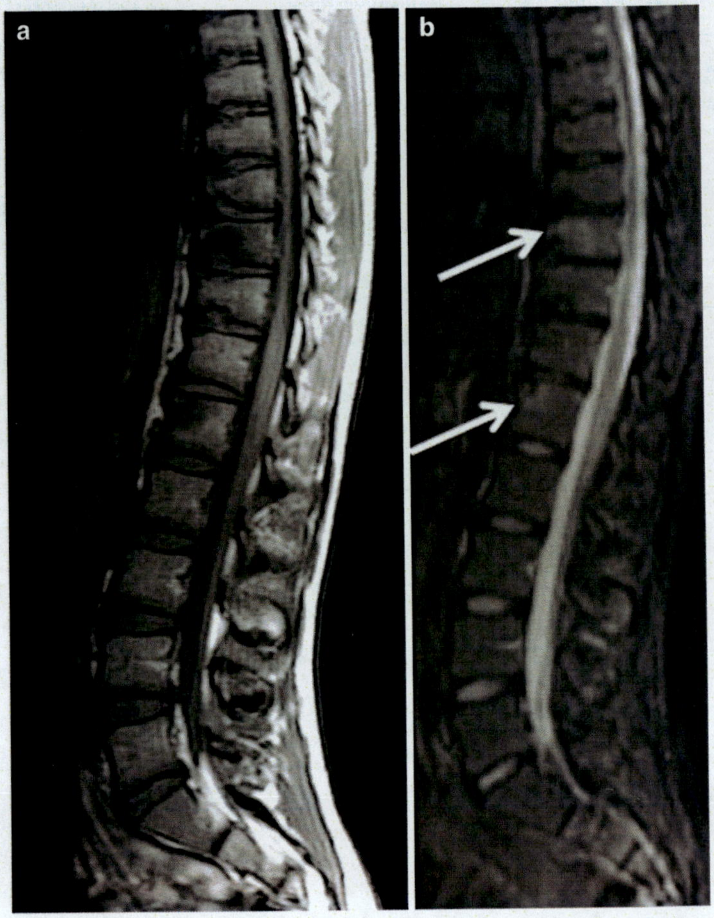

Fig. 30 The sagittal T1-w (**a**) and STIR (**b**) MR images in a 14-year-old female gymnast show anterior wedging of several lower thoracic vertebral bodies and vertebral body L1 with irregularities of the end plates and Schmorl's nodes (**a**). The bone marrow edema of vertebral bodies TH10 and L1 indicate acute Schmorl's nodes formation (**b**, *arrows*)

5 Conclusions

Gymnastics is a physically demanding sport and predisposes to diverse injuries of the musculoskeletal system. The type of injury can generally be related to specific movements, loads or forces, the body part or joint affected and the age of the gymnast or skeletal maturity. Many injuries can be diagnosed with conventional radiographs, but for more detailed information, MR imaging and multi-detector CT are frequently required. MR imaging has gained a crucial role in the diagnostic work up of gymnastic injuries and its main advantage is to demonstrate edema. We advocate the use of multi-detector CT complementary to MR imaging to evaluate the integrity of the osseous structures, especially when evaluating the spine and the epiphysis and apophysis of the immature skeleton. By becoming familiar with the spectrum of musculoskeletal injuries and its imaging features, radiologists can provide the clinician the information necessary to plan the proper treatment allowing thus prompt return to the previous level of gymnastic performance.

References

Backx FJ, Erich WB, Kemper AB, Verbeek AL (1989) Sports injuries in school-aged children. An epidemiologic study. Am J Sports Med 17(2):234–240

Banks KP, Ly JQ, Beall DP, Grayson DE, Bancroft LW, Tall MA (2005) Overuse injuries of the upper extremity in the competitive athlete: magnetic resonance imaging findings associated with repetitive trauma. Curr Probl Diagn Radiol 34(4):127–142

Bencardino JT, Mellado JM (2005) Hamstring injuries of the hip. Magn Reson Imaging Clin N Am 13(4):677–690, vi

Berger FH, de Jonge MC, Maas M (2007) Stress fractures in the lower extremity. The importance of increasing awareness amongst radiologists. Eur J Radiol 62(1):16–26

Bono CM (2004) Low-back pain in athletes. J Bone Joint Surg Am 86-A(2):382–396

Bradley JP, Petrie RS (2001) Osteochondritis dissecans of the humeral capitellum. Diagnosis and treatment. Clin Sports Med 20(3):565–590

Caine DJ, Nassar L (2005) Gymnastics injuries. Med Sport Sci 48:18–58

DiFiori JP, Caine DJ, Malina RM (2006) Wrist pain, distal radial physeal injury, and ulnar variance in the young gymnast. Am J Sports Med 34(5):840–849

Garrett WE Jr (1996) Muscle strain injuries. Am J Sports Med 24(6):S2–S8

Grainger AJ (2008) Internal impingement syndromes of the shoulder. Semin Musculoskelet Radiol 12(2):127–135

Karantanas A, Dailiana Z, Malizos K (2007) The role of MR imaging in scaphoid disorders. Eur Radiol 17(11):2860–2871

Kerssemakers SP, Fotiadou AN, de Jonge MC, Karantanas AH, Maas M (2009) Sport injuries in the paediatric and adolescent patient: a growing problem. Pediatr Radiol 39(5):471–484

Koh ES, Lee JC, Healy JC (2007) MRI of overuse injury in elite athletes. Clin Radiol 62(11):1036–1043

Kruse D, Lemmen B (2009) Spine injuries in the sport of gymnastics. Curr Sports Med Rep 8(1):20–28

Lau LL, Mahadev A, Hui JH (2008) Common lower limb sport-related overuse injuries in young athletes. Ann Acad Med Singapore 37(4):315–319

Ring D, Lozano-Calderon S (2008) Imaging for suspected scaphoid fracture. J Hand Surg [Am] 33(6):954–957

Rosenberg ZS, Beltran J, Cheung YY (1994) Pseudodefect of the capitellum: potential MR imaging pitfall. Radiology 191(3):821–823

Roy S, Caine D, Singer KM (1985) Stress changes of the distal radial epiphysis in young gymnasts. A report of twenty-one cases and a review of the literature. Am J Sports Med 13(5): 301–308

Sands WA (2000) Injury prevention in women's gymnastics. Sports Med 30(5):359–373

Shahabpour M, Kichouh M, Laridon E, Gielen JL, De Mey J (2008) The effectiveness of diagnostic imaging methods for the assessment of soft tissue and articular disorders of the shoulder and elbow. Eur J Radiol 65(2):194–200

Shih C, Chang CY, Penn IW, Tiu CM, Chang T, Wu JJ (1995) Chronically stressed wrists in adolescent gymnasts: MR imaging appearance. Radiology 195(3):855–859

Singh S, Smith GA, Fields SK, McKenzie LB (2008) Gymnastics-related injuries to children treated in emergency departments in the United States, 1990-2005. Pediatrics 121(4):e954–e960

Soler T, Calderon C (2000) The prevalence of spondylolysis in the Spanish elite athlete. Am J Sports Med 28(1):57–62

Stabler A, Paulus R, Steinborn M, Bosch R, Matzko M, Reiser M (2000) Spondylolysis in the developmental stage: diagnostic contribution of MRI. Rofo 172(1):33–37

Sward L, Hellstrom M, Jacobsson B, Nyman R, Peterson L (1991) Disc degeneration and associated abnormalities of the spine in elite gymnasts. A magnetic resonance imaging study. Spine 16(4):437–443

Verhagen RA, Maas M, Dijkgraaf MG, Tol JL, Krips R, van Dijk CN (2005) Prospective study on diagnostic strategies in osteochondral lesions of the talus. Is MRI superior to helical multi-detector CT? J Bone Joint Surg Br 87(1):41–46

Index

A.H. Karantanas (ed.), *Sports Injuries in Children and Adolescents*,
Med Radiol Diagn Imaging, DOI: 10.1007/174_2010, © Springer-Verlag Berlin Heidelberg 2011

V

W